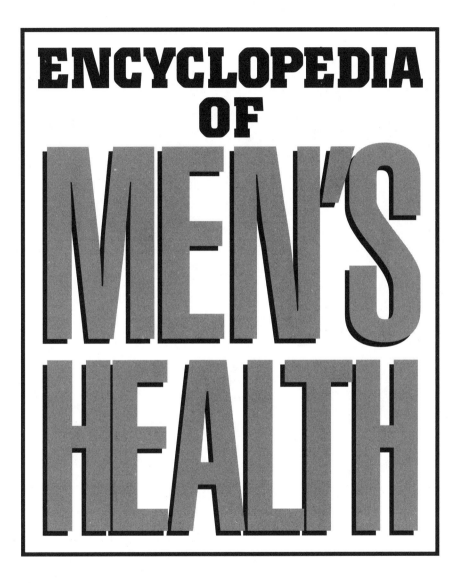

ENCYCLOPEDIA OF MEN'S HEALTH

ENCYCLOPEDIA OF MEN'S HEALTH

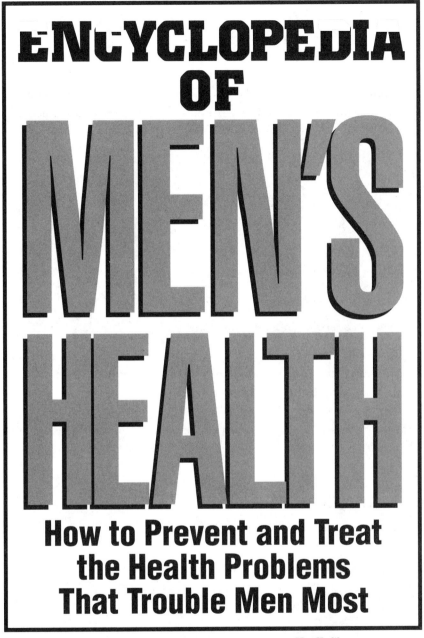

How to Prevent and Treat the Health Problems That Trouble Men Most

Edited by Neil Wertheimer, Managing Editor, Men'sHealth Books

Rodale Press, Inc.
Emmaus, Pennsylvania

NOTICE

This book is intended as a reference volume only, not as a medical manual. The information given here is designed to help you make informed decisions about your health. It is not intended as a substitute for any treatment that may have been prescribed by your doctor. If you suspect that you have a medical problem, we urge you to seek competent medical help.

Library of Congress Cataloging-in-Publication Data

Total health for men:
     Encyclopedia of men's health : how to prevent and treat the health problems that trouble men most / edited by Neil Wertheimer
     p. cm.
     Previously published: Total health for men. Emmaus, Pa : Rodale Press, 1995.
Includes index.
ISBN 0–87596–418–4   hardcover
1. Men—Health and hygiene. 2. Self-care, Health.
I. Wertheimer, Neil. II. Title.
[RA777.8.T68   1996]
613'.04234—dc20   96–8491

Distributed in the book trade by St. Martin's Press

2 4 6 8 10 9 7 5 3   hardcover

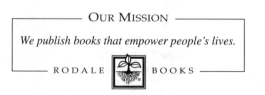

OUR MISSION

We publish books that empower people's lives.

RODALE BOOKS

Contents

Part I

The Basics of Health

The Healthy Man

Ten Steps to a Longer, Better Life

Congratulations on making it to the opening chapter! The fact that you're reading these words means (a) you're ready to take charge of your health or (b) someone who loves you gave you this book and you thought you'd better scan a couple of pages in case you get quizzed later.

If it's (b), give yourself some points for honesty. But stick around for a few more pages. You might find that healthy living is not nearly as oppressive or difficult as you might think. And even if you're not ready for us now, be glad we're on your bookshelf for when you *are* ready.

But chances are most men are already in the (a) category. More than ever, men are being better about their health—and they're seeing some real dividends for their investments. Not long ago, the average life expectancy for men was about 70 years. Now the Bureau of Health Statistics says we can expect to live to at least 72—two extra years of life—and that number will keep rising the earlier we take responsibility for our health and fitness.

But we can't rest on our laurels. Women have an average life expectancy of 79—and don't kid yourself that their seven-year lead is because of some genetic advantage. Fact is, women hang in the game of life longer for one reason: They take better care of themselves.

"For example, when women have a problem, they're more likely to see their doctors and get it checked out," says Kenneth Goldberg, M.D., director of the Male Health Center in Dallas and author of *How Men Can Live as Long as Women*. As Dr. Goldberg explains, what we dismiss as overly cautious behavior can turn out to be a lifesaver. "The more attention they pay to their health, the sooner they will nip problems in the bud. Men, on the other hand, are more likely to ignore some very obvious signs and put off seeing a doctor as long as possible. But this 'manly' view of things is what causes men to die sooner."

So consider *Encyclopedia of Men's Health* your playbook, your game plan for greater health. To write it, the editors of *Men's Health* magazine polled the leading experts in every field—from neurology to urology. We've packed this volume with thousands of tips for dealing with—or getting rid of—mental and physical ailments.

Top Ten Tips for Total Health

Like most game plans, you'll notice that *Encyclopedia of Men's Health* is based firmly on some core strategies—tenets of good health and fitness that will pop up in just about every chapter. It's not that we're trying to brainwash you—but good advice always bears repeating.

So as you read further, keep in mind these Top Ten Tips for Total Health, organized in order of importance based on a survey of some of our most trusted health experts. If you do nothing else for your health, try following these ten commandments. Not only could they help you live longer, they might actually be easier to follow than you thought. And before you know it, you will be taking better care of yourself and tacking years of quality time onto your life.

1. Quit smoking—now.

If you knew performing a certain activity would kill you, probably in an ugly and painful way, and stopping that activity would add years to your life, what would you do?

It sounds like a no-brainer—except that roughly one out of five men keeps making the killing choice by continuing to smoke. Once and for all: If you smoke, or spend a lot of time around someone who does, sooner or later it can kill you.

"It's poison, pure and simple," says James A. Pantano, M.D., a cardiologist in Allentown, Pennsylvania, and author of *Living with Angina*. According to Dr. Pantano, cigarette smoke contains carbon monoxide as well as radioactive particles. The main ways smoking may kill is by heart disease, lung disease or cancer—three of the top five killers of men.

But first, smoking will make your life miserable. You'll suffer the mood swings associated with nicotine addiction; you'll break into embarrassing coughing and retching fits in front of family, friends and colleagues; food will lose its taste. Meanwhile, the smoke will damage your lungs and pollute your blood with carbon monoxide. This in turn will make your heart work harder and faster, raise your blood pressure and sap your energy. Eventually that smoke might start a reaction in your body that causes cancer cells to grow.

On the other hand, you could kick the habit. And here's your incentive: You'll live longer, no matter how long you've been smoking. One study showed that if middle-age men would just kick their smoking habit, they'd prolong their lives by an average of four years—and the sooner they quit, the longer they'll live. There are dozens of organizations, plans and techniques just waiting to help you stop smoking. Your doctor can prescribe medications to help you get the nicotine monkey off your back, too.

The Wild Man's Creed

Sex, drugs and alcohol can be good for you. In fact, they may be essential to your health.

Of course, a statement like that screams for a qualifier. So, as a coda to our Top Ten, we offer the following:

- Sex: As a basic form of physical exercise, sex can be aerobic, and is good for the heart and lungs. But beyond that, experts say that a healthy sex life can help boost your immune system, ward off serious diseases and put the screws to stress. Plus, the more sex you have, the more you can have. "Getting erections helps your ability to have more erections," says Irwin Goldstein, M.D., professor of urology at Boston University School of Medicine. Regular erections keep the tissues of the penis flexible. Use it or lose it.

- Drugs: In this case, we're talking about aspirin. "It's extremely helpful for men with heart problems, and can reduce heart attack risk in men with no coronary disease," says James Pantano, M.D., author of *Living with Angina*. Studies indicate that taking just one 325 milligram tablet every other day may prevent dangerous blood clots from forming, cutting heart attack risk by at least 30 percent. Plus, some studies indicate that aspirin can inhibit the growth of certain types of cancer. But don't self-prescribe aspirin; you may have conditions that could be made worse by taking aspirin. Many doctors argue that it is not very sound to take drugs as a preventive measure. Talk to your doctor first.

- Alcohol: There's been plenty of evidence to show that moderate drinking—no more than one or two drinks per day—can protect against heart disease. But the operative term is moderate. More than two drinks a day is just asking for health problems, particularly in the heart, brain and liver.

One big caveat: Aspirin and alcohol don't mix well with different medications—or each other. Taken together, alcohol and aspirin can cause internal bleeding or worse. So if you're on the aspirin program, take your pill with your meals in the morning or afternoon, have your wine in the evening—and have sex with your partner whenever you can.

2. Eat less fat.

Fat clogs our arteries and causes heart attacks and strokes—it can even prevent us from getting erections. Yet men still gorge themselves on it.

"Foods high in saturated fats are the worst offenders," says Dr. Pantano. That's because these foods also tend to be high in cholesterol and do some of their damage by building up as plaque on the walls of our arteries. These buildups are what lead to heart disease, the top killer of men in the United States.

Plus, the more our blood vessels are narrowed by fat and cholesterol, the less oxygen will be circulated in our bodies and the more fatigued we'll feel.

To get the calories we need to sustain ourselves, experts say we should stick with carbohydrates, which are better sources of fuel for our body than fats. A good low-fat daily diet should include 6 to 11 servings of high-carbohydrate grains as well as 3 to 5 servings of vegetables and 2 to 4 servings of fruit. Keep fats to an absolute minimum. The American Heart Association recommends getting no more than 30 percent of our daily calories from fat—the less the better.

"Meanwhile, if you don't know your cholesterol count yet, find out," says Dr. Pantano. That will give you some idea of how much you need to concentrate on trimming the fat out of your life.

3. Anchor yourself to a doc.

We spend more time picking a mechanic to take care of our cars than we do choosing a doctor to do preventive maintenance on our bodies. That's if we pick a doctor at all.

"It's part of man's bulletproof mentality—going to a doctor is somehow seen as a weakness," says Dr. Goldberg. It's not all our fault—many men feel vulnerable in a doctor's office and so have a strong impulse to avoid one. Instead, Dr. Goldberg says to try thinking of the doctor as your coach taking you through the game of life—a trained professional who knows how to help keep you healthy. "The two of you should be in a kind of health partnership," he says. That means picking a regular doctor and then seeing him as needed—at least once a year.

To do this, you first might have to make a few calls and visit one or two doctors, paying attention to some basic qualities. For instance, you want a doctor whose office hours are convenient to your schedule and who won't keep you waiting more than 30 minutes after your scheduled appointment (and even then he should offer an explanation for the delay).

And when you're in the examination room, note the doctor's style. Does he encourage your spouse or your partner to join you? Does he explain his findings to you to help educate you about your health? Does he believe in trying the safest,

Top Ten Killers of Men

1. Heart disease	6. Pneumonia
2. Cancer	7. Suicide
3. Accidents	8. HIV infection
4. Stroke	9. Diabetes
5. Lung disease	10. Homicide

least-expensive options first? Most important, does he listen to you?

"These are all important questions to ask when you're choosing a doctor," says Dr. Goldberg. "You need the right mix of comfort and confidence in this person. The more time you spend at the front end choosing a doctor, the more likely you'll see him regularly and stay healthier."

4. Get a good workout.

For general physical well-being, nothing tops regular exercise. It helps you fend off heart disease, improves your sex life and enables you to live longer. How many other activities do you know that come with such nifty perks?

You don't have to pump iron to see the benefits of exercise, either. In fact, just 30 minutes of aerobic exercise at least three times a week can keep your heart and lungs healthy, prevent sprains, strains and day-to-day injuries, improve your circulation, increase your stamina and even help fend off colds and flus. Doctors recommend walking, swimming and cycling as especially good aerobic activities.

Aerobic exercise also helps burn off excess fat, which many men would benefit from. "Carrying those excess fat cells around will only put more of a burden on your heart," says Dr. Pantano. That spare tire also puts a strain on your body, particularly your back, which has to do most of the support work.

5. Know thyself.

Like indicator lights on a dashboard, your body has its own system to alert you to problems. But instead of red beacons, you get signs like headaches, fever, vomiting or diarrhea, says Dr. Goldberg. You don't have to be a doctor to know these symptoms—if they persist more than a few days, it usually indicates a problem.

"It goes back to this bulletproof mentality men think they need," says Dr. Goldberg. "They think they should tough it out, or ignore symptoms. They shouldn't."

So listen to your body. Physically check yourself every month or so for unusual

Top Ten Reasons Why Men Are Hospitalized

1. Cardiovascular operation
2. Digestive system operation
3. Musculoskeletal operation
4. Arteriography and angio-cardiography
5. Urinary system operation
6. Cardiac catheterization
7. CAT scan
8. Ultrasound
9. Respiratory system operation
10. Skin and tissue operation

lumps, moles that have changed size or color—anything that strikes you as unusual. And be thorough. "For example, don't be embarrassed to check your testicles for lumps or changes in size," says Dr. Goldberg. He points out that testicular cancer is a significant killer of men, and it frequently goes undetected.

The second part of knowing your body requires some familiarity with the previous models it was based on—such as your parents and their parents.

"It's vitally important for men to have a family history of medical conditions—this is the clearest roadmap you can get for problems you might face later," says Dr. Goldberg. For instance, if both your dad and your grandfather suffered heart attacks, that should be a clear signal to be more careful about your own heart. "It's a very commonsense notion, but so few men take advantage of their family history," says Dr. Goldberg. Don't be one of them.

6. Get out of the sun.

Cancer doesn't need any help from you. Yet many of us spend time working and playing outdoors, and we love basking in the glow of the sun, especially as we get older.

Well, knock it off.

Skin cancer is the most common kind of cancer around, says Dr. Goldberg. "And sun exposure is the main cause of skin cancer," he adds.

Good as the sun may feel, unfortunately, it's also throwing off plenty of radiation, cooking us like so many wieners in a microwave oven. As a rule, Dr. Goldberg advises staying out of the sun between 10:00 A.M. and 2:00 P.M. If you must be outdoors then, be sure to wear plenty of sunscreen with a sun protection factor (SPF) of at least 15 and wear a hat and light-colored clothing. "And stay away from tanning parlors," he says. "They give off the kind of ultraviolet light that can cause skin cancer."

7. Get away from it all.

Our workaday, dog-eat-dog world primes us for stress aplenty. And when the job's done, there are always domestic chores, be they bills, home maintenance or family politics.

No one's suggesting you should shirk your manly duties, but you ought to get a breather from them now and again. That means more than an annual vacation (though you should take one of those, too). Rather, take time out of every day to remove yourself from your hectic life.

"A man needs his own territory where he has time to go and be by himself," says John Dintenfass, M.D., professor of psychiatry at Mount Sinai Hospital in New York City. According to Dr. Dintenfass, that private time gives men a chance to reflect on the day's events and recharge their mental batteries. "That time is essential for your own identity—otherwise you lose your sense of self," he says.

If you don't have a den or shop to retreat to, make some other private space for yourself. This could be as elaborate as designating a certain room in the house at a certain time of day as your "quiet room" or as simple as walking around the block by yourself before you walk through the door. "It requires discipline," says Dr. Dintenfass. "But if you don't do it, life and work will control you, instead of you controlling them." Some men realize years too late that they have no sense of identity and wonder who they are, he adds.

8. Go to sleep.

Food and rest are the two fuels that allow you to live. Guys almost never miss a meal. So how come we're always scrimping on sleep?

"Proper rest is a very commonsense thing to get," says Dr. Goldberg. Sleep gives your mind and body a chance to perform day-to-day maintenance and repairs. But studies have shown that roughly half of all men sleep less than the eight hours a night most of us need. So sleep already. Shoot for eight or nine hours. And to ensure proper rest, try to go to sleep and get up at the same time every day.

9. Laugh once a day—at least.

If laughter was really the best medicine, clowns would be earning M.D.'s. That said, a smile can still be a handy umbrella against a possible downpour of health problems.

"Just the act of laughing can be beneficial from both an emotional and physiological perspective," says Joel Goodman, Ed.D., director of the Humor Project in Saratoga Springs, New York. "Physically, respiration and circulation are both enhanced through the act of laughter. We oxygenate the blood, which energizes us

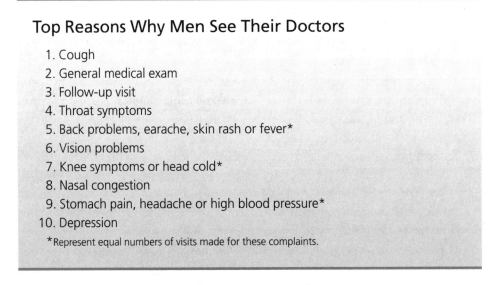

Top Reasons Why Men See Their Doctors

1. Cough
2. General medical exam
3. Follow-up visit
4. Throat symptoms
5. Back problems, earache, skin rash or fever*
6. Vision problems
7. Knee symptoms or head cold*
8. Nasal congestion
9. Stomach pain, headache or high blood pressure*
10. Depression

*Represent equal numbers of visits made for these complaints.

and helps us think more clearly." Plus, Dr. Goodman says, research shows that laughter stimulates chemicals in the brain that actually suppress stress-related hormones. "Stress in a man's life is inevitable, but humor helps us tickle stress before it tackles us. You shouldn't stifle your sense of humor; you should let it out," says Dr. Goodman.

10. Stay moist.

One of the simplest ways to stay healthy is to drink plenty of water. Water is the oil that lubes the mind and body. On top of that, it helps regulate our temperatures, protects our joints, keeps our sexual equipment functioning at peak condition and even helps ward off certain types of cancer. And we almost never drink enough of it.

"There's not much nutritional value—it has zero calories—but we wouldn't last long without it," says Dr. Goldberg. He suggests drinking at least eight to ten eight-ounce cups per day. "Keep some near you during the day and sip it regularly. You'll be surprised how much better you feel," he says. And when you're sick, drink even more. You'll replace the fluid you're losing and help your body cleanse itself of whatever you've caught.

Nutrition Basics for Men

How to Eat Right, Every Day

Flash back to fourth grade. As the teacher chatters about nutrition, you stare at a huge chart on the blackboard. It illustrates your body as a factory, like U.S. Steel. Shovel coal and iron in the front door, add heat, and out rolls steel. Same for you: Shovel raw materials down your maw—beans, green salads and endless glasses of milk—and, marvel of marvels, out comes a healthy you.

Turns out a man's body is a lot more complex than that. What, when and how much to shovel—that equation is more complex than anything encountered by a shop foreman. To stay healthy you need to consume dozens of nutrients in various amounts and concentrations. Consuming 90 percent may not cut it. You need them all. What's more, every man's needs are different, so there's no perfect template you can follow.

"Nutrition is not a black-and-white field and never will be," says Martin Yadrick, R.D., spokesperson for the American Dietetic Association. "People would like it to be much simpler, and the average consumer wishes it were, but it isn't. It's a multifactor thing."

And it's a vital thing. More and more experts believe that most medical problems can be traced, at least in part, to nutritional shortfalls or excesses.

Fortunately, good nutrition is on everyone's minds these days—not only in doctors' offices but in top corporations as well. Even fast-food chains have begun taking strides toward providing healthier meals. No matter how busy or intense your lifestyle, eating well has never been easier.

Understanding the Nutrient Soup

While scientists have identified more than 50 essential nutrients, all fall into one of two groups: macro and micro.

Macronutrients are things you need a lot of, like fats, carbohydrates, proteins and water. The body breaks down proteins into amino acids, which are used to build muscles, organs and blood. Fats provide a concentrated source of calories, help regulate satiety and transport certain vitamins into the body. Carbohydrates,

11

which include sugars and starches, can be stored in muscle and provide the raw material you burn for energy.

Unlike macronutrients, the micronutrients, which include most vitamins and minerals, are good things in small packages. You don't need a lot of them, but you can't afford to run short, either. A severe shortage of micronutrients, although rare, can lead to devastating diseases, like scurvy. But even a slight shortfall over time can result in conditions such as osteoporosis or anemia. Because vitamins and minerals are such a hot topic, we've written a separate chapter on them. So when you're done here, page ahead.

Not getting enough macronutrients can be even more serious—the stuff of newscasts from drought-stricken nations. Children who don't get enough proteins or fats may fail to reach their full size or have trouble healing. Not getting enough carbohydrates can lead to a serious dearth of energy and loss of vital body tissue.

Preventing the Drain

While there's no perfect one-a-day male superhealth cocktail that will keep you in top shape, there are ways to get the right mix. Here are a few ways to make sure you never fall short on the Nutritional Hit Parade.

Fear no food. All that stuff about food groups and food-guide pyramids and mandatory servings per day is a lot of mental baggage to carry around. (Just for the record, the U.S. Department of Agriculture recommends that every man eat 6 to 11 servings of grains, 3 to 5 servings of vegetables, 2 to 4 servings of fruit, 2 to 3 servings of milk, yogurt or cheese and 2 to 3 servings of meat, poultry, dry beans, eggs or nuts. Got it?)

Rather than trying to memorize food groups or numbers of servings, just think "variety and moderation," many experts advise. Over the course of a few meals, be sure to mix and match some low-fat milk and cheeses, some vegetables, lots of breads, some fruits and so on. Have a simple pasta dish today and a fish main course tomorrow. If you eat a variety of healthful foods every day, you'll be ahead of the game even when the exact numbers don't match up.

Get more fiber. In our grandparents' day, fiber was called roughage. Since it's hard to sell breakfast cereals with big banners that say "high in roughage," today we use the more marketable, less graphic term, *fiber*. There's soluble fiber and insoluble fiber, each of which has various sources and a number of health benefits. But don't get hung up on the different types. Eat more cereals, whole-grain breads, pastas, legumes, vegetables and fruits—consuming a wide range of foods with fiber will guarantee you get both types.

A high-fiber diet fills you up without filling you out, keeps your plumbing in working order, helps lower your cholesterol level and may help reduce the risk of colon cancer. Nutritionists recommend you get at least 20 grams per day. How? Try starting out with a breakfast of oatmeal, whole-wheat toast and two pieces of fruit—that'll get you halfway there.

Cut down on fat. Getting too much fat in the diet has been linked to a wide variety of male diseases: heart disease, stroke, cancer and diabetes, to name a few. But many men are confused about dietary fat because it comes in three different forms: saturated, polyunsaturated and monounsaturated. While it's true that some of these fats do some good, experts agree that you get more benefit from limiting fats of all kinds.

Your diet should consist of no more (and preferably less) than 30 percent fat. (Most American men eat about 37 percent of their total calories as fat.) Not only will this help improve your overall health profile, you might also notice something visible start to happen: You'll begin losing weight. That's because the body burns carbohydrates—the type of calories you get from grains, pasta, fruits and vegetables—more quickly than it does fats. Cut down on the fat you put in your belly and you'll cut down on the fat you put on it.

Cut your cholesterol. In the past, men compared cholesterol readings like box scores, in which low numbers were the clear winners. It's more complicated than that. More important than your total cholesterol number is the ratio of total cholesterol to the "good" kind, high-density lipoprotein (HDL), which can help keep blood vessels clear. Ask your doctor if your ratio is 3.5 to 1 or less. If it is, you're in good shape. If it's higher, you'll want to get to work.

Getting regular exercise and eating a low-fat, low-cholesterol, high-fiber diet should be part of your prescription. Studies also show that getting hooked on fish, specifically cold-water fish—to the tune of one serving a day—may raise HDL significantly.

Graze on healthy foods. No one believes anymore that the traditional three squares a day are necessary or even optimal for good nutrition. By all means, munch between meals. But don't add snacks—rather, divide what you'd normally eat throughout the day. And be sure that you munch on healthy things: a piece of fruit, for example, or a serving of cottage cheese or pretzels.

Start the day right. In this hectic age of late nights and hour-long commutes, keeping regular mealtimes—or even *having* meals—can be a challenge. But if you're only going to eat one real meal a day, make sure it's breakfast. After eight or more hours in bed your body is running on empty and needs a fill-up. "Of all the time-honored adages regarding food, perhaps the wisest is: 'Eat breakfast like a king, lunch like a prince and dinner like a pauper,'" says Joanne Curran-Celentano, R.D., Ph.D., associate professor of nutrition and food sciences at the University of New Hampshire in Durham.

Can't stand the thought of scrambled eggs first thing in the morning? Then heat some of last night's stew or boil up a plate of pasta. It isn't against the law to eat "dinner" foods at dawn, and they'll get your engine revved as well as traditional "breakfast" foods.

Adapt to the situation. The days are long gone (if indeed they ever existed) in which men could count on sitting down to dinner at the same time every day and being served a healthy variety of meat, potatoes and vegetables. Today work and meals are often commingled, and not always under the best circumstances. But you can still eat well.

Attending a business reception? Don't hover over the chips like an upright vacuum. Instead, think raw vegetables: carrots, broccoli and celery. And go easy on the dips; they're generally loaded with unhealthy fats. If you're going to be in the car all day, toss a few apples on the seat. You can even keep a bag of pretzels in a desk drawer. The goal isn't necessarily to eat perfectly every day but to eat well enough that you don't get desperate and turn to fatty, high-calorie snacks instead.

Eat everything—in moderation. Experts agree that as long as you don't stuff yourself silly, there are no "bad" foods. "All food is health food in moderation," says Victor Herbert, M.D., professor of medicine at the Mount Sinai Medical Center and Bronx Veterans Affairs Medical Center, both in New York City. "Any food is junk food in excess."

Consider insurance. Research shows that taking some vitamins in doses higher than the current government dietary guidelines may help ward off cancer and heart disease, boost immunity, regulate blood sugar levels and perhaps even prevent the onset of Alzheimer's disease. How do you ensure that you're consuming enough vitamins to gain all those benefits? With vitamin and mineral supplements. Your doctor is probably taking them. Why aren't you?

A basic daily supplement should give you 100 percent of the Recommended Dietary Allowance (RDA) for the following nutrients: beta-carotene (or vitamin A), the B vitamins (thiamin, riboflavin, niacin, biotin, pantothenic acid, folic acid, B_6 and B_{12}) and vitamins C, D, E and K. In addition, it should also contain 100 percent of the RDA for magnesium, selenium and zinc and at least 100 micrograms of chromium, all of which are needed for a man's good health. An even better supplement is one that's labeled antioxidant-rich—in other words, loaded with vitamins C and E and beta-carotene.

Follow the family tree. Experts agree that many chronic diseases—diabetes, heart disease and cancer, to name just a few—are genetically programmed. That is, the "blueprint" for trouble is already written. But it often takes a "trigger" for the disease to occur—and that trigger, in many cases, is diet, says Dr. Herbert.

the male file

The average person eats the following junk food per year.

- 300 containers of soda
- 200 sticks of chewing gum
- 100 pounds of refined sugar
- 63 dozen doughnuts
- 55 pounds of fats and oils
- 50 pounds of cookies and cakes
- 20 gallons of ice cream
- 10 pounds of candy
- 5 pounds of potato chips

So make careful notes of all the health problems in your family. Then ask your doctor what dietary changes you need to make that will do the most good. For example, if every man in your family has had a heart attack by age 60, you're going to want to be particularly vigilant about not getting too much dietary fat, says Dr. Herbert. Be proactive. If your doctor can't answer all your questions, ask him where to go for more information, says Dr. Curran-Celentano.

Vitamins and Minerals

What's New in Food Research

Eating. Sleeping. Having sex. As long as there have been people, there's been lots of this stuff happening. You gotta figure a few trillion pounds of food, hours of sleep and tumbles in the hay have gone down since two-legged talkers took up residence on the planet. Which brings up two questions:

1. With so much practice, why do men still struggle to do these things right?

2. Why is it that science has yet to figure out what they're all about?

Our topic here is food, and more specifically, what the latest research shows regarding your nutritional needs. While it's easy to question the point of all the research going on, you shouldn't: Scientific exploration into nutrients is unquestionably translating into longer, healthier lives for men. Including you. What follows is what you need to know—and need to do—to benefit from what's being discovered.

Staying Healthy with Antioxidants

It used to be considered normal for a man's body to go downhill with age. Today, researchers have traced much of this damage to free radicals, highly reactive molecules that your body produces during normal metabolic processes.

Short on electrons, free radicals scavenge them from your body's tissues, leaving damaged cells behind. As you age, this damage shows up in the form of clogged arteries, cataracts and other acts of terrorism going on inside your body.

Enter the antioxidants—substances produced by the body or found in your diet that wipe out free radicals before they can do their dirty work. They include the nutrients vitamin C, vitamin E and beta-carotene.

"It's very important that we take in enough antioxidants to neutralize free radicals," says Joanne Curran-Celentano, R.D., Ph.D., associate professor of nutrition and food sciences at the University of New Hampshire in Durham. "If we don't get enough, the result is oxidative damage."

Here's more on the big three antioxidant nutrients.

Vitamin C. The star of countless orange juice commercials, vitamin C can help prevent a slew of health problems, from minor infections to heart attacks.

And what about vitamin C's fabled ability to ward off the common cold? "Some

16

the male file

The average person's body contains 65 percent oxygen, 18.5 percent carbon, 9.5 percent hydrogen, 1.5 percent calcium, 1 percent phosphorous and 0.35 percent potassium, sulphur, sodium, chlorine and magnesium. It also has some trace elements, including iron, iodine, zinc and fluorine.

Translated, this means the average person's body has enough iron to make a three-inch nail, enough carbon to make 900 pencils, enough fat to make seven bars of soap, enough water to fill a ten-gallon tank and enough phosphorous to make 2,200 match heads.

studies show it can decrease the severity of colds, and some don't," says Dr. Curran-Celentano. "But even though the studies aren't conclusive, so many people swear by it that it's certainly worth trying."

The Daily Value for vitamin C—60 milligrams, the "full day's supply" found in a glass of orange juice—is certainly enough to prevent a deficiency but probably not enough to reap the preventive benefits, says Dr. Curran-Celentano. "Many people take supplements that contain 500 to 1,000 milligrams a day routinely, which is perfectly safe," she says.

Vitamin C is also abundant in citrus fruits and some vegetables, including peppers, tomatoes, broccoli and cauliflower. (Eat them raw or lightly cooked, though, since vitamin C is destroyed during cooking.)

Vitamin E. This vitamin prevents the oxidation of low-density lipoprotein, the "bad" cholesterol—a process that seems to lead to arterial plaque gunking up your arteries, making you a candidate for a heart attack. Unfortunately, vitamin E is found mostly in vegetable oils, which the heart-conscious man would do well to limit, says Dr. Curran-Celentano. Why? Vegetable oil is a type of fat.

"My feeling—and it's backed up by many studies—is that the levels of vitamin E that seem to be protective are very hard to get through diet alone." She suggests men take a daily supplement of about 100 international units.

Beta-carotene. A form of vitamin A, beta-carotene is another powerful antioxidant with preventive benefits. "Studies show that people with a high intake of beta-carotene—between five and six milligrams a day—have a lower incidence of heart disease and cancer, especially colon cancer," says Dr. Curran-Celentano. "It's easy to get that much if you eat the recommended five servings of fruits and vegetables a day." Go for orange fruits, such as cantaloupe, mangoes, peaches and apricots, and vegetables, such as carrots, squash and sweet potatoes.

Rounding Out the Picture

Antioxidants aren't the only nutrients that keep men healthy. Here are some others that are being found to have important benefits for your health.

Vitamin B$_6$ may help prevent kidney stones—a matter of consuming interest to any guy who's ever had one. There are so many good sources of B$_6$, including soybeans, tuna, beef, pork and chicken, that the average Joe gets plenty. If you're prone to stones, though, consider asking your doctor to prescribe a supplement. (This is one vitamin you shouldn't self-prescribe, since it can be toxic in high doses.)

Potassium's claim to fame is its effect on blood pressure. Studies show that some people can control high blood pressure with less medication once their potassium intake is increased. Experts recommend a minimum of 2,000 milligrams per day—an amount that's easy to get if you eat enough fruits and vegetables, says Richard Wood, Ph.D., associate professor at the Tufts University School of Nutrition in Boston. Good sources of potassium include spinach, bananas, tomatoes and milk.

Magnesium is essential for a healthy metabolism. Researchers claim that getting enough magnesium may reduce asthma symptoms, help people with chronic fatigue syndrome, control blood pressure and even protect you against heart disease. Men need 350 milligrams a day; good sources include spinach, seafood, oatmeal, beans, potatoes and brown rice.

Zinc plays an important role in insulin storage in the pancreas, and low levels of it have been linked to a depressed sex drive. Zinc is plentiful in beef, oysters and wheat germ, but if you're cutting back on red meat and never knew wheat had a germ, you may be coming up short. Make sure your multivitamin contains 10 to 15 milligrams of zinc or take a separate supplement, says Philip Reeves, Ph.D., supervisory research chemist at the U.S. Department of Agriculture Human Nutrition Research Center in Grand Forks, North Dakota.

Calcium is best known for preventing osteoporosis, the "brittle bone" disease. Contrary to popular belief, this isn't just a woman's problem, says Dr. Wood. "Men have naturally heavier bones and slightly higher calcium intakes, which give them some protection," he says. But a lot of men have avoided osteoporosis because something—usually a heart attack—put them out of commission first, and you don't have to worry about osteoporosis when you're dead.

"Men's life expectancy is increasing, so young men today are more likely to end up in a nursing home with a hip fracture than their fathers were," says Dr. Wood. That may seem pretty far in the future to a guy in his thirties or forties, but "the time to build bone is when you're young, so all men should make sure they're getting at least 800 milligrams of calcium a day," says Dr. Wood. Loading up on low-fat dairy products—about three servings a day—is the best way.

Part II

An A-to-Z Guide to Health

Acne

Ending Breakouts Isn't Hard to Do

So you woke up this morning with a zit in the middle of your forehead. What do you do now?

Well, you could bravely venture forth, looking upon this as an exercise in humility, a chance to prove that you can transcend the merely physical. Or you could cancel all your appointments, pull the blinds and pray that this epidermal abomination disappears as quickly as it arrived.

Whichever course you choose, you're likely to wonder why your acne didn't disappear with your youth the way it was supposed to. The answer is fairly simple.

Glands beneath your skin excrete oil to keep the skin's surface smooth and creamy. Hair follicles carry the oil up and out through your pores. Sometimes, though, the follicles, especially those in the face, chest and back, get clogged by dead skin and other debris. When that happens, bacteria begin to grow, the follicle becomes inflamed, and trouble results. Be it a whitehead, a blackhead, a cyst or a good old-fashioned pimple, it's not a pretty picture.

Your complexion goes bonkers during puberty because male hormones stimulate the production of the skin's lubricating oil. As you get older, your hormones settle down, but they don't disappear entirely, and neither may your acne. But fortunately, for most men acne is just a faded memory. Only between 5 and 10 percent of men over 25 still do regular battle with acne.

Despite the myth that chocolate or greasy foods are the cause of adult acne, doctors now believe heredity overwhelmingly dictates whether or not your pores have a tendency to clog.

Zit Defense 101

While nothing will remove acne from your life once and for all, there are plenty of things you can do to minimize the damage.

Stay calm. "Genetic predisposition is what causes acne, but it worsens with stress," says Daniel Groisser, M.D., a dermatologist in private practice in Montclair, New Jersey. Exactly why stress exacerbates acne isn't known—it's thought that it stimulates the adrenal glands, which then raise the level of hormones in the blood.

Wash gently. Because oil is at the heart of acne, it helps to keep the skin clean—but don't overdo it. "People still think acne is a disease of dirt, and so they tend to wash too often and too vigorously," says Alan R. Shalita, M.D., chairman of the Department of Dermatology at the State University of New York Health Science Center in Brooklyn. "That tends to exacerbate the condition by irritating the follicles."

Michael Ramsey, M.D., an associate in the Department of Dermatology at Geisinger Medical Center in Danville, Pennsylvania, recommends washing twice a day with lukewarm water and a mild cleanser, using your fingertips, not a washcloth. Look for labels that have the words "sensitive skin cleanser" or "foaming facial cleanser" on them. Avoid soaps that have astringents, fragrances or moisturizing creams.

Stay dry. Just as you should avoid oily soaps, don't put oily lotions, tonics or creams on your hair or face. "Those things can lead to a buildup of oil in your pores," says Thomas D. Griffin, M.D., a dermatologist at the Graduate Hospital in Philadelphia. "You don't want to do anything that can contribute to clogging." When you buy a sunscreen, he says, look for one that says it's "noncomedogenic," which means it won't form the follicle plugs that cause acne.

Watch your diet. Although scientific evidence indicates otherwise, dermatologists concede that people's individual physiologies might make their skin sensitive to some foods, including anything from shellfish to milk to nuts. "In all the studies, we've never proven that foods have any effect," says Dr. Ramsey. "If patients, however, say that certain foods cause them to develop acne, which they often do, the majority of dermatologists will encourage them to avoid those foods."

Stay healthy and fit. One of your most effective weapons against acne is staying in shape, which includes getting plenty of rest, eating a balanced diet and exercising. "All measures that are good for general health are good for the skin," says Dr. Shalita.

Shave safe. For men with acne, shaving can present something of an obstacle course. "What I do personally is use one of the foaming cleansers, then put on shaving cream," says Dr. Ramsey.

"If it's painful to shave, you might go with an electric shaver rather than a razor. It won't cut quite as close to the skin." Dr. Shalita adds that antibacterial shaving creams are available by prescription.

Have patience. Acne, depending on its severity, can take weeks or months to heal, even under the care of a dermatologist. Be patient, and don't squeeze or pick your pimples—you'll only make them worse.

Help in a Tube

If you do have acne, especially consistent, pervasive acne, modern science has provided a number of products that, together, can come pretty close to curing it.

FAST FACTS

How common: One study found that 34 percent of American men between the ages of 15 and 44 have had acne, but roughly 90 percent of all acne cases disappear by age 25.

Risk factors: Heredity, stress, possibly some foods.

Age group affected: Because male hormones promote acne, we get it most when we're teenagers and least as our hormone levels decline, usually in our fifties or thereabouts.

Gender gap: No one keeps good statistics on adult acne, but dermatologists say it is more prevalent in women than men. Some speculate it has to do with higher stress levels.

Who to see: Dermatologist.

The first line of defense is the topical, nonprescription medications available in drugstores that contain either benzoyl peroxide or salicylic acid. Follow the directions on the tube. They help dry up oily skin and loosen clogged pores. If those don't do the trick, see a dermatologist.

A professional treatment is likely to start with a round of oral antibiotics in combination with tretinoin (Retin-A), says John F. Romano, M.D., clinical assistant professor of dermatology at New York Hospital-Cornell Medical Center in New York City. Retin-A is a prescription-only cream that, unlike most topical medications, actually penetrates hair follicles, helping prevent acne formation at its roots.

If the acne persists, your doctor may suggest heavy artillery: isotretinoin (Accutane), taken by mouth, is a powerful drug that has proven to be remarkably effective in clearing up the most severe cases of acne—so much so that you simply don't see the sort of acne-ravaged face today that was fairly common 20 years ago.

If taken by pregnant women, Accutane can cause birth defects. For men the side effects may include dry skin, eyes and lips, and sometimes inflammation of the nose and burning, redness or itching of the eyes. Accutane can also raise your cholesterol, something you and your doctor should check on a monthly basis.

AIDS

Prevention Is Your Best Hope

$\mathbf{B}$y now, too many of us know at least one guy who has died from AIDS. As you helplessly watch the disease sap the life out of brothers, fathers, drinking buddies or mere acquaintances, you have to wonder: Could I be next?

That's largely for you to answer.

Unlike many life-threatening heredity diseases that are beyond your control, you can take easy steps to prevent AIDS—and prevention is the only certain defense against this prolific killer.

Unfortunately, a lot of men still needlessly risk losing their lives to acquired immune deficiency syndrome, because they're either confused, misinformed or just plain foolish.

"I think guys underestimate their risk," says David Herrell, director of the National AIDS Hotline, a toll-free information and referral service. "They make the assumption that the people they're having sex with aren't likely to be infected. Even when they realize there is a risk, once they get into the heat of passion, they forget about it."

A Brutal Rise

Men account for eight of every ten cases of AIDS in the United States. In 1992 it was the leading cause of death among men ages 25 to 44, surpassing accidents, heart disease, cancer, suicide and murder.

Since it erupted into an epidemic in 1981, 61 percent of those who have gotten the disease have died. Overall, AIDS has claimed 243,423 American lives, and it continues to spread at an alarming rate. From 1992 to 1993, for example, the number of new AIDS cases jumped 124 percent, according to the Centers for Disease Control and Prevention (CDC) in Atlanta. By 1994, 347,767 American men had AIDS, and the CDC estimated that one million people were infected with human immunodeficiency virus (HIV), the virus that causes AIDS, but were not yet showing symptoms of AIDS.

Intravenous drug use, homosexual sexual practices and a combination of these two risk factors accounted for about 80 percent of the AIDS cases in the United

FAST FACTS

How common: By 1994 the Centers for Disease Control and Prevention (CDC) in Atlanta estimated a million Americans were infected with HIV, and 401,749 cases of AIDS had been diagnosed. Of those, 347,767 were men. By 2000 up to 110 million people worldwide will be infected.

Risk factors: Risky sex practices, intravenous drug use, exposure to tainted blood or blood products.

Age group affected: All ages, but it is the leading killer of men ages 25 to 44.

Gender gap: In most countries in Africa and some in the Caribbean and South America most HIV infections occur through heterosexual contact—so men and women are almost equally likely to be infected. But in the United States HIV still affects far more men than women. As of 1994, according to the CDC, men were infected six times more than women.

Who to see: Infectious disease specialist, or call the National AIDS Hotline at 1-800-342-AIDS (Spanish-speaking hotline: 1-800-344-SIDA and deaf hotline: 1-800-AIDS-TTY) for a specialist in your area.

States in 1994. But AIDS isn't a "gay" or "junkie" disease. In fact, a growing number of young heterosexual men and women are getting the disease in the United States. Worldwide, the vast majority of AIDS infections have been contracted through heterosexual intercourse.

The Nuts and Bolts of AIDS

Almost the only way you can contract the virus that causes AIDS is through some risky behavior that leads to an exchange of body fluids.

"If you avoid risky behaviors, your chances of getting AIDS are pretty slim," Herrell says.

To set the record straight, you *can't* get AIDS from casual, nonsexual contact—from mosquitoes, toilet seats, pools, hot tubs or phones. Or even from repeated contact with an infected family member, including the sharing of utensils.

So how do you get AIDS? Through blood transfusions or exposure to HIV-infected blood or blood products. You can get it by using HIV-infected needles. Babies whose mothers are infected can get it via their shared bloodstream. And you can get it through risky sexual practices—far and away the most common mode of transmission.

Once the virus enters the body, it gradually dismantles the immune system. Initially, disease-fighting white blood cells are able to fight back and antibodies are made against the virus (when a man tests HIV-positive it means those antibodies have been found in his blood). But when the virus is inside a cell, it cannot be attacked by the antibodies. HIV-infected cells congregate in the lymph nodes, where they become virus factories, churning out new versions of HIV.

A man who is HIV-positive can remain healthy for many years. But almost always, HIV persists in cell membranes, lying silently until—sometimes more than ten years after the initial infection—the viruses burst out of the lymph nodes, renew their assault on the immune system and cause AIDS. Ultimately, the virus triumphs and the man succumbs to a crushing array of opportunistic diseases such as pneumonia, tuberculosis and Kaposi's sarcoma, a rare form of cancer, that take advantage of the body's weakened defenses.

Slashing Your Risk

Fortunately, as we mentioned before, there are plenty of ways to protect yourself from getting AIDS. Here's how.

Be faithful. Abstinence or maintaining a mutually monogamous relationship with a person who has tested HIV-negative are the only absolutely certain ways to avoid sexually acquiring an HIV infection, according to Michael Saag, M.D., director of the outpatient AIDS clinic at the University of Alabama School of Medicine, Birmingham.

Keep a condom handy. The next time you even think about having unprotected sex with someone new in your life, remember HIV—as in "Hey, I'm vulnerable"—then reach for a condom.

Lubricated latex condoms are best because the lubrication protects against rips and the latex is an effective barrier against HIV. As an added precaution you can buy latex condoms that are coated with nonoxynol-9, a spermicide that has been shown to kill HIV on contact.

If you use a lubricant, be sure it's a water-based product, such as K-Y Jelly, or spermicidal cream. Oil-based products like baby oil, cold cream or petroleum jelly can disintegrate latex condoms.

You also should absolutely avoid using lambskin condoms, because they are perforated with microscopic holes large enough to let HIV slip through.

Try to keep dry. Because HIV can be transmitted through body fluids such as blood, semen and vaginal secretions, some experts advocate having sex without exchanging any body fluids at all.

Sometimes called manual sex or mutual masturbation, it is a concept that few people could have imagined before the age of AIDS. But there are a lot of things we're all having to get used to, says F. Douglas Scutchfield, M.D., director of the Graduate School of Public Health at San Diego State University.

Kiss carefully. Theoretically, there's no risk in a smooch on the cheek. But, in theory, deep, wet French kissing may pose a very low risk. If there were HIV-infected blood in the mouth of one kisser, the virus could potentially be absorbed directly through the mucous membranes in the mouth of the other kisser.

It is also possible—but highly unlikely—to get infected simply through oral sex. For that reason, it's best to use a condom or a dental dam (a latex covering over the vagina) when you have oral sex. It's best, though, to avoid this type of sex unless you're sure your partner is HIV-free.

Keep the back door shut. Unprotected anal intercourse is by far the riskiest sexual practice, particularly if you're on the receiving end of it. That's because trauma to the anal mucosa, which isn't naturally lubricated like the vagina, opens a pathway directly into the bloodstream. Even wearing a condom might not protect you, since it can easily be broken by anal walls, Dr. Scutchfield says.

Know your blood supply. Sterilization and testing for HIV have virtually eliminated the risk of contracting AIDS through a blood transfusion in this country. But that's not true in many parts of the world. Of course, it's unlikely that you'll need a blood transfusion while traveling, but if you do, it's important to know if the blood supply is safe before you consent to receive one. If it isn't and you feel even remotely well enough to travel, you might consider returning to the United States for treatment, Dr. Scutchfield suggests.

Don't share syringes. Because AIDS is transmitted through the blood, you can easily contract the disease by injecting yourself with a needle previously used by another person.

Get Tested

If you're worried about AIDS, you can find out if indiscretions of six months past or more will come back to haunt you (it takes that long for the antibodies to show up in the blood). Anonymous screening tests for HIV antibodies are available at many health departments, hospitals and clinics. Although some places offer free tests, prices can range up to about $40.

For information on testing, treatment and support groups in your area call the CDC's National AIDS Hotline at 1-800-342-AIDS (Spanish-speaking hotline: 1-800-344-SIDA and deaf hotline: 1-800-AIDS-TTY).

Alcoholism

A Thinking Guide to Drinking

You knew your dad finally considered you a man the day he tossed you a cold beer. You knew you'd be accepted into your fraternity after you outdrank everyone at the freshman kegger. You knew your career was taking off when you had your first three-martini lunch with your boss.

From toasting a birth to mourning a death, alcohol is an integral part of the rites of passage in virtually every man's life. But one passage no man wants to make is the slippery slide from a casual drinker to a man who has serious alcohol problems.

If you think an alcohol problem couldn't ever corral you, think again. Alcoholism is an insidious disease—it often takes years to develop—and no one is immune from its devastating effects, says Donald Damstra, M.D., an addiction medicine specialist and substance abuse consultant in Phoenix.

"The distinct minority of alcoholics are skid row bums," says Peter E. Nathan, Ph.D., provost at the University of Iowa in Iowa City and former director of the Center of Alcohol Studies at Rutgers University in New Brunswick, New Jersey.

In fact, there is no typical man who abuses alcohol. It could be your boss, your minister, your son's Boy Scout leader or even you.

If you are among the 12 million American men who have serious drinking problems, you should know that the dark side of alcohol is far bleaker than passing out with your head slumped over the toilet. Alcohol abuse can lead to cirrhosis of the liver, heart disease, stroke, cancer, high blood pressure, pneumonia, diabetes, gout, insomnia, impotence, brain damage, ulcers, malnutrition and premature aging of the skin and bones. It can spark depression, increase stress, destroy friendships, ruin your marriage and derail your career. Alcohol abuse also is linked to nearly half of all traffic, boating and drowning fatalities and one in five deaths caused by disease, accidents and murders.

Crossing the Line

At any given moment, about 10 percent of American men older than 18 have problems controlling their drinking. But if you include recovering alcoholics who no longer imbibe, then the number of guys with drinking problems swells dramatically. Studies suggest, for example, that 23 percent of men have been or will become

FAST FACTS

How common: About 12 million American men have drinking problems.

Risk factors: Heredity, sex, religion, self-esteem and peer pressure are among the factors that contribute to alcoholism.

Age group affected: All age groups. The highest consumption rates and the greatest risk of abuse are found in men ages 18 to 24, followed by men ages 30 to 40.

Gender gap: Traditionally, statistics suggest that men are twice as likely as women to abuse alcohol. But some experts believe women hide their drinking better than men, and so the numbers of men and women who abuse alcohol actually may be close to equal.

Who to see: Family doctor, certified self-help groups, counselors and psychologists.

dependent on alcohol at some point in their lives, says Dr. Nathan. Often those problems occur early in a man's drinking history, such as during college. As he matures he drastically cuts back or quits drinking altogether. But some men don't. In fact, most active alcoholics are between the ages of 35 and 55, according to the American Medical Association.

Certainly there are men who drink heavily—meaning they suck down three or more alcoholic beverages each day—without developing dependency. But how much or how often you drink probably isn't the best way to define alcoholism. A man who never drinks during the week but passes out every Saturday night from drunkenness probably has more problems with alcohol than a man who has a drink every night of the year with his dinner.

The real line between choosing and needing to drink is this: If a man continues to drink alcohol even though it is destroying something critical to his well-being—health, career, relationships, legal status—then he is an alcoholic and should seek help, says Dr. Damstra.

Why some guys abuse alcohol and others don't remains a mystery. Some experts suspect a genetic link, since men with family histories of alcoholism are more likely to become alcoholic. But alcoholics come from all types of family histories, so it's likely that several other factors—peer pressure, self-esteem or religious attitudes, for example—also play key roles in making an alcoholic, says Dr. Damstra.

Look Out Body, Here It Comes

Even if you have yourself convinced that heavy drinking won't get in the way of your family or career, chances are you're still destroying your body. "Alcohol has a negative physiological effect on every human tissue," says Max A. Schneider, M.D., clinical associate professor of psychiatry and human behavior at the University of California College of Medicine at Irvine.

Ready to get depressed? Here's a partial tour of how excessive drinking can damage your body.

Blood. Alcohol suppresses the production of platelets and red and white blood cells. As a result, heavy drinkers are more susceptible to anemia, infections and bleeding.

Brain. Heavy drinking can cause brain damage by slowing blood circulation and oxygen flow to the brain cells. In addition, drinking disrupts communication between nerve cells in the brain and actually can make them crave alcohol. There's more: Excessive alcohol can impair memory. And heavy drinking increases the risk of stroke.

Heart. Although there is some evidence that one or two drinks a day may lower your risk of heart disease, more than two drinks a day can raise cholesterol and blood pressure and cause myocardiopathy, a swelling of the heart muscle that can lead to sickness and death.

Intestines. Alcohol abuse actually changes the structure of cells in the small intestine so they can't properly absorb nutrients and trace minerals. That's one reason that many heavy drinkers develop malnutrition.

Liver. It's the liver that often suffers the most damage from alcohol abuse, since about 95 percent of the alcohol that enters your body is detoxified by it. Alcohol abuse can cause hepatitis (an inflammation of the liver) or cirrhosis (scarring of the liver), which reduce the organ's ability to destroy dead red cells and to manufacture bile and other vital chemicals. Untreated, either can cause death.

Pancreas. Heavy drinkers are ten times more likely to develop diabetes than nondrinkers, because alcohol gradually destroys the pancreas, the organ that produces insulin.

Skin. Alcohol abuse can make you look older because booze decreases the elasticity of the skin, causing it to age faster. Drinking also makes you more susceptible to frostbite and burns.

Stomach. Alcohol decreases the production of mucin, a chemical that protects the stomach lining. Without enough mucin, powerful acids inflame the stomach, causing ulcers.

"Clearly the physical disruption from heavy drinking potentially can have a massive and destructive effect on the body," Dr. Damstra says.

Beating the Beast

Subduing an alcohol problem is a daily struggle that is seldom easy, says Dr. Damstra. Be prepared for setbacks, emotional strains and occasional temptations.

But with persistence, determination and the support of other recovering alcoholics, you can enjoy a lifetime of sobriety. Here's how to get started.

Admit you have a problem. Acknowledging that you have a problem is the first step. The sooner you realize that alcohol is your enemy, the more likely you can repair the physical and emotional damage it has done to your mind and body. Unfortunately, most alcohol abusers don't realize or are unwilling to admit they have serious drinking problems.

"If you suspect you may be an alcoholic, you probably are," says Dr. Damstra.

A couple of things make it difficult for a guy to face reality. First, alcohol abuse often sneaks up on a man so slowly he doesn't even know he has succumbed to it. In fact, it takes most men about six years to make the plunge from social to problem drinking. By then, his emotional defenses are well-established, and it's easy to deny that alcohol is ruining his life. Second, there's the ego. Men simply don't like to admit that they have any weaknesses, Dr. Schneider points out.

"It doesn't take a 'man' to drink. It does take a 'man' to recognize he has a problem and will do something about it," Dr. Schneider says.

Find some helping hands. "The first line of defense for an alcoholic is a qualified self-help group," says Dr. Nathan. "In my experience it's the rare alcoholic who will stop drinking without involving himself in a self-help group like Alcoholics Anonymous."

More intensive treatment such as counseling and psychotherapy also might be helpful, but they're useless if you don't stop drinking. Ask your doctor for help or contact an alcohol treatment center in your area. Or, for confidential information, write to Alcoholics Anonymous, P.O. Box 459, Grand Central Station, New York, NY 10163, or the National Council on Alcoholism and Drug Dependence, 12 West 21st Street, New York, NY 10010.

Let your family in on it. If you suspect you have a drinking problem, odds are those closest to you noticed it quite some time ago. Talk to your family. They may provide enthusiastic support.

Ask your spouse to attend counseling sessions with you. Be wary if she refuses, because it could be a sign that she also has an alcohol problem or is unwilling to admit that your drinking is out of control, says Dr. Damstra.

Avoid temptation. For the same reason Imelda Marcos should avoid shoe sales, guys shaking alcohol should avoid hanging out in the neighborhood bar with their old drinking buddies.

"It's a lot easier to slip back into old habits if you're still doing the same things you were doing when you were drinking," says Eric J. Devor, Ph.D., professor of psychiatry at the University of Iowa Hospitals and Clinics in Iowa City.

Find friends in your recovery group, church or gym who will support your

Cirrhosis: Don't Pickle Your Liver

Most men know more about needlepoint than they do about cirrhosis, a bit surprising considering cirrhosis of the liver is the third leading cause of death for men between the ages of 25 and 65.

Cirrhosis results when liver cells die, permanently scarring the soft liver tissue. Unfortunately, the liver is not an organ you can do without—it's responsible for the storage and filtration of blood and the secretion of bile; it plays a key role in breaking down carbohydrates, fats, proteins, minerals and vitamins; and it converts potentially toxic substances into harmless ones.

"Alcohol is the most prevalent cause of cirrhosis by far," says Vlado Simko, M.D., Ph.D., associate professor of medicine at the State University of New York Health Science Center at Brooklyn, New York. Cirrhosis has other causes. But for men in this country, alcohol is the culprit to watch.

What really makes cirrhosis so dangerous is the way it sneaks up on you. Experts cite a wide range of warning signs—deep fatigue and weakness, nausea, yellowish skin, small spider-like blood vessels that may appear just under the surface of the skin—then in the next breath admit that most of them appear only after liver damage has become extensive.

"Probably the earliest sign of liver disease is weakness," says Paul S. Pickholtz, M.D., a gastroenterologist in private practice in Yonkers, New York. "But you don't usually have any of the other symptoms until you're already in trouble."

Given the insidious nature of the disease, experts recommend you adopt a simple approach. "You shouldn't get to the point where you have cirrhosis because once you do, you're in trouble," says Dr. Pickholtz.

So avoid steady drinking. Cirrhosis isn't brought on by the occasional weekend binge—it's the result of daily drinking over 10 to 15 years.

"The liver has a remarkable potential for regeneration," says Dr. Simko. "If you give enough time between bouts of drinking, even if there's damage to a significant amount of liver cells, other liver cells will regenerate and replace the damaged cells. But if the damage occurs every day, that's difficult to recover from."

Outside of watching your drinking, probably the best thing you can do to prevent cirrhosis, says Dr. Simko, is to get a hepatitis B vaccine. Next to alcohol, hepatitis is the largest cause of cirrhosis. A hepatitis B vaccine works simply—it will stop the disease before it starts. Talk to your doctor if you don't remember ever having received a vaccine.

Am I an Alcoholic?

Unless you're a confirmed teetotaler, taking this quick test might be helpful, since many men are unaware or unwilling to acknowledge that they have an alcohol problem. Be honest, because if you don't face the problem, you can't solve it. If you answer yes to any one of these, you need help.

- You drink in the morning.
- You drink excessively without really feeling any ill effects.
- Alcohol is interfering with other parts of your life.
- You can't enjoy social activities without alcohol being involved.
- You get drunk alone.
- You experience repeated withdrawal symptoms—nausea, sleep disturbance, tremor, irritability and anxiety—only relieved by drinking.
- You are losing control of your drinking and you still can't stop.
- Drinking has become more important than job, family and friends.

quest to stay sober. Try new activities that don't involve alcohol like running or volunteering at a community organization.

Keep it light. Humor is a terrific weapon because it will help you keep your battle against drinking in perspective, says Dr. Schneider.

So if you're at a dinner party, for example, and the host asks you what you'd like to drink, tell him, "I'm too young to drink booze, so what else do you have?"

"It's a joke that will get more chuckles as you get older," the 73-year-old doctor says. "Laugh at yourself and you'll find that it will help you. Keep a positive attitude about your recovery."

Maintain constant vigilance. Between 50 and 70 percent of all alcoholics recover, but it's crucial to remember that alcoholism is a chronic disease—in short, it's always with you.

That's why it's important to remind yourself every day that sobriety isn't just a goal, it's an attitude.

"Sober just doesn't mean that you're dry. It means that you're comfortable being free of alcohol. It's a state of mind," says Dr. Schneider.

See also Drug Dependency

Allergies

Ducking the Sneezes and Wheezes

Our brains may believe in democracy, but our bodies practice more barbarian politics. Without provocation, our immune systems sometimes launch wars against perfectly friendly foreign substances—things like shampoo or pollen, strawberries or shrimp—whose only crime is being there.

Welcome to the coughing, sneezing, itching, swelling battlefield of allergies, where your immune system goes on the attack against imagined enemies and you suffer the consequences.

But allergies needn't make you a victim; there is much you can do to diminish the discomfort they cause. "A normal or very nearly normal life is possible for nearly every person with allergies. It shouldn't be a disabling disease if treated properly," says Philip Norman, M.D., professor of medicine at the Johns Hopkins University School of Medicine/Francis Scott Key Medical Center in Baltimore.

What Causes Allergies?

Almost any substance can trigger an allergic reaction. These substances, known as allergens, are mistaken for harmful foreign invaders by your immune system. Why this happens is still a mystery, although some researchers suspect that some men may inherit a tendency to make antibodies that are extremely sensitive to allergens. In any case, once your immune system identifies an allergen as an invader, it floods your body with powerful defensive chemicals to subdue the substance.

Most allergies are mild, causing no more than sniffles, headaches, watery eyes, a minor rash or weariness. But in rare cases allergies can cause stomach cramps, nausea, vomiting and even death. Bee stings and food allergies, for example, may cause anaphylaxis, a severe allergic reaction that can result in suffocation.

Allergies are lumped into three broad categories—contact allergies, caused by things such as shaving creams, drugs or clothing; food allergies, in which eating a food such as strawberries causes a reaction, and airborne or inhalant allergies, which are caused by substances such as pollen.

Inhalant allergies are by far the most common, namely because the four biggest causes—house dust, pollen, pet dander and mold—can be hard to duck. Inhalant-caused allergies affect 15 percent of all Americans—25 to 30 million people—and they can crop up at any age. Few men, however, develop inhalant allergies after age 30 unless they're exposed to a new allergen such as a pet.

But if you have allergies now, odds are you're stuck with them for many years to come. Allergies can disappear during childhood. If they follow you into adulthood, however, they often get worse. Fortunately, allergies also tend to dissipate in the midfifties as the immune system becomes less vigilant.

Heal Thyself

Allergies may be annoying, but unlike some diseases that resign you to little more than helpless spectating, the battle against allergies rests largely in your hands. Here's what you can do.

Identify the culprit. You can't effectively treat your allergy unless you know what causes it.

"You need to identify what you're allergic to," says William H. Ziering, M.D., an allergist and asthma expert in Fresno, California. "That way you can attack the allergens directly rather than just take medication and globally throw the animals out, throw grandpa out because he's a smoker, pull the drapes down and pull the carpets up."

About 90 percent of inhalant allergies are caused by 10 to 15 different allergens, such as dust mites, cockroaches, dogs and cats, grass and ragweed, says Thomas Platts-Mills, M.D., Ph.D., head of the Division of Allergy and Clinical Immunology at the University of Virginia School of Medicine/Medical Center in Charlottesville. So targeting the allergens that affect you may not be as difficult as you might suspect.

The best way to see what irks you is with a skin test. Using a pin, your doctor or an allergist pricks different allergens into your skin. If a red welt appears, presto! You've found the offending allergen. Of course, you may be allergic to more than one thing, so you may need to raise several welts before you've targeted all the offenders.

Steer clear of what ails you. Once you've identified the offending allergens, the best first step is to get away from them.

"The best treatment for allergies is avoidance of the offending materials," says Franklin Adkinson, M.D., professor of medicine and co-director of the Division of Allergy and Clinical Immunology at the Johns Hopkins University School of Medicine/Francis Scott Key Medical Center. "It's effective without having any side effects, and it's often the most economical way to treat allergies as well. For mild allergies, avoidance and an over-the-counter antihistamine may be all that's necessary to keep the allergy sufferer comfortable."

Create your own inner sanctum. "The most important thing you can do around your home to ease allergy problems is to focus on making the bedroom an allergy-free environment," says Dr. Adkinson. "We probably spend a third of our lives in our bedrooms; plus, when we're sleeping, a lot of our defense mechanisms are not at their peak."

If you're allergic to dust, the best place to start your war on allergens is in your bed.

"The average man in bed has 2,000 dust mites accompanying him, and they're alive," says Dr. Ziering. It's not the mites (tiny relatives of ticks and spiders) themselves that are the root of dust allergies, it's their droppings.

You can eliminate this microscopic problem almost entirely. Use polyester pillows that can be washed in hot water, encase your box spring and mattress in zippered vinyl coverings and wash your sheets in hot water once a week, says Dr. Ziering. These precautions can eliminate 90 percent of the mites.

Be sure to wipe down your dresser tops and windowsills regularly and get rid of clutter (stacks of magazines, books, office folders and any other knickknacks that collect dust). If possible, replace carpeting and curtains—both places where mites can dig in—with throw rugs and window blinds.

Become Mr. Clean. If you suffer from dust or other airborne allergies, you can't stop cleaning at the bedroom.

On average, men spend roughly 95 percent of their lives indoors, of which 60 percent is in their homes, says Dr. Platts-Mills, so controlling indoor allergens is important.

This means frequent (with more severe allergies, daily) dusting, vacuuming and spraying with commercial cleansers—floors, couches, curtains, carpets, everything that is home to the dust mite. Dr. Platts-Mills suggests you ask your allergist about allergy supply companies so you can order cleaning products by phone. Two such companies are National Allergy Supply (1-800-522-1448) and Allergy Control Products (1-800-422-3878).

Remember that cleaning kicks up a dust storm of its own. So wear a filter mask when you clean or find a nonallergic person to do it for you.

Keep cool. Spring and summer are prime allergy seasons, namely because the plant world is busy pollinating itself in an orgy of rebirth. Keeping pollens out of the home during these steamy seasons is a simple matter.

"Air-conditioning will really help you reduce your exposure to pollens," says Dr. Norman. "The air conditioner's filtration system takes out most of the pollen."

Smaller particles like mold spores can be filtered out by installing superfine air filters in your central air and heating systems. Air-conditioning also keeps humidity low, discouraging dampness and the proliferation of molds.

If you don't have air-conditioning, sleep with the windows closed during pollen season. Remember, when you sleep, your defense mechanisms are at a low ebb.

Say hi to dry. Mold, and its allergy-causing spores, are the Freddy Kruegers of allergens.

Wipe down mold-prone areas with bleach or a fungicide, available at most drugstores, and keep your home as dry as possible. Dehumidifiers help, especially in dank places like basements and garages.

Develop a sense of timing. Exercise is fine, but avoid doing it at dawn or dusk, when pollen counts soar. If you insist on getting outside when pollen counts are high, focus on your breathing.

"Try to breathe more with your nose than your mouth," says Dr. Ziering. "The nose has a wonderful intrinsic filter system."

Give food a thought. Allergic reactions to food are often prompt and attention-getting—hives, nausea, difficulty breathing, headaches and diarrhea.

Common food allergens include scallops, eggs, corn, milk, white fish and peanuts. Skin tests can help ferret out the culprit. You also can try to eliminate the symptoms by cutting the suspected food from your diet.

Don't pet your pet. If you suspect that your pet is responsible for your allergies, remove the animal from the house to verify it. Unfortunately, studies have shown that it takes at least six weeks to rid a house of pet dander and other particles of hair, fur, feathers and skin. Keep in mind that pet dander can still sneak into the house on the hands and clothes of your family.

Dust Busters

How bad are the allergens in your house?

You can now get a far more accurate measure of the common allergens lurking in your home. Researchers at Johns Hopkins University in Baltimore can perform a "house dust aero-allergen analysis" that can give you a precise measure of the allergen levels hanging about your house.

If you're interested, ask your allergist about the analysis. The procedure is simple. A small collector is attached to your vacuum. The dust sample is then analyzed by a laboratory, which can then tell you what allergens you have in the home and how concentrated they are.

"Basically, this analysis allows you to assess your indoor environment and really decide whether you have a problem or not," says Robert G. Hamilton, Ph.D., associate professor of medicine at the Johns Hopkins University School of Medicine/Francis Scott Key Medical Center in Baltimore. "Based on this you can either elect to clean the house more vigorously or not worry about it." Current cost—about $25 for each allergen analysis.

If getting rid of Fido will cause a family insurrection, then at least keep him out of the bedroom and wash him regularly.

Bee aware. About 2 percent of men are allergic to bee stings. If you're one of the unfortunate few who are, keep your guard up and don't make yourself an inviting target. Keep your shoes on, don't leave food out, skip cologne or aftershave and avoid wearing bright colors.

If you are stung and develop hives, swelling, dizziness, difficulty breathing or tightness in the chest, seek medical attention immediately.

Don't run away. Some guys believe allergens can be left behind. But packing up and moving does little good if you're allergic to mold or dust mites.

"If you're allergic to dust mites in the United States and you go to another country and visit a home that has a high level of dust mites, you could still experience symptoms," says Robert G. Hamilton, Ph.D., associate professor of medicine at the Johns Hopkins University School of Medicine/Francis Scott Key Medical Center in Baltimore.

Moving may help you sidestep your allergy, but you may pick up new allergies when you move. So your best bet may be to stand your ground and fight off the allergy.

Give Drugs a Chance

If these precautions don't completely eliminate the problem, allergy medications may help. Here's a sampling.

Antihistamines. "The first line of defense for pollens as far as medications are concerned are antihistamines," says Dr. Norman.

Available over the counter or by prescription, antihistamines work by blocking the action of the histamine flood your body orders up when it encounters an allergen. In the past, antihistamines also made you slower than Times Square on New Year's Day, but manufacturers have developed nonsedating antihistamines that won't dope you up. An important note: For best results, take the antihistamine before your allergies flare.

Oral decongestants. But they can also cause unpleasant side effects like insomnia and elevated blood pressure. You may need to experiment to see how they work for you.

Shots. Immunotherapy, a series of gradually more potent injections of the allergen(s) that ails you, is the last line of defense in the allergen war. Immunotherapy doesn't work for food allergies, but studies have shown it is effective in dealing with allergies caused by dust, bee venom, cat dander, ragweed and grass.

"We usually think about immunotherapy for patients who suffer through more than just a single season and in cases where avoidance and first-line medication just don't seem to be working," says Dr. Adkinson.

But be prepared for a long haul. You'll likely be given one to two shots a week for the first 8 to 16 weeks, then one shot every 2 weeks for the remainder of the first year. After that, shots are suggested every 2 to 3 weeks.

Even if you do undergo immunotherapy, you will still need to take medication and avoid allergens.

Alzheimer's Disease

The Race for a Cure

You saw the signs in an elderly friend, but for a long time you couldn't figure out what was going on. He was forgetting simple things, like the names of friends or punch lines to his favorite jokes. Later he began forgetting entire conversations—or even that he'd *had* the conversation. Ordinary tasks, like shopping or balancing the checkbook, became progressively more difficult. Eventually, the man you thought you knew was simply gone—taking with him his charm, wit and boundless consideration.

The cause was Alzheimer's disease. Its most infamous—and terrifying—symptom is a progressive loss of memory, a wasting away of the ability to retain and recollect information that eventually leaves its victim a prisoner of an eternal present. Then, inevitably, comes death. Alzheimer's disease is now the fourth leading cause of death among mature Americans, a silent and mysterious plague that has been called the disease of the century.

If you are under age 60, Alzheimer's likely isn't a near-term threat to you. And given that there is nothing you can do to prevent the disease, it's not worth fretting much over. But chances *are* good that the disease touches someone in your life. And given that you intend to grow old, it's wise to be an active spectator to one of the most prominent battles the medical research community is currently waging.

Disintegration of the Self

Alzheimer's disease is the breaking down not just of memory, experts say, but of the brain itself. Seen under a microscope, the brain of someone with Alzheimer's shows accumulations of abnormal deposits, called plaques, that have infiltrated normal tissue. Over time, the buildup of plaques is believed to cause "the death of neurons, the brain cells that communicate and process information," explains Leon Thal, M.D., chairman of the Department of Neuroscience at the University of California, San Diego. Normal brain functions are crippled and eventually destroyed.

Experts aren't sure what causes Alzheimer's disease. One suspect is beta amyloid, a misshapen splinter of protein that may accumulate and begin jabbing holes in brain cells. Other theories have looked at the role of getting too much aluminum

40

FAST FACTS

How common: Alzheimer's disease is a growing threat. Estimates range from 10 percent of Americans ages 75 to 85 to as high as 50 percent of Americans over age 85. It's estimated that Alzheimer's causes 100,000 deaths a year.

Risk factors: Mostly unknown. Some evidence suggests that it runs in families; that those with less education and fewer career achievements are more susceptible; and that too much aluminum or too little zinc in the diet might play a role.

Age group affected: Primarily the elderly. The older one gets, the more susceptible one becomes.

Gender gap: Men and women are equally susceptible.

Who to see: A family doctor may be able to render a preliminary diagnosis, but it may be advisable to seek a specialist in neurology or gerontology.

in the diet, or too little zinc. But what is increasingly clear, experts say, is that Alzheimer's disease may have many causes and not just one.

It's Not Just Memory Loss

Lose your keys all the time? Forget where you parked? Can't remember a colleague's name? It has to be Alzheimer's, right?

Probably not. For one thing, Alzheimer's is unusual in that people with the disease generally don't suspect that anything's wrong. "If you think you have the disease, then it is likely that you don't," says Dr. Thal.

What's more, while Alzheimer's has become increasingly common, it's *not* a normal consequence of aging. On the other hand, some degree of memory loss is. "Everybody forgets, and a lot of us become aware of that as we get older," says Victor Henderson, M.D., professor of neurology, gerontology and psychology at the University of Southern California in Los Angeles.

So if you've begun forgetting "normal" things, like where you put the keys, you can probably relax. But if what's "missing" are entire conversations or even days, you need to see a doctor, says Dr. Thal. While Alzheimer's disease occasionally strikes men as young as age 40—doctors call this form of the disease presenile Alzheimer's—it almost always occurs in the elderly. "It's very common among older people, and up to 50 percent of people over age 85 have it," says Dr. Henderson.

There's some evidence that Alzheimer's runs in families, experts say. In addition, those with less education and fewer career achievements seem to be more at risk. Experts aren't sure why this is. Perhaps the more you "exercise" your brain, the better it's maintained. Or perhaps those with more education and accomplishments are simply better able to develop strategies for coping with the disease, thus delaying the diagnosis.

Nailing It Down

While getting a correct diagnosis is always important, it becomes critical when Alzheimer's is suspected. This is because there are a number of curable diseases—like small strokes or nutritional deficiencies, like pernicious anemia—that can cause symptoms that mimic Alzheimer's.

Alzheimer's can only be diagnosed with 100 percent accuracy following an autopsy. Doctors, however, can be nearly as accurate using brain scans, interviews with family members, psychological evaluations and a number of lab tests. In addition, Harvard researchers have reported that a simple eye test—in which drops used to dilate the pupils cause a greater amount of dilation in people with Alzheimer's—may help detect Alzheimer's in many cases.

An early diagnosis not only would reduce uncertainty for patients and their families but also would give patients a chance to slow or minimize symptom development by taking part in experimental treatments.

Hope on the Horizon

While there is currently no cure for Alzheimer's, there are a number of treatments that show promise. Approximately 20 different medications are under study, for example. One of these, called tacrine, has already been used in treating patients with mild to moderate forms of the disease.

Tacrine is thought to work by boosting the levels of a brain chemical involved in cognitive functioning. In a 12-week trial of 468 patients with mild to moderate forms of the disease, those taking daily doses of tacrine showed measurable improvement. In real terms they were able to recognize their caregivers more, perform more of their chores and improve their short-term memories.

"This is a potentially useful drug, with a small number of patients actually experiencing much larger improvements than expected," says Martin Farlow, M.D., professor of neurology at Indiana University Medical Center in Indianapolis.

Studies also suggest that the female hormone estrogen may play a role in taming Alzheimer's disease. After reviewing the histories of 8,881 women in a retirement community, researchers found that those who had taken estrogen were 40 percent less likely to develop the disease than women who had never taken estrogen.

"If other studies validate that estrogen can reduce the incidence or slow the development of this disease—or be used as a treatment—then the impact on Alzheimer's could be tremendous," says study author Annlia Paganini-Hill, Ph.D., professor of preventive medicine at the University of Southern California School of Medicine in Los Angeles.

In addition, provocative research from Columbia University in New York City hints that staying mentally stimulated may help stave off the disease. In a study of 593 people over age 60, researchers found that those with higher education and job attainments had about a third of the risk of developing Alzheimer's than did people with low occupational attainments and less than eight years of education.

Researchers speculate that people who are mentally the most active may build a reserve of brain synapses. This means they may experience less of a loss when the disease starts claiming them. "These results suggest to me that this building is a life-long process," says Alzheimer's researcher Yaakov Stern, Ph.D., associate professor of clinical neuropsychology at Columbia College of Physicians and Surgeons in New York City.

The Disease of the Future

First identified by Alois Alzheimer around the turn of the century, the disease has nonetheless become increasingly common, affecting approximately one in ten people between the ages of 75 and 85 and costing upward of $90 billion nationally in health care.

"There's a tremendous amount that's known now about Alzheimer's disease that was not known five or ten years ago," adds Dr. Henderson. "I think with the way things are going, sooner or later there will be a breakthrough in therapeutics. It's too bad it isn't here yet."

If you're caring for someone with Alzheimer's, experts recommend you call a local chapter of the Alzheimer's Association for guidance. To find a group in your area, call the organization's national headquarters at 1-800-272-3900.

Anal Ailments

Eradicating Problems Down Under

Take two small rubber bands. Wrap one around a brick and drag it from one end of the brick to the other. Wrap the second rubber band around an overripe banana and drag it from one end to the other. Now, which rubber band would you rather have for an anus?

The rubber band that got the brick treatment probably has tiny cracks in it. The same thing can happen to your anus when you pass a brick—a large, hard stool—in real life. While such cracks (called anal fissures) are small, you may feel like you've been torn asunder.

Fissures are only one example of an anus gone astray. Anal abscesses are painful, boil-like infections that burrow through the muscle. And then there is the garden-variety pain in the tush—*pruritus ani,* also known as itchy anus. While all of these maladies can temporarily upend your life, you can do a lot to comfort your personal ring of fire.

Fissures: The Terrible Tear

Anal fissures are little tears in the skin around the anus—painful reminders that you ought to eat right.

"Fissure is basically a crack, and you get those either from having a stool that's too hard or a stool that's too watery," says David E. Beck, M.D., chairman of the Department of Colon and Rectal Surgery at Ochsner Clinic in New Orleans. "The hard stool overstretches the anus—it just causes a crack right at the outside of the anus. And that's why it hurts so much, because the outside skin has nerve fibers that sense pain. The inside doesn't."

Diarrhea causes similar tears when it bursts through the anus. "When the diarrhea comes down, it kind of opens the muscle very quickly—it doesn't have time to gently stretch out," says Dr. Beck, who has edited two textbooks on colon and rectal surgery. "A lot of times the perianal burning that patients complain of after having diarrhea is because of a small fissure, and not so much because the diarrhea burns."

A person with a fissure will experience two kinds of pain—a knifing pain at the

FAST FACTS

How common: Nearly everyone encounters some transient anal problems at some time in their lives. Statistics are difficult to find since many people don't talk about it.

Risk factors: Poor diet, poor hygiene or overzealous hygiene can lead to fissures or abscesses. Too much moisture can lead to itching.

Age group affected: Anal itching is more common in children and the elderly. Other problems can occur at any time in one's life.

Gender gap: None.

Who to see: Family doctor, proctologist or colon and rectal surgeon.

time of a bowel movement and then a dull pain caused by spasms of the underlying sphincter muscle. The latter pain can last for hours.

"Everybody attributes any sort of pain in the bottom to hemorrhoids. But probably about a third of those are going to be fissures," says Olaf B. Johansen, M.D., a colorectal surgeon in private practice in Indianapolis.

Anal fissures can produce as much as a tablespoon of bright red blood, appearing in the toilet or on tissue paper during a bowel movement. The bleeding should stop quickly, and nothing needs to be done about it. Men over age 40 in particular, however, should alert their doctors to rectal bleeding because it can be a sign of colon cancer.

Here's how to cope with these unkind cracks.

Eat yourself healthy. "The initial treatment is to get the stool normal," says Dr. Beck. "And for that we add fiber to the diet." So to produce those squishy-banana stools, you have to *eat* bananas—and carrots, apples, bran cereal, whole-wheat bread and any other high-fiber foods. Try for five one-ounce servings of fruits and vegetables a day.

Supplement your fiber. If you're struggling to get enough fiber in your diet to normalize your stools, consider fiber supplements such as Metamucil, Citrucel or FiberCon. "Ideally, you want to get about 25 to 30 grams of fiber a day," says Dr. Johansen.

Get juiced. To prevent constipation, drink six to ten eight-ounce glasses of liquids a day.

Soak it. Soaking your bottom in a tub or sitz bath of plain, warm water helps soothe muscle spasms and cramps caused by hard, dry bowel movements. Experts recommend several times a day, 20 minutes at a time.

Be sure the water is not painfully hot. But remember that the warmer the water is, the greater and longer the pain relief will be. That's what doctors discovered at Cairo University in Egypt, where they tested 18 patients with fissures and 10 patients with hemorrhoids. The patients soaked in water at 104°, 113° and 122°F. Although the higher temperatures provided the greatest pain relief for those patients, test your water for your own personal comfort level.

Some guys with fissures can develop a king-size fear of sitting on the throne and recreating the agony. "I usually advise people who have a fissure to actually draw a hot bath before they have a bowel movement," says Dr. Johansen. "Have the bowel movement and then sit in the bathtub for 20 to 30 minutes. That relieves the spasms and really does a very good job."

Let it slide. Say your diet slips while you're on the road. You're in a Boulder, Colorado, hotel facing a scary, rocklike bowel movement. You know straining to pass it will risk injury, but what else can you do? "You ought to give yourself a small enema," says Dr. Beck. "There are some on the market that have water and mineral oil in them, available over the counter. That will provide some fluid, and the oil tends to soften the stool."

If that doesn't work, try using a finger to break up the stool before it passes—yes, you can do it (doctors recommend you first put on a latex glove and trim your fingernail), or ask a doctor or nurse to help. (With friends like these, who needs enemas?)

If necessary, operate. In 10 percent of fissure patients, scarring or sphincter spasms will prevent a fissure from healing. A 15-minute outpatient operation called sphincterotomy can correct a fissure that continues to bleed or cause pain. More than 90 percent of such patients have no further fissure problems.

Abscess: Boils and Trouble

Maybe you've found a tender, red lump near your anus the size of a nickel or quarter. It's incessantly painful, and you might feel sick and have a fever. After two or three days you're in too much pain to sit or walk. That's an anal abscess rearing its ugly head.

Abscesses start when one of the small lubricating glands around the anus gets infected. The infection creates a cavity that fills with pus, says Dr. Beck. The infection spreads through the sphincter muscle and usually surfaces one to three inches from the anus. In some cases, the abscess moves in reverse and never surfaces.

Fixing an abscess is usually simple, but you need a doctor to do it because of its out-of-sight location. "You just lance it," says Dr. Johansen. "It can usually be done in the office by injecting some local anesthetic, and then you open up the abscess. You drain it out and that will take care of about 60 percent of abscesses." Forty percent of abscesses will leave a small tunnel, called a fistula, leading from the rectum to the skin. Fistulas can run with pus, blood and even feces. When necessary, they are repaired with surgery to remove the infected gland.

Merely taking antibiotics for an abscess is a mistake, says Richard M. Burg, M.D., a colon and rectal surgeon in private practice in White Plains, New York. "As soon as a person has been diagnosed with an abscess, provisions should be made to drain it," he says, "because it will only progress and damage more tissue and cause more pain. An antibiotic can help with the surrounding inflammation of an abscess, but it won't ever cure it."

There is no proven way to prevent abscesses, although there is some evidence that maintaining a normal stool makes having one less likely, says Dr. Beck. Inflammation of the intestine, such as colitis, increases your odds of getting one.

Soaking in a warm tub will provide temporary pain relief.

Itchy Anus: How to Get Relief

Maybe your anus is tired of following you around a sweltering golf course. Maybe it's tired of the rough toilet paper at the clubhouse. Maybe it's tired of being compared to your boss.

Whatever the reason, your anus is irritated and itchy, a condition the doctors call *pruritus ani*. Miss Manners be damned, you've gotta scratch.

"I tend to see a lot more men with that," says Dr. Johansen. "I don't know if it's a lot more common in men or if women just don't come in with it."

The causes are varied but usually involve moisture inflaming the skin around the anus. "Normally your anus is supposed to be dry," says Dr. Beck. "If it gets wet, some changes develop, and it's very akin to having your hands soak in dishwater all day, or a soldier standing in water and getting trench foot."

The rectum may secrete the irritating moisture, it may come from hemorrhoids or diarrhea, or sweat may be the culprit. Too little cleaning can create a rash, as can too much scrubbing. Sometimes soap or toilet paper irritate the skin. Other causes include diet and skin disorders such as eczema or psoriasis.

If your symptoms don't respond to treatment for two or three weeks, call your doctor. Rare skin conditions, such as Paget's disease and Bowen's disease, can cause an itchy anus, as can pinworms and some sexually transmitted diseases.

Here are ways to bring peace to the valley.

Keep it clean. "First thing I tell people is try to keep the area clean, but don't overscrub," says Dr. Johansen. After a bowel movement clean yourself gently with wet toilet paper. If it's practical, get in the shower and wash with plain water—no detergent soap. Then pat yourself dry.

Clean with lotion regularly. Dry toilet paper can be abrasive enough to damage the skin. "I usually recommend that patients clean with a lotion such as Balneol or Prax," says Dr. Burg. "These are very soothing. Do this on a routine basis—not just when you need it—because itching notoriously tends to recur. I make an analogy: It's like brushing your teeth."

He also recommends mild treatments like pramoxine cream (Anusol, Tronolane). Light creams, as opposed to ointments, are less likely to trap moisture against the skin.

Cream it with steroids. If your symptoms are severe, one of the over-the-counter steroid creams, like hydrocortisone, might provide relief, says Dr. Johansen. "The steroid can break that scratch-itch cycle," he says. "Take away the itching and presumably people will stop scratching it. And then it will heal. That's the one role where some of these creams will have some short-term utility." The steroid content is often indicated by "HC" (for hydrocortisone) in the product name.

Powder your bottom. After a shower apply cornstarch or other powder to keep your anus dry. To further absorb moisture, place a small wad of cotton near your anus. Leave it there, and change it several times a day.

Dress for the occasion. If you're sweating a lot, change your underwear several times a day, suggests Dr. Beck. "And well-ventilated clothes tend to keep the area drier, too—loose-fitting jeans as opposed to tight biking shorts, something that'll breathe a bit," he says.

Change soap and paper. Perfumed and deodorant soaps and toilet papers can contain chemicals, like formaldehyde, that irritate the skin. Stick to two-ply toilet paper, soft and plain—and go easy on yourself, because rough rubbing can irritate you as well. Also, avoid commercial cloth wipes. "The cloth they use is too strong—you can scrub too hard," says Dr. Beck. "Second, many of them contain chemicals such as alcohol or witch hazel, which also irritate the skin."

Pass on the pepper. Spicy cuisine and highly acidic foods such as tomatoes and citrus fruits can cause irritating anal secretions. Other suspect foods are beer, milk, chocolate, nuts and popcorn.

Turn off the gas. "Anything that causes a person to pass a lot of gas rectally will also bring out moisture and contribute to itching," says Dr. Burg. So cut back on the broccoli, cabbage, carbonated beverages, or anything else that toots your tuba.

Go easy on the drink. Your behind doesn't take kindly to more than six glasses of caffeine, alcohol or carbonated fluid a day, according to the American Society of Colon and Rectal Surgeons. Caffeine and alcohol actually remove fluid from the body and carbonated sodas give you gas you don't need.

Angina

Avoiding the Worst Kind of Heartache

Y̵ou're on your way to work when the radio reports a bottleneck on the highway up ahead. What do you do?

When it comes to traffic jams, most men would heed that report and go out of their way to prevent slowing down. Well, your first angina attack is a radio report, too—an urgent bulletin, in fact—of traffic problems on the oxygen highway to your heart.

The problems in question are fatty deposits building up as plaque inside your arteries, a condition called atherosclerosis. Ultimately, the plaque narrows the vessels providing oxygen-rich blood to the heart muscle. When your heart needs more oxygen but can't get it, the heart sends out a warning signal that men feel as a crushing pressure or pain in their chests, arms and necks. An angina attack isn't a heart attack, but it is an important warning sign of the biggest killer of men—coronary heart disease, a problem worth going miles out of your way to avoid.

Plague of Plaque

Most men suffer angina attacks during exercise or moments of stress, times when the heart needs more oxygen, says James A. Pantano, M.D., a cardiologist practicing in Allentown, Pennsylvania, and author of *Living with Angina*.

"It's like trying to rev an engine with a blocked fuel line," he says. "They're only going to have angina symptoms during physical or emotional stress. They won't have it just sitting still." That's the essence of what doctors call stable angina: The plaque has created a constant narrowing of the arteries, a regular bottleneck instead of a sudden pileup. For many men, that means they may expect an angina attack every time they perform certain activities such as running up a flight of stairs or having an argument with their wives. But with proper medication, Dr. Pantano says most men can learn to live with it.

What you need to watch out for is unstable angina, meaning you're prone to sudden, unexpected angina attacks—for example, when a piece of plaque comes loose and jams in the bloodstream. "It's a whole different ball game," says Dr. Pantano. "Often the plaque will unclot, but if it doesn't and it clots all the way across the artery, then it will cause a heart attack."

Anyone with angina, or even the hint of it, should be talking to a doctor. If you don't have angina, here are some ways to keep from getting it.

Forfeit fat. Those fatty deposits that close off the bloodstream don't get there by themselves—most of them come from the fats we eat with our daily meals.

"One of the clear-cut things people really need to do is reduce the amount of fat intake in their diet," says James Reed, M.D., professor of medicine at Morehouse School of Medicine in Atlanta and president of the International Society of Hypertension in Blacks. "They need to watch out particularly for saturated fats, along with cholesterol." That means going light on animal sources of fat—red meat, dairy products and cheese especially. Experts recommend that men get no more than 30 percent of their daily calories from fat.

Cease smoking. Nothing puts a burden on your heart or your health like smoking. Studies show time and again that men who smoke increase their risk of coronary artery disease and triple their risk of heart attack. Smoking also robs your heart muscle of oxygen, narrows arteries and can be absolutely deadly for angina patients, says Dr. Pantano.

Get your fatty acid in gear. While you're lowering your fat intake, crank up your consumption of omega-3 fatty acids, a type of fat that actually helps protect arteries and lowers cholesterol in the body. The best source for omega-3's is fish, says Dr. Reed.

"There's a lot to be said for fish. It has a reduced fat content and much less cholesterol, and the fatty acids do appear to retard or impede the progression of atherosclerosis," he says. Mackerel, tuna and cod are all heavy hitters in the fatty-acid department. Most experts recommend at least two servings of fish per week.

Take an aspirin a day. Aspirin, it seems, can do as much for heartaches as it does for headaches. Aspirin essentially makes your blood less sticky and therefore less likely to cause dangerous clots, says Dr. Pantano. "It's a very simple, helpful thing to take every day," he says. "It reduces angina and decreases plaque risk." Many doctors suggest taking one regular-strength tablet—about 325 milligrams—per day as a preventive measure for angina and other heart problems. Aspirin can be harsh on the stomach or interfere with other medicines, though, so be sure to talk with your doctor before taking it daily.

Exert yourself. To keep your heart healthy, getting exercise is just as important as watching your diet. Regular exercise increases overall circulation. Plus, frequent aerobic exercise—cycling or jogging for 20 minutes a day, three to five times a week, for example—will help you burn off excess fat, which might otherwise end up lining the walls of your arteries.

FAST FACTS

How common: Over three million men in the United States suffer from angina and the effects of coronary artery disease.

Risk factors: Men who smoke, have high blood pressure, high cholesterol or a family history of coronary problems are at special risk for angina. Obesity and diabetes also are risk factors.

Age group affected: Men between the ages of 50 and 70 tend to suffer angina the most.

Gender gap: Men are twice as likely to develop coronary problems as women.

Who to see: At the first sign of chest pain, immediately see a cardiologist or get to an emergency room.

If you already have angina, you're probably thinking exercise is the worst thing you could do, since that's what triggers the angina. But if you're careful, exercise might be the best thing for you.

"I've seen people who are sedentary, who've had bouts with angina, start exercising . . . and they've gotten better," says John A. Lombardo, M.D., medical director of the Ohio State University Sports Medicine Center in Columbus. By adopting a gradual exercise plan, he says, you can increase circulation to the heart muscle, as well as increase your amount of physical activity without getting angina.

"But remember that different people can do different levels of exercise," Dr. Lombardo cautions. "That's why, when you have angina with exercise, it's so important to be under the care of somebody who's guiding you through an exercise program." And if you're planning any physical activity, take your anti-angina medicine a few minutes beforehand rather than at the first sign of angina symptoms. "Chances are, if you're taking short-acting nitrates, you'll be able to increase your exercise tolerance by 30 percent," says Dr. Pantano.

Squash stress. Emotional stress, day-to-day tension, even mild annoyances can put a strain on your heart and trigger angina in men who suffer it. Take some time every day to relax. Close your eyes and meditate. Listen to some soothing music. Talk to your doctor about getting on a stress reduction program; less stress on you means less stress on your heart.

Angina Antidotes

If you have angina, the most important thing to remember is: It doesn't have you. In addition to prevention and coping strategies, you can manage angina med-

Sex: Still Safe

Of all the exercises men with angina still want to be able to tolerate, sex probably tops the list. Unfortunately, it's the one subject they least want to broach with their doctors, according to James A. Pantano, M.D., a cardiologist practicing in Allentown, Pennsylvania, and author of *Living with Angina*. "But they're all thinking about it," he says.

And they should be. After all, sex is a form of exercise and can be a source of both physical and emotional stress. Dr. Pantano says sex with new partners or in unfamiliar settings can be especially hard on the heart. "But sex between familiar partners in a comfortable setting is equal in exertion to walking up one flight of stairs," he says.

If that level of exertion is likely to bring on angina, take your medication before jumping into bed. Also, plan your liaisons before or at least two to three hours after a meal. Otherwise, you'll be putting an extra burden on your heart.

ically with a regular prescription. "Once you have coronary artery disease, you have to deal with it for the rest of your life," says Dr. Pantano. "There are any number of medications that can help you learn to live with it."

The most common of these is nitroglycerin, which is dynamite against an angina attack because it temporarily dilates, or opens, narrowed blood vessels. Nitroglycerin is available in pills, sprays and skin patches, under the brand names Deponit or Nitrol.

Another type of drug, the calcium channel blocker, also increases the supply of oxygen to the heart. These drugs, which include diltiazem (Cardizem), nifedipine (Adalat) and verapamil (Calan), are often prescribed in addition to nitroglycerin.

The third major group of angina fighters are beta-blockers, such as the prescription drugs metoprolol (Toprol XL) and propanolol (Inderal). Unlike the other drugs, beta-blockers slow the heart down, reducing its need for more oxygen. These drugs are very effective against angina, but they're slower-acting than nitrates.

See also Heart Attack, Heart Disease, High Cholesterol

Anxiety and Fear

Make Adrenaline Work for You

Think of anxiety as the robot from the 1960s TV show *Lost in Space*. The one that would spin around, berserkly flailing its mechanical arms while screaming, "Danger, Will Robinson! Danger!"

That's the function anxiety serves in each of us. It lets us know when we're threatened, an internal "fight or flight" alarm system that served our ancestors well when faced with a voracious saber-toothed tiger. "Anxiety is a normal emotion that enables us to perform to the best of our abilities," says Michael R. Lewin, Ph.D., a researcher in the Anxiety Disorders Behavioral Program at the University of California, Los Angeles.

In these modern times the perceived threat is more likely to stem from an overbearing boss or even that attractive woman who just moved into your building. The one you're dying to ask out but just can't summon the nerve. Every time you think about knocking on her door and asking her for a date, you suddenly find yourself short of breath, your heart beating like a drum machine, adrenaline pumping through your system, your hands turning clammy, your mouth feeling like it is stuffed with cotton.

"The role of anxiety is to turn the person inward and outward to look for danger. That's what anxiety's all about," says C. Barr Taylor, M.D., professor of psychiatry at Stanford University's Medical Center in Palo Alto, California. "So it makes sense that you try to interpret things as though they are more dangerous than they really are. What you have to do is counter that."

Being nervous about asking a woman out for the first time is perfectly natural. But if you're a 40-year-old man who hasn't dated in 20 years because of acute anxiety—as was the case with one of the participants in a social phobia study conducted by Dr. Taylor—you need help.

As a general rule, when your anxiety interferes with your social life, family or work, then you have a problem. And in extreme cases, studies have found that high levels of anxiety can greatly increase the risk among middle-age men for serious health problems such as high blood pressure and even sudden death from heart attack.

Mind Your Body

For years, whenever someone admitted to feelings of anxiety, the likely response—from physicians as well as family and friends—was, "There's nothing to be afraid of. It's all in your head." Research, however, has shown that anxiety can affect the whole body.

"Clearly, in the long term there's going to be physiological damage," warns Linda Welsh, Ed.D., director of the Agoraphobia and Anxiety Treatment Center in Bala Cynwyd, Pennsylvania.

Ichiro Kawachi, M.D., Ph.D., assistant professor at the Harvard School of Public Health's Department of Health and Social Behavior in Boston, led a study to determine if there was a link between phobic anxiety and heart disease. Nearly 34,000 participants filled out questionnaires to measure their anxiety levels. During a two-year period, researchers found that middle-age men who reported high levels of anxiety were 2½ times more likely to die from heart disease than those who reported lower levels. Even more alarming, though, was the finding that the risk of sudden death from heart attack was six times higher for middle-age men who reported high anxiety levels than for those who reported lower levels.

Similarly, a study led by Jerome H. Markovitz, M.D., assistant professor in the Division of Preventive Medicine at the University of Alabama at Birmingham, found a link between high levels of anxiety and high blood pressure among middle-age men. In his study middle-age men who responded affirmatively to five of seven anxiety-related questions were more than twice as likely to develop high blood pressure than their calmer counterparts. "The major thing here is that it's not so much how much stress you're under, it's how anxious you are, how you respond to it," Dr. Markovitz says.

How to Cope

Such research does not necessarily mean that men are more anxious than women. Rather, Dr. Welsh says, it suggests that men don't cope as well with it. "Men are more likely to grin and bear it, or fight it, rather than acknowledge it."

Dr. Markovitz agrees. "Men are supposed to be repressors of emotions and, essentially, the only emotions that we manage to express are on Saturday and Sunday afternoons in football," he says. "It may be that if we dismiss those feelings and do not address them, then they will have adverse effects on our health."

Those who subscribe to the macho maxim "when the going gets tough, the tough get going" may find themselves going straight into a downward spiral of increasing anxiety. Dr. Taylor says the "tough, stoic, silent sufferer" who thinks he can gain control over his anxiety by ignoring it will end up frustrated. "Men who want

FAST FACTS

How common: Some 23 million Americans, or about 13 percent of the population, suffer from anxiety disorders. But less than one-quarter are ever treated.

Risk factors: Experts believe we each have a biological predisposition toward anxiety, and our psychology can heighten or dampen that anxiety.

Age group affected: All age groups are affected, though anxiety usually peaks in adolescence. Studies have shown that middle-age men are particularly prone to serious health problems as a result of acute anxiety.

Gender gap: Women are at twice the risk for anxiety and anxiety disorders as men. Anxiety and anxiety disorders, however, tend to be more severe and disabling in men.

Who to see: Family doctor, psychiatrist, psychologist.

to get control over their lives find it very disconcerting because, by definition, you can't control a lot of these events. And sometimes the harder you try to control it and still have anxiety and panic, the worse you feel because you feel like your usual coping skills aren't working."

Here are some tips to help you hone effective coping skills.

Take a breather. Often, anxiety will bring on shortness of breath and even hyperventilation. When feelings of anxiety start washing over you, make a conscious effort to breathe slowly from your diaphragm, the muscle at the bottom of the lungs near the stomach. To practice, put one hand on your chest, the other on your stomach. If you're breathing correctly, your lower hand should move out as you breathe in, while your upper hand shouldn't move at all.

Relax your muscles. "Relaxation is not something you can just do," Dr. Lewin says. "It's a skill you need to practice before you can utilize it effectively."

One relaxation skill you might want to consider honing is called progressive muscle relaxation—tensing and then relaxing each muscle in your body, moving from head to toe. Dr. Lewin recommends you practice progressive muscle relaxation daily.

Make a note. Write yourself positive reminders on note cards that will help turn off the faucet when the adrenaline starts rushing through your system. It could be something simple, such as "Remember your breathing." Or it could be a word or phrase that has a calming influence. Dr. Welsh says one of her patients jotted down a saying from her childhood: "What you do today is how you live your life."

Face your fears. Like boxing immortal Joe Louis put it, you can run, but you

Phobias: When Fears Get out of Hand

"I don't like spiders and snakes," sang Jim Stafford in a hit from the 1970s. Most people would agree. But some cross over the line into phobias—an intense, consuming, irrational fear.

Linda Welsh, Ed.D., director of the Agoraphobia and Anxiety Treatment Center in Bala Cynwyd, Pennsylvania, explains the difference between fear and phobia this way: "When you're fearful or anxious, you're in a situation feeling uncomfortable, but you don't go out of your way to avoid it. If you have a snake phobia, you may not go in the woods because there are snakes there. If you're just anxious, you'll go in the woods, but you'll be alert. It's to what extent it impacts your life. And if you're to the point of avoiding things because of it, then it's considered a phobia."

There are about as many phobias as there are things to be afraid of. Among the most common are claustrophobia, fear of enclosed places such as elevators, and acrophobia, fear of heights. Dr. Welsh calls fear of flying "probably the most frequent we see." But patients also come in complaining of fears of crowds, bridges, tunnels, open spaces, highways and dogs, among other things. These all fall under the umbrella of "simple phobias" because they involve fear of one specific thing.

One of the more unusual phobias Dr. Welsh has encountered involved a woman who was afraid of taking showers. "The idea of being in the shower, and the shower head, for some reason, terrified her," she recalls. Dr. Welsh also has had patients who feared vomiting and germs.

"A germ phobia is a pretty common one, bordering into the obsessive-compulsive disorders," Dr. Welsh says. "People who have germ phobias won't go to hospitals."

If your fear of spiders, snakes or anything else has reached the phobic stage, don't be overly anxious. With help from a therapist, you can reach the point where you face your fears, rather than run from them. In addition to the breathing and relaxation techniques used to treat anxieties, treatment for phobias involves exposing patients to whatever it is that makes them uncomfortable, eventually desensitizing them to it.

Chances are you still won't like spiders and snakes, but you might be able to go camping or take a hike in the woods.

can't hide. "Each time you avoid a situation, the next time you're going to have an even harder time," says Alexander Bystritsky, M.D., director of the Anxiety Disorders Program at the University of California, Los Angeles. The only way to overcome your anxiety is to stay in a situation that makes you anxious.

Start gradually. Karin Gruber, a Stanford doctoral student from Germany who worked with Dr. Taylor on the social phobia study, had the 40-year-old man who hadn't dated in two decades start by just making small talk with females. Once he was comfortable talking to women, he had to ask them to join him for coffee or in some other nonthreatening social situation. Within a few months, he was dating.

Get into exercise. Studies have shown that exercise can lower anxiety significantly. "Regular exercise is a critical component to managing anxiety because it allows you to discharge stressful buildups in the body," Dr. Lewin says. "If you constantly work under stress without some kind of physical release, the effect is increased anxiety."

If you booze, you lose. One of the most common—and destructive—outlets men turn to for relief from anxiety is alcohol. The Anxiety Disorders Association of America in Rockville, Maryland, estimates that nearly one-third of Americans with anxiety disorders drink to ease the discomfort. "When the effects of the alcohol have worn away, the anxiety tends to still be there," Dr. Taylor says. "It may even be a little bit exacerbated as a slight rebound effect. One of the biggest problems we see at my clinic are men—middle-age men in particular—who drink in part to cope with anxiety. Bad idea."

Unplug the coffeemaker and hit the sack. It's also a bad idea to guzzle coffee or to stay up late. "These are all things that people do to cope with anxious situations, and they are the worst possible things to do," says Peter Roy-Byrne, M.D., professor of psychiatry at the University of Washington in Seattle.

Caffeine's stimulants will wind you tighter than a drum, and sleep deprivation will only make it more difficult to deal clearly with whatever is causing your anxiety.

Talk about it. Share your feelings of anxiety or stress with a family member, friend or professional.

When to Get Help

When anxiety interferes with your life, you need to see a therapist experienced in dealing with anxiety disorders. Through therapy and, if necessary, medication, even serious cases can be effectively treated.

Dr. Taylor says that with a combination of therapy and medication 70 percent of his patients with panic disorders reported few or no panic attacks and little or no disability in their daily lives.

Arthritis

How to Keep the Pain at Bay

Most everyone has accidentally pounded a finger with a hammer. It's an excruciating moment. But after a primal scream, a spastic dance and some expletives, the hurt begins to fade and you go on with your work.

But imagine that pain being a daily reality, waking up every morning feeling like someone had taken a hammer to your knuckles, knees, elbows, ankles and hips. It's a drain on your pain threshold; a constant agony that stays and stays.

Sounds like a bad science fiction movie called *The Pain That Wouldn't Leave*. But arthritis is all too real. Nearly 40 million Americans suffer from the connective tissue disease. The pain can range in severity from minor aches up to the rare case of life-impairing, hammer-hitting disability.

You have some control over arthritis, however. Early diagnosis and treatment coupled with regular exercise can go a long way toward diminishing the disease's impact, says Gary Gilkeson, M.D., assistant professor of medicine at Duke University School of Medicine in Durham, North Carolina.

"The earlier you start moving and the more components of your body you use, the better off you are. That keeps things lubricated," he says. "If the muscles weaken, you can't use them as well, and limitation sets in."

Zeroing In on a Culprit

There are more than 100 variations of arthritis. The most debilitating type is rheumatoid arthritis, which affects roughly 600,000 American men. The main symptom is swelling and inflammation of the joints, says David Pisetsky, M.D., co-director of Duke University Arthritis Center in Durham, North Carolina, and medical adviser to the Arthritis Foundation in Atlanta. Other signs include fever, weight loss, anemia and nodules on the joints.

"People have classic signs of inflammation: swollen, tender, red and hot-feeling joints. They have trouble moving, especially in the morning, and are stiff all over," says Dr. Pisetsky. "Rheumatoid arthritis usually involves the fingers, wrists, elbows, hips, knees, neck, ankles and small joints of the feet."

FAST FACTS

How common: Roughly 600,000 American men have the more debilitating form of arthritis known as rheumatoid. Estimates on the number of men who have osteoarthritis, the most common variety, range as high as one in every seven.

Risk factors: The causes of most types of arthritis aren't known. But the following likely play some role: heredity, aging, obesity, injuries to joints at an early age and lack of exercise.

Age group affected: Since osteoarthritis is a degenerative disease, your chances of getting it increase with age. It is the most widespread chronic disease in people over age 45. Men, however, are susceptible at any age.

Gender gap: Women are three times as likely to get rheumatoid arthritis. Men and women are equally susceptible to osteoarthritis.

Who to see: Consult your family doctor if you are experiencing chronic joint pain. You might be referred to a rheumatologist.

The pain sets in when the joint's lining, called the synovium, becomes inflamed. That lining invades and damages bone and cartilage.

Just what causes rheumatoid arthritis is a mystery. But if left untreated, it can destroy your body's joints, eventually leading to confinement in bed or a wheelchair. Fortunately, that scenario is played out in only about 10 percent of cases. On the other extreme, 10 percent of folks with rheumatoid arthritis will go into spontaneous remission in the first year.

More common—in fact, the most common form of arthritis—is osteoarthritis, which affects anywhere from 16 million to 35 million people. It's less serious than rheumatoid and often involves just one joint, says Richard Pope, M.D., chief of the Division of Arthritis and Connective Tissue Diseases at Northwestern University Medical School in Chicago.

Although rheumatoid arthritis strikes women three times more often than men, osteoarthritis hits either sex about equally, Dr. Pope notes.

The condition results in the breakdown over time of cartilage, which acts as a joint's cushion at the end of a bone. The fluid-filled membranes that act as grease in the crankcase of our joints become inflamed and painful.

If you tore a ligament or damaged cartilage as a high school running back, you're especially vulnerable to osteoarthritis. The disease likes to target previously injured joints—oftentimes knees, says Dr. Pope.

But jocks aren't the only ones susceptible to osteoarthritis, warns Dr. Gilkeson. Heredity also plays a big role.

"If your father has an inherited form of osteoarthritis, the chances you'll get it are one in four," he notes. "It all depends on how strong the cartilage is."

Simply living to a ripe old age is another cause. The majority of us will develop osteoarthritis in our sixties and seventies, says Dr. Pope. That's because age reduces the ability of cartilage cells to regenerate.

Easing the Agony

Being diagnosed with arthritis can be as mentally painful as physically, knowing that the ache will probably be a permanent part of your life. Arthritis and depression often go hand in hand.

But for putting a kibosh on pain, a diagnosis is just what the doctor ordered.

Dr. Pisetsky says early recognition of the disease is the first step to getting proper treatment. "Rheumatoid arthritis can cause joint damage within the first couple years. If you treat it early, you can prevent that," he says. "Some folks delay seeing a doctor because they think joint pain is an inevitable sign of aging."

A doctor diagnoses rheumatoid arthritis based on symptoms, a physical and a blood test that determines the presence of rheumatoid factor, an abnormal substance found in the blood of about 80 percent of adults with the disease. Osteoarthritis is diagnosed through symptoms and a physical, with x-rays used only to confirm the diagnosis.

Once you know for sure arthritis is the culprit behind body pains, there's plenty you can do to slow it down. Whether you have the rheumatoid or osteo brand, take these steps to stay in tip-top form for as long as you can.

Keep the joints hoppin'. In medical minds the sentiment is nearly unanimous: Exercise is the most important weapon in your fight against arthritis.

Non-weight-bearing exercise, like bike riding, swimming or even light walking, strengthens the muscles and in return takes stress off arthritis-burdened limbs. That eventually lessens swelling and pain, says Dr. Gilkeson.

One study compared 51 patients with osteoarthritis of the knee who weren't in a walking program with 51 patients who were. After an eight-week program of 24 90-minute walking and education sessions, the results were clear. Those in the walking program showed a 70-meter increase in the maximum distance they could walk in 6 minutes, as well as a 27 percent decrease in pain. The nonwalkers showed a 17-meter decrease in how far they could walk in 6 minutes.

Battle the bulge. Being overweight when you have arthritis is like being a two-pack-a-day smoker who's been diagnosed with lung cancer: It can only make a bad situation worse. The repetitive trauma that joints sustain from walking is magnified a hundredfold when you're overweight, says Dr. Gilkeson. "The best thing you can do is lose as much weight as you can and stay as light as you can," he notes.

For every ten pounds you're overweight, your chances of getting osteoarthritis double, he notes. "Even after you get arthritis, there's still a big benefit to losing weight," Gilkeson says.

Control the inflammation. Folks with rheumatoid arthritis need a pain-killing, anti-inflammatory drug like ibuprofen, which is easier on the stomach than aspirin, says Dr. Pisetsky. For osteoarthritis, Dr. Pisetsky recommends taking acetaminophen as a first therapy, with the dose controlled by the amount of pain. Talk to your doctor first rather than self-prescribing yourself to painkillers.

Look on the bright side. The way you deal with pain plays as big a role in your well-being as treating the disease itself, says Dr. Gilkeson. The current trend in arthritis treatment is to teach coping skills, he notes.

"When they experience pain, some people have a panic-attack reaction," he says. "But therapy teaches them to say, 'I've had this before and I know it'll get better.' The nervous and immune systems are innately tied to one another."

Heat things up. Arthritis can cause muscle tightness, so applying a hot water bottle or heating pad to stiff joints is a real pain reliever, says Dr. Pope. "You should put heat on for about 15 minutes before starting exercises." Another soother is a hot bath or shower, he notes.

Eat fish for relief. Fish oil has been shown in clinical studies to cut down on the swelling of arthritis, says Dr. Pope. "It works by altering the inflammatory mediators in the joints," he notes. One of the best sources of polyunsaturated fat is cold-water fish such as salmon, sardines and herring.

Move cautiously. With arthritis you should be careful not to make already weak joints worse. Don't try deep knee bends or go for a brisk jog, which can put undue pressure on the joints, says Dr. Pope.

In fact, certain occupations such as mechanics, farmers and schoolteachers are more prone to osteoarthritis simply because of the repetitive stooping and crouching they do, notes Dr. Pisetsky.

Down the Line

So what happens when even your best efforts at exercise, weight control and pain relief don't do the trick?

In the case of rheumatoid arthritis people might need to go on more powerful, slower-acting drugs, like gold salts, hydroxycholoroquine (Plaquenil) and sulfasalazine (Azulfidine).

Stretching Away the Pain

It's an especially bad arthritis day, and your achy breaky joints are in an up-roar. Do you (a) lie down on the couch and watch football for three hours or (b) get on the floor and *move* those muscles?

Guess the answer. Here are four range-of-motion exercises recommended by the Arthritis Foundation that you can do three to ten times, once or twice a day, to help you stay limber.

Shoulder. Lie on your back with your arms at your sides, raise one arm straight over your head and touch the floor, then return it to your side. Repeat with the other arm.

Hip. Lie on your back with your legs straight, about six inches apart, toes pointing up. Slide one leg out to the side and return. Repeat with the other leg.

Knee and hip. Lie on your back with one knee bent and the other straight. Bend the knee of the straight leg and raise it toward your chest. Push the leg into the air and lower it to the floor. Repeat with the other leg.

Shoulder. Place your hands behind your head. Move your elbows back as far as you can while also moving your head back. Repeat.

Methotrexate (Rheumatrex), an immunosuppressive drug taken orally, also slows down the disease, says Dr. Gilkeson. "It's effective in anywhere from 50 to 75 percent of patients," he notes. "It certainly doesn't cure the disease but there's less pain and less swelling and it slows down the progression of the disease."

A last resort is surgical replacement of the joint, says Dr. Pisetsky.

"You can get terrific relief and mobility from surgery," he says. "People with os-teoarthritis can do especially well, and could be perfectly healthy after the operation."

Asthma

No Need to Wheeze on the Sidelines

After just one 40-yard sprint, the five-foot-ten, 180-pound would-be linebacker was wheezing and gasping for breath. Although the coach mercifully invited him to be team manager, asthma had dashed his hopes of making the high school squad.

That kid may have been your brother, next-door neighbor or even you. But times have changed, and guys with asthma aren't relegated to the sidelines anymore. Better understanding of the disease and vast improvements in its management now allow asthma sufferers to elbow onto life's field of play.

In many cases, "you can maintain a high quality of life and perhaps be as active as a guy who doesn't have asthma," says William H. Ziering, M.D., an allergist and asthma expert in private practice in Fresno, California. World-class athletes such as former mile record holder Jim Ryun, Olympic cross-country skier Bill Koch and professional basketball star Danny Manning have gone on to greatness after learning to keep asthma under control. So can you.

It Takes Your Breath Away

During an asthma attack the bronchi and smaller bronchioles—the tubes that pass oxygen to your lungs—suddenly clamp down, slowing air flow. At the same time, the lining of these airways swells and releases mucus, blocking air flow even more. Having an asthma attack is like sprinting 100 yards, then trying to catch your breath by sucking through a straw.

It's not always clear what causes asthma to occur. Men with this condition typically have a variety of "triggers," from smoke, pollen and air pollution to pets, dust mites or even medications. Anxiety, viral infections and exercise have also been known to spark attacks.

About five million American men have asthma and nearly 2,000 will die of asthma-related causes each year. And for reasons that aren't quite clear, both the number of men who get asthma and the number who die from it have increased over the past decade. Some experts suspect this increase is partly from patients and even physicians not taking the disease seriously enough.

63

"Asthma isn't episodic. It's really a chronic inflammatory condition that is never turned off," Dr. Ziering says. "Neither patients nor some physicians have appreciated the implications of that enough."

Without treatment asthma can permanently narrow the airways and cause exposed nerve endings to become even more sensitive to asthma triggers. The result, of course, can be even more frequent—and debilitating—attacks in the future.

Gaining Control

Children who develop asthma may spontaneously cease to be troubled with it as their airway enlarges. But often it becomes a lifelong condition. Still, it can be controlled with treatment in most cases, experts say. And men who keep a close eye on symptoms and take decisive action can often avoid attacks entirely, says Franklin Adkinson, M.D., professor of medicine and co-director of the Division of Allergy and Clinical Immunology at the Johns Hopkins University School of Medicine/Francis Scott Key Medical Center in Baltimore.

"Asthma is now much easier to control than it was ten years ago," says Dr. Adkinson. "Asthma is a disease which shouldn't interfere with a normal lifestyle and normal life span if you get appropriate therapy and learn to cope with the disease."

To keep asthma from taking the wind out of your sails, here's what experts recommend.

Don't pull the trigger. Experts agree that the first and best step in preventing asthma attacks is to stay out of the line of fire. "If you know what your triggers are and it's possible to avoid them, you always begin with prevention," says Robert B. Mellins, M.D., director of the Pediatric Pulmonary Division at Columbia Presbyterian Medical Center in New York City.

Avoid allergic reactions. Although pollution and respiratory infections like colds and flu account for the bulk of asthma attacks, about half of the men with asthma also have one or more allergies that contribute to the problem. Skin sensitivity tests can help you and your doctor identify allergens that may be triggering your asthma.

Once you know what these allergens are, it will be easier for you to make the necessary changes in your life to avoid them. That could range from covering your mattress and box spring with an allergy-free encasing to washing your pets more often.

Take control of the air. Breathing cool, dry, winter air will often send lungs into overdrive. When going outdoors be sure to wrap a muffler over your mouth and nose to help warm and moisten the air before it reaches your lungs.

But don't go overboard and crank up the heat and humidity in your home, adds Dr. Mellins. Air that's too moist can encourage mold growth, which will often make

FAST FACTS

How common: About five million American men currently have asthma, although the numbers seem to be increasing.

Risk factors: The causes of asthma aren't clear, but the condition is usually brought on by some kind of trigger unique to each sufferer: smoke, pollen, air pollution, dust mites, even exercise.

Age group affected: Occurs most often before age 25.

Gender gap: Asthma is twice as common in young boys than girls. In adults aged 30 and over it occurs equally in men and women.

Who to see: Family doctor, allergist.

asthma worse. "The best thing you can do is simply keep your indoor environment comfortable, neither too dry nor too moist," he says.

Be a smart city slicker. "In this country most people live in areas where the air is unhealthy, and pollution is often enough to set off many men's asthma," says Dr. Ziering.

Breathing through your nose instead of your mouth will help filter out harmful airborne particles, he says. It's also a good idea not to be outside at times of peak pollution—taking a late afternoon run in some areas is akin to wrapping your mouth around a muffler. Many cities issue a daily air pollution index that's listed in the weather section of the newspaper. As a rule, the air is generally cleanest in the early morning or after a hard rain.

Be wary of indoor pollution. Experts estimate that one in seven cases of adult-onset asthma may be caused by workplace allergens. Maybe you can't quit work, but you can move your desk closer to an open window or other source of fresh air, or away from something that's making you wheeze—like that bearskin rug that's hanging on the wall. You also might want to politely ask the higher-ups when the filter system was last cleaned or inspected.

Keep the air clean. At home, opening windows and airing out rooms at least once a week can help remove particles that may cause problems. You should also regularly clean and replace furnace and air conditioner filters according to manufacturer's recommendations, says Dr. Ziering.

Work up a sweat. Studies have shown that men with asthma who are aerobically fit are less likely to suffer attacks because they're better able to exert themselves without taxing their systems, says Stephen Rice, M.D., Ph.D., a pediatrician and sports medicine specialist at the University of Washington in Seattle and an asthmatic himself.

It's important, however, to take your medicine (assuming you use it) before exercising, he adds. Inhaled mists are very effective at preventing attacks when taken 20 minutes before working out.

Warm up slowly. Plunging straight onto the playing field—be it a basketball court, soccer field or bicycle track—without an adequate warm-up may increase your risk of attack. It's better to start slowly, says Dr. Ziering. If you're running a 10-kilometer course, for instance, walk for the first quarter-mile, then start jogging at a 12-minute-mile pace, picking up speed as you go, he suggests. Also, using an inhaler 5 to 15 minutes before you exercise often can prevent exercise-induced asthma.

Take the plunge. Swimming in an indoor pool ranks high on the anti-asthma exercise list because the air directly above the water's surface is warm and moist and less likely to irritate "twitchy" airways, Dr. Rice says.

Go with the flow. One of the most important advances in asthma care is the peak flow meter. This is a simple mechanical device that can give you an accurate measure of how much airway obstruction and lung capacity you have at any given moment.

Once you and your doctor have determined your maximum flow volume, the peak flow meter will give you an idea of whether you can push yourself or if you should ease up for a while. If your lungs are operating between 80 and 100 percent of your maximum ability, then you're doing well. If you're only managing 50 to 80 percent of your max, however, you should proceed carefully.

Experts recommend measuring your lung capacity at least twice a day, particularly if you plan to exercise or do other strenuous activities.

Take time to relax. Experts aren't sure why but tension and stress can intensify and aggravate asthma. So if you are susceptible to asthma, try practicing a relaxation technique (stretching or yoga, for example) and do what you can to avoid panic, Dr. Mellins says.

Making the Most of Your Medicine

Most men with asthma will need to use prescription drugs to help keep their symptoms under control. In most cases asthma medications are used to reduce lung inflammation and relax bronchial spasms that trigger attacks. Used correctly, the drugs can virtually eliminate attacks, allowing you to live a normal, wheeze-free life.

Men with mild asthma—those who have symptoms once or twice a week—typically use medications called beta agonists (Ventolin, Brethaire) before doing anything that could stress the airways. These medications, which are also known as bronchodilators, can also be used to clear the airways after an attack has occurred.

"The beta agonist inhaler is a rescue medicine," explains Dr. Ziering. "It opens up your bronchial tubes and it does it within seconds or minutes. If you have asthma, you should carry an inhaler with you at all times so you can use it when needed."

Men who have moderate asthma require daily treatment with an inhaled anti-inflammatory drug like beclomethasone (Becloven, Vanceril) or cromolyn sodium (Intal).

While asthma can usually be managed with medication, sometimes it gets worse. See your doctor if you're starting to use your bronchodilator more frequently or if you're refilling your inhaler more than once a month. You should also get help if routine tasks make you feel out of breath or if you're awakening short of breath more than three times a month.

See also Allergies

Athlete's Foot

How to Save Your Sole

If your foot is itching, burning, stinging or peeling, you may have a case of the most common fungal infection in the world. Scratch if you must, but don't panic. Athlete's foot is annoying but generally harmless and usually fairly easy to do away with.

And yes, active guys like you are prime candidates. That's why it's called athlete's foot. "Active people get it more frequently, probably because they sweat more," says Paul Lazar, M.D., professor of clinical dermatology at Northwestern University Medical School in Chicago. Athletes also tend to run around barefoot in public showers and locker rooms, which tend to be fashionable fungus hangouts.

The fungus that most often causes athlete's foot can attack any part of your foot, wherever it—literally—gets a toehold. But most frequently, athletes foot affects the area between the last two toes. A severe case may make your foot look like it's wearing a blister moccasin. The fungus has also been known to slither under the toenails.

Sidestepping the Fungus among Us

How can you keep this predator of the feet from assaulting *your* feet?

"It's a greenhouse inside your shoe—warm and wet. Fungi are plants; like all plants, they like greenhouses," says Dr. Lazar. So the first step to fighting athlete's foot, he says, is to create an environment less hospitable to the fungus. That means keeping the environment around your feet as Sahara-like as possible.

Here's how.

Towel your hooves. For obvious reasons this is more important after a bruising tangle with your tennis pro, an eight-mile run or a shower in a public gymnasium, but it is nonetheless important for the less active as well, since normal perspiration is a major contributor to the problem, says Dr. Lazar.

Take a clean towel and wipe the feet dry before putting on fresh, dry socks, paying particular attention to the spaces between the toes—particularly the last two on the outside edge of your foot. "If you have the time, it's not a bad idea after towel drying to let your feet air dry for five or ten minutes," says Keith Schulze, M.D., a dermatologist in private practice in Wharton, Texas.

FAST FACTS

How common: An estimated 70 percent of Americans develop athlete's foot at least once.

Risk factors: Wet feet, dirty feet, feet in tight shoes.

Age group affected: All age groups are affected, but it rarely develops before adolescence, which is when the skin begins producing oils that provide nutrients for the fungus to grow.

Gender gap: Studies show that more than twice as many men as women get athlete's foot. Some experts speculate that men, for whatever reason, are simply more vulnerable to this form of fungal infection.

Who to see: Dermatologist.

No time to air dry? Use your hair dryer to speed the process—and to dry your shoes out, too, suggests Rodney Basler, M.D., a dermatologist and assistant professor of internal medicine at the University of Nebraska Medical Center in Omaha.

Powder your paws. Powder acts as a drying agent by absorbing sweat, says William Dvorine, M.D., chief of dermatology at St. Agnes Hospital in Baltimore. But avoid powders that contain cornstarch. Sometimes yeast organisms can contribute to athlete's foot, and cornstarch is like caviar to hungry yeast. Also, think twice about using medicated antifungal powders if you don't have signs of athlete's foot—it's not likely but you could be breeding a superfungus with genetic resistance to the active ingredient that makes those powders effective, Dr. Dvorine says.

Wear socks that wick. They fight athlete's foot by carrying moisture away from the feet. Cotton is most frequently recommended, but the current crop of miracle fibers that wick water away from the skin should also help keep your feet dry. Avoid fabrics like polyester and nylon, which will actually trap perspiration in the sock and on your foot (unless the weave is very loose indeed).

Choose shoes that breathe. Leather, Dr. Schulze says, is the most commonly recommended material, but canvas sneakers breathe well also. Sandals—if you can stand the slams from your buddies—are best for keeping your feet dry. But Dr. Lazar points out that a wet sandal can harbor athlete's foot organisms almost as well as a wet foot.

Wash your feet. Pay special attention to the areas between your toes, and make it a habit. "Soap will kill most of the organisms that produce athlete's foot," says Dr. Schulze. But remember to thoroughly dry your feet afterward.

Switch shoes a lot. Ideally, wear a different pair each workday, Dr. Schulze says. Rotating footwear permits individual pairs to dry out thoroughly between wearings.

Stomping Out Unwanted Guests

If, despite your better efforts, you fail to keep the athlete's foot fungus at bay, you may need tougher action.

Visit your pharmacy. In many cases athlete's foot preparations available in your local drugstore will finish the job. Active ingredients in these preparations include clotrimazole (Lotrimin), tolnaftate (Tinactin), miconazole (Micatin) and undecylenic acid (Desenex). Powdered versions are preferable for the obvious reason—they help dry your feet.

Check with your doctor. Even though you don't need a prescription for most antifungal medications, it still makes sense to visit your dermatologist. You probably won't die if you don't, but so many things (such as bacterial infections) can produce the symptoms of athlete's foot that a visit makes sense. Otherwise, you could wind up fighting a fungus that isn't even there and missing the real culprit. Plus, athlete's foot can have more serious consequences if you have certain other medical conditions as well, such as diabetes or poor circulation.

Time to Dig Your Feet In

If you're one of the unfortunates who develops blisters, gets a case that wraps your foot in an inflamed "moccasin" or gets it under your toenails—all indicators of a major fungal assault—then you have no choice: See your dermatologist. He's the only one who can provide you with the "big guns" you'll need—potent oral antifungals—that will be necessary to control the infection.

"A severe case with involvement of the toenails can take a year-and-a-half to resolve, even with the oral medications," Dr. Schulze says. "There are newer drugs that offer promise of resolving it in three to six months, such as fluconazole (Diflucan) and itraconazole (Sporanox), but they're too new to say for sure. Griseofulvin (Fulvicin P/G) is what we use the most, and that *will* require about a year-and-a-half."

Warning: These drugs have been known to interact with others and do produce unpleasant side effects in some. Ask your dermatologist about possible drug interactions with medications you're taking.

Back Pain

Best Bets for a Bedrock Back

As symbols of male strength and bravery go, few are as powerful as the back. Consider this: When a man's contributions at work make him so important as to be indispensable, he's the "backbone of the operation." And any man who fears risks, can't make decisions and doesn't command attention is labeled "spineless."

It's no wonder, then, that having a backache elicits a unique kind of dread. After all, that bony column of vertebrae, disks and cartilage, with its attached muscles and nerves, is the secret behind our strength and mobility. A sudden backache means more than an onslaught of pain—it's a loss of power as well.

Problem is, most men don't take very good care of their backs.

But they should.

Backing Away from Pain

"Back pain is one of the most common ailments of mankind," says Louis Sportelli, D.C., a Palmerton, Pennsylvania, chiropractor who has worked with bad backs for more than 30 years. In fact, experts estimate that roughly 80 percent of men will experience back pain at some point in their lives. Not surprisingly, backache is among the most common conditions doctors treat.

The vast majority of back problems are caused by sprains in the muscles or tendons. You don't have to lift massive weights to wrack your back. Just dragging out the garbage can do it, or bending over to pick up a paper clip. Even sleeping wrong can send your muscles into painful spasms.

In some cases back pain may occur when the slick, gliding surfaces between vertebrae (the facet joints) get inflamed and irritated. Pain can also occur when spinal disks—those tough, shock-absorbing cushions between the vertebrae—crack open and ooze their gelatinous insides against a nearby nerve. This condition, commonly called a pinched nerve, typically sends shooting pain into the arms or legs.

While serious disk problems can be frightening, they're also quite rare. Even when a disk does rupture, the pain will often disappear on its own. On the other

71

hand, even minor back sprains can cause major league problems. That's why prevention is so important.

"If everyone were to do the right things for their backs, the incidence of back pain would decrease significantly," says Edward A. Abraham, M.D., assistant clinical professor of orthopedics at the University of California, Irvine, and author of *Freedom from Back Pain*. "If you're a person who hasn't had any pain yet and you follow a smart program, there's a good possibility you may not have any back pain ever."

Here are a few suggestions to help keep your back on track.

Go for the back stretch. "It's crucial to be limber. A flexible back will go a long way toward protecting your back from injury," says Roger Minkow, M.D., co-medical director of the San Francisco Spine Center and founder of Backworks, an exercise and therapy program used nationally.

Here's a basic back stretch: Facing a wall, spread your arms and legs and lean forward until your hands are touching the wall. Slowly pull your stomach toward the wall, arching your back inward, then relax. Repeat five times. Experts recommend doing this stretch before exercising or any other time you want to limber up.

It's important to remember, however, that stretching can be a double-edged sword, cautions Dr. Minkow. A lot of people hurt their backs by stretching improperly. If you already have back problems, you should see an expert who can recommend stretches that are right for you.

Get strong. "If you're interested in preventing lower-back pain, exercise is a must," says Dr. Abraham. He recommends aerobic exercise—swimming, cycling or cross-country skiing, to name just a few. Swimming may be the ideal back exercise because it strengthens crucial support muscles. But any exercise is good as long as you enjoy it and it gets blood flowing and stretches muscles with a minimum of stress.

Hold tight and light. "The biggest cause of back injuries is lifting too much and lifting improperly," says Dr. Sportelli. Stretching out your arms when you lift throws you off balance and puts unnecessary strain on your back muscles. Instead, be sure to hold things close to your body when picking them up. Bend at your knees, keep your back straight and try to let your leg muscles do most of the lifting.

Watch your spinal sleep. Even when you're resting, your back may not be. Sleeping on your belly, for example, forces you to twist your head to the side, placing both the neck and back under tremendous tension. Instead, try sleeping on your side, suggests Dr. Sportelli.

"If you're sleeping on your side, you should be able to draw a level line from the middle of your skull down through your neck and all the way down your spine," says Dr. Sportelli.

Add some padding. Sleeping with a pillow tucked between your knees will help

FAST FACTS

How common: Roughly eight out of ten men will have back problems at some time during their lives.

Risk factors: Back injuries in men are mostly the result of muscle strain caused by lifting heavy objects, improper lifting, playing too hard or having weak back supports, such as undertrained abdominal muscles.

Age group affected: Back problems become more frequent in the late thirties and beyond as a lifetime of lifting begins to take its toll.

Gender gap: Men tend to suffer back pain more often than women because they are more likely to put physical strain on their backs.

Who to see: When pain is severe or prolonged, see your family doctor. You might be referred to an orthopedist, chiropractor or physical therapist.

keep the legs parallel to the hips, helping to relieve the strain on the lower back and hips.

Move your butt. Most of us spend an inordinate amount of time sitting, which puts even more stress on your spine than standing does.

"Change positions," advises Dr. Abraham. If you spend your days working at a desk, get up every hour or so and walk around, he recommends.

Get a leg up. If you stand a lot and don't have the opportunity to sit, Dr. Abraham advises shifting your weight frequently. "You can just take a book, maybe a few inches thick, and put one foot up on the book," he says. "That shifts your pelvis around and affects how your weight is distributed on your back."

If you're standing for long periods of time and can't find a handy curb or bench to prop your foot on, just shifting your weight from one foot to the other can bring fast relief.

Sit back and relax. Experts agree that stress is a major cause of back pain. "We're not even aware of how we tighten our bodies and backs in response to stress," says Dr. Abraham. But that kind of tightening on a regular basis can cause muscle spasms and soreness that could eventually lead to more serious back pain.

"You need to find some time during the day to allow your body to relax," says Dr. Abraham. Just taking a five-minute break to clear your mind will help clear your back of tension. For more serious back pain, your doctor may even recommend meditation or biofeedback to help keep the tension levels down.

Find the proper chair. Sitting in a good chair can go a long way toward easing back woes, says Dr. Minkow, who has designed seats for both airline and home use.

Despite what the salesman may tell you, what you need in a chair is pretty simple. Your feet should rest flat on the floor when your back is flush against the back of the chair. Also, the curve of the chair's backrest should reach its apex right around your belt line. If it doesn't, your lower back isn't getting the support it needs.

Get shoes with sole. Every step you take sends shock waves straight up the back. To cushion the blow, try wearing a light shoe with a thick sole instead of a hard-soled loafer or workboot. Back pain sufferers have reported rapid and significant relief upon switching to lightweight, flexible shoes with a shock-absorbing cushion in the soles.

After the Damage Is Done

If you already have back pain, you ought to be talking to your doctor, especially if the pain seems to travel into your buttocks and down the backs of your legs. This is often a symptom of a ruptured disk, in which displaced material from between the vertebrae begins exerting painful pressure on the sciatic nerve. In some cases this kind of back pain can only be corrected by surgery.

For the most part, though, back injuries can be effectively treated at home. Here's what you need to do.

Take it easy. Once you've hurt your back, the first thing you need to do is rest—chances are you won't feel like doing much else anyway.

"The best thing you can do for acute pain is to get in bed and lie on your back with a pillow up under your knees," says Dr. Abraham. Or lie on your back on the floor, knees bent at a 90-degree angle and your calves resting on the seat of a chair. This position relaxes key back muscles and puts the least strain on your spine.

Get your back up. While some rest is good, more isn't necessarily better. After a few days muscles will start to weaken with bed rest—and weak muscles aren't the answer to a bad back. "The quicker you can get back to your normal activities, the quicker your back is going to heal," says Dr. Abraham. "But there are no hard-and-fast rules. If your back hurts too much, you're doing too much."

Reach for a painkiller. Virtually any over-the-counter analgesic can help ease back pain. Best are the anti-inflammatories, like aspirin or ibuprofen. (Acetaminophen will help relieve pain, but it won't do much for inflammation.)

Run hot and cold. Using ice and heat can provide excellent relief for bum backs, but they can't be used interchangeably.

In the first few days after an injury, experts say, ice is the way to go. "Ice decreases swelling and inflammation and increases blood flow to the injured area," says Dr. Abraham. Keep a towel or some sort of cloth between your skin and the ice to prevent frostbite. Apply the ice as often as you can for at least 30 minutes each time. After a few days, Dr. Abraham recommends a mix of ice and heat—30 minutes of ice, then 30 minutes of heat.

Once a few days have passed, it's time to turn up the heat, says Dr. Abraham. Heating the back with a heating pad or a hot towel will help relax muscle spasms and provide fast relief.

Get back in training. Once you're standing tall again, be sure to keep your back limber and strong with regular exercise and stretching. If you've suffered a serious back injury, talk with your doctor or an exercise therapist about the best fitness plan for your back.

"Almost all back patients can be helped with proper therapy, and proper therapy has to include an active exercise program," says Dr. Minkow. But be sure to ease into any exercise slowly and spend about ten minutes warming up beforehand.

Shed some pounds. While excess weight doesn't usually cause back problems, it can make them worse. "Once you have back pain, every pound you carry hurts," says Dr. Minkow. "Everyone feels better when they lose weight because it's less extra weight their backs have to lug around."

If you're overweight, you should be on a weight-loss program as well as a fitness routine. Cutting back on fatty foods, especially red meats and dairy products, like eggs, cheese and butter, will not only help reduce the burden your back has to carry but will take a load off your heart and circulatory system, too.

When to See the Doctor

Unfortunately, back pain isn't always caused by tweaked muscles or beaten-up disks. Sometimes backache is a symptom of other diseases, like cancer or an infection of the spinal column. Be especially wary of pain that comes on suddenly for no apparent reason, or pain that shoots down your leg to your knee or foot, or which lingers for a long time.

"If you give a treatment two weeks and it's not making any noticeable difference or you're getting worse, then you have to see a professional," says Dr. Minkow.

Bad Breath

Cleansing the Mouth That Roars

Bad breath could be changing your world and you don't even know it. You may be charming, witty and interesting, but unless you're a mime, you have to open your mouth to prove it—unfortunate if your breath smells like a bay at low tide. People aren't apt to point out that there are terrible odors emanating from your mouth. Ah gee, love to stay and talk, but I've got to run and join the Peace Corps.

"Few people, except maybe your dentist, are going to tell you you have bad breath," says Henry Finger, D.D.S., a dentist in Medford, New Jersey, and a former president of the Academy of General Dentistry. "Many times it may change your relationships and you don't have the faintest idea why."

Bad breath can have three causes—noxious foods and drinks, poor oral hygiene or medical problems like sinus infections, gum disease or intestinal problems. All of these problems are quite common.

How to know if your breath is bad? Dr. Finger offers a simple self-test. Take a piece of gauze or a cotton swab and run it around your mouth, over the top of your tongue and around your gums. Then do what everybody else has to do.

"Smell it," says Dr. Finger. "In most cases if you have offensive breath, you're going to smell that odor."

Begin and End the Battle at Home

How you manage bad breath depends on its cause. If your bad breath stems from a medical problem, you'll have to see a professional for help. But in most cases bad breath can be addressed, and eliminated, at home.

"If you have a healthy mouth and digestive tract, then you should be able to correct your bad breath with routine home care," says Dr. Finger.

Attack plaque. Your mouth can be a haven for plaque, a soft, clear film to which living and dead bacteria glom. At any time there are up to 50 trillion of these odor-causing bacteria in your mouth.

Brushing your teeth after each meal removes this gooey substrate along with the

76

FAST FACTS

How common: Bad breath can afflict anyone who neglects oral hygiene, and a lot of us do. For example, more than half of us have some degree of gum disease—and that's only one cause of bad breath.

Risk factors: Poor oral hygiene, spicy or fatty foods, gum disease, sinus infections, indigestion.

Age group affected: Men of all ages.

Gender gap: In the war on bad breath men and women start on equal ground. But men can be less fastidious about their diet and their oral hygiene, a casual attitude that can have those around them fleeing for cover.

Who to see: Dentist, family doctor.

bacteria and food bits stuck in it. Follow that by flossing between your teeth—especially along the gum line—and you'll get what's left.

"The name of the game is to kill the germs," says David F. Halpern, D.M.D., a dentist in private practice in Columbia, Maryland.

Give your tongue the twice over. A microscopic look at the tongue shows a smooth surface studded with what look like toadstools. The underside of these toadstools is a favorite hiding place for plaque and accompanying bacteria.

"Within those little valleys the bacteria can multiply unaffected unless you go in on a daily basis and actually brush your tongue," says Dr. Finger. "When you're finished brushing your teeth, take your toothbrush and brush all across the top surface of the tongue. That will ensure that there's no remaining bacteria to create any odors."

Don't want to brush your tongue? Wipe it with a teaspoon, handkerchief, tissue or piece of gauze. Anything that will remove the bacteria coating.

Rinse out your mouth. Few of us always have a toothbrush with us, but unless you're a Bedouin, there's usually water handy. "A lot of times bad breath is really a result of a dry mouth," says Dr. Halpern. "The odors just kind of ferment in a dry environment. By swishing your mouth with water, you're flushing away some of the bad residue." Swishing is especially important if you're a coffee or milk drinker. Left to lurk in the mouth, these two drinks are notorious for bad breath.

Suck it up. No water? Suck on a sugar-free lemon drop. Citrus fruits stimulate salivary flow, and saliva, being slightly acidic, helps suppress bacteria. Chewing gum can serve the same function, loosening food bits then flushing them away with saliva.

Avoid problem foods. Spices (onions, hot peppers, garlic) and spicy offshoots (deli meats like pastrami, salami and pepperoni) tend to stay in your mouth and re-circulate for up to 24 hours no matter how often you brush.

Research indicates that a diet high in certain fats may contribute to bad breath. Fats found in cheeses, butter, whole milk and fatty meats may contain certain aromatic substances that we metabolize and then exhale, none too pleasantly. And fatty cheese sticks to your choppers as well as your arteries, making them particularly hard to scour.

Sorry, Charlie. Tuna fish also tends to linger.

Don't skip breakfast. There are things bubbling in your stomach that can re-move the paint from siding at 50 yards. Overnight they have time to fester and in the morning they tend to rise. A morning meal helps to absorb these gases before they leech into the environment.

Try a breath freshener. Go sugarless, and don't expect miracles. Most of the commercial sprays on the market will mask bad breath for only 15 to 30 minutes, says Dr. Finger. "By and large you can't depend on mouth rinses or sprays to mask the odor for longer than that," he says.

Certain natural fresheners work well over the short-term, too. "Parsley and some other herbs like wintergreen and mint have oils that are aromatic, and those aromatic oils can freshen the breath," says Dr. Halpern.

Employ a double-barreled mouthwash. Many commercial mouthwashes are strictly breath fresheners—you want one that kills bacteria, too. Listerine, for exam-ple, has marketed a mint version of the old standard that's not only palatable but also helps battle gum disease.

See your dentist. If you're flossing 12 times a day and avoiding offending food and drink and you still have breath that curls your co-workers eyebrows, your prob-lem has deeper roots.

Bad breath might be a result of gastrointestinal problems. Some diseases like cancer, tuberculosis and syphilis can cause bad breath, too. But the most common medical problem that gives rise to bad breath is periodontal, or gum, disease. As many as 50 to 80 percent of adults have some form of gum disease, and until it's ad-dressed, you'll continue to have bad breath.

Baldness

Stay Ahead of Your Genes

Men prefer to be alone when they lean into the mirror to stare morosely at a hairline retreating faster than commuters fleeing a group of panhandlers. Bald may be beautiful but only on someone else's head.

Actually, you're losing hair as you read this. It's part of a natural process that has the hairs on your head growing, resting and shedding in a continuous cycle. If you have a balance between growing and shedding hairs, you have a full head of hair. If you don't, you probably have androgenic alopecia, or male pattern baldness.

Here's the pattern—a hair enters the resting phase of the cycle at a normal rate, sheds at a normal rate then balks when it comes time to re-enter the growth cycle. The rebel hair follicle either stops production entirely or produces a truncated, emaciated version of the original hair, a fine nonpigmented thing known as a vellus hair. It's a hair by definition but no deterrent to people who want to use your noggin to admire their reflections.

Hair loss can have other causes—severe stress, major surgery, a serious illness—but male pattern baldness is at the root of most shiny domes. The cause is the hormone androgen. Androgen is common to every man, but some men have a sensitivity to it in the scalp where, for reasons that aren't entirely clear, it throttles hair growth. This androgen sensitivity is genetically inherited and it's not unusual—by age 50 half of all men go markedly bald, no secret to anyone who has ever looked down on a rush hour sidewalk from a third-story window. Nothing can stymie this androgen assault either, though researchers have discovered that men who are castrated before puberty won't go bald even if they are genetically predisposed.

Castration being a painful solution and puberty being a thing of your past, there's no stopping male pattern baldness entirely. But if you're losing your locks, there are things you can do to ease, and in some cases halt or even reverse, the spread of shine.

Man's Role

There's little you can do about the hairs that have already jumped ship. But you can make the most of the hair that's still there and, done properly, that's often enough to maintain the appearance of a youthful hairline.

Make use of creative cuts. This isn't news, but it's often done wrong—witness the chromedome who grows one strand of hair aberrantly long and wanders through life looking like a firecracker with a long fuse.

The best rule for thinning hair: Less is more.

"If the hair is kept shorter, it actually appears to be fuller," says Anthony Palladino, owner of the Beverly Hilton Barber Shop in Beverly Hills, California, whose work has helped disguise the balding pates of such luminaries as Jack Nicholson and Bruce Willis.

Short hair helps ease the signs of hair loss at both the front and the back, says Palladino. If you have a bald spot at the back of your head, long hair there will pull down and away from that shiny crown, making it more visible than it already is.

Get a perm. No kidding. A mild perm increases hair volume.

"A perm takes one hair and curls it up so that it takes up more space and makes your head look bushier," says Guy Webster, M.D., Ph.D., associate professor of dermatology and director of the Center for Cutaneous Pharmacology at Jefferson Medical College of Thomas Jefferson University in Philadelphia. "You can make things look a little better by getting a perm."

Wash your hair every day. Freshly shampooed hair, says Palladino, looks fuller. Go easy on conditioning, though—once a week is enough. Overly soft hair is harder to style. Don't sweat the type of shampoo, either. "No shampoo on the market makes hair fall out," says Dr. Webster.

Don't overdo, though. "The more you fool with the hair, the worse it is for your hair," says Dr. Webster. "The more you style it, the more you tug on it, the less happy it is."

Dr. Webster is all for daily shampooing if needed and the occasional perm. But you don't want to be constantly brushing, combing and plucking at your hair. This doesn't mean you have to treat your hair like 15th-century Ming china. Just be reasonable.

What Modern Medicine Can (and Can't) Do

With the possible exception of Congress, no arena is as rife with confusion and outright misconception as treatment for male pattern baldness. In pursuit of hair men have placed all manner of ridiculousness on their heads, from small bowls discharging electrical currents to liquid nitrogen, the latter growing hair in some men but also turning their noggins bright red. A word from the wise.

"If a claim seems too good to be true, it probably is too good to be true," says Steven Greenbaum, M.D., chief of dermatologic surgery at Jefferson Medical Col-

How common: Every man experiences some degree of hair loss with age. Marked hair loss from male pattern baldness affects roughly half of all men by age 50.

Risk factors: This one's strictly genetic.

Age group affected: Male pattern baldness can begin any time after the onset of puberty.

Gender gap: Why don't women generally bare their scalps to the world? Because they're short on androgen, the hormone that's responsible for shutting off hair growth. When women do lose hair, they tend to lose it evenly over the entire scalp rather than developing the "halo" look so common among older men.

Who to see: Dermatologist.

lege. "There's no product available now that can completely regrow men's hair." Nevertheless, doctors do have options.

You've heard no doubt of minoxidil. It's the first and only government approved hair restoring drug on the market, and there's a reason for this—minoxidil does work. Studies have shown that a twice daily daubing with this cream (marketed commercially as Rogaine) can sometimes jolt hair back into the growth phase. In tests minoxidil has produced noticeable hair growth in a third of balding men, fuzzy hair growth in another third and nothing at all in the remaining third.

Tests have shown that minoxidil seems to work best on younger men who are just starting to lose their hair and men who still have a dusting of fine vellus hairs. It won't grow hair on a slick bald head.

Minoxidil has its drawbacks. It takes an average of four to six months to see if it works. Dermatologists usually have their patients try it for a year, at roughly the cost of your first car (a year's supply is about $600). The drug is fairly new, approved by the U.S. Food and Drug Administration in 1988, so if there are any long-term side effects, they aren't known. And if minoxidil does work, it only does so as long as you use it—quit the twice daily applications and the hair you've grown will disappear in a few months.

Another medical option is the hair transplant. There once was a time when a hair transplant looked more like a home for crows than a refuge for a beautiful woman's fingers. No more.

"Hair transplants have improved tremendously from the days where they looked like a bunch of corn stalks," says Dr. Greenbaum. Done correctly, says Dr. Greenbaum, a quality hair transplant is virtually impossible to distinguish from a real head of hair.

How do hair transplants work? For some reason, hair on the side of the head is naturally resistant to hair damning androgen. So dermatologists simply remove plugs of hair from the side of the head and seed them in bald spots, where they grow unaffected by the androgen beneath them.

Drawbacks? Hair transplantation is a time consuming process. Transplanting several hundred plugs of hair can require a half-dozen surgical sessions spanning as much as a year. It's expensive, too. At roughly $50 per plug (about 8 to 12 hairs) a massive reforesting effort can cost around $15,000.

A third medical option is scalp reduction. Since skin is elastic, your dermatologist can remove as much of your bald skin as possible then fill the gap by stretching hair-bearing sections of your head over it.

Scalp reduction is often used in conjunction with a hair transplant. Again, don't expect to restore your teenage hairline, there's only so much hair to stretch.

Most scalp reductions run $1,500 to $3,000. It's an outpatient procedure that should have you in bandages only for a day or so.

Keep Your Head Up

With so many potential customers, research into a cure for male pattern baldness proceeds at a frantic pace. One exciting option in the works is a drug that could keep the hormone androgen from damaging the hair follicle, effectively blocking baldness before it starts. Whatever the means, many experts are convinced that the end of male pattern baldness isn't far off.

"Researchers are working on other tricks and better medicine," says Dr. Webster. "I'm optimistic that within 10 or 15 years there will be, if not a cure for male pattern baldness, an incredibly effective treatment."

Here's one last option for you to consider—let nature take its course. Everyone's hair thins with time, a receding hairline doesn't make you the Elephant Man.

"About 99.9 percent of the time the problem is perceived as being worse than it really is," says Dr. Webster. "This isn't to say you're not going bald. But other people don't really care as much about your appearance as you do."

Belching
The Art of Managing Excess Air

In certain cultures belching is seen as perfectly acceptable behavior. In some instances it is even viewed as flattery. In many parts of Asia, for instance, an after dinner burp by the guest indicates to the host that all went down swimmingly.

Fine in Beijing, but pressing back and airing your clams on the half-shell is usually frowned on in our society.

Unfortunately, burping can't be eliminated entirely—the mathematics of existence preclude it. A man's gastrointestinal tract is capable of accommodating slightly less than one cupful of air and other gases. But a man generally takes in and produces close to ten cupfuls of gas in a day. You do the math.

Proving that your tax dollars aren't going to waste, researchers have analyzed belches and found that they are comprised of nitrogen, oxygen and a trace of carbon dioxide. In short, air. The burp may be a social gaffe but it serves an important purpose—what goes in must eventually come out, and your body often accomplishes this with a burp. Perfectly normal. One study showed healthy young people belch an average of 11 times in 20 hours, mealtimes not included.

Exhaust Control

There's no cure for belching, but this is certainly no cause for alarm.

"It's often a protective measure when you belch," says James Cooper, M.D., chairman of the Department of Medicine at Fairfax Hospital and professor of medicine at Georgetown University School of Medicine in Washington, D.C. "You get that air out of there and relieve your discomfort."

You can't—and don't—want to do away with belching. But you can keep it to a civilized minimum. Here's how.

Watch your manners. You can easily swallow a pint of air during a meal. Shoveling down a hamburger and a soda while debating the merits of the full-court press will have you sucking in air like a humpback whale. Listen to your mother. Don't talk while you eat. Chew slowly and thoroughly, with your mouth closed. Don't drink and eat at the same time. Don't eat on the run.

"People who eat quickly or drink while they're eating tend to swallow more air," says Dr. Cooper. "You need to watch how fast you eat."

Eschew gluttony. Simple cause and effect here. "Don't overload your stomach at any one meal," says Dr. Cooper. "If you overeat, you'll belch."

Watch what you eat and drink. Carbonated soft drinks and beer are quick to set you popping, worse still if you suck them out of a can. Certain foods have a high air content, too, like ice cream, soufflés, omelets and whipped cream.

Other major belching provocateurs include foods that loosen the lower esophageal sphincter—a little valve at the base of your esophagus that normally keeps food and gas from coming up from the stomach. Fried foods, high-fat meats, poultry skins, fatty salad dressings, chocolate, caffeinated drinks and peppermints all can cause this trap door to wilt on its hinges, allowing trapped air to rush up from your stomach with a vehemence, and a scent that can surprise both you and everyone else in the immediate zip code.

Of course, if you *want* to belch, change your strategy. "If you eat a seven course dinner at a fancy restaurant you might feel a little distended," says Steven Peikin, M.D., head of the Division of Gastroenterology at the Robert Wood Johnson Medical School and Cooper Hospital in Camden, New Jersey, and author of *Gastrointestinal Health*. "So you take a peppermint and it acutely relaxes the lower esophageal sphincter, allowing you to belch and feel relieved."

Avoid the water fountain. Water is wonderful, but sucked from a fountain it's also largely air.

Avoid chewing gum and sucking on hard candies. These result in much saliva and air swallowing. Plus, chocolate and fat-containing sweets loosen the lower esophageal sphincter, making it even easier for all the surplus air to come right back up, says Dr. Cooper.

Don't smoke. "Sucking on a pipe, a cigar or a cigarette can cause excessive stomach gas," says Dr. Peikin, "and that gas has to have a place to go. Plus, nicotine relaxes the lower esophageal sphincter, which can cause belching and heartburn."

Let nature take its course. "Don't force yourself to belch. It won't help," says Michael Oppenheim, M.D., who practices in Los Angeles and is the author of *The Complete Book of Better Digestion*. Forcing a belch often makes things worse, says Dr. Oppenheim. In trying to force up trapped air, you suck down more air.

Cool out. Anxiety tends to set you swallowing, no secret to anyone who has ever gone to the altar or driven over 50 miles per hour in a Yugo. Research shows that you can gulp quite a bit of air every time you swallow.

"A lot of people tend to gulp air when they're nervous," says Dr. Peikin.

Exercise and relaxation techniques can help reduce anxiety over the long haul.

FAST FACTS

How common: Everyone belches.

Risk factors: Swallowing too much air, eating the wrong foods.

Age group affected: All age groups.

Gender gap: Men are no more prone to belching than women.

Who to see: Most belching requires no treatment, but excessively heavy belchers might benefit by consulting a family doctor or gastroenterologist.

For a quick fix during tense situations try clamping down on a pencil or (a bit more gently) your finger. Keeping your mouth open makes it difficult to swallow.

Don't get upset. If you belch a lot, don't be too concerned. Probably the worst thing you may have is an incompetent lower esophageal sphincter, cause of heartburn in some 40 million Americans.

"That's the most common disease that's associated with belching and it's rarely serious," says Dr. Peikin. "Belching is more of an embarrassment than anything else."

Blisters

Don't Get Rubbed the Wrong Way

You can't wait to wear that new pair of shoes on the basketball court, even though you haven't worn high-tops in years. Or maybe you have to rake leaves all day, even though you haven't gripped anything bigger than a pen since last year's raking. Your reward? Blisters: nature's way of mocking your newfound ambition and enthusiasm.

Blisters crop up when friction causes the top two layers of skin to separate and the space in between fills with fluid. Most occur on the feet, the result of ill-fitting shoes or a sudden increase in activity level. They can also appear on the hands after a gripping encounter with a bat, racket, tool or anything else you can get a handle on.

Living in the Friction-Free Zone

There is no bliss in blisters. They hurt, they annoy and they keep you from doing what you want to do. The best course of action is to prevent them by keeping your skin free of friction.

Step into the right shoes. You're obviously asking for trouble if your shoes are tight. But too loose is also a problem. "Even a small amount of sliding can cause enough friction to form a blister," says Glenn Gastwirth, D.P.M., deputy executive director of the American Podiatric Medical Association, "especially if you're athletic."

A finger's width of space between your longest toe and the end of the shoe is ideal. But there's more to it than length. Make sure the toebox is high enough for you to easily wiggle your toes. To protect your heel make sure the rear of the shoe is cut neither too high nor too low.

Shop for shoes late in the day, when your feet are their largest size. And wear the kind of socks you'll be wearing when you wear the shoes.

Do the last thing first. Every manufacturer has a template from which they design their shoes. This is called a last. "Flip the shoe over and draw an imaginary line down the middle," says Allen Selner, D.P.M., a podiatrist at the Medstar Foot and Ankle Center in Studio City, California. "If there's an equal amount of shoe on both sides it's a straight last. If it's unequal, it's either an inflair or an outflair." The shape of the last should match the shape of your foot. "If your foot curls one way and your

FAST FACTS

How common: Just about everyone will get a blister at some point over the course of their lifetimes.

Risk factors: Ill-fitting shoes; foot abnormalities; excessive walking, running or gripping of objects.

Age group affected: Blisters favor people of any age who lead an active lifestyle.

Gender gap: Women get foot blisters more often than men; men are more likely to get them on their hands.

Who to see: Most blisters can be self-treated. But if you are having recurring or intense blister problems, see a podiatrist or a dermatologist.

shoe curls the other," says Dr. Selner, "something has to give."

Break them in slowly. Although new shoes should feel comfortable right out of the box, don't wear them for long stretches of time. Instead, wear them an hour or two the first day and increase gradually from there.

Cover the area. "As a precaution with new shoes, wear a small moleskin patch on the area that's vulnerable to blisters," advises Dr. Gastwirth. The idea is to transfer friction and pressure to the moleskin rather than *your* skin. Dr. Gastwirth prefers moleskin to adhesive bandages because it doesn't slide around and cause friction of its own. He recommends the moleskin be slightly larger than the area that might blister.

Wear the right socks. For athletics, wear dual layer socks, says Joseph Ellis, D.P.M., a podiatrist in La Jolla, California, and author of *Running Injury Free*. "The two layers are made of different materials," he says. "The part against the skin shunts moisture to the outer layer. This keeps the skin cooler and reduces friction."

Do some sole searching. To prevent blisters on the bottom of your feet, Dr. Ellis recommends wearing inner soles. "Spenco makes a neoprene inner sole that provides a good cushion," he says. "It gives a little bit and reduces the friction."

Get a grip. The same principle applies to prevent blisters on the hands: avoid friction. If you're taking up bowling, biking or a racquet sport, or if you're about to use hand tools, wear protective gloves. "There are gloves specially designed for different sports," says Ronald Moy, M.D., assistant professor of dermatology at the University of California, Los Angeles.

Ease into it gradually. The best way to start a blistering activity is to toughen your skin slowly and gradually. "Build up a callus," advises Dr. Moy. "That's the body's response to repeated friction and pressure. The skin builds up thickness to protect itself."

Pop Goes the Blister

Once you get a blister, three things are essential: maintain comfort, promote healing and prevent infection. Here are some specifics.

Burst the bubble. "The best thing to do is to poke a hole and drain it yourself within the first couple of hours," says Dr. Ellis. "It will reduce the pressure and let you get back to activity quicker."

Popping the blister leaves you vulnerable to infection so do it only under the right conditions, not between innings of a softball game. "Put alcohol on the blister to kill any bacteria that's on there," says Dr. Ellis. "Heat a pin or needle over a flame and poke a hole to let the fluid drain."

Dr. Gastwirth advises holding the needle parallel to the skin surface, not pointed down. "Pierce it a couple of times between the edge and the middle, where the blister is raised by fluid, and be careful not to pierce healthy flesh."

Afterward, keep the area pristine clean. "Don't remove the roof of the blister," says Dr. Gastwirth. "If it's open, dust and dirt can get in. Apply antiseptic and cover it with a sterile bandage. But don't make the bandage so thick it becomes a new source of irritation."

Get to the source. To prevent a recurrence, check your shoes and socks for points of friction. "See if the shoe is excessively worn," says Dr. Gastwirth, "or if there's a torn seam or lining." Look at your socks, too, he adds. "Friction can be caused by an irregular stitch, a tear, a seam or wadding up."

Check your mechanics. If you keep getting blisters on your feet, you might have a biomechanical problem. High or low arches, for example, or a Charlie Chaplin walk—with the legs turned out. Dr. Selner suggests you check your gait. "Stand normally and start walking in place. Then let your feet stop. Look at the angle of your feet to the line you're walking. If your foot is turned out more than 15 degrees, you may have a problem."

A podiatrist might recommend arch supports or an orthotic device to correct the problem or alleviate the discomfort it's causing.

See also Foot and Heel Pain

Body Odor

Masking Man's Manly Scent

Some scientists believe body odor once served an evolutionary function. Scents wafting from certain areas of the body may have advertised a man's sexuality. A fine thing in prehistoric times, but today smelling like a mastodon is no longer considered an aphrodisiac.

What creates body odor? Actually, it's not as simple as you may think. There are two kinds of sweat glands—the eccrine sweat glands, which are present all over the body, and the apocrine sweat glands, which cluster primarily under your armpits and around your groin. It's the apocrine glands that are the main culprits in body odor, although it's not their secretions which produce the problem.

"The glandular secretions are sterile and they don't have any smell," says R. Kenneth Landow, M.D., clinical professor of medicine and dermatology at the University of Southern California School of Medicine in Los Angeles. "It's when they persist on the skin and can be acted on by bacteria that we get the smell."

Left unattended, bacteria feed on the apocrine oils. As the oils are broken down they become rancid and smell.

A Clean Machine

Body odor can vary depending on your body chemistry, how much sweat and odor you're genetically inclined to emit, your activities, your mood and the time of year, but the most effective plan of attack always remains simple and constant.

"The body odor battle," states Dr. Landow, "centers on good personal hygiene."

Wash regularly. Simple enough, and step number one in the fight against body odor. "Remember the odor principally comes from the bacteria working on the oily secretions," says Dr. Landow. "If you wash off the secretions, you shouldn't have an odor problem."

For most men, says Dr. Landow, one shower a day is enough. If you're a longshoreman, a Chippendales dancer or a roofer in Death Valley, you'll probably need to shower more.

When you're in the shower, there's no need to assault yourself—you want to wash off oil and bacteria, not sand to the bone. "You don't want to overwash to the point that you irritate the skin," says Dr. Landow. "When the skin gets irritated, you can get more bacteria growing on it, so that defeats the purpose."

Use an antibacterial soap. With an antibacterial soap, not only do you wash away the secretions, says Dr. Landow, you kill off the scent-producing bacteria, too.

There are dozens of antibacterial soaps on your supermarket shelf—most common deodorant soaps, like Dial and Zest, contain substances that help kill bacteria. Stronger antibacterial soaps, including scrub soaps used by surgeons, are also available. They're available over the counter at most drugstores. Ask your pharmacist for his recommendation.

Use a deodorant. Deodorants mask underarm odor by leaving chemicals on the skin that help to kill off bacteria and have a pleasant odor of their own.

"For most men, using a good deodorant is quite sufficient for managing body odor," says Dr. Landow.

Use an antiperspirant. If your deodorant doesn't seem to work, try adding an antiperspirant to your arsenal. The antiperspirant reduces the amount of sweat the body produces so the bacteria have fewer oils to work on. Many commercial products now contain both a deodorant and an antiperspirant—delivering a one-two punch that's usually very effective.

Try a topical antibacterial cream. Some men get irritations from deodorants and antiperspirants, which contain aluminum salts and other drying agents that may be too strong for sensitive glands in the armpits. Since skin irritation can exacerbate body odor, annoying your underarms isn't the best approach.

If commercial deodorants bother you or they don't seem to be working, try an over-the-counter topical antibacterial cream, like Neosporin, suggests Randall Hrabko, M.D., a dermatologist in private practice in Los Angeles. These creams won't stop you from sweating, he says, but as their name implies they do kill bacteria.

Hammer the underarm. Plain old sodium bicarbonate, more universally known as baking soda, can do the same thing under your arms that it does in your fridge—kill odor-causing bacteria and absorb moisture. As an alternative to commercial deodorants try sprinkling a generous amount of baking soda into your bath or mix it with a little talcum powder to slap under your arms.

Watch the wash. Men tend to view washing machines as mechanized black holes, a single machine capable of absorbing a month's worth of laundry. Most washing machines in the home, especially the smaller units, don't work that well to begin with, and stuffing your entire ensemble into a single load doesn't help matters any.

"If you don't clean your clothes properly, they'll retain the odor because the bacteria and the body oils are still present on the clothes," says Dr. Landow. Don't overload the washer. And if your machine at home doesn't seem to be doing the job, consider getting a new one or sending your clothes to a professional cleaner.

Shave your armpits. This may sound trendy at best and effeminate at worst, but the fact is underarm hair serves as a sort of fly strip for secretions and bacteria. "If you shave the hair, you can get rid of a lot of the places where the bacteria can get trapped," says Dr. Landow.

Watch what you eat. Foods and spices, like fish, onion, garlic, cumin and curry, produce extracts of proteins and oils that can seep back out through your pores. What set your mouth watering the night before can leave you smelling like a back alley the next day.

Don't Sweat It

Not all body odor is easily managed. If you've tried all the tips above and you still smell like last month's socks, then it's time to see your family doctor or a dermatologist. He can prescribe something stronger. He can also look for other potential causes of body odor. Skin diseases, like eczema, can cause body odor; so can diseases, like diabetes. Such cases, however, are rare. In most instances, with a modicum of planning, body odor is one worry you shouldn't sweat.

"For most men," says Dr. Hrabko, "bathing regularly and using an underarm deodorant is enough to handle body odor."

Boils

Solutions for a Complex(ion) Problem

Boils are to complexion problems what Hulk Hogan once was to professional wrestling: bigger, meaner and higher-profile than the rest.

Why? While pimples are more of a surface problem, boils start as an infection inside a hair follicle, meaning they have much deeper roots.

And a boil is a lot bigger than the standard pimple: usually about a centimeter in diameter (roughly the width of your small fingernail) or larger, says George Murphy, M.D., professor of dermatology at the University of Pennsylvania in Philadelphia.

"The nodule feels like a marble or a pea that you can actually move under the skin," says Dr. Murphy. "They can come on very rapidly, in two or three days, and enlarge quickly. Suddenly the patient feels it because a boil can be very, very painful."

The typical boil hangs around for several weeks, fading away only after the body's white blood cells conquer the inflammation inside the follicle, says Dr. Murphy. A sign of your white blood cells' battle with the inflammation is the yellowish pus you'll often see at the head of the boil.

Because of its hair follicle roots, the bothersome red bump, also known as a furuncle (a cluster of furuncles is known as a carbuncle), is most likely to crop up where the hair is: on the neck, face, buttocks and groin.

Most boils are caused by a bacteria called *staphylococcus aureus*. It's found on most people's skin, but for unexplained reasons the bacteria only causes boils to form in some cases, says Dr. Murphy.

"Those who tend to get boils may carry the bacteria in their nasal secretions, and chronically inoculate themselves," Dr. Murphy notes.

Sometimes, medical problems such as diabetes or immune system deficiencies make a person more susceptible to the painful skin eruptions, says Stephen Webster, M.D., chief of dermatology at the Gunderson Clinic in LaCrosse, Wisconsin. Folks with skin disorders, like atopic dermatitis and eczema, are also at bigger risk.

FAST FACTS

How common: About 5 percent of the population will suffer from a boil this year.

Risk factors: Men with diabetes, men who are overweight, those with compromised immune systems, men who sweat heavily and those on long-term steroid use are all more susceptible than the general public. Also, men with severe anemia or those who suffer from atopic dermatitis or eczema.

Age group affected: Boils are uncommon before puberty but age doesn't seem to play a role beyond that.

Gender gap: Men get boils slightly more often than women, primarily because men have more hair, but also since men perspire more because of their sweatier work and exercise routines.

Who to see: Family doctor or dermatologist, especially if the boil lingers for several days and is painful. If the boil is accompanied by fever, that's a sure sign of infection and it should be treated right away.

Boil Prevention

Even if you are prone to boils, there are things you can do to keep them away.

Stay in touch with soap. Good hygiene makes a big difference, says Amit Pandya, M.D., assistant professor of dermatology at the University of Texas Southwestern Medical Center at Dallas Southwestern Medical School. "Use an antibacterial soap. If you can decrease the number of bacteria on your skin in the first place, you'll have less chance of getting a boil," Dr. Pandya says.

It's also important to bathe shortly after exercise, when the number of bacteria on the skin is increased, he notes.

Loosen up. Tight-fitting clothing that doesn't let the skin breathe could be a boilmaker, Dr. Murphy says. "With men, that's one of the most common causes. They'll be out playing golf wearing tight-fitting clothing where the sweat isn't vented properly."

No close shaves. If you cut a facial hair too close to your face, the hair will retract under the skin surface and get trapped, says Dr. Murphy. "That sets up the initial inflammation that could lead to a boil."

Wash your hands. Especially if you're a grease monkey. Oils that contact the body will irritate the hair follicles and cause a boil or acne, says Dr. Pandya. "Try to minimize contact and protect yourself with some type of coat or jacket. And wash your hands often."

Boiling It Down

Once you're sure you have a boil, it's the doctor's call whether you'll face the "knife" or not.

"If the boil is soft and there's obviously a collection of pus, it's ready to be lanced," Dr. Webster says. "But if it's an early boil, we tend to treat it with heat and antibiotics."

And just when should you see a doctor about your boil from hell? "Any acute, painful swelling of the skin that doesn't resolve in a couple of days should be evaluated by a physician," says Dr. Murphy.

Here are a few treatment tips.

Compress it. You can speed up the healing process by applying hot, wet compresses to the boil every two hours to bring it to a head and hasten drainage. The heat can also lessen pain from the pressure inside the follicle.

Don't pick on yourself. Keep your hands off, says Paul Zanowiak, Ph.D., a pharmacist and professor of pharmacology at Temple University School of Pharmacy in Philadelphia. If you try to squeeze the boil yourself, it's possible the membrane in the pus sac could break down and multiply your problem. "The lining of the boil bursts and sets up another boil, which can come out in clusters called a carbuncle," he says.

Dr. Murphy adds that self-lancing could be deadly. "That could send bacteria into the bloodstream, and in rare instances could cause infection of the heart, brain or bones," he says.

Attack with antibiotics. If your boil seems to have taken up permanent residence, or if you have a recurring problem with the painful bumps, a doctor may prescribe antibiotics, says Dr. Murphy.

"People with severe boils could be put on a treatment of systemic antibiotics," he says. "Chronic carriers may be treated with a 12-week course of antibiotics to eradicate the staph from the nose."

Bronchitis

Opening the Airways

After days of fighting off what seems to be a simmering cold or flu, you erupt in a thunderous explosion of moist, gagging coughs that make you sound like your neighbor's sputtering lawn mower.

What's going on? Chances are you have bronchitis, an inflammation of the bronchi—the air passages in the lungs—caused by a bacteria or virus. In response to the inflammation, the body produces secretions to protect the lining of these airways. As these secretions build up, they interfere with breathing and you begin to cough in order to clear out phlegm, mucus and other lung gunk. Bronchitis also can cause shortness of breath, wheezing, fever and pain behind the breastbone.

In most cases the inflammation is caused by the same viruses that cause colds and flus. These acute or short-term bouts of bronchitis are common and usually clear up within a week. If phlegm is yellow or green, the bronchitis is likely caused by bacteria and will require antibiotics.

In fact, acute bronchitis is so prevalent that almost every guy will tangle with it at least once, says Norman H. Edelman, M.D., a pulmonary specialist in New York City and scientific affairs consultant to the American Lung Association.

"If you've ever had a cold that extended into your chest, then you probably have had acute bronchitis," Dr. Edelman says.

Chronic bronchitis, unlike the acute kind, can last for months or even years. Air pollution may be a risk factor, but smoking is by far the most common cause of chronic bronchitis. In fact, at least 90 percent of men who have it are smokers, says Ronald Greeno, M.D., co-director of respiratory therapy and pulmonary function at Good Samaritan Hospital in Los Angeles. Smoking harms the bronchi because it increases mucus production and gradually thickens and narrows the walls of the airways. That makes breathing difficult and increases the risk of infection. Unchecked, chronic bronchitis can lead to emphysema and even heart failure.

Forestalling Trouble

Simply living a healthy life can drastically slash your risk of bronchitis, says Dr. Greeno. Here's how.

Snub the smokes. As we mentioned, smoking is the number one cause of chronic bronchitis and greatly increases your chances of getting the acute kind. So if you smoke, quit, suggests Dr. Greeno.

Avoid the passive stuff, too. "Passive smoke is clearly one of the most serious forms of air pollution that we're now exposed to," Dr. Greeno says. "It predisposes children and many adults to episodes of bronchitis." Avoid smoky bars and restaurants. If someone in your household smokes, consider creating a well-ventilated smoking area away from the frequently used rooms of your home.

Chill out. Stress saps your immunity and may make your lungs more vulnerable to bronchitis and other respiratory infections, says Dr. Greeno. So practicing relaxation techniques such as meditation and progressive relaxation may help.

Eat the right foods. A balanced diet can help your immune system prevent bronchial infections. Try to eat at least five servings of fruits and vegetables, like apples, oranges, beans and carrots, six servings of grains such as cereals and whole-wheat breads, two servings of dairy products, like cheese and yogurt, and a couple servings of fish, poultry or meat each day, says Dr. Greeno.

Keep in shape. Taking a brisk 20-minute walk three times a week and regularly doing other aerobic exercise such as swimming also can help keep your immunity in tip-top shape and prevent bronchitis, Dr. Greeno says.

Protect yourself from the flu. Bronchitis often is a complication of the flu. An annual flu shot can help prevent that and is particularly recommended for certain high-risk groups: those age 65 or older or those with chronic heart or lung problems, diabetes or other chronic health problems, says Dr. Greeno.

When the Lungs Have It

If bronchitis sets in, the first question is whether to see a doctor. The answer is yes if you have a temperature of 101°F or higher, chest pain, shortness of breath or vomiting, or if you are coughing up blood or thick yellow-, green- or rust-colored sputum. You should also consult a doctor if you have a history of respiratory ailments such as asthma or emphysema.

Being a man, you might be tempted to tough the symptoms out. But doctors say that is probably the worst thing to do, since untreated bronchitis may lead to pneumonia.

"Guys, particularly those in their thirties and forties, are terrible about seeking proper medical care. They think it's undignified or not a male thing if they go to the doctor. If they do come, they often bring their wives who do most of the talking while the guy just sits there and nods occasionally. So guys really need to know that it's okay to seek help for bronchitis and other ailments," says Eric G. Anderson, M.D., a family physician in La Jolla, California.

FAST FACTS

How common: About 4 to 5 million American men get acute bronchitis annually. Another 6 million have chronic bronchitis.

Risk factors: Smoking, recent cold or flu, history of underlying respiratory disease such as asthma or emphysema. Possibly air pollution.

Age group affected: Acute bronchitis is most common among children younger than age 5 and men older than age 45. Chronic bronchitis is most prevalent in middle-age and elderly men.

Gender gap: For every four men who have acute bronchitis, five women get it. But men are three times more likely to have chronic bronchitis as women.

Who to see: Family doctor or internist.

Before your appointment collect sputum in a cup. It may speed your office visit since the first thing your physician will want is a sputum sample, and you may not be able to cough it up on demand, Dr. Greeno says.

If you have chronic bronchitis or acute viral bronchitis, your doctor may prescribe an aerosol inhaler to temporarily relax the walls of the airways, and to decrease the cough and shortness of breath. If you have an acute bacterial infection, antibiotics will help. Here are a few other things that may speed your recovery.

Keep the water flowing. Drink an eight-ounce glass of water or juice every waking hour, Dr. Greeno says. It will help prevent dehydration and break up phlegm, so it will be easier to clear out your lungs and airways.

But stay booze-free. Some guys think a cold beer will cure anything, but not in this case. Alcohol slows your metabolism, suppresses the immune system and increases the amount of time it will take you to recover, says Dr. Greeno.

Don't push yourself. A few men mistakenly believe that a good, hard workout at the gym will help clear up bronchitis by forcing the gunk out of the lungs. But exercise—or even dragging yourself into the office—does more harm than good. Not only can you infect others, you'll probably get dehydrated, and that weakens your body's natural defenses. So get plenty of rest and postpone your racquetball match until you feel better, suggests Dr. Greeno.

Lose the phlegm. The more sputum you cough up, the fewer problems you have in your respiratory tract. If you have difficulty producing sputum, consider using a cough medicine that contains guaifenesin, such as Robitussin PE, an expectorant that will help you expel phlegm from your lungs, Dr. Greeno says.

Licorice lozenges also are a good expectorant, says herbal expert Varro E. Tyler,

Ph.D., professor of pharmacognosy at Purdue University in West Lafayette, Indiana.

Control the coughs. "You want to do some coughing to keep your airways clear, but excessive coughing isn't good because it's just going to make your throat sore and inflame your airways even more," says Bradley M. Block, M.D., a family physician in private practice in Winter Park, Florida. "I tell bronchitis patients to use an over-the-counter cough suppressant that contains dextromethorphan, such as Robitussin-DM. Of course, follow the manufacturer's directions."

Keep a humidifier humming. Moist air—it doesn't matter if it is warm or cool—may help loosen up phlegm and decongest your airways, Dr. Block says. If you use a humidifier, however, be sure that it is cleaned and dried after each use to prevent disease-causing molds from growing in it.

Bursitis and Tendinitis

Maintaining Your Body's Moving Parts

On that first brilliant autumn Sunday, you trot onto the field like John Elway for a spirited game of touch football. You throw deep, just like Elway. You get bumped and knocked down, just like Elway. And when you wake up the next morning, you still feel just like the Denver Broncos quarterback—only it's the way he felt during the 1988 season, when his right elbow hurt so bad he could barely play.

Or on that first warm weekend of spring, you decide to play Hercules to the Aegean Stables, otherwise known as your garage. After a day of heavy lifting you can hardly lift your arm because of the excruciating pain in your left shoulder.

The simple truth is that your joints are like the moving parts of any other machine. Eventually, they wear down. And in the human machine, that usually happens about the time you turn 40. The result is often tendinitis and bursitis, the two most prevalent types of joint ailments.

"I don't know of any answer other than to die young," quips James Richards, M.D., an orthopedic surgeon at Matthews Orthopedic Clinic in Orlando, Florida. "If you live long enough, you're going to have some of those things. That's one of the prices of survival."

Joint Resolution Needed

Tendinitis is most common in the shoulder, wrist, elbow, knee and ankle. Bursitis strikes most frequently in the shoulder, elbow, knee and heel. Both involve inflammations in the joints, where muscles and tendons work in close proximity to bones.

"Most of the time, it's part and parcel of the same problem," says Kent Pomeroy, M.D., a physiatrist, or doctor of physical medicine, one who treats injury or disease with physical agents such as light, heat, cold, water and exercise, in Scottsdale, Arizona, and past president of the American Association of Orthopedic Medicine. "Most of the time, it's hard to separate the two out."

Bursae—tiny, thin-walled sacs of fluid—serve to cushion the body's moving parts. There are about 150 bursa sacs scattered throughout your body. "When you get an inflammation of a bursa sac, the walls of the sac, which are usually paper thin, thicken and the sac fills with fluid," explains Steven Habusta, D.O., an orthopedic surgeon in private practice in Toledo, Ohio. The swelling that results can cause extreme pain.

Similarly, tendinitis—which is far more common than bursitis—is an injury where the tendon attaches to the bone.

By the time you hit your midthirties, those little bursa sacs and tendons have a lot of mileage on them. One overly ambitious weekend of work or play may be all it takes for your body to mimic a 1930s Hollywood tough guy and say, "Let's blow this joint." But for many, it's merely a case of deterioration from years of normal use. "The vast majority of people I treat have no specific history," Dr. Richards says. "It just comes on all of a sudden."

Men between the ages of 35 and 50 are most susceptible to the problems associated with bursitis and tendinitis. W. Ben Kibler, M.D., medical director of the Lexington Clinic Sports Medicine Center in Kentucky, says that most of what is commonly thought of as tendinitis "is actually more of degeneration than inflammation."

Moderation, Protection, Prevention

What causes bursitis and tendinitis isn't always clear, but it's often the result of overuse. Don't think weekend warriors are the only ones at risk, though. Sedentary workers can develop bursitis merely by resting their elbows on the desk. And anyone who works all day at a computer terminal or typewriter can find themselves with a painful case of tendinitis in their wrists.

Here are steps you can take to help avoid becoming a sad sac with a tendon-cy to get hurt.

Pad it. Bursae are closest to the surface in the knees and elbows, and that's where they take the most abuse.

"If you're involved with any activity that would be putting any kind of repeated banging on the ends of the elbows and knees, you should pad them," Dr. Habusta says.

Roofers and carpet layers, for example, should wear knee pads.

Warm up. Before diving into strenuous exercise—whether it's a friendly game of touch football or lifting weights at the gym—take time to warm up your body.

"Men try to go full-bore into exercise," Dr. Pomeroy says. "They're more likely to aggravate their bursae, not to mention their muscles and tendons. Getting the body warm before getting into the exercise softens the tissues and relaxes them so that they're more pliable and have a better blood supply. In short, they're more likely to respond without injury."

You don't need much warm-up, says Dr. Pomeroy. Five minutes of running in place, calisthenics or stretching is enough. Also, it's a good idea to cool down for several minutes after exercise, Dr. Pomeroy says.

FAST FACTS

How common: Bursitis and tendinitis account for more than one-quarter of the patients for any active, orthopedic practice. Among men ages 35 to 50, bursitis and tendinitis are involved in as many as two-thirds of complaints of rheumatic woes.

Risk factors: Overuse, physical activity. Repetitive movements and biomechanical problems such as uneven leg length also can be contributing factors.

Age group affected: The risk of bursitis and tendinitis increases with age. Men in their thirties and forties are especially likely candidates since—as a group—they tend to overreach their physical capacity more than other age groups.

Gender gap: Women are equally prone to bursitis and tendinitis. Being primarily overuse injuries, they may be slightly more common among men since men are generally more physically active.

Who to see: Family doctor, rheumatologist, physiatrist, who is a doctor of physical medicine, one who treats injury or disease with physical agents such as light, heat, cold, water and exercise.

Learn from baseball. If you work in a job that requires repetitive movements—whether it's typing at a computer keyboard or lifting heavy objects—take a brief time-out each hour to stretch. "In baseball the seventh-inning stretch serves a purpose," Dr. Richards says. "Sitting at a ball game, you get stiff and sore. Standing up and stretching makes you feel better."

Stay relaxed. If you're under stress, the odds increase dramatically that you'll do something to injure yourself. "One of the most common injuries I see is when a person is moving from one house to another," Dr. Richards says. "That's one of the most stressful things in the world. And when you do things under stress, you're more apt to hurt yourself." So take a deep breath and relax before tackling that moving job or yard work.

Play the right angles. If you work at a computer, try to keep your arms and wrists level with the keyboard. That will avoid putting strain on the wrists that can cause tendinitis. "If you can have a keyboard at lap level instead of up on a desk, you can avoid some of those problems," Dr. Richards says.

Once You Have It

The classic symptoms of bursitis and tendinitis—pain, redness, swelling and heat around the affected joint—are usually quite clear. Your options are equally straightforward.

Rest. Take time off. "Hurting is a natural splint," says Dr. Habusta. "The body's telling us not to use that part. The biggest problem with men is they try to be over-aggressive sometimes. If the body says 'Don't use it,' don't use it."

How much time should you take off? If there's pain at rest, says Dr. Habusta, then you need complete rest. Once your bursitis or tendinitis stops hurting at rest, you can gradually—and that means gradually—ease back into exercising the affected part.

One exception: If the pain is in your shoulder, you must keep some flexibility—even if it's painful. "A shoulder will freeze up in three days if it isn't moved," warns Dr. Pomeroy. "The biggest problem then is getting movement back. That's a bigger problem than bursitis or tendinitis."

Take an anti-inflammatory. Aspirin and ibuprofen will decrease the swelling and pain for immediate relief. But Dr. Kibler cautions that relieving painful symptoms is not the same as curing the problem.

Ice it. Ice reduces pain and inflammation by decreasing swelling, precisely what you need for bursting bursae or tender tendons. For acute pain Dr. Habusta recommends you ice the affected area three times a day, 20 minutes at a pop. Put a towel between the ice and skin to keep from burning your skin.

Heat it. Once the swelling goes down, heat can help heal the injured area, says Dr. Pomeroy. Warm compresses, damp, hot towels or a soak in the hot tub should do the trick.

Seek help. Acute bursitis or tendinitis is often easily addressed, disappearing in a matter of days. But if two weeks pass and the inflammation hasn't eased, you need to see a doctor.

"If the pain and swelling doesn't go away, don't ignore it," cautions Dr. Habusta. "You need to have it checked out."

Again, if the pain is in your shoulder, don't wait that long. Dr. Pomeroy recommends seeing your physician within 72 hours if shoulder pain is severe.

Carpal Tunnel Syndrome
Avoiding the Top Occupational Hazard

It starts with aching pain in the upper arm or forearm. Then comes tingling in the fingers, an odd numbness or buzzing in the hands, a feeling that your arms are heavy and tired. Gradually, it gets worse, especially at night; you start waking up because of intense tingling in your wrists. After a while, holding a screwdriver or knotting a tie becomes a major challenge.

Welcome to the weird world of carpal tunnel syndrome.

Not for Computer Users Only

Carpal tunnel syndrome and related problems have been called "the occupational illnesses of the decade," in part because of the growing prevalence of keyboards attached to personal computers. Contrary to popular belief, though, carpal tunnel is neither new nor limited to computer users. There are references in medical writings to symptoms that were probably carpal tunnel as far back as the 1700s. More recently, carpal tunnel has been known to afflict everyone from carpenters, mail sorters and bricklayers to dairy farmers, supermarket checkers and sign-language translators. Assembly-line workers such as those in the automobile industry are especially susceptible, as are meatpackers and others who work in chilly conditions.

Ergonomists, who study the sometimes troubled interface between man and machine, blame the current attention on the fact that more people are spending day after day doing one small task over and over again. Especially if that one task is executed with the wrong posture, or if the wrong equipment is used, it can add up to what one ergonomist calls "thousands of tiny traumas" to the hands and wrists. The trouble comes when those tiny traumas aren't allowed to heal.

"Cumulative trauma disorders, of which carpal tunnel syndrome is one, are basically a question of lack of repair," says Chris Grant, Ph.D., a research fellow with the Center for Ergonomics at the University of Michigan in Ann Arbor. "The body doesn't have the time or the resources to repair itself."

Repetition is only one of several risk factors. Others include holding one position for long periods, extreme joint positions, excessive force, cold temperatures and vibration.

Nine's a Crowd

The carpal tunnel is a roundish bracelet of bones and ligament at the base of your hand. Through it runs nine finger tendons and a major trunk of your cerebral wiring called the median nerve. The median nerve conducts impulses to the brain from the thumb, forefinger, middle finger and ring finger.

Too much repetitive movement of the wrist and fingers, or exertions that are too severe, can irritate the tendons, their sheaths or the median nerve. That can cause swelling, scar tissue and increased friction in the carpal tunnel, especially if no time is given for healing. When the median nerve gets compressed or rubbed, it gets impaired. That interrupts the impulses it carries, causing the tingling, the numbness and, eventually, the pain.

Fortunately, there are plenty of steps you can take to keep carpal tunnel from becoming a painful part of your life. The first and most important of these is to heed the early-warning signs and get professional advice. "Pain is an indication that you may already have a problem," says David Thompson, Ph.D., professor emeritus of industrial engineering and engineering management at Stanford University. "A lot of workers try to macho their way through it by self-medicating with whatever nighttime television tells them will work. They don't want to make waves and maybe get laid off, but they end up with a serious disorder."

The Inner Man

Even when pain is present, carpal tunnel syndrome is for many men a manageable malady. Here are some suggestions for taking the syndrome by the horns by taking care of your body.

Take a break. The obvious cure for an injury that results from repetitive stress is to stop the activity causing the stress, giving damaged tissues time to heal. Of course, you can't always stop working, but you can try to rotate troublesome tasks with other, less troublesome tasks. You can also take rest breaks. Several studies have shown that short, frequent breaks—Dr. Grant calls them microbreaks—are more beneficial than longer but less frequent breaks. "These 30-second breaks have been reported to decrease fatigue and increase endurance if taken frequently," she says.

Stay in shape. Overall physical conditioning can play an important role in avoiding carpal tunnel syndrome. One study found that overweight people were four times more likely than slender people to develop symptoms of carpal tunnel syndrome. The same study found that those who didn't exercise frequently were seven times more likely to develop carpal tunnel than those who did. Gout, diabetes, thyroid and kidney conditions have also been shown to increase the risk of developing carpal tunnel syndrome.

FAST FACTS

How common: Very common and getting more so. Figures vary widely, but conservative estimates are that some 300,000 Americans have carpal tunnel syndrome.

Risk factors: Any activity that requires prolonged repetitive movement or "fixed" position of the wrists, hands and arms. Extreme joint positions, excessive force, cold temperatures and vibration also can cause problems.

Age group affected: All ages get carpal tunnel syndrome. Most physicians agree that people are more likely to develop the syndrome as they get older, perhaps because of nerve deterioration, perhaps because of longer straining on the job.

Gender gap: More than twice as many women develop carpal tunnel syndrome as men. Why is a mystery. Some physicians suspect hormones are to blame, others think women tend to occupy more jobs than men that require repetitive movement, like typing.

Who to see: If you work for someone else and you think your pain is job related, start with your boss: Many businesses have detailed procedures regarding work-related medical problems. Otherwise, see your family doctor, an internist or a physiatrist, who is a doctor of physical medicine, one who treats injury or disease with physical agents such as light, heat, cold, water and exercise. If you're not getting better in a few months of therapy, you might get referred to an orthopedist, hand surgeon, occupational medicine specialist or a rheumatologist.

Circulate. Part of the problem is inhibited blood circulation—that's why people who work with their hands in refrigerated environments such as meatpackers are especially prone to getting carpal tunnel syndrome. "Circulation is everything," says Robert E. Markison, M.D., a hand surgeon and associate clinical professor of surgery at the University of California, San Francisco, School of Medicine. Therefore, anything that helps improve circulation, including stopping smoking and getting some aerobic exercise, can help prevent the condition.

Warm your hands. You can give your circulation an extra boost by warming up your hands with some gentle rubs before you start work. Another way to warm up cold hands is to wear fingerless gloves, says Dr. Markison.

Eat right. A healthy diet helps the body stave off carpal tunnel syndrome in any number of ways, according to Emil Pascarelli, M.D., professor of clinical medicine specializing in cumulative trauma disorders at Columbia-Presbyterian Medical

Center/Eastside in New York City and co-author of the book, *Repetitive Strain Injury: A Computer User's Guide.* Vitamin C, found in many fruits and vegetables, may help heal the tiny traumas that can lead to carpal tunnel syndrome, he says. Vitamin E, found in vegetable oils, whole-grain cereals and eggs, has been shown to reduce muscle damage. While still controversial, several studies have shown that vitamin B_6, found in bananas and whole-grain cereals, among other foods, may help reduce the pain associated with carpal tunnel syndrome.

Dr. Markison recommends consuming the "natural anti-inflammatories" found in fresh produce and fresh fruit juices, including the carotene in carrot juice and the bromelains in pineapple juice. Vitamin B_6 is toxic in high doses so supplements should not be taken without approval from your doctor.

Think right. Dr. Pascarelli believes that keeping a healthy attitude can play a major role in avoiding the syndrome. "Stress and unhappiness tend to produce tenseness in the muscle groups," he says, setting the body up for repetitive motion injuries.

Pump it up. Beyond overall conditioning, Dr. Pascarelli recommends taking some of the strain off your hands and wrists by building upper body strength. Baseball pitchers work their upper bodies to help them throw fastballs. Working your upper body can help you pound nails or a computer keyboard. Use weights or calisthenics to beef up those shoulders and arms.

Go with the flow. Keeping your body limber also helps keep injury at bay. Many therapists recommend yoga or other stretching exercises. Concentrate on moving with as much fluidity and with as little rigidity as possible, Dr. Markison says. A jazz musician as well as a surgeon, Dr. Markison practices sleight-of-hand coin tricks to help keep his own carpal tunnel pain at a manageable level.

The Outer Man

No matter what type of work you do, a plethora of practical techniques can also help you avoid carpal tunnel syndrome. Of them all, probably the most important is how you hold your body.

Whether at a desk or on an assembly line, it's important to keep your wrists in a neutral position, not flexed up or down. If you work at a desk, therapists recommend sitting with your back straight, your shoulders facing straight ahead and your elbows held close to the body with your elbows approximately at 90 degrees. According to Dr. Pascarelli, your wrists should be suspended in air, not resting on the edge of your desk or even on a wrist rest. If you stand at work, make sure the height of your work area doesn't force you to constantly lean over or reach up, and don't make your arms and wrists consistently bear all the weight of the work at hand.

What's That Syndrome?

When it comes to carpal tunnel syndrome, there's a mass of confusion out there. It is but one of a number of upper-body problems grouped under the umbrella headings repetitive strain injuries, cumulative trauma disorders or, in sports, overuse syndromes.

Besides carpal tunnel syndrome, other injuries included in those broad categories include tendinitis, bursitis, tenosynovitis (irritation of the sheath around a tendon), DeQuervain's disease (tenosynovitis at the base of the thumb), epicondylitis (otherwise known as tennis elbow) and cubital tunnel syndrome (damage to a nerve passing through the elbow).

The confusion comes when one type of repetitive strain injury is mistaken for another. Over and over again doctors who study carpal tunnel syndrome make a point of mentioning how often this happens. Different repetitive strain injuries tend to have similar symptoms, and doctors or physical therapists with too little experience—not to mention the average Joe who's trying to figure out why his arm hurts—frequently misdiagnose them. That's why it's important to seek informed advice from a specialist.

Some other favorite ways to avoid carpal tunnel syndrome mentioned by ergonomists and physicians.

Spy on yourself. Taking a good long look at your work habits should be a starting point for avoiding job-related repetitive strain injuries. For ongoing monitoring of your work posture, try putting a mirror in view of your work station.

Use soft machines. Any tool you use regularly should be examined for the stress it puts on your wrists, arms and hands. Avoid tools that require bent wrists to operate; pistol grips are best. Also try to avoid small tools such as screwdrivers that have to be pinched to be held. Pinching is hard on hand and wrist muscles.

Handle with care. Handles that provide a comfortable grip are important, too. Margot Miller, a physical therapist and director of national programs for Isernhagen Work Systems in Duluth, Minnesota, says that the best grip width for most men is approximately 2¼ inches in diameter. Thick or large-barreled pens are a good idea for this reason. Miller also recommends rubberized or texturized grip surfaces that are easy to hold—slippery surfaces that force your hands to bear down create unnecessary strain. And don't forget to alternate tasks between hands whenever possible.

Avoid bad vibrations. The vibration from tool handles should be reduced as much as possible. Miller suggests wrapping hollow tool handles with a vibration-dampening product (such as those made by Viscolas or Sorbothane). For those who work with vibrating tools all day, she also suggests wearing gloves filled with gel inserts available at ergonomic suppliers or safety-equipment stores. Ask for gloves which contain a viscoelastic polymer.

Employ office helpers. Computer jockeys who use a mouse all day might want to investigate the trackball, a stationary mouse with the cursor-controlling ball on the top. With either tool, you should have it positioned for use so you needn't stretch. Other tips include switching between mice and trackballs, relaxing your arms while using them and adjusting your mouse-driving software for least effort.

Other strain-saving devices include headsets and automatic dial telephones, keyboard macros (programming several steps into a single key function) and, for the truly serious, voice-command computers.

Consider your play time. Just because you're playing instead of working doesn't mean you can't do damage to your wrist. According to Dr. Pascarelli, gardening, painting, lifting weights, playing music, playing video games, even gripping the steering wheel on your car are all activities that need to be pursued prudently lest they cause or contribute to repetitive stress injuries.

When Sterner Measures Are Necessary

If, despite your better efforts, you do develop serious pain, several phases of conservative treatment are available before contemplating the last resort—surgery.

Get massaged. Physical therapists can give you deep tissue massages that will help break down scar tissue and restore freedom of movement. Dr. Markison performs his own version every morning by massaging his fingers and forearms with lotion, paying special attention to the joints.

Be active. Various stretching exercises can also help promote flexibility, but caution is recommended here: A study conducted for the National Institute for Occupational Safety and Health showed that many of the exercises commonly used to combat carpal tunnel syndrome hurt more than they helped. Check with your doctor or physical therapist before embarking on any exercise program.

Employ fire and ice. Alternating an ice pack treatment with soakings in a hot bath can help reduce inflammation and pain (unless you have circulatory problems, in which case ice treatments should be avoided). Dr. Pascarelli recommends rubbing the ice in a stroking motion along the wrist and forearm in intervals of 40 to 60 seconds, just long enough to let the skin get numb and red, repeating the process as often as 10 to 15 times a day. Heat packs, heating pads and warm baths will also help reduce pain, Dr. Pascarelli says, although he feels these are more appropriate for long-term therapy rather than short-term pain relief.

Use inflammatory tactics. Ibuprofen, taken as needed for pain and inflammation, is the first line of defense for many men with carpal tunnel syndrome. For more advanced cases physicians may prescribe injections of cortisone, a steroid. It's important to be aware that these drugs only mask the symptoms temporarily and are not to be considered treatments apart from other remedial efforts.

Splint it. Hand and wrist splints can ease symptoms, especially at night, when the pain is usually at its worst. They work by keeping the wrists straight, thereby avoiding the repetitive irritations that cause the pain. Your therapist or doctor may use an off-the-shelf model or custom design one specifically for you. In either event Dr. Pascarelli strongly advises against becoming overly dependent on splints. If they are used too long, he says, they can cause some muscles to atrophy from underuse while others are subject to strain from trying to pick up the slack.

When All Else Fails

Surgery for carpal tunnel is a last resort, but an effective one. It's a relatively simple, brief procedure, usually not requiring an overnight stay in the hospital. In short, a small incision is made near the palm of the hand in order to free some of the pressure on the median nerve. Assuming the nerve hasn't already sustained permanent damage, relief is virtually immediate.

Doctors caution, however, that unless the habits that caused the condition in the first place are changed, odds are the problem will return, in many instances more severely than before.

Cataracts

Clearing the Cloudy Vision

Sooner or later—but usually much later—it happens to almost all of us. Colors lose their punch, paling against what we remember them to be. The summer sky loses its brilliance, the panoramas darker than those in memory.

And finally, the faces of those we love grow indistinct, out-of-focus cameos seen through a poorly made window glass.

Cataracts, we call the cause—that filming of the lens of the eye that for thousands of years was something that inevitably accompanied aging.

But enter the twentieth century, modern surgery techniques and the technology of ultrasound, and this ancient bane of the aging is becoming a thing of the past.

"We don't do a single thing today, not a single step, the same way we did when I was trained as a resident," says Richard Bensinger, M.D., an ophthalmologist in Seattle and spokesman for the American Academy of Ophthalmology.

"The results with the older procedures were so unpredictable that it was customary to wait to perform the surgery until the patient's vision was just so bad that even an imperfect result was better than what he had.

"Today, within a matter of weeks the average patient can see as well as he could when he was young."

Proof of the improvement in treatment: Cataract surgery today is the most frequently performed operation in the United States.

The Age Factor

The primary cause of cataracts is something we'd all like to avoid but can't—getting older. Men and women in their fifties and older make up the vast majority of those seeking treatment—and the incidence increases enormously with age. Cataracts would appear in everyone if they lived long enough.

But saying that cataracts come with age is like saying the sun causes light—it tells you nothing about the why of it all. The reality is that no one really knows precisely why we develop cataracts as we get older.

"A lot of things can cause cataracts," Dr. Bensinger says, "trauma, infection, dia-

110

betes, measles. But we really don't know exactly why they develop with age. It could be a breakdown in the systems that manufacture the proteins in the lens, or it could be something else. But in any event the vast majority of cataracts are in fact directly associated with only one thing, and that's getting older."

Similarly, cataracts normally develop in both eyes. But no one knows why one eye is almost always significantly worse than the other. "That's typical for most body systems that occur in pairs, but again, no one really knows why paired organ systems degrade this way," says Dr. Bensinger.

Which leads to the single sad reality of cataracts—and it's not very sad: There's not much you can do to prevent them. "A very large number of people develop them in their sixties, and by the time you're in your seventies, it's a race to see whether death or cataracts will strike first," Dr. Bensinger says.

Alternative Theories

A small body of evidence suggests that alcohol and tobacco use may be linked to earlier onset but not to cataract formation itself.

Some evidence also exists—based on studies of fishermen—that heavy exposure to sunlight can accelerate onset and increase incidence in given age groups. For that reason, ophthalmologists recommend regularly wearing sunglasses outdoors.

As for the value of nutritional intervention, there is no hard evidence there either. One theory suggests that cataracts are caused in part by oxidation of the lenses caused by so-called free radicals. Beta-carotene, vitamins C and E and the minerals zinc and selenium are known antioxidants, so some doctors suggest taking a daily dosage.

The Surgical Solution

Through the mid-1970s cataracts were treated by surgical excision—cutting the clouded lenses out of the eyes and correcting the eyesight with a pair of very thick glasses. The treatment, although commonly effective, did have a rate of imperfect results that would be unacceptable by today's ophthalmic surgeons.

Modern technologies, however, have vastly changed the method and the manner of cataract treatment.

In the most popular surgical procedure, an ophthalmologist will make a cut about three millimeters (roughly one-tenth of an inch) long in the surface of the eye. This incision is so small that sutures aren't normally required to close it; it heals well without them.

Your eye surgeon will then insert a device that uses ultrahigh frequency sound waves to literally liquefy the clouded lens within its capsule. The doctor then vacuums out the old lens and inserts a small plastic replacement—individually cut and ground to restore the focusing ability of a particular patient's eye.

Bingo—end of operation and welcome back to the land of the sighted. "The typical patient has usable vision the very next day and normally can see quite well within a matter of one or two weeks," says Colman Kraff, M.D., director of the Kraff Eye Institute in Chicago and clinical instructor in ophthalmology at the Northwestern University Medical School in Chicago.

"The procedure we use today will restore excellent vision to about 95 percent of all patients," Dr. Bensinger says. This also means the multiyear wait for vision to get bad enough to justify a surgical intervention is a thing of the past.

"If you're uncomfortable with your vision as a consequence of cataracts, in most cases there's just no need today to wait to do something about it," says Dr. Bensinger.

Chronic Fatigue Syndrome

Illness or Illusion? An Answer Is Emerging

In December of 1985 Mark Schneider, a 36-year-old apprentice building mechanic in Northport, New York, got the flu. Gradually it developed into bronchitis, then mononucleosis. The symptoms never went away.

Years later, Schneider still takes at least two naps a day. His ability to concentrate is so poor that he doesn't trust himself to drive distances; his memory is so spotty that he's virtually given up reading. He can't hold a job, so he lives with his parents; his social life is nil. Still, he feels he's improved. "My day used to be 45 minutes long," Schneider says. "I would get out of bed, eat and go back to bed. Now my day's six hours long. But I'm still going to bed when most people are going out to enjoy themselves."

Like thousands of other men, Schneider has been diagnosed with chronic fatigue syndrome (CFS), an overwhelming sense of exhaustion that seems to have no underlying cause.

Sorting Out the Symptoms

Exactly what causes chronic fatigue syndrome is one of the great medical mysteries of our time. Even how it first reveals itself is the topic of debate and research.

The problem sometimes begins, as it did for Schneider, with what seems to be an ordinary bout of the flu. Instead of going away after a few weeks, the symptoms—which can include fever, sore throat, swollen lymph nodes, sore muscles and diarrhea—linger. Other symptoms can develop, too: headaches, difficulty sleeping, difficulty concentrating, forgetfulness. True to its name, though, the overriding symptom of CFS is a bone-crushing fatigue.

"You can hardly get out of bed when it hits you. It never goes away; it waxes and wanes," says Pat Hopkins, a volunteer with the National Chronic Fatigue Syndrome and Fibromyalgia Association in Kansas City, Missouri, who has had CFS for 23 years. "You may have one day that's pretty good and the next day you can't move."

While the most dramatic cases of CFS often begin with a case of the flu, there is evidence that the condition is more likely to begin insidiously. "Studies have found a wide range of abnormalities in CFS patients, from immunological to psychological

113

and sometimes infectious," says Keiji Fukuda, M.D., an epidemiologist with the Centers for Disease Control and Prevention in Atlanta. "The problem with these findings is that a lot of them conflict with each other. It becomes very confusing trying to integrate all of these findings into one theory that makes sense."

Because research can't pin down a CFS smoking gun, skeptics are only more inclined to believe CFS is less an illness and more a form of a psychiatric syndrome. It doesn't help that there are few hard facts about CFS sufferers. Experts do believe that two-thirds of the CFS sufferers are women, but this estimate may be skewed because women are more likely to seek a physician's help for CFS symptoms. Schneider is sure that there are more men with CFS than the researchers recognize. "Men are trying to be masculine about it—they're trying to hide," he says. "They're ashamed of the diagnosis."

And no wonder. There's nothing wrong with feeling worn out after a hard day's work, but most men feel that being tired for no apparent reason makes them look like slackers. Take heart: CFS is a recognized problem, and there are ways to spot its elusive symptoms and beat it.

Taming Chronic Fatigue

Because the symptoms of chronic fatigue syndrome are similar to some of the early symptoms of so many other conditions—everything from kidney disease and anemia to AIDS and leukemia—the first step for anyone who thinks he may have it is to rule out those other possibilities. That means getting an evaluation by a doctor who is familiar with the CFS guidelines set out by the Centers for Disease Control and Prevention.

And if you are one of the men diagnosed with chronic fatigue syndrome, here are some steps you can take to make your battle with it as short and as easy as possible.

Slow down. Stress is one of the common denominators for guys with chronic fatigue syndrome—so many overextended young professionals came down with CFS in the go-go 1980s that it became known as the yuppie flu. Thus, the universally recommended treatment for CFS is simple: Get plenty of rest, eat a balanced diet and exercise moderately.

"Look at your lifestyle," says Peter Manu, M.D., director of medical services at Hillside Hospital in New Hyde Park, New York. "Rearrange your priorities, cut down on the pressure. You have to start drawing the line somewhere."

Stay active. Becoming sedentary or being groggy from too much sleep are both common side effects of CFS. "We find most CFS patients sleep too much," says Dr. Manu.

With CFS you won't feel like working out, and vigorous exercise only makes the fatigue worse. Nevertheless, do try to get aerobic exercise, even if that means no more than getting up and walking around the house—even minor activity will be better for your body in the long run. "If you don't have muscle fatigue already, you're going to get it by spending three months in bed," warns Dr. Manu.

Don't label yourself. Hopkins urges that you keep yourself open to admitting that you may have something besides CFS. Many patients who thought they had CFS have recovered after being treated for everything from sleep disorders and sinus problems to hyperventilation. Depression is often mistaken for chronic fatigue syndrome, too. Dr. Manu, among others, reports that a high percentage of CFS patients respond favorably to antidepressants.

Beware the quacks. Any disease, especially one as mysterious as CFS, is bound to bring out the hustlers. "The way people treat CFS ranges from practices that make a lot of sense to practices that are a bit scary," says Dr. Fukuda.

There's a long list of megavitamins, minerals and natural supplements—everything from magnesium and zinc to garlic and black currant oil—that are rumored to relieve the symptoms of CFS. None of these have been proven to be of any value, according to a study conducted by the Harvard School of Public Health. The same goes for any number of specialized diets. The Harvard study analyzed the diets that five self-help books claimed would cure CFS, including several that eliminated yeast, sugar and carbohydrates. Again, no proof was found that any of these diets are effective. Worse, the study warned, such diets may actually be harmful because they're nutritionally unbalanced.

Syndrome Symptoms

Chronic fatigue syndrome shares many of its symptoms with other diseases, so it can be tricky to spot. Persistent fatigue would be your biggest clue. In addition, if you have at least eight of the following symptoms for more than six months, see your doctor:

1. Mild fever.
2. Sore throat.
3. Painful lymph nodes.
4. Muscle weakness.
5. Muscle aches or pains.
6. Fatigue that lasts longer than a day after exercise that you used to be able to do with little or no fatigue.
7. Headache.
8. Aches and pains in your joints.
9. Change in sleep pattern.
10. Sudden development of many of these symptoms.

Adopt a diet. Studies aside, many CFS patients have found special diets or vitamin regimens that seem to work for them. In fact, Pat Hopkins says, diets that eliminate sugars and caffeine are especially popular because people with fatigue have a tendency to overindulge in those substances, only to come crashing down again when the rush wears off.

Dr. Manu feels that, if nothing else, such diets can have therapeutic value. "There is no scientific evidence that these things work," he says, "but there is a lot of anecdotal evidence. If there's nothing harmful in the diet, I say go ahead. Patients need to feel they have some sense of control, that there's something they can do."

Cold and Canker Sores

Avoiding Lip Service

You can be in the most suave of tuxedos, your physique chiseled from years of exercise, your conversation honed from reading the most important journals. But have an open sore on your lip, and all confidence melts away as you cower in the shadows, hand cupped over mouth.

And many of us have been there. Canker and cold sores rank among the most common of human afflictions. They've been a problem as long as humanity has been around, says David Fairbanks, M.D., an otolaryngologist and spokesman for the American Academy of Otolaryngology-Head and Neck Surgery.

While their causes are different, cold sores and canker sores have much in common. Both are painful lesions that develop on the lip or inner mouth. Stress is the top trigger for both. And with both, outbreaks occur infrequently for most, continuously for a few and last anywhere from 10 to 14 days.

The rare guy with constant cold sores might be suffering from some underlying disease related to the immune system and should see a physician. For the rest of us, occasional outbursts of either canker or cold sores aren't serious, will almost always heal with time and don't require a doctor's visit.

Similar But Different

Cold sores, which appear on the outside of lips, come from a type of herpes virus chemically distinct from the genital sort. Most people develop immunities to cold sores as young children. But for some unknown reason 33 percent of us never acquire those immunities, meaning occasional cold sore outbreaks as adults. We're not catching a new virus; rather, the old virus lies dormant in a facial nerve until something—stress, sunlight, certain foods, fever, a cold—weakens the body's defenses, causing the sore to rear its ugly, oozing head.

Many know an outbreak is imminent when a tingling sensation in the mouth begins, usually 24 to 36 hours before the sore erupts in blisters about half the size of a pencil eraser. The blisters swell and rupture, oozing colorless fluid that forms a yellowish crust. The pain from a bursting blister can match that of a hard bite to your lip.

Like cold sores, canker sores usually pop up the day of a hot date, big meeting

117

or crucial exam, but thankfully, they're a lot less visible. They lurk inside the mouth on wet, moist surfaces, most often on the tongue, soft palate and inner cheek.

Canker sores usually begin as tiny blisters or painful red spots. Within a couple days the blister becomes an inflamed, woundlike ulcer. Exposed nerve endings in the canker sore are irritated by whatever in the mouth is salty, sour or scratchy— spicy dogs, cherry Slurpees, salted peanuts—and the contact can cause excruciating pain for some. "Some people have a pinpoint on their tongue and they complain so much you'd think they'd had major surgery," said Louis Abbey, D.M.D., professor of oral pathology at Virginia Commonwealth University School of Dentistry in Richmond. "Others have a mouthful of sores and they say they don't hurt too badly."

To prevent both canker and cold sores, doctors recommend reducing stress in your life. "People free of stress hardly ever get canker or cold sores," Dr. Abbey notes. He recommends devising a stress management program—preventing sores is just one of many health benefits that could result.

Containing Cold Sores

Given time, even the most painful cold sore will disappear on its own. But a combination of preventive steps and fast responses can greatly diminish the problem. Here are things to do.

Remember the sunscreen. Exposing your lips to sun may trigger cold sores, so consider giving up the bronzed-god look. No matter how unhip you think it is, always wear a broad-brimmed hat and lip protection outside.

Consider medicinal solutions. If cold sores are a persistent problem, ask your doctor about whether the prescription drug acyclovir is appropriate for you. A daily dose of the drug, known by the brand name Zovirax, will significantly reduce the number of outbreaks, according to a study. Subjects taking 400 milligrams of acyclovir twice daily for four months had 53 percent fewer cold sores than those given a placebo.

Protect others. After an outbreak the chances of infecting another adult with the cold sore virus are slim. But avoid passing it on to that rare adult who has yet to be exposed by foregoing kissing and oral sex during an outbreak. If you touch the sore and then rub yourself, you may transfer the virus to another part of your body. Although it's rare, cold sores can form on the inside of the mouth, on the nostrils, fingers, genitals and eyelids.

Keep it moist. Use petroleum jelly, lip balm or an over-the-counter antibiotic ointment as often as needed after the blister breaks. Avoid picking at the sore; it only invites the possibility of developing a secondary bacterial infection. If you notice swelling and pus or if the sore fails to heal in two weeks, see your physician.

FAST FACTS

How common: Canker and cold sores rank among the most common of human afflictions, attacking almost everyone at some time or another.

Risk factors: Excessive and prolonged stress for both canker and cold sores. Exposure to sun can also trigger cold sores. Mouth wounds and certain foods may trigger canker sores.

Age group affected: All ages.

Gender gap: Men and women are equally likely to have canker and cold sores.

Who to see: If the sore becomes infected or doesn't heal, see your family doctor.

Corralling Canker Sores

Like cold sores, stress can trigger a canker sore outbreak. Some people also get canker sores from eating too many nuts—including peanut butter and coconut—or from sweets, chocolate or acidic fruits such as pineapples, grapes and plums. Here are some preventive measures.

Protect your mouth. Any mouth trauma can trigger a canker sore, from hot pizza to a tooth or filling rubbing against the inner lining of your cheek to biting the inside of your mouth.

Avoid the food foes. Certain chronic canker sore sufferers report recurrences after eating sweet, spicy or acidic foods. Keep track of what triggered the canker sore and eliminate it from your diet. If the food is gone but the canker returns, look for other causes.

Avoid the pain. Once a canker appears, sour, salty or acidic foods will burn or otherwise exacerbate the sore.

Make a medicine mix. A "K & B cocktail" helps numb the mouth once the sore appears. Mix equal portions of Kaopectate and Benadryl Elixir (both can be bought over the counter). Before meals, hold a mouthful for a couple of minutes. Afterward, spit it out or swallow it. Eating should be less painful afterward.

Try other medicine techniques. Antacid tablets neutralize mouth enzymes that aggravate the sores. Also try anesthetic lozenges and mouthwashes to deaden nerves.

Colds and Flu

Keep the Bugs from Getting You

This morning you felt like the race horse of the professional world, ripsnortin' through your duties a mile ahead of the pack. But by midafternoon you feel more like an aching, dragging, dripping nag. Clearly, you're not going to win by a nose today—not one that's this runny.

While colds and flu are unlikely to land you in intensive care, they can keep you in the stable for a few days. What's more, they're extremely difficult to avoid. Colds can be caused by more than 200 rhinoviruses—the word literally means nose viruses—and are among the most common illnesses people get. In addition, about one in four Americans gets the flu every year. Among the elderly and infirm the infection rate is even higher, approaching one in two.

What Is It—Cold or Flu?

Although colds and flu share some of the same symptoms—coughs, sore throats, nasal congestion and muscle aches—they're caused by entirely different viruses, and flu symptoms are usually more severe. "A cold tends to be more upper respiratory, with nasal congestion, sore throat and earache," says Susan Debin, M.D., a family doctor in private practice in Orange, California. "When you get into the flu, it tends to be more in the chest."

Fever is another tip-off. With flu, your temperature may shoot up to 101°F or higher within a few hours, while a cold may not cause much of a fever at all. In a study of 139 adults with colds, for example, fewer than 1 percent had fevers above 99.6°F. (Maybe that's why they call it a cold.)

Perhaps the main difference between colds and flu is the severity of the illness. Flu tends to be far more uncomfortable—and dangerous, experts say. According to the Centers for Disease Control and Prevention in Atlanta, flu in this country is responsible for about 15,000 deaths a year. In addition, some flu strains have been frighteningly "hot." In 1918, for example, a supervirulent strain of flu killed about 21 million people worldwide.

If you're in otherwise good health, of course, getting a cold or flu is unlikely to have dire consequences. The worst of the illness will pass within a few days, although you may have some residual pain and fatigue for a week or two longer.

Cold War Defenses

Given the huge number of cold viruses out there, preparing an effective vaccine is virtually impossible. But because flu has only three main strains—types A, B and C—it makes an easier target.

The principle behind a vaccine is simple. When you take a serum that contains inactivated viruses, your immune system is stimulated to make antibodies to kill that same type of virus in the future—*without* making you sick in the process. Studies have shown that an annual flu shot will prevent about 70 percent of flu cases.

Doctors typically recommend flu shots for people over age 65 or those with long-term, serious conditions, like asthma or diabetes. But even young people who are high risk, such as smokers or those who work in high-exposure areas like schools or hospitals, should consider getting vaccinated, says Dr. Debin.

After you get the shot, it will take your immune system about two weeks to marshal its defenses. So don't wait until the flu's already swept through the office before seeing your doctor. It's best, experts say, to get vaccinated between October 15 and November 15—before the flu season peaks.

Practical Prevention

Although the viruses that cause colds and flu are everywhere, there are some simple ways to lower your risk. Here's what experts recommend.

Scrub-a-dub, Bub. Cold and flu viruses are often spread by hand-to-mouth or hand-to-eye contact. Washing your hands several times a day will wash away the chance of secondary bacterial infections. If someone at home is already sick, cleaning surfaces will also help prevent germs from spreading.

Stay far from the sniffling crowd. December through February is flu season—not a good time to pack into that trendy new bistro. After all, one hearty sneeze can launch virus-laden nose droplets 12 feet. So it might be a good idea to stay away from cramped social settings, at least when the virus has been cutting a swath through your community.

Stop smoking. Cigarette smoke paralyzes the protective, hairlike cilia in your airways that help sweep virus-laden mucus from your body. This is why smokers are far more likely to catch colds than nonsmokers. So don't smoke, and if someone else lights up, light out.

Address stress. You got married, your sports car died and you just moved 500 miles to a new job. The effects on your body of all this stress are nothing to sneeze at. In one study researchers at Carnegie Mellon University in Pittsburgh asked 420 people about the stress in their lives. Then they exposed them to cold viruses. The more highly stressed a person was, the more likely he was to catch a cold.

Scientists suspect that stress releases hormones that suppress your immune system, making you more vulnerable to colds and other infections. Studies, however, also show that even simple relaxation techniques, like slow, deep breathing or just hanging out with friends, can help the immune system work more efficiently.

Finding Comfort

Even if you take an active role in trying to head off colds and flu, at least three to four times every year or so your nose is likely to be transformed into a nasal Niagara. Although there isn't a cure for these viral interlopers, there are ways to make yourself more comfortable.

Bring out the big guns. When your flu is caused by the type-A virus, your doctor may recommend a prescription drug called amantadine (Symadine, Symmetrel). Taken within two days of the onset of symptoms, amantadine can cut the duration of your illness in half, says Michael Fleming, M.D., a family physician in private practice in Shreveport, Louisiana. But fast action is critical: If you wait a week before taking the drug, it probably won't be effective.

Drink up. This is the best way to keep virus-fighting mucus thin and flowing. When you're sick, "the mucus secretions can get very thick," says Dr. Debin. "And when they're thick they're going to obstruct airways—that's when pneumonia can set in." Drinking eight to ten eight-ounce glasses of water a day should help keep things fluid. Warm liquids are usually more soothing than cold ones, she adds.

Go easy on the booze. Alcohol can suppress your immune system and make you even more uncomfortable by drying out mucous membranes. So lay off the libations until after you're feeling better, says Dr. Fleming.

Eat well. Good nutrition—lots of fruits, vegetables and whole grains, along with protein sources, like beans, dairy products and lean meats—makes for a stronger immune system, research shows. While a well-rounded diet won't prevent all colds and flus, it will improve your odds for staying healthy, adds Dr. Fleming.

Exercise a cold. Regular exercise can help prevent colds by strengthening your immune system. But research also suggests that exercise *during* a cold also might help you get over it. But there are several "buts". Wait until the acute symptoms have passed—usually three days—and go easy. Do not exercise if you are experiencing chest congestion, aching muscles, a hacking cough or a fever. You could slow your recuperation if you do, says Bryant Stamford, Ph.D., director of the Health Promotion and Wellness Center at the University of Louisville.

FAST FACTS

How common: Colds and flu are among the most common causes of illnesses worldwide. Each year in the United States they cause 26 million days of missed school and 23 million days of missed work.

Risk factors: Seasons (fall, winter and early spring), stress, allergies, smoking, poor nutrition, being close to an infected person.

Age group affected: Kids younger than age five average 6 to 12 respiratory illnesses a year. In adults, who gradually accumulate protective antibodies, the average is 3 to 4.

Gender gap: Women get more colds than men, possibly because they're likely to spend more time with children or in healthcare settings.

Who to see: For a difficult cold or flu, talk to a pharmacist or your family doctor. If you have hoarseness, pain in the chest, breathing difficulty or extended vomiting, be sure to get to your family doctor.

But rest the flu. While regular exercise may be good for colds, it's not so great for flu. Experts say that overexerting yourself can allow flu viruses to do even deeper damage such as invading muscles. Before returning to your exercise routine, it's best to wait two weeks after your symptoms are gone.

If you're not sure you're ready to resume your usual activities, then you're probably not. "Most of these illnesses respond to rest," says Dr. Fleming. "So if you get sick, if you feel bad, then rest—stay down. Rest is much better than being active."

Wet the air. In winter when the furnace is cranked up and the humidity's low, your throat, nasal passages and lungs can get dry and scratchy. Adding moisture to the air with a vaporizer or moisturizer will help keep your airways lubed.

Give them the brush-off. Viruses can survive for hours outside the body, as can bacteria. Both can linger on your toothbrush. "It's not the virus but the bacterial infection that can make a cold or flu last longer. I encourage individuals to throw out their toothbrush if they've had an illness," says Dr. Debin. "Get a new toothbrush so you're not reinfecting yourself."

Soothe your sore throat. While over-the-counter medicated lozenges will help relieve sore throat pain, just sucking on hard candy, which stimulates the flow of saliva, can also be helpful. Experts also recommend gargling with a solution made from one to three teaspoons of salt in a glass of warm water. Drinking warm liquids, like tea with honey and lemon, can help, too, says Dr. Fleming.

Turn up the heat. Hot peppers contain a fiery substance called capsaicin, which will cause the mucous membranes to secrete more liquid—one of the body's ways of eliminating viruses. So when illness strikes, make your favorite cuisine extra hot.

Try chicken soup. All over the globe, hot chicken soup is the home remedy of choice for colds. While any hot liquid can help cut through congestion, chicken soup seems to do the job best. Not only does it get mucus flowing, but researchers at the University of Nebraska Medical Center found it also inhibits the action of neutrophils, blood cells that cause nasal congestion and discomfort.

Blow gently. Remember, it's a nose, not a trombone. If you honk with all your might, you could blast the infection back into your ears or sinuses, making a minor illness even worse. Instead, blow your nose gently, one nostril at a time.

Take to the C. Scientists have long debated whether or not vitamin C is helpful in combating colds. In a summary of 18 scientific studies, however, the *British Journal of Nutrition* concluded that vitamin C may in fact help shorten a cold's duration and help reduce the symptoms.

It's not clear how much vitamin C is the optimal dose. Subjects in the studies typically took 1,000 to 3,000 milligrams a day. A more conservative approach is to increase the amount of vitamin C in your diet. Drinking about five glasses a day of juice—orange, tomato, grapefruit or pineapple—will provide 500 milligrams of vitamin C—a safe and effective amount, says Dr. Fleming. Other high-C foods include broccoli, brussels sprouts and strawberries.

Over-the-Counter Relief

Although there are more than 800 cold remedies on pharmacy shelves, all contain one (or more) of just a handful of medications commonly used to relieve cough, congestion and other cold and flu symptoms. They won't cure the illness, experts add, but they can make you more comfortable while nature runs its course.

In the belief that if one is good, more must be better, many drug companies include several ingredients in each product—a practice doctors refer to as the "shotgun" approach. While these shotgun remedies hit many symptoms at once—like pain, cough and congestion—why take drugs for symptoms you may not even have?

Keep it simple, advises Dr. Debin. Decide which symptom you want to treat, then look for the medication that will hit just that one. Ask your doctor or pharmacist for guidance. In the meantime here's a breakdown of the medications you're most likely to need.

Decongestants. Medications such as oxymetazoline (Dristan 12-Hour Nasal Spray, Vicks Sinex 12-Hour Nasal Spray) and pseudoephedrine (Afrinol Repetabs, Sudafed), taken as pills, drops or sprays, help open stuffy nasal passages, giving your beleaguered schnozz some much needed relief. While decongestants are generally safe, using a spray for more than three days in a row can cause "rebound" congestion, in which your nose may be stuffier than it was before.

Antihistamines. Medications such as diphenhydramine (Aller-med, Benadryl) can help dry up a drippy nose by causing the mucous membranes to secrete less fluid. These medications also cause drowsiness, however, so doctors often recommend taking them at bedtime.

Cough suppressants. If you're suffering from a dry, hacking cough, products containing dextromethorphan (Benylin DM) will help calm things down by damping the "cough center" in the brain. For colds that have phlegm, using an expectorant, like guaifenesin (Robitussin-PE), will moisten and loosen the gop, making it easier to cough up. Be sure to see a doctor if phlegm is excessive.

Anesthetics. For short-term relief of sore throat pain, sprays or lozenges containing benzocaine (Chloraseptic Sore Throat Lozenges) or menthol (Luden's Original Menthol Throat Drops) can be a big help. But be sure not to inhale while applying the spray, as that will make it less effective.

Analgesics. Over-the-counter painkillers, like acetaminophen, ibuprofen and naproxen can help relieve muscle aches and fever that accompany colds and flu. While some people start taking aspirin at the first sign of colds or flu, doctors urge caution. In very rare circumstances aspirin can put adults who have flu symptoms at risk of developing Reye's syndrome, a life-threatening neurological illness (the risk is far greater among children). Phone your doctor if you have concerns about aspirin.

Colon Cancer

How to Launch a Pre-emptive Strike

Only two types of cancer in men can be detected and stopped *before* they become cancer. Colon cancer is one, skin cancer is the other. The difference between the two? Men are four times as likely to get colon and rectal cancer, and once they do, they find themselves face-to-face with the third top cancer killer of men. Only lung and prostate deaths exceed the number of colon cancer deaths among men.

Lots of men dying who don't have to—what's wrong with this picture?

"Part of the problem is that neither gender owns this cancer," says Richard Billingham, M.D., clinical associate professor of surgery at the University of Washington School of Medicine in Seattle. "Because it affects both men and women, it hasn't become an issue like prostate or breast cancer and doesn't get much press. This drives us doctors crazy because it is *highly* preventable if people only knew how to deal with it."

One big reason colon cancer can be so readily prevented is that before it forms, it's red-flagged by growths known as polyps. These are small bumps with big heads and skinny necks that generally range in size from about one millimeter to four centimeters. They're not cancerous at first, but depending on their type, 5 to 40 percent of polyps become tumors. Still, it typically takes about five years for this malignant change to take place, leaving a window of opportunity for doctors to remove the polyps, nipping the cancer in the bud.

Getting It in Your Sights

Polyps can be detected in a number of ways. Waiting for symptoms is not one of them. "For the most part the patient can't see them, and they don't hurt and they don't bleed," says Dr. Billingham. "There's no way to know they're there unless a physician actively looks for them."

The most common way that's done is with a flexible sigmoidoscope, a thin, bendable, 24-inch tubelike device with a tiny light and lens that goes inside the body, allowing a doctor to see what's inside you through a viewing port. It's inserted in the rectum for a five-to-ten-minute procedure that allows a doctor to examine the entire lower third of the colon, where more than 50 percent of tumors occur.

The American Cancer Society recommends that all men over age 50 get a flexible sigmoidoscopy every three to five years. It's not an exam to look forward to, but it is effective. In one study of 100 mostly male subjects with no history or hint of colon cancer, sigmoidoscopies turned up polyps or tumors in a quarter of the cases.

If polyps are found with a sigmoidoscope, there's a 50 percent chance that more polyps are growing upstream, deeper in the colon. The next step is a procedure using a colonoscope, an instrument that's similar to a flexible sigmoidoscope except it's three times longer, to go further into the colon. A colonoscope not only views polyps, it snares and removes them, generally during a single procedure. Routine colonoscopies every three to five years are recommended for men at high risk for the disease—for example, if colon cancer struck a parent or sibling. (If you get a colonoscopy, a sigmoidoscopy isn't necessary.)

If polyps have already turned cancerous, there are more methods of detection. For one thing, symptoms may develop such as changes in bowel habits—more diarrhea or constipation or a change in the frequency of bowel movements, for example—or blood in the stool. A simple fecal test for detecting blood can help with diagnosis, although the test is unreliable. Reason: Not all cancers bleed, plus results can be thrown off by, for example, the juice from a rare steak. Bottom line: Scope screenings are the best form of detection. Dr. Billingham estimates that 95 percent of colorectal cancers could be prevented through routine screening alone.

The Power of Diet

Detection isn't the only way to prevent colon cancer, however. You can also avoid things that raise your risk and take up things that reduce it. In the case of colon cancer a lot of factors appear to make a difference, most of them dietary. The three major principles are these:

Cut fat. One of the most consistent findings in colon cancer research is that a diet high in fat (especially animal fat) raises the risk of disease. Population studies, for example, find that people in countries with low-fat diets such as Japan have lower rates of colon cancer—until they move to the West, when their rates go up. In one research review 11 of 13 studies confirmed this connection between fat, meat, animal protein and colon cancer rates.

Recommendation: Reduce fat intake to 30 percent or less of total calories from the 35 to 40 percent most Americans eat. Every little bit helps, says Moshe Shike, M.D., director of the clinical nutrition program at Memorial Sloan-Kettering Cancer Center in New York City. "We're not sure that cutting back fat intake by only 5 percent will make a difference by itself, but it's a good start," he says. "The idea is to start cutting a little, then try to progress."

Bulk up. Equally important as cutting fat, eating a diet high in fiber (which few Americans do) also substantially lowers risk of colon cancer. A review found this connection in 12 of 13 studies. One report suggests that colon cancer risk in the United States could be cut 31 percent if everyone got 13 more grams of fiber per day over and above the 11 grams that's typical. Depending on the brand, high-fiber breakfast cereals contain between 5 and 11 grams of fiber per serving. Other good sources of fiber include beans, lentils, dried pears, apples and whole-wheat spaghetti.

Eat lots of fruits and vegetables. These foods are both low in fat and generally high in fiber, so it stands to reason eating lots of them will reduce colon cancer risk. No fewer than 23 studies bear this out. Beyond that, however, compounds in foods such as broccoli, brussels sprouts, onions, leeks and garlic may positively affect the activity of cancer-controlling enzymes, says Dr. Shike.

A Prevention Lifestyle

In addition to these basic guidelines, there are other options that may be worth acting upon. These include:

Drink alcohol moderately. That's always good advice, but here's another reason why: In one of many studies that link spirits with colon cancer, imbibing three drinks of wine or liquor each day raised risk by more than two times.

Ask your doctor about aspirin. Numerous studies have found that people who take aspirin regularly have lower rates of colon cancer. Still, there's reason to ask if seemingly healthy people should take drugs as a preventive measure. Check with a physician before embarking on any medication program.

Get active. Physical activity has consistently been associated with lower risk of colon cancer. But the cause-and-effect equation is unsolved. "It may be a question of lifestyle," says Bruce Wolff, M.D., professor of surgery at Mayo Medical School in Rochester, Minnesota. "People who are most likely to exercise are also more likely to have a low-fat diet."

Treatment: It's No Treat

Even when colon cancer gets beyond the point where removing polyps will cure you, there are still options. "Surgery is almost always the first step," Dr. Wolff says. For all but the lower rectum this involves taking out the cancerous section of in-

FAST FACTS

How common: The 75,000 new cases of colon and rectal cancer in American men each year make it the third most common tumor in men.

Risk factors: Primary risk appears to be genetic. If a parent has had it, your risk triples. You're also at higher risk if you've had ulcerative colitis, an inflammatory condition of the colon, for ten years.

Age group affected: Ninety percent of colorectal patients are over age 40.

Gender gap: Virtually none. Although there are about 1,000 more new cases of colorectal cancer in men than women every year, out of a population of 280 million, the numbers are virtually the same.

Who to see: Gastroenterologist or colon/rectal surgeon.

testinal piping and splicing it back together again. It's major surgery that takes two to three hours and requires three to four weeks to recover. If the cancer is low in the rectum, particularly the lower two inches, treatment may require a colostomy, in which an artificial tube must be installed to excrete wastes into a pouch worn under clothes—"a last resort," says Dr. Billingham. Radiation or chemotherapy may be prescribed to keep the cancer from recurring.

If colorectal cancer lesions are caught in their early stages, surgery results in a five-year survival rate of about 90 percent, according to Dr. Billingham. With more advanced lesions, however, that figure drops to 50 percent—another reason that early detection is the best course.

Constipation

How to Be a Regular Guy

Imagine a formula that would virtually eradicate one of the most common, embarrassing and downright uncomfortable medical complaints in the United States. If you could bottle it and stick a price tag on it, you would be wealthy beyond your wildest dreams. The product would jump off the shelves, as the advertising campaign hyped it as a miracle cure.

But this is no snake oil—or even mineral oil. The cure for constipation exists, and has been known for some time. The three-part formula is so simple you can make it at home. Increase the amount of fiber in your diet, drink more water and exercise regularly.

That's it. Follow that advice, the experts say, and you'll be a regular guy. Robert S. Sandler, M.D., associate professor of medicine at the University of North Carolina School of Medicine at Chapel Hill, estimates that following that formula would prevent constipation in 95 percent of people in the United States. Even among those who go to a physician or specialist for constipation, Dr. Sandler estimates that 80 percent would see their discomfort decrease with that simple diet and exercise plan.

And we're talking about a lot of people here. Constipation strikes commoners and kings alike. Heck, even The King—Elvis Presley—suffered from chronic constipation. It's *the* most common digestive disorder in the United States, the complaint of at least 4.5 million people. And 7 percent of American males say it's a chronic problem.

But you never saw Elvis—or any other performer—host a celebrity telethon for constipation research. "The problem with constipation is that it's not sexy like cancer, doctors don't like to study it because it's not glamorous and patients are embarrassed to talk about it," Dr. Sandler says.

"Constipation is not well-understood," adds Edward Feldman, M.D., clinical professor of medicine at the University of California, Los Angeles, School of Medicine. "In the last five years we've been learning more, but the basic truth is that there are many different forms and multiple reasons."

FAST FACTS

How common: The most common digestive complaint among American males. About 7 percent say it's a chronic problem.

Risk factors: Failure to eat sufficient amounts of fiber (20–35 grams per day), not drinking enough water (six to eight eight-ounce glasses daily) and lack of regular exercise account for the overwhelming majority of constipation cases. Delaying going to the bathroom also can cause constipation.

Age group affected: All age groups can be affected, but it grows more common the older you get.

Gender gap: Twice as many women are likely to complain of constipation.

Who to see: When constipation is interfering with your day-to-day life, see a family doctor. You might get referred to a specialist in gastroenterology or to a special program in digestive motility.

Are You Constipated Tonight?

Men have trouble on the can from time to time. But that doesn't mean there's a constipation crisis.

The real medical concern with constipation, say doctors, is whether there has been a dramatic, prolonged change in your regular bowel habits—not whether a single trip to the can left you wincing in pain.

"When somebody has a change in their regular habits, it needs to be readily explainable," says Timothy R. Koch, M.D., chief of the gastroenterology section at the Veterans Administration Medical Center and associate professor of medicine at the Medical College of Wisconsin, both in Milwaukee. "A change in a regular pattern means something has happened. And if it's persistent, you have to see a physician."

When it comes to bowel movements, the most common definition of "regular" is at least three stools a week. But bowel movements vary widely, and regular means what you do and not what the guy in the next stall says, nor what they suggest in TV ads.

So if you have a generally healthy output system and there hasn't been a sudden change in your habits of late, don't worry if you have a rough time occasionally.

Then when is constipation a problem? Either when bowel movements become so infrequent that the discomfort interferes with your daily life, or when your waste is so hard that it's truly debilitating to pass it.

How to Loosen Up

For the vast majority of men, intestinal traffic jams will be a thing of the past if they follow these preventive steps.

Did Constipation Kill The King?

Dan Warlick was there when they carved up The King. As chief medical investigator for the state of Tennessee that fateful year, Warlick took part in the autopsy the night of August 16, 1977, to determine what caused the death of Elvis Aron Presley. The official verdict was that the entertainer died from a heart attack. In their book, *The Death of Elvis*, investigative reporters Charles C. Thompson II and James P. Cole reviewed suppressed autopsy documents and concluded that Elvis died of an accidental drug overdose.

Warlick, however, has a different theory that he believes conforms to what he witnessed at Graceland—where Presley's body was found on the floor of his lavish, master bathroom—and in the autopsy room at Baptist Memorial Hospital. Warlick believes Presley's chronic constipation—the result of years of prescription drug abuse and high-fat, high-cholesterol gorging—brought on what's known as Valsalva's maneuver. Put simply, the strain of attempting to defecate compressed the singer's abdominal aorta, shutting down his heart, Warlick theorizes.

"At the time of Elvis's autopsy, I was there when we did what we call 'run the gut,' when you take some scissors and open the full length of the intestine," Warlick recalls. "He had this horrendous impaction."

Warlick says the physicians and experts assembled for the autopsy were astounded by what they saw. "Dehydrated feces that were claylike and went all the way up his descending colon and halfway across his transverse colon . . . He really was backed up." Apparently, that was not unusual. "He was commonly and constantly impacted, I believe," Warlick says.

Add fiber to your diet. So you think that real men eat cheeseburgers, pizza and Buffalo chicken wings. Maybe. But chances are, regular guys don't. Start working fruits, vegetables, legumes, beans, cereals and whole grains into your daily diet.

It seems everyone's harping on you to eat fiber nowadays, and with good reason. In the early 1970s a study done in Africa among people who ate a high-fiber diet found they had more bowel movements and less constipation than low-fiber eaters in Europe and America. Although it was clear that a lack of fiber didn't cause constipation, extra fiber certainly seemed to help. The reason: The body can't digest most fiber. As it passes through your gut it soaks water up like a sponge, making stools softer and larger. The large intestine then works harder to get rid of the waste faster.

It's no secret that Elvis kept odd hours. "He got his sleep and rest whenever he could. So if it was two o'clock in the afternoon and he wanted to go to sleep because he was going to go to the movies at 3:00 A.M., he took downers. Then, if he was up at 1:30 A.M. and needed to be more awake, he took uppers. That starts and stops the action in your intestines. If you take a lot of downers . . . it tends to allow your colon to fill up and become more distended. If you do that chronically, eventually you're going to mess up your gastrointestinal tract, its rhythm and how it works," says Warlick.

And his eating habits only made matters worse. "He had a diet that was high in fat. He liked all these things like greasy cheeseburgers, burnt bacon and peanut-butter-and-banana sandwiches fried in butter and ice cream by the half-gallon. I mean, it just knocked the bulb out of the cholesterol meter," says Warlick, now an attorney in private practice in Nashville who counts among his clients George C. Nichopoulos, M.D., Elvis's embattled personal physician.

It was not unusual for Elvis to spend hours at a time in the bathroom. "His constipation certainly played a significant part in his discomfort," Warlick says. That helps account for the fact that even though he entered his bathroom, book in hand, at 8:00 A.M. on August 16, 1977, nobody checked on him until about 2:00 P.M. Officials believe he died at about 9:00 A.M.

Elvis may have been able to swivel his hips like nobody before or since, but he couldn't move his bowels to save his life. That may be why The King was on his throne when he was fatally stricken.

In addition, fiber eaters have lower rates of colon cancer and heart disease, perennial killers of men. No one's sure why exactly, but the betting is on the increased substitution of low-fat, high-fiber foods for high-fat, low-fiber fare.

There's nothing bad associated with too much fiber except that it can cause gas or diarrhea, especially when you add extra amounts too quickly. So the recommendation is to eat more than you have been but increase your intake gradually. Experts recommend 20 to 35 grams a day, but the average American only eats about 11 grams daily.

Some high-fiber breakfast cereals have as much as 10 to 14 grams of fiber per serving. A cup of strawberries will add 3.9 grams, while a half-cup of boiled black-

If It's So Bad, Why Do We All Want It?

For some reason lots of us claim to be constipated even when we aren't. In a survey of more than 15,000 people by the National Center for Health Statistics nearly one in ten said they were constipated even though they had a daily bowel movement. And more than three in ten people who had bowel movements four to six times a week claimed to suffer from constipation.

What this says is that a lot of people who have regular bowel movements still experience symptoms—straining, gas or perhaps just a general sense of being bloated.

eyed peas will give you 8.3 grams. There's your daily recommended amount. It can be done.

Drink up. Drink plenty of water (or juice or liquid), six to eight eight-ounce glasses a day. One thing you should know about fiber: It absorbs many times its weight in water. So to help keep the added fiber from clogging you up, drink water.

Exercise. If your bowels aren't moving, they may be taking the cue from you. Once again, it's a simple equation: Regular exercise helps keep you regular.

Avoid the fat. A National Center for Health Statistics study found that people who eat dry beans, peas, fruits and vegetables report less constipation. Dr. Koch says the common denominator was the lack of fat. Low-fat diets help avoid constipation, and colon cancer as well.

Just go. The single worst thing a man can do to make himself constipated is not to go to the bathroom when his body tells him to. A guy might not want to use a public toilet, or maybe he's just in a hurry and ignores the urge.

It's these modern times, according to Henry C. Lin, M.D., director of the G.I. Motility Program and Section of Nutrition at the Cedars-Sinai Medical Center in Los Angeles. "If you're in an 8-to-5 job and happen to have a call of nature at 10:30 during a group meeting, it's more difficult to act on that urge than if you were working out in a field," Dr. Lin notes. "That's a fact of life since the industrial revolution."

The problem is that when we put off sitting on the toilet, the gut reabsorbs water from the stool that wants out, and what was soft and easily expelled becomes hard and pebblelike, making it difficult to expel. So when you gotta go, go.

For Instant Relief

Like Scrooge on Christmas morning, you swear that you're a changed man. From now on you'll have bran cereal for breakfast, fruit with lunch and beans with dinner. You'll also drink water throughout the day and jog in the afternoon. But right now, you need relief. It's been days since your last bowel movement, and your intestines feel like somebody poured cement in them.

Most people head for the nearest drugstore to buy over-the-counter laxatives when they're badly blocked. Constipation is big business: Over $685 million is spent each year on over-the-counter laxatives. But doctors warn that laxatives are addictive and can actually make constipation worse by weakening the muscles in your intestines.

Occasional use of laxatives is safe, doctors say. But they are no substitute for a sensible and healthy diet. If you need relief *now*, keep in mind that bulk-forming laxatives, like psyllium (Metamucil)—which draw water into the stool, making it larger, softer and easier to pass—are preferable to stimulant laxatives that contain senna (Senokot) or phenolphthalein (Ex-Lax). "Avoid the ones that whip the colon, which can lead to inflammation," warns Dr. Feldman.

An enema or suppository is the quickest route to relief, but once again, doctors warn that they should be used sparingly. Overuse can result in a lazy colon, making matters worse. With enemas use only clear water or saline solutions. And with suppositories stick with glycerin ones.

Other Causes of Clogging

A very small percentage of constipation cases are symptomatic of nastier conditions. A tumor or growth in the colon can block things up. Constipation also can be a symptom of diabetes, Parkinson's disease, various nerve disorders and thyroid disease, to name a few.

More often, a minor bout of constipation is the result of external forces. Here are a few to be aware of.

Travel. A lot of people get constipated when they travel. There's no good reason why this happens, although as Dr. Lin points out, "We're conditioned animals, conditioned to use the facilities near our home. When you take a laboratory animal into a strange environment, it wouldn't follow its regular routine. We're really not very different."

Drugs and medications. Any kind of medication, from pain relievers to high blood pressure medicine, can cause fits and spells of constipation. Ask your pharmacist about any drugs you are taking.

Stress. Years ago research confirmed stress can alter the functions of your gut. But while trying to take it easy is always a good idea, constipation is definitely not just a mental thing. Says Dr. Koch: "There's a lot of physician bias about this problem. Most physicians think it's just something that happens. But you can't explain it away by saying it's all psychological."

Corns and Calluses

Smoothing Over the Hard Spots

Clever thing that it is, the skin knows how to protect itself. It piles up layers of its own dead cells over areas that are exposed to repeated pressure and trauma. That's what corns and calluses are.

You can afford to be callous about calluses; They're usually not painful. But there's nothing corny about corns. Unlike calluses, they have an inner core that reaches into the skin and presses on nerve endings. They hurt.

The hard kind are firm and shiny. They form on the tops of the toes where a bony prominence rubs against the ceiling of a too-small shoe. Soft corns—so-called because they're mushy in texture—form *between* the toes, usually when narrow shoes cause the digits to scrape together. Corns make it hard to live an active life, so don't go soft on them. Here are the right steps to take.

Choose Your Shoes Well

Like the vegetable they're named for, corns grow only under suitable conditions. Wear the right shoes and you'll probably never see one.

Make sure they're long and tall. Hard corns are signs that you don't have enough room in front of your toes or above them. "You should be able to freely wiggle all your toes," says Carol Frey, M.D., associate clinical professor of orthopedic surgery at the University of Southern California, Los Angeles. "There should be half an inch between the end of your longest toe and the end of the toebox." She notes that your longest toe might not be the *big* toe.

Height also matters, says Glenn Gastwirth, D.P.M., deputy executive director of the American Podiatric Medical Association. Some designs have low toeboxes, causing your toetops to scrape the leather. "Make sure the shape is right," he says. "Don't just go by your usual size."

Eschew narrow shoes. If your corns are the soft type, chances are your shoes are not wide enough. As a rule, advises Dr. Frey, avoid pointy tips. "Wear shoes with a rounded toebox."

Ask for sole custody. "Most toe problems are because of the volume of the shoe, not the length or width," says Allen Selner, D.P.M., a podiatrist at Medstar Foot and Ankle Center in Studio City, California. "If you can remove the inner sole or replace it with a thinner one, you'll have more volume. Most athletic and walking shoes come with removable soles."

Get it right, right away. "Shoes should be comfortable the moment you buy them," says Dr. Frey. She advises shopping at the end of the day when your feet have expanded somewhat. And get fitted while standing, not sitting down. Dr. Gastwirth suggests walking around the store as much as possible.

Check out your old shoes. It's not just tight new shoes that can rub the wrong way. Your comfy standbys could be the problem. "There might be a frayed seam or a tear in the lining," says Dr. Gastwirth. If that's the case, get rid of the shoe or have a cobbler repair the offending part.

Sock it to your socks. The culprit might not be your shoes at all. Your favorite pair of socks might have a hole in the wrong spot, Dr. Gastwirth points out, or those tube socks you bought for jogging might have a prominent seam. If so, toss them.

Harvesting Your Corns

Once corns crop up, you might need to do more than step into the right footwear. Here are some expert do's and don'ts for dealing with them.

Pad them. You can get relief from hard corns by shielding them from your shoes. "You can get doughnut-shaped pads at a pharmacy," says Rock Positano, D.P.M., co-director of the Foot and Ankle Orthopedic Institute at the Hospital for Special Surgery and Lenox Hill Hospital, both in New York City. "They fit around the corn and protect it from pressure and friction."

File it away. You can reduce the pressure on a hard corn by cutting it down to size. Dr. Positano suggests this method: "Soak the foot in warm water for about 15 minutes to soften the corn. Then file it gently with a pumice stone." Make sure you don't rub the normal skin next to the corn and underneath it.

Put it in a splint. If you have a history of hard corns, the toes themselves might be deformed. Thanks to either heredity or repeatedly squeezing into tight shoes, the bones can curl up and the toes can begin to resemble claws. The middle knuckle sticks up like a mountaintop, making it susceptible to close encounters with leather. To correct this, Dr. Frey recommends hammertoe shields. "They have loops that go over the toe and a pad that goes under the foot," she says. "They pull the toe and straighten it out."

Keep your toes apart. If you have soft corns—the kind that grow between the toes—the little bones on the sides of the digits are probably banging into each other. To protect them from each other, Dr. Frey recommends foam toe separators, which

FAST FACTS

How common: According to one survey, 15.9 percent of men complain of corns and calluses.

Risk factors: Ill-fitting shoes, mechanical irregularities, an active lifestyle.

Age group affected: Beginning in adulthood, the rate of incidence goes up steadily with age.

Gender gap: Twice as many women complain of corns and foot calluses, probably because of the difference in shoe styles. Because of their sports, jobs and hobbies, men are more prone to calluses on the hands.

Who to see: If corns keep coming back or don't go away with self-treatment, see a podiatrist.

can be purchased at a pharmacy. Or, you can place a wad of cotton or lamb's wool between the two toes.

Don't slice them. If you're tempted to perform bathroom surgery, give it up. Experts agree that cutting-edge self-treatment is not too sharp.

Don't reach over the counter. You'll find lots of products for softening corns and calluses. "They can be very dangerous," says Dr. Positano. "Most of them contain salicylic acid. It will kill devitalized tissue, but it can also burn the normal skin adjacent to or underneath the corn." Any form of self-treatment, he adds, is especially dangerous for anyone with diabetes or circulation problems.

When to Trim Your Callus

"Calluses are good," says Joseph Ellis, D.P.M., a podiatrist in La Jolla, California, and author of *Running Injury Free*. "They protect your skin. But problems can arise because the body thinks if a little protection is good, a lot must be better. It keeps building up the callus." A callus that grows big enough can become its own source of pressure. If it happens to grow on the bottom of your foot, it can feel like you have a rock in your shoe.

If it gets to that point, Dr. Ellis advises trimming the callus. "Use a pumice stone, an emery board or even sandpaper," he says. "Don't try to cut them out with a knife or scissors."

Cramps

The Key to Staying Unlocked

Cramps are a sudden and anguishing way to end a workout. But be glad you get them.

Muscles that are straining too hard sense when damage is about to occur, and essentially lock up before that can happen. "When you cramp up, you shut down," says Joe Gieck, Ed.D., head trainer at the University of Virginia in Charlottesville.

Muscle fibers operate by contracting and expanding, but when a cramp occurs, the fibers freeze into a prolonged contraction. This can happen in any body part that contains a muscle, but cramps are most common in the legs, particularly the calves—a problem often referred to as a charley horse.

Overexertion is just one cause of cramps, actually. Well-known and despised is that nocturnal leg cramp that wakes you up screaming. Its cause: A calf muscle getting stuck after a turn or stretch in your sleep. In addition, a sharp blow can cause a muscle to lock up—its way of telling the body not to use it for a while.

Virtually every man will get cramps at some point, says Michael Ciccotti, M.D., an orthopedic surgeon specializing in sports medicine at the Rothman Institute at Pennsylvania Hospital in Philadelphia.

Usually the cause is overuse, but cramps can also be caused by such things as arteriosclerosis or a ruptured back disc, says James Richards, M.D., an orthopedic surgeon at Matthews Orthopedic Clinic in Orlando, Florida. Consult your doctor if muscle cramps are lingering without clear reason.

Curbing Cramps

Cramps may seem unpredictable, but in fact, overuse, injury, dehydration and low blood flow all predispose muscles to the problem. So here are steps to take to avoid cramps.

Pace yourself. Overexertion is the leading cause of cramps, so the answer is obvious: Take it easy, particularly when doing something new. If you're waterskiing for the first time, for example, don't spend three hours zooming across Lake Minnehaha. Instead, build up to it slowly, advises Dr. Ciccotti. "If you want to run three miles, begin at half a mile, then increase to three-quarters of a mile. You're increas-

140

FAST FACTS

How common: Virtually everyone will occasionally get a muscle cramp.

Risk factors: Cold weather, overexertion, not stretching or being out of shape, a sharp blow, a turn or stretch in your sleep.

Age group affected: Muscle cramps don't discriminate by age, although men over age 65 are more likely to experience cramps because of other medical problems.

Gender gap: Men and women are equally prone to getting a muscle cramp.

Who to see: For cramps during exercise it's not necessary to see a doctor. If you frequently get nighttime cramps, however, you'll want to see a family doctor or internist.

ing the ability of muscles to withstand the microtrauma of the exercise," he says.

Hydrate to the hilt. Another common cause of cramps is exercising without taking in enough water. As a rule, experts say, you should plan on drinking a minimum of eight eight-ounce glasses of water a day, and more if you're exercising regularly. "If you wait until you're thirsty, you're already dehydrated," adds Todd Molnar, M.D., sports medicine specialist at the Southern California Orthopedic Institute in Van Nuys, California. To prevent cramping during heavy workouts, he recommends taking three or four swallows of water every ten minutes.

Replace electrolytes. Sweating makes you lose more than just water. Your stores of electrolytes—minerals, like potassium, calcium and magnesium—can also be depleted. Since electrolytes are responsible for carrying electrical charges to the nerves that signal muscles to contract and relax, a shortage can cause muscles to "misfire."

While electrolyte depletion isn't likely to be a problem for weekend warriors, it can be serious in hard-core athletes, like marathoners. "They should try to remain hydrated with something with replacement ions in it, like Gatorade or another sports drink," he says.

Think before drinking. While it's never a good idea to overimbibe, doing so before a workout can particularly cramp your style. "People who drink alcohol the night before will be more dehydrated," says Dr. Molnar.

Stretch out. Stretching for five minutes before and after exercise will help relax tightness in muscles and is an excellent way to put a crimp in cramps.

To stretch your calves—perhaps the most common site of cramps—stand a few feet from a wall, facing it. With your left foot in front and your right leg behind you, lean forward with your hands against the wall. Press your right heel downward until you feel a good stretch. Hold for five seconds, then relax. Repeat five times. Then switch sides and repeat the stretch in your left leg.

Put on some heat. Just as cold weather can make it difficult for your car's engine to turn over, it also makes muscles less limber. That's why runners tend to get cramps more often in fall and winter, says Dr. Ciccotti. So before going out for a chilly-day workout, be sure to dress warmly, he advises. You can always shed a few layers once you've had time to warm up.

Kick the nic. If you are a smoker, you may be more prone to muscle cramping, adds Alan Mikesky, Ph.D., an exercise physiologist at Indiana University-Purdue University at Indianapolis. Nicotine can restrict blood flow to the muscles and trigger cramps.

How to Slack It

When a cramp occurs, fast action usually means fast relief. Here's what to do.

Drink up. As the above points out, a cramped muscle is often dehydrated. Quickly guzzle some fluids.

Stretch it. The goal is to unlock the contraction. If you can, stretch the cramped muscle with one hand and alternately squeeze and release it with the other. Or stretch the muscle by contracting the opposing muscle. For example, pulling your toes toward your chin will stretch the calf, or straightening your elbow will stretch your bicep.

Massage it. Once the muscle is released, massage it to stimulate blood flow.

Cool it. If you can't get the muscle to release and the pain is great, use ice to numb the area. Just be sure to keep the ice moving so you don't hurt the skin. Three to five minutes should be enough.

Use common sense. Sometimes the solution is deceptively simple. Like standing up if you have a foot or leg cramp. Or loosening your covers if you're having nocturnal cramps. One expert even suggests pinching your upper lip; either it's a pressure point that helps relax the muscle or it's merely a good distraction until the muscle releases on its own.

Dandruff

Keep Those Specks in Check

The typical commercial for dandruff shampoo goes something like this: Handsome guy walks into room wearing blue business suit, his broad shoulders covered with what appears to be half the annual snowfall of Aspen. Dandruff is pointed out by some tactless dweeb in accounting. Handsome guy is roundly embarrassed. Co-workers are disgusted, especially the attractive woman who looks at him as though he just clubbed baby seals.

Truth is, those folks in the office shouldn't be so quick to point a condemning finger. After all, they need their hands to wipe off their own scalp-produced specks.

"Everybody has a little dandruff," says Guy Webster, M.D., Ph.D., associate professor of dermatology and director of the Center for Cutaneous Pharmacology at Jefferson Medical College of Thomas Jefferson University in Philadelphia. "You can stir up dandruff on even the healthiest scalp just by scratching it with your finger."

Getting Flaky—And Getting Over It

While it may be embarrassing and is certainly unsightly, dandruff is anything but serious. It won't lead to baldness or thinning hair and isn't the result of poor hygiene, bad habits or some family curse.

What dandruff is, pure and simple, is dead skin cells. Everyone has 'em, since they flake off as new cells are pushed from deeper skin layers—one reason why everyone has dandruff to some degree (including bald men). But for some reason unknown to doctors, skin cells on the scalp proliferate—form, die and flake off—at a faster rate in some men than others. And that's one reason why some men may have just an occasional flakeout, while others can dump a veritable blizzard on their shoulders day after day.

Of course, there's another reason why you may be among the latter: Your very maleness. While everyone gets dandruff to some degree, guys tend to get it worse than women because hormones like testosterone lead to an oilier scalp, which can result in increased flaking. Statistics show that at least four in ten men will develop "problem dandruff" at some point in their lives.

That's not to say that what you consider to be problem dandruff may even be dandruff at all. A profusion of flaky, itchy head scales that appear thicker and greasier than the usual flaky snow job may be the result of seborrheic dermatitis. One clue: Dandruff usually stays on the scalp, while seborrheic dermatitis can also affect eyebrows, ears and other parts of the body. Psoriasis, another case of skin cells going hyper, is also confused with dandruff. It's marked by thicker yellowish or silvery scales or "plaques" that itch like the dickens and leave your scalp red and inflamed.

Wash Away Your Cares

"Having dandruff is a little bit like going out in the rain," says Steven Greenbaum, M.D., chief of dermatologic surgery at Jefferson Medical College of Thomas Jefferson University in Philadelphia. "You can't stop the rain, but you can put up an umbrella so you don't get wet. There's no cure for dandruff, but you can totally arrest it with proper treatment."

And what's that? A good first step is to simply try to wash your cares away with a daily shampooing. "The first thing I tell my patients is, 'just wash your hair more,'" says Dr. Webster. "Washing is a great way to remove scales. Most of the time, shampooing once a day with a nonmedicated shampoo is enough to control dandruff." But if you've been hitting the shower more often and are still avoiding dark-colored shirts, then try some of these steps.

Take five to do it right. *How* you shampoo can be as important as how often you do it—especially if you're using one of those special medicated "dandruff" shampoos. Most experts recommend lathering and then leaving the shampoo in your hair for at least five minutes. "The thing to remember with these medicated shampoos is you're treating your scalp, not your hair," says Dr. Greenbaum. "You want the medication to come in contact with your scalp. The longer you leave it on, theoretically, the more it gets absorbed into your scalp."

So what should you look for in a medicated shampoo? Dr. Greenbaum says the best over-the-counter brands contain selenium sulfide (Selsun Blue) or pyrithione zinc (Head & Shoulders). Tar-based shampoos (T-Gel) also work well, especially for particularly stubborn dandruff and problems associated with seborrhea or psoriasis. Medicated shampoos are safe enough to use daily, but if you notice your dandruff is returning, try switching to a new brand. Sometimes your skin develops a tolerance to the active ingredient, and it loses its effectiveness.

Lose the mousse. There's another self-inflicted cause for flakes that often goes overlooked. Hair products, like mousse, styling gels and hairsprays, says Nelson Lee Novick, M.D., associate clinical professor of dermatology at Mount Sinai School of Medicine of the City University of New York. Some of these produce flakiness that's

FAST FACTS

How common: Everyone has some dandruff.

Risk factors: Anyone with androgenic hormones, like testosterone, which includes all men. Anyone whose skin cells reproduce—again, all of us. Cold weather and stress can trigger outbreaks. Mousse, styling gels and hairsprays can dry up and flake as well.

Age group affected: It can start in infancy—just look at any newborn with cradle cap—but it usually doesn't become a serious problem until those postpuberty years when vanity kicks into high gear.

Gender gap: While it affects both sexes, men are more likely than women to have "problem dandruff"—thicker scales and more frequent flakes—because of the male hormones.

Who to see: If you can't control your dandruff, see a dermatologist or your family doctor.

often mistaken for dandruff—especially when used to excess. The answer: Avoid them if you notice more dandruff after using them.

Wear a hat in winter. Keep your head covered when you're out in the cold, advises Dr. Webster. The dryness of winter air is murder for the dandruff-prone scalp, and leaning into a blustery wind bareheaded will worsen inflammation—and hence, dandruff.

Chill out. Like other skin conditions, dandruff seems to get worse during times of stress. "Relaxing can help," says Dr. Greenbaum. Good ways to manage stress and ease your emotional burdens include listening to music, exercising regularly or practicing deep breathing or yoga.

Take some thyme. If oil isn't your thing, try another helper from the kitchen cabinet. A potion made with the herb thyme is believed to help control dandruff when rinsed into the hair after shampooing, says Louis Gignac, a New York City hairstylist and author of *Everything You Need to Know to Have Great-Looking Hair*. His recommendation: Boil four heaping tablespoons of dried thyme in two cups of water for ten minutes. Strain it and allow the brew to cool. Then pour it over your damp, just-shampooed hair and massage in gently. You don't need to rinse it.

See also Dermatitis and Eczema, Psoriasis

Delayed Ejaculation
No More Waiting Game

Let's say you and your partner are making love and you're 5 minutes into it. Time ticks away and soon you near the 15-minute marker with no sign of tiring. Atta boy, you think.

After 30 minutes your lover is duly impressed. At 45 minutes your lover's impressed and a bit sore. Then again, so are you—but it's worth it because 45 straight minutes of lovemaking might be history in the making.

More time passes and the clock keeps ticking. Now it feels like forever. You're both dripping with sweat, panting like dogs and feeling as romantic as a funeral. Your lover has had multiple orgasms, but you still haven't had your first. Your eyes glaze over as you suddenly think of quitting this exhausting exercise in futility—you'd rather run the Boston Marathon on your hands.

What's going on here? It doesn't happen like this in the movies.

It sounds like a case of delayed ejaculation, and it's not something you'd normally see in a movie—or anywhere else for that matter.

The "Other" Dysfunction

Delayed ejaculation is a condition that occurs when a man can't ejaculate during lovemaking. It's usually caused by psychological factors, like stress or fear. But it also can come with age as your penis becomes less responsive than it was in your youth. It can even be caused by diabetes or abdominal surgery.

You don't often hear much about delayed ejaculation because it isn't as common as, say, premature ejaculation or impotence. And don't confuse it with priapism, a medical condition in which a man *can't* lose his erection whether he ejaculates or not.

Often the psychological cause for a case of tardy titillation is a matter of trust, says Marilyn K. Volker, Ed.D., a sexologist in private practice in Coral Gables, Florida. Or, more specifically, a lack of trust.

"In these situations it's usually a case where a man has learned not to trust his partner. He feels he needs to be in control, and he can't let go and relax during sex," Dr. Volker says.

FAST FACTS

How common: Not very, but your chances of experiencing delayed ejaculation can increase with age.

Risk factors: Caused mostly by psychological factors, like stress or fear. Some medications, particularly antidepressants, can be the culprit, too, as well as age, diabetes and abdominal surgery.

Age group affected: Any man, though most likely to occur in men in the over-50 age group as a sign of aging.

Gender gap: Men only.

Who to see: Sex therapist, unless you suspect a physical cause or have a physical symptom, like pain—then see a urologist.

Fear, stress and anger can also take your mind off The Mood regardless of how horny you think you feel. For example, a man who's deathly afraid of getting his partner pregnant might be so preoccupied with that thought that he never loosens up enough to enjoy intercourse.

Even some medications might inhibit ejaculation, including some antidepressants and anti-inflammatory agents.

Defining the Delay

Having an erection that lasts all night sounds good from a distance. Up close, it's not nearly so enticing.

"Some men say they wish they had this problem, but the truth is you don't want it because it means the whole sexual experience is controlling you," says Dr. Volker.

"Sex under these conditions can be frustrating for a man's partner as well," adds Arlene Goldman, Ph.D., coordinator of the Jefferson Sexual Function Center at Thomas Jefferson University in Philadelphia.

How can you tell when your lovemaking has crossed the line from unparalleled performance to overdue orgasm? Listen to this advice from Durwood E. Neal, Jr., M.D., associate professor of surgery, microbiology and internal medicine at the University of Texas Medical Branch in Galveston.

"Most people would probably say that if intercourse lasts for greater than an hour or an hour-and-a-half without you climaxing, it's delayed," he says.

If you're delayed once in a blue moon, it's probably nothing to worry about—play it off as great endurance. But if you're consistently failing to ejaculate—or it's causing problems for you or your lover—see a sex therapist or urologist.

And for the record: Despite what you told your dates in high school, your testicles will not horribly explode if you don't ejaculate, says Marc S. Cohen, M.D., associate professor of surgery and urology at the University of Florida College of Medicine in Gainesville.

"Your body will reabsorb the fluid naturally. You won't get an abundance of fluid, a pressure buildup or anything like that," Dr. Cohen says.

Don't Stay Up All Night

If you're suffering from an occasional or first-time bout of delayed ejaculation, try these tips to help you climax.

Make a list. "For a man who's never had this problem before, I usually recommend that he run through a mental checklist to help identify the cause," Dr. Goldman says.

Ask yourself if you're taking any new medications; if you've been under extra pressure or stress lately; if you're fatigued or tired; if you're angry with your lover or someone else; if you've had too much alcohol to drink; or if your feelings for your lover have changed. All of these can annihilate your amour.

Limit the libations. A common cause for delayed ejaculation is simply drinking too much alcohol.

"Studies have shown that ejaculation may be depressed by the general depressive effect of alcohol. Some guys will drink a lot and feel like He-Man and think they can go forever, but that's not quite the case," Dr. Neal says. "In fact, someone who's acutely intoxicated may not be able to get an erection at all."

So when it comes to swigging the swill to pump up the passion, do what Socrates advised and practice moderation in all things—keep your limit at about a drink or two an hour.

Practice together. If you're able to ejaculate by masturbating but not while fully engaged with your lover, Dr. Volker suspects it might be a lack of trust that's keeping you from ejaculating. To overcome this, she suggests you practice masturbating with your partner to build this trust. (Masturbation will also help teach you good ejaculatory control, meaning you'll be better able to achieve orgasm when you want to.)

"When you're comfortable masturbating in front of your lover, your partner should then put a hand over your penis," Dr. Volker says. "When you're comfortable with masturbating together, you can insert yourself in your partner at the point before you feel like climaxing."

Let fantasies unleash your lust. Some men fail to ejaculate because they feel guilty about what turns them on, and as a result, the guilt buries their arousal—and

orgasm. But exercising your imagination might be just what the doctor ordered.

"Many men with retarded ejaculation problems don't fantasize enough to really arouse themselves. The key to them ejaculating is that they have to be really aroused, and fantasies can help them do this," says Dr. Goldman.

Tune into what turns you on. It might be provocative pictures, adult movies or thoughts of having a fling with the sexy secretary at work or your lover's sister. Don't be afraid of these fantasies if they turn you on—there's a difference between fantasizing about them and acting them out. Sometimes just indulging yourself in these thoughts will be enough to help you reach orgasm.

"Realize that they're only fantasy," Dr. Goldman says. "Most of us have fantasies that are a bit aberrant, but that's part of what makes them exciting."

Try some manual control. Sometimes a man just isn't getting enough sensation out of his lover, particularly if his lover is a woman with a vagina that's overly re-laxed, perhaps after childbearing says Harold M. Reed, M.D., director of the Reed Centre for Ambulatory Urological Surgery in Bay Harbor, Florida.

"Sometimes the vagina may not provide enough frictional sensation, and some men need this frictional contact and stimulation more than others in order to ejac-ulate," Dr. Reed says.

If vaginal intercourse is doing wonders for her but not you, ask your lover to give you a hand—or a mouth. Other sexual acts may provide more stimulating con-tact on the sensitive parts of your penis.

Dental Problems

Taking Care of the Adult Tooth

More than a few of us can remember watching granddad remove dental hardware from his mouth at night and laying the device—a creepy-looking thing with metal hooks and false teeth stuck into flesh-colored plastic—carefully on a towel on the bathroom counter. Most of these granddads offered us the same advice. "Take it from me, bud. You don't want to lose your teeth."

Fortunately, dentures on the counter will be a far rarer sight for today's generations thanks mainly to fluoridated water, toothpaste and better dental care. There's a problem that comes with keeping our teeth longer, though. Ralph Burgess, D.D.S., the former head of preventive dentistry at the University of Toronto Dental School, sums it up nicely. "We have," he says, "more teeth and gums to take care of."

Don't get us wrong, it's a nice problem to have. Toothlessness is a major disadvantage, and not only because dentures are clumsy and embarrassing. According to Joel M. Boriskin, D.D.S., an adviser to the American Dental Association who practices in Oakland, California, the health of many senior citizens who have lost their teeth is seriously compromised by the difficulty they having eating nutritious foods. "It's true that when we retain our teeth longer, we retain the added costs of regular dental care and of the other procedures that may be necessary to keep those teeth healthy," he says. "But you're exchanging major problems for far less significant problems."

Enemies of the Adult Mouth

The two biggest threats to your smile are cavities and gum disease, and the same culprit—plaque—is responsible for both. Plaque is a sticky residue that is formed on the teeth and gums by the bacteria that thrive in the dark, moist environment of your mouth. Those bacteria feed on the bits of food, microscopic and otherwise, that get caught on your teeth and gums as you eat.

By cleaning your teeth thoroughly you starve the little buggers. "Get those food particles out of your mouth," says Richard Price, D.M.D., clinical professor of dentistry at Boston University's School of Dentistry and an adviser to the American Dental Association. "The less time bacteria have to work on the food debris, the less damage to your teeth."

According to Barry Dale, D.D.S., a cosmetic and family dentist in Englewood, New Jersey, kids and teenagers tend to get cavities on the top and sides of their teeth. Older adults, by contrast, tend to develop cavities at the base of their teeth, near the gum line. That's because we're more prone to gum disease, and unhealthy gums can recede—you literally get longer in the tooth. These freshly exposed parts of your teeth are more accessible to bacteria, making them more vulnerable to cavities.

Dr. Dale says the art of filling cavities has greatly improved over the years, especially with the addition of sophisticated porcelain-like resins to the standard gold and silver fillings in the dentist's arsenal. The newest filling available, Dr. Dale says, releases minute amounts of fluoride to help prevent future decay.

Wear and Tear

Another common problem for the adult tooth is a filling that's past its prime. "Temperatures in your mouth can go from freezing when you have some ice cream to boiling when you have hot coffee," says Dr. Dale, "and we know what changes of temperature like that can do to a car over a few seasons. The seasons in your mouth change several times a day, so fillings break down, they erode, they can get damaged in any number of ways." What you'll notice if a filling is beginning to go, if you notice it at all, is an increased sensitivity to temperature and/or sweets, a tendency for bits of food to get caught on the filling's deteriorating edges or perhaps a rough sensation when you pass your tongue over it.

Emergency Repairs

For the clumsy among us it helps to know what to do if you ever chip a tooth or get one knocked out altogether. According to Barry Dale, D.D.S., a cosmetic and family dentist in Englewood, New Jersey, advancements in the manufacture of porcelain-like resins have made cosmetic repairs easier, more attractive and more durable than they used to be.

When a tooth is chipped, these resins are molded to replace what's missing and bonded to the remaining base of the tooth. There's a small chance your dentist may use the chipped portion of the tooth in the restoration, Dr. Dale says, but most likely it will be discarded. "You have nothing to lose by bringing it in," he says, "but I wouldn't waste a lot of time looking for it."

Dr. Dale adds that these patch jobs can usually be taken care of in a single visit to the dentist's office, although for your back teeth, which handle the heavier chewing, a metallic filling or a multiple visit for a cap manufactured in a laboratory may be required.

When the tooth is knocked clear out of its socket, you need to get both the tooth and yourself to a dentist's office quickly—within an hour or so, according to Dr. Dale—if you're going to have any chance of successfully reattaching it. After reinserting the tooth, a dentist likely will anchor it to adjoining teeth with a bonding material until the gum tissue surrounding it reattaches. Even with successful reattachments, the nerve of the tooth may not recover, so a root canal may be necessary, either at the time of the reattachment or later.

The likelihood of a successful reattachment will be greatly enhanced if you don't clean off the fragments of gum tissue that still cling to the tooth, Dr. Dale says. That's because the tissue cells on the tooth will grow together with their brothers in the socket like two sides of a cut healing back together.

Another critical hint when you pop a tooth: Keep it wet, preferably in milk, until you get to the dentist.

Like fillings, teeth themselves can give way after a while, which means you're more likely to develop cracks in your teeth as you get older. Part of the reason for that, according to Dr. Price, is tension: People under stress often clench or grind their teeth and that pressure can cause an aging tooth to develop a hairline fracture. Here again, you may not notice anything other than an increased sensitivity to cold, but you may feel an occasional stab of pain when chewing.

Healthy Teeth Basics

The best way to keep your mouth healthy is to follow the same routines you were supposed to follow as a kid: Brush at least twice a day, floss at least once a day and visit your dentist at least twice a year. "Don't neglect the fundamentals," says Dr. Price. "It's the fundamentals that win ball games."

Here are some pointers on how to make the fundamentals work best for you.

Go shopping. Virtually every company in the oral hygiene business has introduced new, improved toothbrushes in recent years. The new designs range from brushes with rippled bristles, making them more efficient at getting in between teeth, to brushes with small, angled heads, making it easier to reach back molars, to brushes with flexible handles, which help you avoid putting too much pressure on your teeth and gums. There's also a new generation of electric toothbrushes that move the bristles significantly faster than the electric toothbrushes of old.

The goal of all these new products, of course, is to better clean away both food particles and the sticky plaque that causes gum disease and cavities. According to the Journal of the American Dental Association (ADA), early studies indicate that several of the new designs do appear to do the job better than the old-fashioned models, but long-term research is needed to confirm those findings. The ADA's report adds, however, and several dentists we interviewed agreed, that the old soft-bristle brushes work fine if they're used right, and used frequently. Ask your dentist for a lesson in proper brushing.

Get a timer. Research has shown that most of us spend an average of 51 seconds brushing our teeth. That's not nearly long enough to clean them thoroughly. Triple that is more like it. "The most important item you can have in your bathroom," Dr. Price says, "is a three-minute egg timer."

Stick with it. Do real men floss? Christine Dumas, D.D.S., an adviser to the American Dental Association who practices in Los Angeles, thinks not. "Men perceive it as a girl thing," she says. Too bad, since many dentists consider flossing even more important than brushing. Dr. Dumas recommends a one-month training regimen. "Research shows it takes 28 days to develop a new habit," she says. "Make sure you floss every day for 28 days and you'll be on your way."

Just as new toothbrush designs are flooding the market, so are new varieties of dental floss. There are new flavors, new widths, new fibers that slide more easily between the teeth and new devices to hold the floss more easily in position.

Dentists say that people with extensive dental work may find waxed floss less prone to shredding than unwaxed, but beyond that most agree it isn't the type of floss that's important. "Use the one that's easiest for you to use," says Judith S. Post, D.M.D., a dentist in private practice in Montclair, New Jersey, "because that's the one you'll use more often."

Rinse before bed. Most dentists think the basics of oral hygiene are all you need to worry about, but some, including Dr. Dumas, are staunch advocates of fluoride rinses. "Rinsing with a fluoride rinse has been shown to decrease cavities by up to 40 percent more than just brushing alone," she says. Listerine mouthwash also helps control the bacteria responsible for plaque, she adds.

Clean before you irrigate. Irrigators are those appliances that shoot a stream of water at the gums to wash away food particles. Except when they're used with a fluoride rinse, many dentists consider irrigators to be of questionable value; some, in fact, believe irrigators may do more harm than good by actually driving debris deeper below the gum line. For that reason, Dr. Dumas suggests that if you like using one, make sure to clean your teeth thoroughly before you do. And, adds Dr. Price, go easy on the hydraulic power. "This is not a fire hose," he says. "Irrigators are meant to wash the debris out, not blast it away. Use it on a low or medium setting."

Stay off the ice. One way to avoid developing cracks in your teeth, Dr. Price says, is to avoid eating ice, especially at the same time you're eating something hot, like pizza. Extremes of temperature cause tooth enamel to contract, which can lead to fractures. "Ice cubes belong in your soda, not in your mouth," he says.

Depression

Banishing the Blues

Women's magazines practically burst with articles on how to ward off the blues. Men, of course, tend to write off such advice. Imperatives like "Have a good cry," "Record your worries" or "Connect with others" seem impractical to us—not to mention potentially embarrassing. But the premise of much of this advice is right on.

"The best way to manage the blues is to get off your butt and do something," says Michael D. Yapko, Ph.D., a clinical psychologist in private practice in San Diego.

Climbing Out of the Valley

Of course, not all depression is amenable to self-help. Serious clinical depression—often the result of a chemical imbalance in the brain or a traumatic experience—strikes about 5 percent of us each year. Uplifting articles aren't likely to help.

The good news is that depression—whether it's serious and long-lived or just a temporary case of the blues—can usually be relieved.

"Even among serious clinical depressions, at least 80 to 90 percent of them can be treated and people can get back to their lives," says Matthew A. Menza, M.D., assistant professor of psychiatry and neurology at the Robert Wood Johnson Medical School in New Brunswick, New Jersey.

Granted, the successful treatment of clinical depression may involve a serious armory of specialists and drugs. Meanwhile, the everyday blues we all get from time to time can often be successfully fought by a single warrior—you.

"In cases of mild depression, with a few changes in your life you can resolve the problem on your own," says Dr. Menza. Here are a few ways to get started.

Get some perspective. Men who always see the glass as being half-empty are more prone to the blues than those who see it as half-full. In many cases depression is less a biological illness than a direct result of how you view the world. The mistake is when you think negatively and actually believe yourself, says Dr. Yapko.

For instance, let's say you make a business call that isn't returned. Do you assume the person is busy and will call you as soon as possible? Or do you automatically fret that he won't call back because he's too busy to talk to the likes of you? This

155

Moods in a Bottle

These days, it seems like treating depression involves capsules as much as couches. Although there are a number of powerful antidepressant drugs that act on chemicals in the brain, preventing moods from spiraling downward, they are by no means cure-alls. These drugs have strong side effects and should only be taken in cases of serious depression. Here's a short list of the most common antidepressant medications.

• Tricyclic antidepressants: Medications such as imipramine (Tofranil) and amitriptyline (Elavil) help keep pleasure-inducing chemicals, like serotonin, bouncing around the brain longer. Side effects include dizziness, vision problems and dry mouth. In some cases they may cause heart problems or interfere with ulcer medications.

• Monoamine oxidase (MAO) inhibitors: Known by brand names like Nardil (phenelzine) and Marplan (isocarboxazid), these powerful drugs counteract enzymes that interfere with natural mood-lifting chemicals in the brain. They may have powerful side effects as well. MAO inhibitors can cause sudden high blood pressure when used with alcohol, over-the-counter cold medicines and even caffeine-containing foods and beverages, like chocolate and cola. They can also cause serious reactions when taken in combination with tyramine—a chemical found in some wines and aged cheeses.

• Serotonin reuptake inhibitors: Also known as new-generation antidepressants, these medications feature such happy-sounding brand names as Zoloft (sertraline hydrochloride), Prozac (fluoxetine hydrochloride) or Wellbutrin (bupropion hydrochloride). Like the tricyclics, these newer antidepressants help prevent the dissipation of mood-lifting brain chemicals. Generally, they are considered safer than older generations of drugs. Side effects may include anxiety, insomnia and decreased sex drive.

sort of self-deprecating, and self-centered, speculation is common among men in their thirties and forties—products of the "Me" generation, says Dr. Yapko.

"The baby boomers are at the highest risk for depression because they tend to be the most self-absorbed," says Dr. Yapko. "You start going through all these speculations about why someone doesn't call you back and your mood fluctuates with your interpretation."

How to Get Happy Again

Dr. Yapko's advice? Don't speculate so much on what *could* be. Focus on getting facts and try not to take impersonal things personally. Devote your attention to things that are in your control, then do your best to make them happen. Some other thoughts:

Have realistic goals. It's fine to dream, but don't let those dreams wander into the realm of delusion. "We all have expectations about life, and to the extent that those aren't met, we may feel some frustration and depression," says Dr. Menza. "It's important to have goals, but men need to be realistic or they're setting themselves up for depression."

Blow off the blues with exercise. The less active you are, the more likely you'll be depressed. Some experts believe exercise is as good a treatment for depression as psychotherapy.

"Studies show that all but the most severely depressed people who begin to exercise do as well as those who get standard psychotherapy," says Keith Johnsgard, Ph.D., professor of psychology at San Jose State University in California and author of *The Exercise Prescription for Depression and Anxiety*. According to a study at Stanford University School of Medicine in Stanford, California, the benefits are the same regardless of your weight and fitness level, how vigorously you exercise or whether you choose to exercise alone at home or in a crowd at the gym. The bottom line, researchers found, was that individuals who exercised regularly reported fewer depressive symptoms than those who were inactive.

Experts aren't sure how exercise combats depression. It may be that physical activity increases brain activity and releases natural chemicals called endorphins that deaden pain and lift our moods. But the important point is that exercise works and it works well.

"Certainly exercise is not the treatment for severe depression—though it certainly wouldn't hurt—but in terms of battling the normal everyday ups and downs that people have, it's extremely important," says Dr. Menza. "Exercise keeps down anxiety, it keeps down weight, it makes us feel healthy and it helps us sleep better."

Don't sleep it off. When you're feeling down, try getting up a little earlier in the morning, suggests Dr. Menza. "If you spend a couple of nights sleeping a little bit less than normal, strangely enough you may find your mood perks up a little bit," he says.

But don't neglect your sleep either. It's hard to see the world in a bright light when your eyes are half-shut all the time. "A lot of men burn the candle at both ends. They're up early and they go to bed late," says Robert Jaffe, Ph.D., a marriage and family counselor in private practice in Sherman Oaks, California. "If you're not getting enough sleep, that alone can cause depression." Though sleep needs vary, as a rule most of us need between eight and nine hours of sleep a night. Try to get it.

Beware of stimulants. Thanks to their stimulating ingredients, coffee and cigarettes are among the biggest legal pick-me-ups around. Unfortunately, what goes up must come down.

"These are powerful drugs," says Dr. Jaffe. "They bring you to an artificial high and then drop you right down, which can make you feel low."

In addition, while a cocktail or two may give you a happy glow initially, the feeling doesn't last. Alcohol is actually a powerful depressant, so if you're already depressed, drinking will probably make it worse. So give up the cigarettes, and keep your caffeine and alcohol intake to a moderate level—no more than one or two drinks a day, experts say.

Talk it out. While communication is a powerful tool for coping with depression, many men's communication skills lean more toward Clint Eastwood than Phil Donahue, especially when something is troubling them.

"Men to a large extent are loners in our society," says Dr. Jaffe. "A lot of times when men are going through something, they don't really have anybody to talk to about it."

The next time you're blue, try approaching your partner or a close friend— odds are you'll find they're more than happy to listen.

Have a friend, be a friend. "Unless you're connected to something greater than yourself," says Dr. Yapko, "you're at a higher risk for depression." So get involved. Take an interest in other people. Cultivate friendships. Offer a hand to a philanthropic organization—there are plenty of them that could use it.

Don't be shy to cry. It's not the first remedy we think of, or the most comfortable, but men need to shed a few tears now and again.

"Women can release their sadness with tears a lot easier than men," says Dr. Jaffe. "Being able to cry is really important. Feelings of sadness need to come to the surface and be expressed. The more they're kept under the surface, the more likely they are to cause depression."

Find what you like. No man lives for work alone. Having a variety of interests will help keep life interesting. "Anybody who's bored with life is going to find it a lot easier to be depressed," says Dr. Menza. "Having something to look forward to each day is very important in life."

Check your medicine cabinet. Many common medications, including sedatives, blood pressure drugs and antihistamines, may contribute to depression. If you suspect medications you're taking are getting you down, talk to your doctor or pharmacist about alternatives.

Living in the Great Depression

There's a lot you can do to lift the blues, but when it comes to serious depression, you're going to need an expert's help.

FAST FACTS

How common: Every man experiences the blues now and then, but roughly 10 percent of men will be diagnosed with major depression at some point in their lives.

Risk factors: Diseases, medications or a chemical imbalance in the brain can lead to depression. Experts also believe that heredity plays a role: If one of your parents has experienced major depression, your risk is three times greater than someone who doesn't have the family history.

Age group affected: Depression can hit at any age. Men usually are affected for the first time in their thirties.

Gender gap: Women are twice as likely as men to experience major depression.

Who to see: Family doctor to rule out other diseases, psychiatrist to explore the possibility of medications and a psychologist for ongoing psychotherapy.

"Being moody for a day isn't a problem, but if you're having persistent symptoms of depression, you need to see a professional," says David Dunner, M.D., professor and vice-chairman of the Department of Psychiatry and Behaviorial Sciences at the University of Washington in Seattle. "Men in particular tend to write off serious depression and not get treatment for it—and that can have serious consequences."

Experts aren't entirely sure what causes serious depression. It may be caused by changes in body chemistry. Depression may have psychological roots as well: memories of abuse, for example, or reactions to traumatic events.

When it comes to serious depression, stoicism is more than just foolish. It can be deadly as well. Men with depression are twice as likely to commit suicide as their female counterparts, says Dr. Dunner. That's why it's so important to recognize the danger signs. See your physician if you're experiencing several of the following.

- Feeling down or low most of each day
- Losing interest in almost all activities
- Experiencing significant weight gain or loss
- Inability to sleep
- Feeling agitated
- Feeling fatigued
- Experiencing inappropriate guilt or feelings of worthlessness
- Inability to concentrate or make decisions
- Having suicidal thoughts

Dermatitis and Eczema

How to Avoid Rash Behavior

Any man who does weekend carpentry or gardening knows the scratchy feeling of dry skin. Soaking your hands under a faucet at the end of the day can be a true moment of ecstasy.

But when skin gets so dry and inflamed that it reddens, flakes, blisters or swells—a condition called dermatitis—it can be discomfort worthy of your crustiest language.

Dermatitis is quite common; nine out of ten men experience it at some time, doctors estimate. "Think about it. Have you ever had a rash? That's dermatitis," says Hillard H. Pearlstein, M.D., assistant clinical professor of dermatology at Mount Sinai School of Medicine of the City University of New York.

Technically, dermatitis is an umbrella term for many skin problems, including psoriasis and dandruff. But when a doctor tells you you have dermatitis, he's probably referring to one of two types: Atopic dermatitis, better known as eczema, a chronic inflammation of uncertain origin, or contact dermatitis, when the skin has a bad reaction from contact with a specific substance.

Contact dermatitis is the far more common of the two, but eczema is more troublesome, primarily because of its longevity but also because of its intensity. Some men have it their entire lifetimes and are never sure when the next outbreaks will occur or what part of their bodies it will hit. It ranges from sudden, short-lived dry patches to perpetually crusty, inflamed, unsightly skin.

Eczema often is triggered by sensitivities to materials, like pets, dust, plants, soaps or wool. Dry air, stress and cold weather also can cause an outbreak. In addition, eczema runs in families. "There's some commonality between hay fever and asthma and atopic dermatitis. They're all inherited on the same gene. So patients may have asthma, too. Or their sister has asthma and their father has hay fever," Dr. Pearlstein says.

While contact dermatitis can be as uncomfortable as eczema, contact dermatitis is more like an allergic reaction: When the cause goes away, so does the problem. Both eczema and contact dermatitis have similar symptoms, however, and also similar cures.

160

FAST FACTS

How common: Up to 90 percent of the population has had an outbreak of dermatitis.

Risk factors: Heredity, allergies. Common irritating substances are wool, rough fabrics, pets, strong soaps and detergents, nickel (your watchband, for instance) and ragweed.

Age group affected: Birth to death. Even babies get a form of eczema called cradle cap.

Gender gap: Men and women are equally affected. Ragweed may affect more men than women.

Who to see: Dermatologist or your family doctor if you have a rash that won't go away after a week or so.

Work is Cruel

Dermatitis flourishes in the workplace because the skin gets exposed to so many potential irritants.

"Cutting oils irritate machinists' skin. Outdoor workers are exposed to airborne ragweed—a common skin irritant," says Bruce Bart, M.D., chief of dermatology at Hennepin County Medical Center and clinical professor of dermatology at the University of Minnesota in Minneapolis. Cement, turpentine, chemicals of all formulations, even the rubber gloves healthcare workers wear can drive a sensitive guy to scratch. In fact, it's estimated that 2 percent of the total population breaks out in a rash if you put a latex rubber glove on them.

Whether it's the workplace or something at home that irritates you, "the first thing to do to prevent a rash is to avoid the irritant—and the second and third things, too," says Guy Webster, M.D., Ph.D., associate professor of dermatology and director of the Center for Cutaneous Pharmacology at Jefferson Medical College of Thomas Jefferson University in Philadelphia.

But some of us can't avoid all of our irritants. Others don't even know what they are. Be it a chronic medical condition or a rare reaction, however, dermatitis can be subdued through smart behavior.

Bath Behavior

You hop in the shower. You lather up your hide until it stings. Then you rinse off with hot water you can barely stand and towel dry as if you were sandpapering a cabinet. That bathing technique was okay when you were 17. At 37, though, it's time to learn a new one, particularly if you are prone to rashes or eczema.

Go gently into the soap aisle. "You don't want soap that's advertised as being deodorant soap, that says, 'We clean ya!' It's too harsh," says Dr. Webster. "And stay away from anything that smells weird or is a funny color. Go for the stuff that says it's gentle, like Dove or Neutrogena," he adds.

Take a cool bath. Dry skin loves to soak in moisture. But keep the water cool. Not only does hot water make your skin itchier by increasing blood flow to the surface, it also cuts away the natural oils that moisturize and protect.

Get down and dirty. Beware the cold-weather seasons, when cold outdoor air dries your skin and heated, moistureless indoor air makes it worse. Bathing can remove the oils that protect your skin, so consider bathing less frequently during fall and winter, advises Norman Levine, M.D., professor and chief of dermatology at the University of Arizona Health Sciences Center in Tucson.

Dry gently. After you bathe, pat yourself dry rather than wiping. You'll save your skin from considerable irritation.

Oil up. "The big thing with dermatitis is to keep the skin well-lubricated, particularly in the winter. Moisturizers keep the skin soft and less itchy," says Dr. Levine.

Experiment and find a moisturizer that feels good to you—it won't necessarily be the most expensive one. In fact, plain old petroleum jelly is an excellent emollient, although some men find it a little too greasy. Hypoallergenic moisturizers (Almay) are good to try, too, suggests Dr. Bart.

Every time you step out of the shower, moisturize. "You gotta get greasy," Dr. Webster adds. Why after showering? Because it's water, not moisturizer, that dry skin really wants. Moisturizing after bathing traps and holds the water in your skin. In fact, drinking lots of water is part of the solution to keeping skin moist.

Mug the musk. Lots of men are sensitive to the musk substance used in musk-scented soaps, aftershaves and colognes, says Alexander Fisher, M.D., clinical professor of dermatology at New York University in New York City. That same substance also makes problem skin even more sensitive in the sun—a condition called photo-dermatitis. "Men can get a pretty bad rash from musk," Dr. Fisher says.

Soothing the Scratchy Beast

You don't know what nasty substance you touched or rolled in but your skin looks like someone left it out on the turnpike and the itch is driving you nuts. Here's how to save that skin.

Visit the drugstore. Over-the-counter remedies may bring relief. Oral antihistamines (Tavist-D or Contac) can reduce the swelling that often accompanies outbreaks. And over-the-counter hydrocortisone ointments (Cortizone-10) may salve the itch.

But avoid your childhood remedy, calamine lotion. It might provide temporary relief but it will end up drying your skin and irritating it more, warns Dr. Webster.

Soak in cereal. A warm five-to-ten minute bath with colloidal oatmeal added can soothe an angry hide. Aveeno is one brand of oatmeal-for-the-bath to look for.

Get frosted. If the rash is confined to an area, like the top of your hand or foot, a cold compress or an ice pack can relieve the itching. "Cold compresses are very soothing," says Ronald R. Brancaccio, M.D., clinical associate professor of dermatology at New York University Medical Center in New York City. "If the rash is on your face, mix a little milk in the cold water," he suggests.

Sit on your hands. Scratching only makes the situation worse. For one thing, it increases the possibility of infection. Plus, it prolongs the healing process. If you just can't keep your hands away, press the spot, don't scratch.

When to Yell Doctor

If self-help hasn't worked within a week or two, give your dermatologist a buzz. He'll probably prescribe a stronger steroid cream or even an oral steroid, like prednisone (Deltasone), for a bad rash.

If you're mystified about the cause of your outbreak and you don't know what substance to avoid, the doctor may give you a series of patch tests to identify the allergen. The patches are called Finn Chambers and they're impregnated with a mix of common allergens. A dermatologist will try about 20 to 80 patches on the quest for the guilty allergen, says Dr. Brancaccio. When one patch raises a telltale rash, it's bingo.

See also Dandruff, Dry Skin

Deviated Septum

Straight Talk about Out-of-Joint Noses

It's the one physical attribute that you, Mike Tyson and Joe Frazier may very well share.

Even if you retired the boxing gloves after your first schoolyard fistfight—or had the finesse to negotiate your way out of them all—you could still be a contender for a deviated septum and the respiratory problems that go with it.

The septum is the ridge of bone and cartilage that divides your nose in half. Your septum would be straight in the best of all possible worlds. But life's inescapable lumps have a way of knocking a septum askew.

It doesn't take a right hook, either. A bad fall can do it. Even the trip through the birth canal can leave you with a deviated septum.

"Babies get their noses crunched in the canal," explains John A. Henderson, M.D., assistant professor of ear, nose and throat surgery at the University of California, San Diego.

Some men inherit characteristics that predispose their septa to straying. People with long, narrow noses are more likely to have trouble than those who grow up to have short, wide ones.

Nearly half of us wind up with deviated septa on the way to adulthood. They're particularly common among men, says Thomas Pasic, M.D., assistant professor of otolaryngology-head and neck surgery at the University of Wisconsin-Madison. Why so? Guys tend to be active. We're still more likely to get the wayward basketball, the errant Frisbee, the badly aimed tennis ball in the face.

Recognizing the Symptoms

Once it's gone astray, your septum can cramp the style of the rest of your respiratory tract. If it tilts far enough to one side it can block an airway, making it hard for you to breathe out of one nostril. If it's been battered into an S-curve, it can obstruct air flow through both sides of your nose. Either way, there's an inescapable feeling of stuffiness and congestion.

A deviated septum also can contribute to snoring and sleep loss. The congestion that accompanies it can force you to inhale with greater effort while you sleep. In

FAST FACTS

How common: By the time American men reach adulthood, roughly half have septa that have gone astray.

Risk factors: Fighting, playing sports, being born, coming from a family of long, narrow noses.

Age group affected: Newborns can have this problem. The older you get, though, the more opportunities you have to get your septum knocked around. A small deviation can grow worse with age as your nose sags and droops.

Gender gap: The problem shows up in men more than women, primarily because men are more likely to get whacked in the face than women.

Who to see: Family doctor. If he suspects a deviated septum, he might refer you to an otolaryngologist.

turn, this can cause your throat and airway to rumble—that's what snoring is. In more extreme cases the clog can cause your throat to constrict, jolting you to near wakefulness. That's called sleep apnea, and nights of that will leave you exhausted.

There's more. A deviated septum can set you up for recurring nosebleeds, Dr. Pasic says. "If there's a jag or a big bend in the septum—an area that sticks out and gets a lot of extra air flow—that area will dry out more quickly," he explains. Once it's sufficiently dry, the tissue can crack and then bleed.

Finally, a septum can get whacked so far out of alignment that it blocks the opening through which your sinuses drain. And that can set the stage for sinus infections and headaches, says C. Thomas Yarington, M.D., clinical professor of otolaryngology at the University of Washington and head of the Mason Clinic, both in Seattle.

Setting Things Straight

The good news is many men with deviated septa have virtually no symptoms, despite all the potential ones.

"A lot of people have a deviated septum and it makes no difference," says David Fairbanks, M.D., an otolaryngologist and spokesman for the American Academy of Otolaryngology-Head and Neck Surgery.

The bad news is that it doesn't always last. An off-kilter septum can lay low for years, then slowly start causing problems. It happens as we age and our noses start looking suspiciously like our grandfathers'.

"The nose becomes longer and droops more with age," says Jerome C. Goldstein, M.D., visiting professor of otolaryngology-head and neck surgery at Johns

Hopkins University in Baltimore and Georgetown University in Washington, D.C. "And as it droops, this can accentuate what was originally a mild deviation."

Even the most deviated septum can be set straight with surgery. But that's your last-ditch option. There are less drastic ones. Here's a rundown:

Wait a week. Congestion and stuffiness don't necessarily mean your septum is out-of-line. You may simply have a cold. If it's a cold, things should clear up in a week or so. Give it that long, advises Lloyd M. Loft, M.D., professor of otolaryngology at New York Medical College in Valhalla.

Play doctor. If you're still congested after a week, Dr. Henderson suggests this simple home deviated septum test. Ask yourself three questions: Do you sleep with a glass of water at bedside? Do you wake with a dry mouth? Do you snore? (Your girlfriend or wife can answer the last one, if she hasn't already.)

If all three answers are yes, odds are you're breathing through your mouth—because your nose is stuffed. A deviated septum and/or allergies may be the culprit. Have your doctor investigate further.

See a real one. Ask your doc to evaluate your septum *and* your sensitivities. Allergies can compound the symptoms that accompany a deviated septum—the stuffiness and congestion. Often, treating allergies provides enough relief so that surgery to repair the septum is no longer necessary.

Tend to your allergies. If you have allergies, do what it takes to get them under control. Simple avoidance may do the trick—say, vacuuming and dusting regularly if you're allergic to dust mites. Your doctor can prescribe antihistamines if you need more help.

"You need a thorough evaluation by a specialist," Dr. Loft says. "It may be that there are other factors inside the nose causing the trouble that can be treated medically. It may be chronic inflammation from irritation or allergy that can be treated with sprays or pills so you don't need surgery."

Consider surgery. Fewer than one of every ten people with deviated septa need surgery, says Graham Boyce, M.D., assistant professor of otolaryngology-head and neck surgery at Louisiana State University in New Orleans.

If you're among that minority, relax. The surgery is straightforward, takes less than an hour and can be done on an outpatient basis, with either local or general anesthesia (your choice). The surgery leaves no visible scar.

Diabetes

Maintaining a Delicate Balance

When you've been working all day and dinner's just a cardboard box away, pizza is more a matter of convenience than actual thought. Let's face it: Many men give little consideration to what they eat.

Fortunately, the digestive system can usually handle a guy's dietary exuberance. No matter how much pizza he shovels in, each slice is soon broken down into its component parts, including a sugar called glucose, the fuel that keeps us alive. At the same time, a hormone called insulin is released into the bloodstream. Insulin works like a key, unlocking receptors on the outside of cells so that glucose can be used as energy or stored for future use.

Guys with diabetes have plenty of glucose. What they lack is sufficient insulin to transport it. Or perhaps the cells won't accept it. Either way, the glucose remains in the bloodstream. Over time, high levels of glucose can be toxic. And because the cells aren't getting enough to eat, you may feel tired and run down. This is what doctors mean when they talk about high blood sugar.

Themes and Variations

There are two major types of diabetes. Type I, or insulin-dependent diabetes, occurs when the pancreas, the gland that produces insulin, is damaged. Though this type of diabetes can occur at any age, it typically occurs during childhood. People with Type I diabetes need daily injections of insulin in order to survive.

Type II diabetes accounts for 85 to 90 percent of diabetes in men. With Type II diabetes, the pancreas does produce insulin. But a problem arises when insulin attaches to the cell receptors that allow for glucose entry into the cell. When this process is impaired, it is called insulin resistance. It appears to be inherited, and in many cases the problem is exacerbated by being overweight. Type II diabetes typically appears later in life, often after age 40. It sometimes, but not always, requires insulin injections.

Spotting the Danger

Obviously, you have to know you have diabetes before you can control it. Alarmingly, many men don't know. Of the 6.5 million American men estimated to have diabetes, less than half—about 3 million—have actually been diagnosed with the disease and most of them were probably quite surprised. "A person can very well start developing the complications of diabetes without knowing he has it," says Richard Kahn, Ph.D., chief scientific and medical officer for the American Diabetes Association based in Alexandria, Virginia.

It's not uncommon, for example, for a man to be dog-tired for weeks or even months without knowing anything serious is wrong. Or he could be excessively thirsty and urinating frequently, says Dr. Kahn. Other symptoms of diabetes include extreme hunger, sudden weight loss, irritability, nausea and vomiting, blurred vision or tingling or numbness in the legs, feet or fingers.

Without proper treatment and careful attention to what you eat and drink, diabetes eventually can lead to serious complications, including nerve damage, blindness, loss of limbs, or kidney and heart problems. That's why it's so important to get medical attention at the first sign of symptoms.

A Controllable Condition

If you do have diabetes, more often than not you can control it—and keep its deadly complications at bay.

"Diabetes is really a hands-on management disease," says George Dailey, M.D., head of the Division of Diabetes and Endocrinology at Scripps Clinic and Research Foundation in La Jolla, California. For a man with Type I diabetes this means regular injections of insulin. For guys with Type II diabetes, however, making a few simple lifestyle changes—along with regular monitoring of blood sugar and sometimes taking oral medications—can usually keep blood sugar at safe levels, Dr. Dailey says.

Vivid proof of this came with the results of the Diabetes Control and Complications Trial, a ten-year government-funded study that involved more than 1,400 people. Those who closely monitored and kept their blood sugar levels under the strictest control with insulin, diet and exercise programs were able to reduce the risk of complications by approximately 60 percent. Here's how you can help control your condition.

Cut fat from your frame. "Men who are overweight have a much greater chance of getting Type II diabetes," says Richard Dolinar, M.D., an endocrinologist at Arizona Medical Clinic near Phoenix.

In fact, about 85 percent of men with Type II diabetes are overweight. The good news is that shedding excess pounds is often enough to improve blood sugar levels.

"Experience has shown us that proper weight control can bring diabetes under control in 80 to 90 percent of the cases," says Dr. Dailey. You don't have to be a fanatic, either. Studies have shown that many people can achieve normal blood sugar

FAST FACTS

How common: As many as 6.5 million American men have diabetes. The odds of developing diabetes are about one in nine.

Risk factors: A family history of the disease and being overweight both increase the risk. Ethnicity also seems to play a role: The prevalence of diabetes among Blacks, for example, is about 30 percent higher than among Whites.

Age group affected: Most men develop Type I, or insulin-dependent, diabetes during puberty. Type II, or non-insulin-dependent diabetes typically strikes men after age 40.

Gender gap: Men and women are equally likely to have diabetes.

Who to see: Family doctor, endocrinologist, dietitian.

levels by losing as little as 10 to 20 percent of their present weight.

Cut fat from your diet. Experts agree that eating less dietary fat is one of the most important weapons in preventing cardiovascular complications of diabetes. Fat is bad for anyone's heart—and worse still for men with diabetes, who are four times as likely to die of heart disease. Dietary fat can make you fat, and being overweight makes the body's insulin work less efficiently.

Try to limit your intake of all fats to 30 percent or less of total calories, with artery-clogging saturated fat—found in meat and dairy products—to less than 10 percent of calories, experts say. The American Diabetes Association recommends substituting high-fat foods with high-carbohydrate fare, like grains, vegetables and fruits. If you've recently been diagnosed with diabetes, you may want to see a dietitian for a complete safe-eating plan.

Graze, don't binge. For men with diabetes how they eat is as important as what they eat. Rather than gorging on one or two big meals a day—which will cause glucose levels to peak and trough—experts recommend eating smaller, more frequent meals throughout the day.

"Spreading out your food intake will help promote better blood sugar values," says Christine Beebe, R.D., a registered dietitian and director of Health and Wellness Programs at St. James Hospital in Chicago Heights, Illinois, and former chair of the National Nutrition Council for the American Diabetes Association. "That means having at least three meals a day and sometimes more. Between-meal snacks can help normalize blood sugar levels as well." She recommends snacking on air-popped popcorn, salt-free pretzels or fruit to maintain blood sugar without filling you up with fat.

Feed on fiber. A common symptom of diabetes is feeling hungry all the time—

and a hungry man is a man who's tempted to overeat on sweets, snacks and food in general, all of which are guaranteed to send blood sugar soaring and contribute to weight gain.

A better bet is to fill up on foods that are high in soluble fiber—like fruits, vegetables, nuts and beans. High-fiber foods will help keep your cholesterol down, and they'll also fill you up so you're less likely to raid the pantry later.

Get chrome-plated protection. Research suggests that one way to help prevent Type II diabetes is to get more chromium in the diet, says Richard A. Anderson, Ph.D., lead scientist in mineral nutrition research with the U.S. Department of Agriculture's Human Nutrition Research Center in Beltsville, Maryland. Good dietary sources of chromium include brans, whole-grain cereals, brewer's yeast, broccoli, spinach and various fruits.

Space your carbs. Nutritionists typically recommend that men eat plenty of carbohydrates—the more the better. But guys with diabetes can't be so cavalier about carbs. While they still should get about 40 percent or more of total calories from carbohydrates, having too much in the system all at once can cause blood sugar levels to shoot up—the opposite of what you're trying to achieve. It's better to eat them steadily throughout the day, says Beebe.

Evidence suggests, however, that people with diabetes may have more trouble metabolizing or utilizing carbohydrates at breakfast than later in the day. In the morning, Beebe says, "you might want to have a lower carbohydrate or smaller breakfast and spread your carbohydrates out to later in the day." Limit portions of fruit juice, in particular, to one-half cup at breakfast, and use whole-grain breads and cereals in modest portions, she advises.

Enjoy the sweet stuff—in small amounts. Researchers agree that the evils of sugar have been overstated. "The concept of sugar being the culprit is really passé," Beebe says. "We now know that a modest amount of sugar is okay in the diet of a person with diabetes."

Still, don't overdo it. "You won't get a lot of nutrients from sugary food," says Beebe. "Plus, most of the time sugary foods contain a lot of fat."

Limit your drinking. Moderate drinking—no more than one alcoholic drink a day—is fine, says Beebe. But be aware that alcohol will lower your blood sugar level, possibly to a level that is too low if you're taking insulin or diabetes pills. Always eat when you drink, Beebe advises, and be sure to consider the calories of alcohol—one 12-ounce can of light beer, for example, contains 96 calories.

Work up a sweat. Since exercise helps cut pounds and increase the body's circulation, it's an excellent way to make insulin work more efficiently and help control blood sugar levels.

"Studies have shown that exercise can reduce insulin resistance," says Dr. Dailey. "Exercise recommendations for men with diabetes really aren't much different than they are for anyone else—three to four times a week for 30 minutes or so a day. But if you're on diabetes medication, low blood sugar may follow exercise." So don't charge out onto the racquetball court without getting a checkup first. Guys with diabetes are also at risk for heart problems, so see your doctor before suiting up.

Beyond Self-Care

While there's a lot you can do yourself to keep diabetes under control, you need to be under a physician's care.

Men with Type I diabetes (and occasionally those with Type II), for example, will require regular injections of synthetic insulin, since they produce little or none of their own. And while Type II diabetes can often be controlled with such things as exercise and careful nutrition, eventually many men will need drugs—usually oral medications, such as Glucotrol, from a class of drugs called sulfonylurea—that boost insulin supplies and make the insulin work more efficiently.

Experts are looking into other treatment options as well. For example, researchers have already devised an insulin pump—a device implanted inside the body that releases the right amounts of insulin and is controlled by the patient.

"It eliminates the need for injections and delivers insulin deep into the abdomen, providing a variable rate of insulin, close to the way a normal pancreas works," explains Christopher D. Saudek, M.D., director of the Johns Hopkins Diabetes Center and professor of medicine at Johns Hopkins University School of Medicine in Baltimore.

Diarrhea

Avoiding a Run of Bad Luck

Diarrhea can hit you like a visit from an unwanted relative: It arrives without warning—always at the least convenient time—and makes two days seem like two weeks.

As gut reactions go, diarrhea is one of the worst. Your body literally dumps the contents of your intestines in response to any one of a hundred reasons—tainted food or water usually, but also illness, allergies or even stress. No matter what causes diarrhea though, the end result is always the same—a sudden urgency to void your bowels, a fast trot to the bathroom, followed by loose stools.

This sort of thing can go on for hours or days, but it shouldn't. Not only is diarrhea painful and uncomfortable, it's also potentially dangerous. During a bout of diarrhea, we lose twice as much fluid as we would under normal circumstances. If the diarrhea persists long enough, you could end up with a serious case of dehydration.

Trotting Out the Germs

Most times, diarrhea is caused by bad luck. Maybe you crossed paths with a viral or bacterial infection; more likely, you consumed food or water contaminated with a diarrhea-inducing germ.

Either way, the bug wreaks havoc in your intestines, agitating your digestive system and triggering muscle spasms. The muscles begin moving food along too quickly for your body to absorb water or nutrients from it, explains Stephen Hanauer, M.D., professor of medicine and clinical pharmacology at the University of Chicago Medical Center. You can guess the result.

"The bottom line is these germs have turned the faucet on," says Charles Ericsson, M.D., professor of medicine at the University of Texas Health Science Center at Houston and an expert on traveler's diarrhea. The best way to avoid diarrhea, Dr. Ericsson says, is to avoid the germ.

Mind your menu. Whether you're out on the town or out on the continent, it's a good idea to make your food choices carefully.

Remember the old adage that revenge is a dish best served cold. In other words, be wary of raw or cold foods, particularly meats and shellfish. Buffets and

172

salad bars are trouble spots, too. "Salads create a nice, cool, moist environment where germs like to grow up," says Dr. Ericsson. And buffet foods can be breeding grounds for gut-wrenching bacteria and parasites because they're not hot enough to kill the germs.

"When it comes to foods, virtually anything that's served steaming hot and freshly prepared is safe," says Dr. Ericsson. And he means hot. "It should be a little difficult to put in your mouth without blowing on it. If it's not hot enough to give you pause, send it back and get it heated up more."

Be finicky about fluids. When traveling, especially in developing countries, be wary of water and other fluids.

"Even if the tourist office says the water is safe to drink, I'd be careful. The water might leave the plant meeting U.S. standards, but by the time it gets to the tap, it may have passed through contaminated pipes," points out Dr. Ericsson. When in doubt, drink bottled water, making sure the container is properly sealed before you buy it.

Carbonated beverages from soda to beer are especially good choices because carbonation kills germs, says Dr. Ericsson. Avoid milk products unless you know they've been pasteurized and properly refrigerated. Drink coffee or tea only if it's steaming. And yes, alcoholic beverages, like wine, are a safe bet, too.

Don't eat and run. Eating followed by physical activity can bring on a case of diarrhea faster than you can round the bases or dribble downcourt. In the world of sports this problem is not so affectionately called runner's trots. Physically, all that jostling speeds undigested food more quickly through your system—and you end up making the 100-yard dash for the bathroom. Try eating a small snack about an hour before you exercise, then eat your meal when you finish.

Be alert to allergies. Food allergies or intolerances are sometimes precursors of diarrhea. Common offenders include milk products, which contain lactose, a sugar many adults can't tolerate.

"Artificial sweeteners, like sorbitol, can also irritate the bowel and trigger diarrhea," says Dr. Hanauer. As he explains, sugars in general are hard to digest and can cause loose stools. If that's true in your case, go easy on sugar-free candy and gum where these sweeteners are often used, and if you must satisfy your sweet tooth, stick to treats with natural sugars such as fruit.

If you think food allergies are causing your diarrhea, pay attention to other allergy symptoms after you eat such as bloating, stuffy nose or a burning throat. Consult an allergist who can help you identify and eliminate the foods or ingredients that bother your bowels. Remember, the more you control what goes in, the better you can control what comes out.

Spot spice sensitivities. Like some sugars, spicy or rich foods also can irritate your bowels and cause diarrhea. Be prudent with pepper and cautious with curry, as well as any other spices that seem to loosen your stools.

Slowing Down the Flow

So you followed all of these expert hints and still got diarrhea. When you're on the receiving end of the runs, you don't care how it started, you just want it to stop. But you're supposed to sit in pain and just let it drain, right? Wrong.

"Most people think—and a lot of doctors still recommend—letting diarrhea run its course, and that's just an antiquated notion," says Carlos Ricotti, M.D., a gastroenterologist at Trumbull Memorial Hospital in Warren, Ohio. According to Dr. Ricotti, using remedies to halt the trots isn't harmful in most cases. In fact, you'll be helping your body fend off dehydration by keeping more fluids in your system.

"Nihilists in the past have argued that you ought to sit there and literally gut it out. But why endure diarrhea? It's not a question of keeping bad bacteria in your body, it's a question of controlling the symptoms of diarrhea until your body naturally takes care of the germ," adds Dr. Ericsson.

If you're feverish, or if your diarrhea is bloody or especially profuse, see a doctor. Chances are you've picked up an infection and may need a medical prescription, advises Dr. Hanauer. Otherwise, here are some ways to keep up your strength and cork up the works.

Drink fluids. First and foremost, increase your intake of fluids at the first sign of diarrhea. Experts say that clear fluids, like water or broth, are best. Sports drinks such as Gatorade are also excellent for keeping up your strength during diarrhea, since they replace important minerals you're otherwise losing. Avoid beverages with caffeine or alcohol, though. These will cause you to lose even more fluids.

Be a B.R.A.T. To keep up your energy, but keep down on heavy foods that will only irritate your intestines more, doctors recommend sticking with the nutritionally packed but easily digested B.R.A.T. diet: bananas, rice, applesauce and toast.

Make a binding resolution. Bananas are also an essential ingredient of this fruit punch: Blend one ripe banana with eight-ounces of orange juice. The two fruits will replace lost vitamins and minerals. Plus, the banana packs the fiber pectin, which absorbs water and keeps it in your system.

Opt for OTCs. When natural remedies fail and you need to be about your daily business, two over-the-counter remedies can help. The most effective is loperamide, the active ingredient in several antidiarrheals such as Imodium A-D, which deactivates the nerves that trigger diarrhea. Bismuth subsalicylate relieves diarrhea, too, and you'll find it in that old reliable standby, Pepto-Bismol.

FAST FACTS

How common: Virtually everyone gets diarrhea at some point in time.

Risk factors: Men who have food allergies or sensitive stomachs are more likely to get diarrhea. Also, guys who travel frequently are more often exposed to the bacterial and parasitic infections of foreign lands.

Age group affected: There is no age restriction on diarrhea, but the very young and the elderly are more prone to the more serious result of diarrhea—dehydration.

Gender gap: Diarrhea affects men and women equally.

Who to see: Family doctor, gastroenterologist.

Both remedies are recommended for temporary use only, so don't take them for more than a day or two. And again, don't use either medication if your diarrhea is bloody or accompanied by a fever. In that case, you probably have an infection, and those antidiarrhea drugs will only prolong your problem.

See also Food Poisoning, Irritable Bowel Syndrome

Diverticular Diseases

How to Prevent Digestive Diversions

The path of digestion, like true love, does-n't always run smoothly. Ideally, it should go in one end and out the other, but detours crop up all too often toward the end of the road.

An estimated one-third of Americans develop dead-end pouches—diverticula—in their colons by age 50. In fact, diverticular disease is one of the most common in Western civilization.

This isn't nearly as bad as it sounds. The mere existence of the pouches—diverticulosis—is no big deal. Most of us can go through life without even knowing they're there. About 20 percent of men who have them, however, suffer some discomfort, and in 5 percent the pouches become infected and inflamed, causing a painful, and sometimes life-threatening, condition known as diverticulitis, which may require urgent medical treatment, even surgery.

An attack of diverticulitis is hard to ignore. Pain, often severe, is usually in the lower left part of the abdomen, but it can be elsewhere (in Asians, for some reason, it's more often on the right side). Diarrhea or constipation often come along.

Diverticulitis is easily confused with other things, however, even by an experienced doctor. The periodic pain and diarrhea of relatively mild attacks can look an awful lot like irritable bowel syndrome. When pain is focused in the upper right part of the abdomen, it may be mistaken for a stomach ulcer; on the lower right side, it can pass for appendicitis. One study found that just 7 percent of right-sided diverticulitis was diagnosed accurately before surgery.

While symptoms of diverticular disease are far more common with advancing years, they are increasing among younger people these days, particularly men. An attack of diverticulitis is likely to be especially nasty—and mistaken for something else—if you're under age 40.

A Dietary Disaster

Although the cause of diverticular diseases is unclear, the leading theory has to do with pressure. The colon moves food and waste matter along by contractions of its muscular wall. These contractions may, in time, push out weak parts of the colon wall, forming those dead-end pouches, known as diverticula.

Along with heart disease, diabetes and certain kinds of cancer, diverticulosis seems to be a "disease of civilization." While it's exceptionally common in the West—two-thirds of American men will have the condition if they live into their eighties and the overall rate of occurrence in England and many other developed regions isn't different from the United States—it's all but unheard of in undeveloped places. Two researchers who worked in Africa for 20 years, for example, reported never seeing a case of diverticulosis.

Could it be something we ate? The critical factor appears to be the content of the digestive tract. Waste matter in the large intestine gives the muscular contractions something to squeeze—thus easing the pressure on the colon walls themselves. What appears to be missing in the Western colon is sufficient bulk to absorb the pressure.

"According to the hypothesis, diverticula arise as the result of the colon's attempt to cope with the hard, desiccated Western stool," suggests Eamonn Quigley, M.D., chief of the Section of Gastroenterology and Hepatology at the University of Nebraska Medical Center in Omaha. It's no coincidence that the rise of diverticular disease in the West came some 30 years after industrialization made a refined diet within the reach of all.

Other parts of the world are seeing the same pattern. People in Singapore, once thought to be immune to the disorder, are beginning to suffer their share—along with other blessings of Western culture. Similarly, while only 1 percent of native Japanese men have diverticular disease, it's considerably more common among Japanese-Americans raised in Hawaii.

Putting fiber back into your diet is the key to diverticulosis risk reduction. And the earlier in life you start, the better.

Bulk up. "Change your diet to unprocessed foods," urges William B. Ruderman, M.D., chairman of the Department of Gastroenterology at Cleveland Clinic Florida in Fort Lauderdale. "The best source of fiber is whole-grain breads and cereal products." Increase other kinds of fiber—fruits and vegetables—in your diet, too.

Add bran. It's hard to get enough fiber (20 to 35 grams per day is the recommendation of experts) if you eat out much or rely on prepared foods for convenience. A dietary fiber supplement, like miller's bran or wheat germ, sprinkled on soups, salads and cereals can ensure sufficient roughage.

But don't take the fast track. "If you've been eating a low-fiber diet for 25 or 30 years, you can't change to a high-fiber diet all at once," says Dr. Ruderman. "You have to do it gradually to avoid cramping, bloating and abdominal distress."

Add water. To be bulky and soft, waste matter in the large intestine draws fluids from surrounding tissues. If you're not drinking enough water—and many men don't—more fiber can lead to dehydration. Six eight-ounce glasses of water (or other noncaffeine drink) daily is usually the recommended minimum.

Get the meat out. Increased consumption of beef and beef fat has also been identified as a potential culprit in diverticular disease. This probably works indirectly—the more meat in your diet, the less room for fiber-filled grains, fruits and vegetables.

Exercise. There's no proof that exercise (or the absence thereof) is related to the development of diverticular disease. "But exercise is important in generally maintaining healthy bowel function," Dr. Ruderman says.

Whole grains, vegetables, fruits, brans . . . less meat . . . more exercise—sound familiar? The same lifestyle that's recommended to reduce men's heart disease and cancer risk is your best bet against diverticulosis. Convenient, isn't it?

Dealing with Diverticular Diseases

Many men who have diverticulosis suffer no symptoms. Or they have some periodic pain, diarrhea or constipation, but it's uncertain whether this has anything to do with the condition. "This should be managed just like irritable bowel syndrome—with a high-fiber diet," says Dr. Quigley.

You may also be advised to strengthen the fiber element of your diet by using a supplement, like psyllium (Metamucil) or a cellulose product (Citrucel).

When a diverticulum has become infected, on the other hand, you need real medical help—usually several days of antibiotics, with a low-fiber diet to let the bowel rest. If it's severe, you may need to spend a few days in the hospital.

Once the attack has subsided, though, it's back to a serious high-fiber lifestyle. One study found that 10 percent of patients who went on a high-fiber diet after a diverticulitis attack experienced a reduction in the frequency of symptoms.

In addition, you'd do well to avoid seeds, popcorn, nuts—"anything that will get through the gastrointestinal tract undigested in particles sufficiently large to lodge in diverticula and act as the focus for infection," Dr. Quigley says.

Surgery is a discouraging word that's often spoken when diverticulitis comes up. The usual procedure is to remove the part of the large intestine that has the troublesome diverticula.

According to Dr. Quigley, it's generally necessary only when things have gotten seriously out of hand—an abscess that can't be drained less invasively, a hemorrhage that doesn't stop spontaneously or a narrowing that obstructs the intestine.

Whether repeated diverticulitis attacks need surgery depends a lot on the indi-

FAST FACTS

How common: Very. More than half of Americans have diverticula after age 40. Twenty percent have some symptoms.

Risk factors: Age, and a refined, low-fiber diet.

Age group affected: Progressively common with age. By the age of 80 more than two-thirds of men have diverticula.

Gender gap: Not much data, but appears equally common among men and women.

Who to see: If you encounter significant abdominal pain, see your family doctor, who likely will refer you to a gastroenterologist.

vidual situation. If the episodes are severe or becoming recurrent, it's time to consider surgery, says Dr. Ruderman. Elective surgery is better than emergency surgery, the latter being more difficult for the doctor and more difficult for you to recover from. If you have the procedure, although the disease has a life of its own, your risk of recurring problems is reduced.

See also Irritable Bowel Syndrome

Drug Dependency
Regaining Control of Your Cravings

Suppose you took an introductory class on producing a television show, and then some trusting person let you take over the control booth of the CBS Evening News. Folks watching at home would get a pretty warped view of the world, right?

Drugs do the same thing. They're impostors in your brain, very similar to the chemicals that your brain cells use to communicate—neurotransmitters. The drugs jump in where your brain's natural stimulants and tranquilizers should be. A drug like cocaine, for instance, gets into your "control room" and starts pushing your pleasure buttons willy-nilly. Unfortunately for you, by the time the "rush" is over, your brain's natural chemicals—the guys who really know what they're doing—have gone on vacation. You're left with an empty, lousy feeling.

Thus begins the cycle of addiction: You crave more drugs to feel good again. You get high, come down and feel bad once more. Even knowing the damage you're doing, you continue taking drugs.

Understanding Addiction

Drug dependency shows up in a complex blend of body, mind and behavior symptoms. You build up a tolerance to your drug, and in the face of withdrawal you compulsively take more—despite the significant problems that develop.

It's important to note that the word "drug" here does not imply "illegal drug." While it's true that illegals, like heroin, are particularly strong and addictive, legals, like nicotine, painkillers, sleeping pills and even caffeine, can hook you as well.

"Any time a person has trouble controlling or limiting his use of a drug, whether it's cough syrup or crack cocaine—whenever he has trouble or 'just cannot give it up'—he is showing a dependency on that drug," says Joan Mathews-Larson, Ph.D., director of the Health Recovery Center in Minneapolis. "When you add in the numbers of people smoking or abusing over-the-counter medications, the numbers are truly enormous."

A large scale study of five U.S. cities showed up to 1 in 14 men abuse or are dependent on drugs, and drug users cost the country nearly $7 billion a year in treat-

Where to Get Help

Check your local telephone book for regional services. Here are some national organizations that also might be of help.

— National Council on Alcoholism and Drug Dependence, 12 West 21st Street, New York, NY 10010. 1-800-NCA-CALL

— National Clearinghouse for Alcohol and Drug Information, P.O. Box 2345, Rockville, MD 20847. 1-800-729-6686

— National Cocaine Helpline, Phoenix House Foundation, 164 West 74th Street, New York, NY 10023. 1-800-COCAINE

— Narcotics Anonymous, World Service Office, P.O. Box 9999, Van Nuys, CA 91409. (818) 773-9999

— Cocaine Anonymous, P.O. Box 2000, Los Angeles, CA 90049. 1-800-347-8998

ment, loss of productivity and other expenses. An estimated 50 million Americans have used cocaine, and 6 million of them still do on a regular basis. Each day, 50,000 people try cocaine for the first time.

"Drug dependency is definitely not only a psychological problem," says Adam Lewenberg, M.D., an internist in private practice in New York City. "The vulnerability is the product of many things—the culture, genetics, an individual's psychology—but the dependency itself is a medical problem."

There are mysteries about susceptibility to drug addiction. "Some people will use heroin a couple of times and will get addicted to it totally. Other people can take it and leave it," says Joseph D. Beasley, M.D., a specialist in treating addiction and director of Comprehensive Medical Care in Amityville, New York. "But anybody who uses it over and over again—I think the same is true of cocaine—will eventually become dependent on it. These drugs are different from booze in that anybody who uses enough of them is probably going to become addicted to them." While some people have built-in barriers to developing alcoholism—75 percent of all Chinese, for instance—there is no such protection from cocaine or heroin, Dr. Beasley says.

And dependency is not peculiar to illegal drugs. For instance, benzodiazepines (Xanax or Valium) have been popular for treating insomnia, anxiety and convulsions since the 1960s. Research shows that nearly a third of the patients taking them four weeks or longer develop dependence.

Are You Hooked?

Maybe you toot a line of cocaine just to kick start the morning, and then a booster snort or two gets you through work. You hide it from your wife mostly—she can get so crabby about a little white powder. Your boss doesn't have a clue, but he *does* grumble about productivity.

Guys like you aren't addicts, right? Think again. You may be addicted if you match these criteria.

- You can't function normally without the drug.

- You've built up a tolerance to your drug of choice. This means you have to take increasing amounts to feel the same effect.

- You feel awful, physically and mentally, if you cut back or stop taking the drug.

- Your drug use is screwing up your family, friendships and job.

Keep Your Nose Clean

Let's face it: Intoxicating substances are available to virtually every American. Your best defense against addiction is to not start using drugs in the first place. Experts in addiction treatment offer these strategies for steering clear of drugs.

Know your family history. If you're more vulnerable to drug dependency than the average Joe, knowing that will keep you alert to trouble. "If you have a parent or grandparent or even brothers or sisters with this disease—the disease of chemical dependence or addiction—then you really have to be very cautious, because there is a hereditary tendency or susceptibility to addiction," says Max A. Schneider, M.D., clinical associate professor of psychiatry and human behavior at the University of California, Irvine, College of Medicine.

Research is demonstrating that some people have a genetic disorder limiting their production of calming neurotransmitters called dopamine and serotonin, says Dr. Beasley. "These are the kids who have the hyperactivity, perhaps attention deficit disorder, the person who is erratic, has trouble concentrating, tends to be nervous and tends to have trouble just sitting down calmly and dealing with one task at a time," Dr. Beasley says. Data show such people run a high risk of developing a problem if they start taking drugs, particularly stimulants. This is especially true of people whose hyperactivity has been treated with methylphenidate (Ritalin).

Take the CAGE test. If, despite all the warnings, you do dabble in drugs, watch for trouble signs. A simple test originally used with alcoholism also applies to drugs, says Dr. Schneider. Ask yourself whether any of these four factors have surfaced.

- Cutting down: Have you ever thought you should?
- Anger: Ever get angry because of what someone said about your habit?
- Guilt: Ever feel guilty about using drugs?
- Eye-opener: Ever need one just to get going in the morning—coffee, another stimulant or more of your drug of choice?

"If you have any one of those things, then you ought to be cautious—you're in trouble," says Dr. Schneider.

Just say, "Ain't gonna." The admonition "Just say no" is an oversimplification. People take risks every day—jaywalking, for example—knowing quite well that it's dangerous. But remember that giving in to drugs means surrendering control of your entire self. "Drugs are stronger than human beings," says Dr. Schneider. "Brain chemistry is affected by the drugs and, knowing that, one has to say, 'Hey, I want to stay in control at all times and I ain't gonna use that stuff.'"

Reach Out for Help

Damn, you're tired of it all. The physical lows and the equally low bank balances, the failed relationships and the embarrassing legal problems. But doing something about the cause—drug dependency—takes determination, and you should expect to encounter certain roadblocks.

Stigma is one, says Dr. Schneider. While medical professionals call drug dependency a disease, much of society still considers it a sign of weakness or depravity. Another barrier is that old devil "group peer pressure," the desire to fit in with the rest of your crowd—and face it, chemical addicts tend to run in packs.

Look inward, and you'll find another stumbling block: denial about your drug use problem. "This is one of the major things that keeps people from reaching out for help," says Dr. Schneider. "Denial consists of several items, and one is our egos: 'I'm bigger than that, I'm stronger than that, I can handle this stuff—it's not going to handle *me*.' Secondly, there is what we call euphoric recall. When we're under the influence of one of these drugs, they work: We get the buzz, we feel good, we are accomplishing our goal of blotting out our pain. We forget that we fall down or we get arrested or we're doing something illegal or that we've hurt our family by word or by deed. We forget that it's hurting our health."

In quitting drugs your goals are twofold. First, you need to detoxify—stop the drug taking and restore the body's natural chemistry—and you may need the assistance of your local hospital or detox center. Second, you need to "stay quit" with the help of an on-going program, because the potential for relapse is enormous. Here's advice from addiction experts on how to get help.

Eat your way clean. Good nutrition will help repair damage done to a drug user's body, says Dr. Beasley, and it will greatly reduce cravings for drugs. He recommends:

Eating a balanced diet and a wide variety of foods.

Eliminating or cutting back on sugar and foods with caffeine. They can cause mood swings, which may lead to destructive cravings.

Eating frequent small meals to keep blood sugar stable. Go no more than three hours without eating.

Cutting back on highly processed foods.

Taking vitamin and mineral supplements.

Go anonymous. When you're first seeking help for your drug problem, says Dr. Schneider, "the easiest, cheapest way is going to a Narcotics Anonymous or Cocaine Anonymous meeting." But be ready to combat a heavy dose of denial. "I can tell you what'll happen if you just walk in," he says. "A good share of the time you'll say, 'Hell, they're worse than I am—I'm not that bad. And I don't need this.' And that's where the ego and the denial come into play."

Consider medications. Some guys manage to kick drug habits on their own. But withdrawing from some drugs without a doctor's care can be deadly. "Particularly with the sedative hypnotics, the pills, the alcohol—people die in withdrawal if they aren't properly taken care of. They have seizures, they have cardiac arrest," says Dr. Schneider. Without medication the first five days of heroin withdrawal is excruciating. With cocaine or amphetamine withdrawal you become irritable and anxious—medications aren't essential in such cases, but they ease the way.

Find the right doc. You need a doctor with specialized training to help you get clean. "First thing I would say to my own doctor is, 'Do you know anything about chemical dependence, and do you know how to help detox somebody?' Because a lot of the docs don't. Or you call somebody from the National Council on Alcoholism and Drug Dependence or your county medical association, and get hold of one of those doctors because they are highly trained."

Beware of pop culture myths. Hollywood is rife with movie heroes who slug down whiskey and then gun down bad guys with the accuracy of a military sharpshooter. As alluring as such story lines are and as much as those images may appeal to your manliness, don't forget that it's all fiction. "You see the good stuff that happens to them," Dr. Schneider says of such movie heroes. "You don't see them when they're arrested, you don't see them when they're sick, you don't see them when they get divorced, you don't see them when they're in trouble and they say or do nasty things at home, and you don't see them when they can't get to work or they're not efficient on the job."

Remember: It's chronic. Just kicking a drug habit isn't enough. The potential

FAST FACTS

How common: An estimated 1 in 14 men in the United States abuse or are dependent on legal or illegal drugs.

Risk factors: Anyone can become dependent on drugs. Heredity, culture and family environment can play a role. Guys who abuse alcohol or have a history of mental disorders are more likely to abuse drugs.

Age group affected: All ages. Even kids get addicted to inhaling solvents.

Gender gap: Men overall are more likely to abuse or be dependent on drugs. Women, however, are more at risk for abusing prescription drugs because they use them more often.

Who to see: Inpatient and outpatient centers help patients detoxify and deal with the causes of their drug dependencies. Local support groups are usually listed in the telephone book.

for backsliding will follow you the rest of your life. "We've always tended to look at this as an acute illness. 'Well, you've sobered up and that's it,'" says Dr. Schneider. "And it's not—it's like diabetes. Who can get diabetes? Anybody, any age group. Who can get chemical dependence? Any age group. What's the cause? Well, we're not sure of the cause, but it's a chronic disease where relapses—like in arthritis, like in diabetes—occur. And I can't stress this strongly enough, because without an ongoing program the relapse rate is tremendously high."

Forget "social use." Drugs are cross addicting, Dr. Schneider says. Suppose you've kicked a cocaine habit, but you figure no harm could come from a couple tokes of marijuana at a party. Wrong. The euphoria will trigger your old craving for cocaine, and suddenly you're in trouble again. "Once a person's been addicted to one mood- or mind-altering drug, one has to be very cautious about using any of them," he says. Even nicotine and caffeine can lead you back to your old habit.

See also Alcoholism

Dry Skin

How to Be a Smooth Operator

A key proviso of the Macho Code holds that, for a man, a weather-beaten face is a desirable thing. Hence we can assume that John Wayne, while he was riding around the desert in all those Westerns, wasn't packing a bottle of Oil of Olay in his saddlebag.

In real life dry skin isn't all it's cracked up to be. "It can be quite uncomfortable, for one thing," says Nelson Lee Novick, M.D., associate clinical professor of dermatology at Mount Sinai School of Medicine of the City University of New York. "If it persists, it can lead to itching, and itching leads to scratching, so you set up the whole itch-scratch-itch cycle.

"Dryness can also lead to cracking of the skin, and that can be very uncomfortable, especially because it can lead to bacterial infection," Dr. Novick adds. "In its most severe scenario dry skin can lead to dermatitis and eczema, which results in a rash, an actual eruption on the skin."

Because so many men are rough on their hands in their work—exposing them to wind, sun and other chafing elements, like chemicals and detergents—that tends to be where dry skin problems develop most. "Dry skin is aggravated by what men do with their hands," says Hillard H. Pearlstein, M.D., assistant clinical professor of dermatology at Mount Sinai School of Medicine of the City University of New York. "Also, when you use your hands a lot, dry skin bothers you more there, and you seek treatment. Plenty of guys may have dry skin on their backs, but we never see them."

Feet tend to be the second-most frequent source of dry skin complaints from men, Dr. Pearlstein says, for the same reason.

What causes dry skin? The answer might surprise you. "There's an erroneous assumption that dry skin results from a loss of oil," says Dr. Pearlstein. "People think they need to use oil on their skin to replace the oil they've lost. In fact, dry skin is the result of a loss of water. So putting oil on the skin works because it helps hold water in."

Water Conservation

Knowing that water is the secret of a supple epidermal environment, it doesn't take a genius to figure out how to prevent dehydration. "Avoid things that take

186

How common: Everybody gets dry skin once in a while, although people with naturally oily complexions will have less trouble than those who don't.

Risk factors: Dry air, whether it be on the ski slopes or in a poorly ventilated office building, is a prime cause of dry skin problems. Athletes who take a lot of showers or baths may develop problems as well.

Age group affected: Our skin tends to be less able to keep itself from drying out as we age, although it doesn't usually cause problems until we're into our sixties.

Gender gap: Men have larger oil glands than women do around their face and shoulder areas, which means they're slightly less susceptible to dry skin in those areas. On the other hand, men still tend to spend more time outdoors than women do and less time moisturizing, which makes them more susceptible.

Who to see: If the problem doesn't go away when you use moisturizers, see a dermatologist.

moisture out of the skin," says Sheryl Clark, M.D., assistant professor of medicine at Cornell Medical Center in New York City. Here's how:

Stay greasy. People are a lot like dirty plates, according to Paul Lazar, M.D., professor of clinical dermatology at Northwestern University Medical School in Chicago. Hold either of them under hot water for a long time and the grease will come off. What's good for dishes, though, is bad for skin. The solution for people with dry skin problems is simple, Dr. Lazar says: "Take fewer and shorter showers or baths, and use lukewarm water instead of hot water."

Pat and slather. Virtually every dermatologist recommends that guys with dry skin use a moisturizer, especially after bathing. So put aside your macho disdain for body lotions and start spreading.

Most also recommend that you pat, rather than rub, yourself almost dry when you get out of the tub or shower. That way, you'll seal some of the dampness in when you moisturize. Ivor Caro, M.D., a dermatologist at the Virginia Mason Clinic in Seattle, stresses that the water you leave on your skin can evaporate rapidly, so it's important to apply the moisturizer quickly. Otherwise, Dr. Caro tells his patients, go ahead and dry off thoroughly, then apply the moisturizer at a more leisurely pace.

Educate yourself. Women seem to learn all about skin care products in grade school, but lots of guys wouldn't know a vanishing cream from a petroleum jelly.

Not to worry, says Dr. Pearlstein. Choosing a moisturizer is more a matter of personal taste than anything else, since they all get the job done. Nor do you need to spend a lot of money; Dr. Pearlstein says Crisco is just as effective a moisturizer as some fancy concoction from the cosmetics counter.

As a general rule, he says, lotions are going to be less greasy than creams, and creams are less greasy than ointments, so you may want to go with a lotion while you have your business clothes on. There's a slight risk of an allergic reaction to the fragrances used in many moisturizers and soaps, so many dermatologists recommend avoiding the scented varieties.

Stop lying. The lye in soaps gets skin clean but also dries it out. Dr. Clark recommends using mild soaps that contain no fragrances or preservatives. Brands that she has found to be effective include Dove (unscented), Neutrogena and Cetaphil.

Shave smart. If you have dry skin, splashing an astringent aftershave on your face is like throwing salt in an open wound. Moisturizing aftershaves are available, says Dr. Novick. Ask your druggist for a recommendation.

Oil all over. One of the best methods of moisturizing your skin, Dr. Pearlstein says, is to put a little bath oil in your tub. Make sure to soak yourself for a few minutes *before* you put in the oil so that your skin gets moisturized, though. "A lot of people make the mistake of putting the oil in first," he says. "Once the oil coats the skin, you've defeated your whole purpose."

the male file

Why does skin wrinkle when you're in water for a long time?
Answer: The wrinkles are caused by the skin absorbing the water.

Ear Pain

Coping with the Pressure

The last time you had an earache you were in a crib, screaming so loud you woke the neighbors. Now here you are, in a grown-up bed, wishing once again that someone would come along and get rid of the stabbing, throbbing pain.

Chances are you have otitis media, an inflammation of the middle ear. It's not the only cause of ear pain—later in this chapter we'll deal with a bunch—but it's by far the most common, and it doesn't afflict infants alone.

Otitis media usually strikes in the winter and early spring, when a cold or sinus infection inflames the eustachian tube, which brings air to the middle ear from the nose and mouth. The infection enables bacteria or viruses to enter the middle ear. Pus builds up behind the eardrum, causing the pain and feelings of pressure and blockage. That's when you wish you were a baby again, so someone would cuddle you.

Sound Advice

Curling up in someone's arms is not a bad idea for grown men either. But then do something for your earache. Here are some tips.

Take your medicine. "Infections in the ear usually need an antibiotic," says Thomas J. McDonald, M.D., chairman of the Department of Otolaryngology–Head and Neck Surgery at the Mayo Clinic in Rochester, Minnesota. If an antibiotic is prescribed, be sure to take the full course of treatment (usually 10 to 14 days), even if the pain goes away before that.

If the pain is accompanied by a cold or allergy, your doctor might recommend an antihistamine or a decongestant. And a pain reliever is always a good idea. "An over-the-counter analgesic can be very effective in reducing the pain," says Dr. McDonald.

Drop in on it. Warm up some mineral oil or baby oil and drop it into the ear canal. That will help relieve the pain, says Dr. McDonald. Don't use drops, however, if the ear is draining pus.

And don't be alarmed by the drainage. "It's a good thing," says Dr. McDonald. "It means the eardrum has ruptured and the pus can leave." If that happens, don't think you'll never hear again. Ruptured eardrums usually heal just fine.

Warm it up. Dr. McDonald recommends applying moist heat to the ear for five or ten minutes every two hours. One way is to place a wet washcloth over the ear. Another is to soak a cotton ball in warm water and insert it in the crevice beside the ear opening. It's okay if the warm water seeps into the ear.

Keep your head up high. Lying flat can make the pain worse. So, stay seated or at least prop yourself up, even if you're trying to sleep. "If your head is slightly elevated, it improves the ventilation of the middle ear," explains Dr. McDonald.

Swimmer's Ear: How to Get Dry

If your outer ear is extremely tender to the touch, chances are you have swimmer's ear. When water gets trapped in the ear canal it creates the kind of soggy environment that bacteria love. An infected canal can swell up, causing pain and a blocked-up feeling. Fortunately, it's easy to avoid and to treat.

Blow dry your ears. Swim plugs can help keep your ears dry, but they tend to leak. "After swimming hold a hair dryer several inches from your ear and blow warm air into it," advises William Slattery, M.D., an otolaryngologist at the House Ear Clinic in Los Angeles. "The temperature should be comfortable, not too hot," he adds.

Use a drop of prevention. After a swim you can restore acidity in the ear canal with antiseptic ear drops. This is especially useful if your ears feel moist. You can get products, like Swim Ear, at a pharmacy, or mix a batch of your own. Dr. Slattery recommends a 50-50 mixture of white vinegar and water. "Fill a bulb syringe with the mixture and gently let it run into your ear," he says. "Or, you can use an eyedropper. Hold your head to the side and place six to ten drops in the ear."

The same procedure will help if you have an infection. But don't use drops if your eardrum is perforated or your ear is draining, warns Dr. Slattery.

Flying: Equalize the Pressure

Know why your ears feel blocked and painful when you fly? The eustachian tube is unable to equalize the change in air pressure. The eardrum gets sucked inward, muffling sound and stretching the membrane. Here are some ways to ensure comfortable ear travel.

Don't fly with a cold. "If you're having trouble breathing through your nose, there's a good chance your eustachian tube is blocked up," says Ronald Amedee, M.D., associate professor of otolaryngology at Tulane University Medical Center in New Orleans. In which case it will have trouble equalizing pressure. "If you have a cold, put off the flight," he says. "If you can't, use a decongestant nasal spray about 30 minutes before boarding. A mild antihistamine, like Actifed, can also be helpful."

How common: About 22 million people a year see physicians for earaches. Four million are over age 15.

Risk factors: Infections, pressure changes, various conditions in the head and face.

Age group affected: Earaches occur mainly to children. But ear pain can affect anyone.

Gender gap: None for infections; men are more likely to encounter impact noise and blows to the head.

Who to see: Family doctor or an otolaryngologist for ear pain related to infections or trauma.

Some antihistamines can make you drowsy and don't mix well with certain other drugs, so ask your doctor first before self-prescribing.

Keep gulping. Swallowing activates the muscle that opens the eustachian tube. That's why it's good to chew gum or suck on a mint, especially during descent.

Swallow and spray. Dr. McDonald recommends this combination just before takeoff and descent: "Put some gum or candy in your mouth, close off one side of your nose and spray decongestant into the other nostril, swallowing at the same time. Then do the same thing on the other side." The spray enters the eustachian tube and opens it up.

Stay awake. We don't swallow as often when we're asleep, hence it's harder to adjust to pressure changes. "Delay your nap until you achieve cruising altitude," Dr. Slattery advises, "and ask the flight attendant to wake you up before the plane descends."

Blow it out your ear. Frequent flyers are familiar with this maneuver for unblocking the eustachian tube: Pinch your nostrils shut; take a mouthful of air; blow out, using pressure from the cheek and throat muscles (not your chest or diaphragm) as if you were trying to force your fingers to fly off your nostrils.

Traumas: See a Doctor

Loud noises can knock you on your ear. While the pain you feel after a rock concert is probably from muscle tension and may go away once you relax, impact sounds, like explosions, gunshots and jet engine blasts, can do greater damage. "The extreme change of pressure can perforate the eardrum," says Michael K. Wynne, Ph.D., associate professor in the Department of Otolaryngology at the Indiana University School of Medicine in Indianapolis. If you feel great pain after a sudden loud noise, see a doctor.

Other traumas can also be a pain in the ear. A blow to the side of the head—from an accident or contact sport, for example—can bruise the cartilage of the outer ear or cause damage inside, or possibly some part of the face or neck that refers pain to the ear. Again, any pain that follows a trauma should be checked by a physician, says Dr. Wynne.

Maybe It's Not Really Your Ear

For a small organ the ear has a huge supply of nerves. That means disorders elsewhere can feel like they're in the ear. This is known as referred pain. The real problem when you feel ear pain might be anything from damaged muscles or joints in the head or neck to an infected sinus to pressure from a throat tumor.

If your physician finds nothing wrong with the ear itself, he will look for other causes and perhaps refer you to another specialist.

Among the more common sources of referred pain to the ear are jaw problems known as temporomandibular disorders, or TMD. Ira Klemons, D.D.S, Ph.D., director of the Center for Head and Facial Pain in South Amboy, New Jersey, recommends that you see a head-and-face pain specialist if you have one or more of the following symptoms along with ear pain: headaches, pain in the face, pain when you compress your jaw, difficulty opening your mouth more than an inch and a half or clicking or grating sounds when you open or close your mouth.

See also Hearing Loss, TMD

Emphysema

How to Breathe Easy

You've seen it somewhere: An emaciated old man in a wheelchair or on a park bench, a little steel bottle next to him, clear tubing running up to a clip on his nose.

Emphysema is not, as the old Dutch immigrants used to say, pretty for nice. It's ugly to see, ugly to have.

But more than anything else, it's sad—sad because the irreparable injury to the lungs that is emphysema is almost always preventable.

"Cigarette smoking is far and away the primary cause—numbers 1 through 26 on the list," says Mark Rosen, M.D., chief of the Division of Pulmonary and Critical Care Medicine at Beth Israel Medical Center in New York City. "If you eliminated smoking in society, you'd essentially eliminate most emphysema along with it."

Emphysema, which normally takes decades to develop, is simply defined as a condition caused by the irreparable destruction of lung tissue—usually more than 30 percent before symptoms become noticeable.

When you smoke, the fumes you inhale destroy the walls of the alveoli, the air sacs in your lungs. Individual alveoli lose their elasticity, and consequently their ability to deflate, according to Barry Make, M.D., director of Pulmonary Rehabilitation at the National Jewish Center for Immunology and Respiratory Medicine in Denver.

"At a certain point, the patient starts to experience shortness of breath during normal activity," Dr. Make says. "He has to work harder to get the same amount of air into his lungs, his heart's working harder and he's burning substantially more calories every day. In severe cases people with emphysema lose weight—these patients are emaciated, they look like cancer victims with huge chests."

The enlarged chest is a consequence of the lungs' lost ability to deflate. Another problem: Because he exhales less efficiently, a man with emphysema may develop higher levels of carbon dioxide in his lungs—the substance which normally triggers the urge to breathe when it reaches a certain level. The result: Desensitized lungs, which do not respond normally to carbon dioxide stimulus.

But the consequences aren't only physical.

"As the disease progresses, his work capacity drops—he just can't get enough air—so employment may be affected," Dr. Make says. "And it really changes the role in the family: Men are conditioned to be the strong ones, and it gets uncomfortable for everyone when he can't perform that role anymore—depression and reduced sexuality are pretty common results."

To make a bad situation worse, there's very little of substance that can be done to improve the situation.

Alvin Teirstein, M.D., professor of medicine and director of the Division of Pulmonary and Critical Care Medicine at Mount Sinai Medical Center in New York City, concurs.

"The damage is irreversible," Dr. Teirstein says. "We can provide some relief for the chronic bronchitis that's usually associated with emphysema, and we can often achieve some improvement by prescribing exercise—they can breath more easily if the chest muscles are strengthened. But short of experimental procedures or a lung transplant—which are the very last things we'll do—treatment is essentially ameliorative."

So what can you do? The answer is obvious. Don't start smoking if you don't now. And if you do smoke—stop.

FAST FACTS

How common: In smokers—very; in others—almost nonexistent. The actual numbers: nearly 2 million diagnosed cases in the United States; more than 16,000 deaths each year.

Risk factors: Smoking, but a small percentage of patients—5 to 10 percent—are at increased risk because of an inherited deficiency in a blood protein called alpha-1 antitrypsin.

Age group affected: Anyone who smokes; secondhand smoke presents little risk to nonsmokers.

Gender gap: None, but incidence is rising among women as the number of women smokers rises.

Who to see: Pulmonary specialists, internists.

Fatigue

Solving the Energy Crisis

Most men talk of fatigue as if it were some kind of cold or flu—something they get in spite of everything they do, not because of it. When that heavy-lidded, heavy-limbed sensation creeps in, stealing your best moves and brightest ideas, you need to blame something. Why not fatigue?

But that's just a tired old excuse. In most cases, fatigue is not the enemy—you are. Especially if you scrimp on sleep and exercise, go head-to-head with stress and pay closer attention to box scores than good nutrition.

Much as we'd like to think otherwise, fatigue is not some external bug we've been infected with—it's usually something we generate ourselves. When our body's physical and mental reserves are exhausted from too much working, playing or worrying, it's only natural that we lose our ability to think and act quickly and efficiently.

But with a few simple moves, you can outsmart fatigue and get a bigger charge out of life.

The ABCs of Zzzs

You don't need a medical degree to understand that you need to sleep. Nevertheless, plenty of men dismiss the value of a good night's rest. One government study found that roughly half of all men sleep less than the eight hours most of us need. We pay the price—in lost energy.

"The root of fatigue in the average American is inadequate or insufficient sleep at night," says Thomas Roth, Ph.D., chief of the Division of Sleep Disorders Medicine at Henry Ford Hospital in Detroit. Because of our increasingly busy lifestyles, sleep times have been steadily decreasing over the past 15 years, Dr. Roth explains.

If your energy level plunges between two and four in the afternoon, you could probably use a few more winks. If you sleep longer on weekends than on weekdays, or if you need two alarms to shake you from your leaden slumbers, odds are you're a certified member of the national zombiefest. But you don't have to be.

"There are a lot of tools you can build into your life to fight run-of-the-mill fatigue," says M. F. Graham, M.D., a Dallas physician and author of *Inner Energy: How*

195

to Overcome Fatigue. "If you get into a pattern that incorporates these tools, you'll find that chronic fatigue is much, much less of a problem." Here's what experts recommend.

Know your needs. Although we often think of eight hours as being the "right" amount of pillow time, every man's needs are different. Whether you need nine hours of sleep or you can get by on six, there's not much you can do to change your essential biology. "I suspect a lot of men in their thirties walk around bragging that they can get by with five hours of sleep," says Dr. Roth. "You cannot—I'll repeat this—you cannot teach yourself to sleep less."

So how much sleep do you need? The next time you're on vacation, see how much sleep you actually get, suggests Rick Ricer, M.D., associate professor of family medicine at the University of Cincinnati. Once you're freed from the tyranny of late-night paperwork and a 5:00 A.M. alarm, your natural body clock will automatically set the pace. Once you know how much sleep you need naturally, you can make sure you get that same amount once you're back on the job and in your normal schedule.

Take a nap. If you can't get the sleep you need at night, you can help make up the deficit with naps during the day. While napping may run counter to our society's 18-hour-day ethic, it's a natural—and respected—refresher elsewhere.

Studies have shown that naps as brief as 30 minutes can help improve alertness and sharpen your ability to perform complicated mental tasks, says Dr. Roth. The best time to nap is generally between one and four in the afternoon—a time when most of us are sleepiest anyway.

Run It Down

It's curious, but the times we feel most tired are often the times we're not exerting ourselves as much. "Regular exercise makes you stronger. You have more endurance so you're able to deal with day-to-day fatigue better," says Bruce Beall, a fitness counselor and executive director of the George Pocock Memorial Rowing Center in Seattle and a member of the 1984 U.S. Olympic rowing team. "Plus, exercise teaches you how to handle fatigue. You learn to persevere just a little bit longer."

Here are a few easy ways to help keep your mind and body at full steam.

Activate with aerobics. While almost any exercise can help fight fatigue, the best is aerobic exercise. It doesn't matter whether you ride your bike, walk briskly around the block or indulge in some half-court one-on-one. Whatever your activity of choice, aerobic exercise, done for a minimum of 20 minutes two or three times a week, will help improve circulation, muscle tone and even your outlook, experts say.

Ditch the deskbound doldrums. Physical activity shouldn't be limited to the

FAST FACTS

How common: With the possible exception of Superman, virtually all men will experience fatigue at some point in their lives.

Risk factors: Stress, inadequate sleep, poor nutrition, lack of exercise.

Age group affected: Men of all ages get fatigue, although it usually gets worse by the time we hit our thirties.

Gender gap: Men and women are equally likely to succumb to fatigue, though men are less likely to deal with it until it becomes a serious problem.

Who to see: Family doctor if fatigue is interfering with your life.

gym. Since sitting at your desk for long periods of time only heaps on the fatigue, give yourself regular breaks. Walk down the hall or up stairs. Do a few push-ups against your desk. Even the shortest bout of activity will help stretch stiff muscles and pump a bit more oxygen to your brain.

"Taking a break every 45 minutes just to stretch out will really help a lot in fighting fatigue," says Dr. Ricer. "It doesn't take long—30 seconds is enough."

Work out, but don't wear out. While adding some exercise to your life is an energy booster, overdoing it just opens the energy drain. So if you're wiped out after playing four sets of tennis, then you should probably cut back to two or three, says Dr. Graham. A more objective measure is to check your pulse rate each morning before getting out of bed. If your resting pulse has gradually increased or if you feel "hungover" or fatigued, you may be overdoing it.

Fatigue-Fighting Fuels

Your body is an elite machine with a high-performance engine. Naturally, it requires premium fuel. "Nutrition is of the utmost importance," says Dr. Graham. "The main thing is to maintain a good, balanced diet." Here are a few other things to try.

Load up on carbs. Nutritionists agree that the highest-energy (and healthiest) diets are packed with complex carbohydrates, like whole grains, pastas and fruits. And since a high-carb diet leaves little room for dietary fats, it will help keep your weight down as well.

Experts recommend striving for a diet with about 15 percent of calories from protein, 55-65 percent of calories from carbohydrates, and no more than 30 percent from fat.

Maximize mealtimes. To get the most mileage from your diet, it's not only what you eat but when you eat that's important. Breakfast is key since it's your body's chance to stoke up when its nutrient stores are at their lowest. A good breakfast includes skim milk or yogurt for protein, plus cereal or whole-wheat toast for the complex carbs.

Forego fatiguing feasts. After packing in a large meal, about the only moves your body makes are those involved in digestion. That's why you often feel sluggish right after lunch or dinner. If big meals leave you stupefied, experts say, try eating smaller amounts more often.

Drink smart. While caffeinated beverages, like coffee and soda, provide quick pick-me-ups, the benefits typically fade after a few cups. The same is true with alcohol. It can be a stimulant in small amounts but a depressant in larger amounts.

"If you want to avoid fatigue, avoid alcohol," says Dr. Graham. Meanwhile, drink plenty of water, since dehydration can cause fatigue. Experts recommend drinking at least eight eight-ounce glasses of water a day. Avoid drinking huge quantities at one time, however.

Swallow some insurance. While a good diet will provide all the vitamins and minerals you need, it may be helpful to supplement your diet with an all-purpose multivitamin. "They're an insurance policy," says Dr. Graham.

Don't Mess with Stress

When we hear the words "stress fatigue," most of us think of collapsing buildings or bridges. But stress can also fatigue much smaller structures, such as men. And unlike buildings, which typically endure until some catastrophic event drops them to rubble, guys can cave in from everyday wear and tear.

"The most common causes of run-of-the-mill fatigue in men are the stresses of regular life—changes in income, marital difficulties or even good stresses, like a promotion or a new job," says Dr. Ricer. "Fatigue is common in a stressful world like ours, and men are certainly not immune."

You don't have to let stress wear you out. Here's what experts suggest.

Work it out. Exercise does more than reduce physical problems that can lead to fatigue. It's also an excellent stressbuster when used wisely and in proper "doses." "The natural outlet for stress is exercise," says Dr. Graham. Have an important meeting at two? Getting in a walk or run at noon will help get your mind and body in fighting trim. As a rule, experts say, breaking a sweat at least three times a week will help keep your energy high and your stress levels down.

Fire up some fun. If all you ever do is sleep, eat and work, don't be surprised if your emotional engine is getting hard to start. "Find yourself a hobby you love," suggests Dr. Ricer. "You'll feel a lot more energized if you have something to look forward to each day."

Take a few deep breaths. Experts have found that a brief bout of deep breathing is a fast way to help clear your mind and body of accumulated stress and fatigue. In fact, experts say one reason you may be fatigued in the first place is that you're breathing too shallowly, causing a reduction in the oxygen supply to your body and brain.

"Just close the office door, put a 'no visiting' sign on it for a few minutes and take some deep, abdominal breaths," Dr. Graham suggests. Be aware, however, that *excessive* deep breathing can also cause problems.

When Fatigue Is Something More

Not all fatigue is caused by stress, poor nutrition or inadequate sleep. It can also be caused by more serious problems, ranging from depression or diabetes to hepatitis, mononucleosis, thyroid disease or chronic fatigue syndrome.

"If your fatigue doesn't go away with simple measures and you're still very tired all the time, then you need to be checked out," says Dr. Ricer. If you're feeling worn out for longer than a week, you should probably see your doctor. But if fatigue is also accompanied by high fever, dizziness, nausea or bloody stools, you'll want to see a doctor right away. "Fatigue can be part of any chronic illness. It's important you see your family doctor," says Dr. Ricer.

Fever

Protection from Friendly Fire

In war foot soldiers who are under attack will call in an air strike. When it's your immune system that's on the front line, your body responds with a fever. The heat may be uncomfortable and bothersome, but ultimately it's on your side, because it creates a hostile environment for the enemy invaders.

While fever is occasionally caused by such things as medications or even a stressful situation, more often it's triggered by infection—viral illnesses such as colds or flu, for example, or by bacterial bugs, like salmonella.

As long as your fever stays below 103°F, experts say, it probably isn't medically necessary to lower it. The heat, after all, may be giving your immune system an edge. But when your forehead feels hot enough to burn toast, and those waves of intermittent, tooth-rattling chills are making you feel like a castanet, you're going to want to turn the temperature down.

Some Like It Hot

Although we're taught early on to respect the onset of fever—if only because all that stood between us and a day home from school was that magical number *98.6*—studies suggest that there isn't one temperature that's "right" for everyone.

"Generally, the range is between 96.5° and 100.5°F," says Thomas C. Rosenthal, M.D., professor of family medicine at the School of Medicine and Biomedical Sciences at State University of New York at Buffalo. "A temperature above 101°F would be considered a fever."

Normally, your body is kept at a more-or-less constant temperature by the hypothalamus, a "thermostat" inside the brain. But when the immune system encounters an invader—a flu virus, for example—it releases a protein called interleukin-1. This in turn trips a series of reactions that cause the hypothalamus to raise its "set point," causing your temperature to rise.

Of course, some guys' engines just naturally run a little hot. A temperature of 100°F that's right for you, for example, could indicate a fever in someone else. If you're curious about what's normal for you, try taking your temperature about every four hours during the day for three days in a row. This will tell you what your normal temperature range is. Once you know this, you'll have a better idea in the future just where fevers begin and end.

How Long Is Enough

It's important to remember that fever, unlike the bugs that caused it, is merely a symptom of some other illness. Keeping yourself healthy should be the first line of defense.

If, despite your best efforts, you still get sick, keep in mind that fever is rarely dangerous. "Generally, in a normal, healthy, nonpregnant individual you would have to go over 104°, 105°F maybe, before elevation in temperature will cause any major problems, and even then it would have to be for a long period of time," says Matthew J. Kluger, Ph.D., director of the Institute for Basic and Applied Medical Research at the Lovelace Institutes in Albuquerque, New Mexico.

But there are exceptions. For guys with heart trouble, for example, even a moderate fever can be troublesome, says Dr. Kluger. This is because as the body's temperature rises—say, from 98.6° to 102°F—your metabolic rate increases by up to 25 percent, putting additional strain on the heart.

In addition, any fever that doesn't go away on its own after a couple of days—or sooner if it's also accompanied by diarrhea, vomiting, severe headache, pain while urinating or other serious symptoms—should be treated by a physician. "I think you really need to see your doctor with any fever that hangs around more than 48 hours," says Michael Fleming, M.D., a family physician in private practice in Shreveport, Louisiana. "You don't need to tough it out."

Bright Lights, Big Heat

Your portfolio is organized, your tie is straight and the board of directors is waiting. So why do you suddenly feel like your head is on fire?

"We call it a stress-induced, or psychological or emotional, fever," says Matthew J. Kluger, Ph.D., director of the Institute for Basic and Applied Medical Research at the Lovelace Institutes in Albuquerque, New Mexico.

While stress-induced fever has not been extensively studied, animal studies indicate it's similar to fever brought on by infection, in which levels of fever-regulating hormones rise, causing the body's thermostat to be temporarily reset.

"There's a German word, *lampenfieber*, which literally means lamp fever," says Dr. Kluger. "That's the German equivalent of stage fright."

Stress-induced fever is not something you need to treat or worry about, Dr. Kluger says. It's probably just one of your body's defenses—part of the fight-or-flight mechanism that prepares the body for action.

"It's speculation, but I would imagine that psychological fever probably has some protective function," says Dr. Kluger. "That is, it enhances or revs up your host defense responses, which would make sense in terms of the possible injury that could be associated with a stressful event, whether it's a bacterial infection or injury."

Quenching the Flames

Even though it's not true that a high temperature can boil your brain, it can make you feel as though something is cooking up there. To beat the heat and keep yourself more comfortable, here's what experts recommend.

Cool off with an OTC. Perhaps the quickest way to turn down the heat is with medications, like aspirin, acetaminophen, ibuprofen or naproxen—nonprescription painkillers that have the additional effect of inhibiting the enzyme that's responsible for turning up the thermostat.

Never, however, give aspirin to children because of the risk of Reye's syndrome, a serious neurological condition. Give them acetaminophen instead.

Stick to a schedule. When taking aspirin or other fever-lowering medications, it's important to take them regularly, following the directions on the package. Otherwise, you may experience uncomfortable temperature swings as your fever drops after you take the medication and then peaks again after its effects wear off, says Dr. Rosenthal.

Stay fluid. When you have a fever, it's not unusual to sweat away two or even three times the usual amount of water. To prevent yourself from becoming dehydrated, drink plenty of fluids. This is particularly true if you're not taking medications to turn down the heat. "For every degree that your temperature is above normal, drink about four glasses or more of water a day," says Dr. Rosenthal.

Take a lukewarm soak. Settling in for a relaxing bath can help relax muscles and generally make you feel cooler. Forget, however, the notion of cooling yourself with a cold bath or by dousing yourself with rubbing alcohol. This will just cause your body to struggle to maintain the feverish temperature, possibly making you even more uncomfortable, says Dr. Rosenthal.

Don't bother bundling. Although the chills that often accompany fever can send you scrambling for your down jacket, you don't want to overdo it by adding layer upon layer of clothing. "If you have a fever, you shouldn't bundle up in a bunch of blankets and take the risk of overheating," says Dr. Rosenthal.

Catch up on rest. "Activity is going to make you feel worse. One of the big things I recommend is rest," says Dr. Fleming. "As I tell people, 'Be a couch potato.'"

Eat carefully. Forget Grandma's advice about feeding colds and starving fevers—or is it the other way around? Either way, it means absolutely nothing. "You should eat whatever you can without forcing foods down," says Dr. Rosenthal. "White rice is a good choice, and toast, juices and generally fruits. They help keep your nutrition up while you're sick and they don't challenge your digestive system any more than it's already challenged by fighting off an infection."

Don't spread the wealth. Think of your nose as a virus-laden aerosol can. One good sneeze can spray droplets as far away as 12 feet. So be considerate and cover your nose with a tissue when Mount Schnozzola erupts.

"Generally, it takes influenza five to seven days to get better, and upper respiratory infections seven to ten days to get better," says Dr. Rosenthal. "So you're going to want to be cautious about exposing other people to your illness, particularly other people that may have their health compromised by taking certain medications, or those with cancer or AIDS, or the elderly."

Flatulence

Be Gone with the Wind

Hippocrates investigated flatulence. Benjamin Franklin, too, lent studious thought to a cure for "escaped wind"—possibly because he spent so much time closeted in stuffy rooms with overfed patricians whose occasional ventings set his wig standing on end. Hippocrates couldn't find a cure, nor could Franklin, and as anyone who has ridden public transportation knows, gas is still very much with us.

Why? Because we're all up against some irrevocable arithmetic.

Normal humans generate between one-half pint and two quarts of gas per day, says Michael Oppenheim, M.D., who practices in Los Angeles and is the author of *The Complete Book of Better Digestion*. That gas has to go somewhere. According to one study, that somewhere is on the other side of your pants. "One study showed that, among a group of young men, passage of rectal gas occurred on the average of 13 times daily," says Dr. Oppenheim. "Twenty-one passages per day was the upper limit of normal."

Most flatulence is produced by bacteria living in your large bowel. These bacteria break down the food you eat, giving off gases of their own. When lots of oxygen is present, this bacterial foodfest exudes three relatively innocuous gases—hydrogen, carbon dioxide and methane. Unfortunately, there isn't much oxygen in the colon, giving rise to complex gases neither science, nor your dinner guests, have been able to fully identify.

There are two things you need to know up front about rectal gas: "Everybody thinks they have too much, and in most cases they don't," says Dr. Oppenheim. "And rectal gas is never the sign of a serious disease."

What Goes Down Must Come Out

There's something else you might already expect—there's no getting rid of rectal gas entirely. Killing off bacteria in the bowels is the most obvious solution. It's been tried with different types of antibiotics, but bowel bacteria have proved resilient, and science remains defeated. Don't let advertisements for commercial products lead you to believe otherwise.

FAST FACTS

How common: Everyone experiences flatulence.

Risk factors: High-carbohydrate and high-fiber foods (like beans) that can't be completely digested. Dairy products if lactase deficient.

Age group affected: All age groups.

Gender gap: Though the fairer sex would have us believe otherwise, men are no more apt to have flatulence than women.

Who to see: Flatulence rarely requires medical intervention. But if it is truly excessive, consider seeing your family doctor or a gastroenterologist.

"Among the triumphs of medical science you won't find a single drug that eliminates gas," says Dr. Oppenheim.

Though you can't eliminate gas, you can cut down substantially on the supply. It's not complicated, either. In short, you tweak what you eat.

"Diet is really the key to treatment," says Steven Peikin, M.D., head of the Division of Gastroenterology at the Robert Wood Johnson Medical School and Cooper Hospital in Camden, New Jersey, and author of *Gastrointestinal Health*. "Restriction of the foods that give you gas is the way to go. If you avoid gas-forming foods, then your gas load is much lower."

Top offenders? Glad you asked.

Beware of lactose. "If you have flatulence the first thing to rule out is do you or do you not have lactose intolerance," says Dr. Peikin.

Lactose intolerance is a low intestinal level of the enzyme lactase. Without this enzyme you can't break down lactose, the sugar common in many dairy foods including milk. Undigested, this sugar rides its way into the large bowel where bacteria break it down into hydrogen.

Unfortunately for the world at large, lactose intolerance is both attention getting and common. By adulthood 10 to 20 percent of Caucasians are lactase deficient. Among Blacks and Asians, the number hops to a whopping 75 percent.

Testing to see if you're lactose intolerant is simple. Avoid dairy products for two to three days and see if your gas subsides. If you want an answer quickly and are bold enough to face the music, drink three to four glasses of milk with a meal. If you're lactose intolerant, says Dr. Peikin, the answer will shortly be quite evident.

If you can't do without milk products, try eating smaller servings. Or turn to fermented milk products, like yogurt and cheese, which have less lactose for you to break down. You can also buy lactose-reduced milk, but it's slightly more expensive. You also might want to buy a lactase enzyme supplement for other foods.

If you choose to avoid dairy products, you need to be careful because your diet will likely be calcium deficient. Dr. Oppenheim recommends one gram of calcium carbonate supplement a day to make up for the loss. Calcium is essential to strong bones and helps control blood pressure.

Be cautious of carbs. Carbohydrates have long been touted as the food source of choice. While it's true that they are the root of few dietary evils, a big cause of flatulence is the digestive system's inability to absorb certain carbohydrates. High on the list of difficult to digest carbs: beans, brans, brussels sprouts, onions and peas.

"The real gas-making food culprit is carbohydrates," says Dr. Oppenheim. "Humans digest fats and proteins very efficiently. But even the healthiest small intestine breaks down only a fraction of the carbohydrates it receives."

And so it ends up in the bowels where the bacteria do their thing.

If you want to turn down the gas, slant your food choices toward easily digested stuff. Foods that cause little or no flatulence problems include fish, fowl, red meat, whole-wheat (versus bran) bread, potatoes, white (versus brown) rice, lettuce, tomatoes and citrus fruits.

Don't add fiber to the fire. Some high-fiber vegetables and fruits may increase gas. Fiber is an important addition to a healthy diet, but if you're new to roughage, drink plenty of water and add fiber to your diet in small doses so your bowels can get used to it.

One of the biggest culprits is, again, beans. Other high-fiber troublemakers include pears, bananas, carrots, cabbage and just about any dried fruit.

Consider charcoal tablets. One product experts recommend to give flatulence relief is activated charcoal tablets. Studies have found that activated charcoal tablets are effective in reducing excess gas.

The gas attaches to the outside of the charcoal and gets carried out of the body, Dr. Peikin explains. "They can reduce flatulence and alter the aroma of bowel gas."

You can buy charcoal tablets without prescription. Two cautions, says Dr. Peikin. Activated charcoal can sweep drugs out of your body as well, so don't take medication and charcoal tablets within two hours of each other. And if you do use charcoal tablets, don't be alarmed by the end result.

"Perfectly harmless," says Dr. Peikin, "but they'll turn your stool black."

Food Poisoning

Avoiding the Belly Dance

News item: Seven hundred are stricken and four die in the Pacific Northwest as the result of eating hamburgers contaminated with bacteria.

News item: More than 600 passengers and crew on a Mexican cruise are felled by eating food infected with shigellosis, an intestinal bacteria that can be transmitted by improper sanitation.

It seems you hear about it a lot: Food poisoning resulting in vomiting, diarrhea, sharp stomach pain, chills, fever—and in rare circumstances, death. The cause turns out to be food or liquids contaminated by one of what seems a bewildering array of dangerous organisms.

Food poisoning, or foodborne illness, may be among the most common illnesses in the United States. "We don't know how large a problem because it is estimated that only 1 to 10 percent are reported," notes Margy J. Woodburn, Ph.D., professor emeritus of nutrition and food management at Oregon State University in Corvallis and co-author of *Food Preservation and Safety*. By some estimates, cases of food poisoning number at least 24 million each year in the United States.

The vast majority of cases amount to short-term nausea, diarrhea and/or vomiting and stomach pain. But in very extreme cases food poisoning does kill—somewhere between 500 and 9,000 people each year in the United States.

More telling is the cost to the nation which, in lost time and medical bills, runs between $5 billion and $6 billion a year.

What to Do When It Hits

The young, the old, those who have AIDS or are HIV-positive and pregnant women are most at risk for food poisoning. For men food poisoning is most serious for those with chronic conditions such as diabetes, liver disease or cancer. These groups should consult a doctor as quickly as possible if struck.

If you're a relatively healthy male, then food poisoning has a pretty consistent profile. The bout usually starts one to six hours after eating the tainted food, and ends roughly six hours after it begins.

Food poisoning actually refers to cases in which the harmful bacteria has multiplied on the food prior to eating. Foodborne infections are when you eat food that has bacteria on it, but the bacterial growth happens in your body; in these cases symptoms may not show up until six hours later, and you may get a fever as well.

In either scenario, the vast majority of cases don't require a doctor—you just gut it out. Here's what to do.

Seek truth in numbers. If you think you've been food poisoned, check to see if whomever you were eating with is also sick. If so, report the problem to your health department.

Liquefy yourself. Prolonged vomiting or diarrhea will drain your body of fluids. So to keep from getting dehydrated, drink water, and plenty of it, spread out over time. Consider adding a bit of salt and sugar to the water to give your body some needed nutrients. Safe alternatives to water include juices, tea with sugar or sports drinks fortified with electrolytes.

Ride it out. Get comfortable and fasten your seat belt—you're in for a bumpy few-hour ride with something that's unpleasant, even nasty, but usually not too serious. On second thought, don't buckle that belt; you're gonna need to make it to the facilities, fast and often.

Let it flow. Unless you have severe diarrhea over a long time or can't get easy access to a toilet, don't take medicine. Diarrhea is just the body's way of getting rid of what ails you.

Talk to a doctor. Call a doctor if any of the following apply: You don't feel better five or six hours after the onset of symptoms and you can't keep food or fluids down; there is a fever of 101°F or higher; there is bloody diarrhea; you are unusually weak; your vision is blurred.

Know Your Enemy

The world of microbes is a complicated place. "One of the things that people have a hard time understanding is that most microorganisms are not harmful. They don't cause disease," says George K. York, Ph.D., professor emeritus of food microbiology at the University of California, Davis. He adds, however, "Many times, organisms we want in one product will spoil another product.

Here are some of our microbe neighbors we would be better off avoiding.

Salmonella. There are more than 1,500 types known. It's widespread in food, water and excrement, and can lead to gastroenteritis and typhoid fever. It grows over a wide range of temperatures, and can survive both freezing and freeze-drying. There are an estimated 42,000 cases of salmonella infection a year in the United States, usually linked to raw eggs and animal products.

FAST FACTS

How common: Very, although it's frequently neither recognized nor reported to health authorities. It's been estimated that one in every ten Americans will get a dose of food poisoning each year.

Risk factors: When eating out, you're at risk when food isn't well-cooked or when supposedly hot or cold food arrives lukewarm. At home you're at risk any time you don't keep cooking surfaces and your hands well-washed and clean. Food stored at room temperature after it's cooked is risky. Highest risk comes in eating raw seafood.

Age group affected: All age groups can be affected. The very young and the elderly whose health is compromised should be especially cautious. Most serious when there's another disorder present, such as diabetes or AIDS.

Gender gap: Food poisoning is an equal opportunity medical problem.

Who to see: If the poisoning doesn't run its course in five or six hours, contact your family doctor if symptoms are unusually severe.

Listeria. A bad one. It can cause meningitis and brain abscesses, although usually only in the vulnerable: the young, pregnant and elderly whose health is compromised. Linked to unpasteurized milk and unripened cheese.

Escherichia coli. Known better as *E. coli*, this is a variety of a bug that lives in the human and animal intestinal tracts. *E. coli* spreads easily; in the most extreme cases it has caused an estimated 400 deaths in the United States among children, the elderly and adults with compromised health. Healthy adults can experience bloody diarrhea. Associated with contaminated ground meat that goes undercooked, but can contaminate many foods.

Campylobacter jejuni. Associated with poultry, beef, swine, sheep and water. There are an estimated 2 million cases a year.

Shigella. Accounts for an estimated 32,000 cases a year. One problem with shigella is that a few food handlers infected by the bacteria may transfer it to food through poor handling practices.

Vibrio parahaemolyticus. Grows in the ocean and is associated with raw and undercooked seafoods such as raw oysters. Certain raw shellfish that have been infected have been known to cause fatal hepatitis infections in people with existing liver problems.

Bacteria and viruses are the most common but aren't the only things that cause serious food poisoning. Chemicals and metals, some naturally occurring and more produced and dumped into the food chain by our fellow human beings, are sources of poisoning as well.

Swordfish, for example, can pick up mercury and pass it along when you bite into a steak.

Another example: Fatty fish, like salmon and herring, pick up nasty chemicals such as PCBs, dioxin and agricultural pesticides that are sprayed by farmers and that eventually wash their way to the sea.

Why We're Getting Bugged

There are a score of reasons why it seems we're getting bugged more and more.

"We're eating more meals away from home," suggests Dr. Woodburn. Plus, nowadays everything is big scale, she adds, "so there would be larger numbers involved in an outbreak, and it would more likely be reported."

Moreover, Mom generally knew how to run a kitchen so as not to make her family sick. Says Dr. Woodburn: "We're getting less education now on basic principles. The age group with the poorest practices are those younger than age 35. We've become complacent." And the most complacent and least knowledgeable are men.

Plus, the human food chain—the system of production and distribution that brings you your dinner via the local fast-food joint or the supermarket—is increasingly international and complex. When food is produced in large numbers in one location, pressure on slaughterhouses and packagers can produce carelessness. All in all, there's just more opportunity for bugs to contaminate food products.

The cry goes up for more federal inspection. But contamination in meat or any food or liquid is hard to spot. It can't be detected by sight, smell or touch.

Seafood poses a similar dilemma. In 1993 Americans consumed an average of 3.2 pounds more fish and shellfish than in 1970. But lots of the fish consumed in the United States is caught by amateurs, so there's rarely professional inspection. On average the Food and Drug Administration inspects every U.S. fish-processing plant every other year. An estimated 20 percent of seafood plants voluntarily submit to separate inspections by the National Marine Fisheries Service.

Lifestyle plays a big part in making men vulnerable to food poisoning. Once upon a time Dad burnt the burgers to a crisp. Nowadays we like medium-rare because it tastes better.

We're in a hurry and grab easily cooked foods such as ground beef, sausage or ground turkey. Fifty percent of the beef consumed in the United States is ground. The grinding process ensures that any bacteria in the meat, instead of remaining on the surface where it might be burned off, gets mixed up into the meat.

Says Dr. York: "We should have a lot more food poisoning than we do because of the crazy things people do." The problem's not just that food gets contaminated in production, but, Dr. York adds, "Most cases occur at the final preparation stage, where people are not careful and don't know what they're doing."

Eating and Not Getting Sick

What can you do? Follow these guidelines.

Says Dr. Woodburn, "Men tend to have less safe practices than women because they often have just started to cook and had less experience in the kitchen and with food handling."

Your protection is in your common sense—and what dietitians calls the four Cs.

1. Cleanliness. Wash your hands before preparing food, after handling raw meats, poultry and fish, and then again before eating. Keep all surfaces clean: utensils, cutting boards, tabletops. In particular, scrub those surfaces that touch food; soap is good to use, chlorine bleach diluted in water even better because it kills bacteria.

2. Cross-contamination. Keeping things clean means not spreading bacteria to other food. "For example, don't use the cutting board that you've cut raw meat on for a salad that's not going to be cooked," says Dr. York.

3. Chill it well. Refrigerate leftovers. Likewise, refrigerate deli foods, meat, milk and eggs as soon as you are done with them. If you've left perishable food out more than three hours, throw it out.

And while you're at it, make sure your refrigerator works: The main compartment should be at or below 40°F and the freezer at or below 0°F.

4. Cook it well. Thorough cooking will kill most microorganisms. For most perishables a food temperature of 145° to 155°F will destroy most microbes. Ground meat should be cooked until the temperature reaches 165°F. (Meat thermometers are available at most supermarkets; just pop it into the middle of the meat and get your reading.) As for microwaving just follow the cooking directions, and be sure to stir afterward so all parts become hot.

Here are a few more points beyond the four Cs.

Monitor where you eat. "Make sure the restaurant where you eat is well-organized and clean," says Dr. Woodburn. "If food should be hot, it should be very hot, and if cold, very cold. If you're served a hamburger pink in the center, send it back, or chicken that's pink. Sending back suspect food "helps educate the restaurant," Dr. Woodburn adds.

Know your foods. Some specific foods to be careful with.

Chicken. It's estimated that 21 percent of domestically produced broiler chickens have some salmonella bacteria. That means always cook it well. And make sure you clean any surface raw chicken touches so that germs aren't lying in wait to contaminate other food.

Milk. Unpasteurized, raw milk is risky. Many men are sold on its having greater nutrition, although this is not really the case. In 1987, 62 people in California died from drinking unpasteurized milk. No matter what type of milk you drink, keep it refrigerated.

Hamburger and beef. Cook it. Steak tartare is great. Also dangerous.

Eggs. The problem is salmonella. Cooking them kills it. That means soft-boiled eggs or sunny-side up are a risk. Safe is a three minute per side fried.

Fish and seafood. Cook it. Says Dr. Woodburn: "If you have problems with liver disease, are undergoing chemotherapy or have a low immunity, avoid raw seafood. Otherwise, decide if you want the risk. If you're healthy, maybe it's okay. If you have impaired health, you should probably decide not to."

Fruits and vegetables. The problem here isn't as much bacteria as pesticide residues. If such chemicals concern you, buy organically grown vegetables, and wash all produce thoroughly.

Foot and Heel Pain

End the Agony of da Feet

Women pamper and pedicure them, keep them moisturized and well-maintained. But guys? Heck, we pay about as much attention to our feet as synchronized swimming.

Too bad, because that's probably why those poor dogs of yours sometimes want to roll over and play dead . . . if they haven't already. The typical man uses his feet to cover more than 100,000 miles in his lifetime—equal to about four times around the Earth. And with every step, the 26 bones, 38 muscles, 56 ligaments and literally yards of nerves and blood vessels of each foot must absorb a heavy load: the force of nearly *four* times his body weight.

The good news is those gunboats of yours are built for battle. If you are experiencing pain, then you are probably to blame by stuffing yourself into ill-fitting shoes. That also means foot and heel pain is easily remedied.

Shoes: An Achilles Heel to Your Feet

For foot relief a good place to start is at the shoe store. "Much of the foot and heel pain that men have results from wearing improperly fitting shoes—especially dress shoes," says Pamela Colman, D.P.M., assistant director of health affairs for the American Podiatric Medical Association. "What men have to realize, but unfortunately many don't, is that like women's shoes, their dress shoes also usually have a narrow toebox—and that can promote foot pain, as well as problems like hammertoes, bunions and ingrown toenails.

"To avoid these problems, make sure you have plenty of room in the toebox by having someone press down on the front of the shoe while you're standing. If you don't have at least a thumbnail's space between the end of your big toe and the edge of the shoe, you don't have enough room."

Some other shoe issues:

Cushion your heel. Time wounds all heels—at least for men. "Heel pain is the biggest complaint among men because they tend to be more active than women, but also because their shoes often don't have good cushioning," says Dr. Colman. "One of the best things you can do when buying shoes is to put your hand inside the shoe and press down. If the sole bounces back, it has good cushioning; if not, get another shoe."

Wear shoes in the right shape. As important as buying the right-size shoes is buying the right-*shape* shoes, says William Van Pelt, D.P.M., a Houston podiatrist and former president of the American Academy of Podiatric Sports Medicine. Basically, feet (and shoes) come in three shapes: curved, slightly curved and straight. Those with high arches usually need a curved shoe; those with flat feet benefit from straight shoes and shoes that are in-between.

Tie one on. Lace-up shoes usually provide more support in the top of the shoe, which helps lessen the effects of fallen arches, says Philip Sanfilippo, D.P.M., a podiatrist in private practice in San Francisco. Experts say that men who wear "tie" shoes are less likely to get fallen arches than those who mainly wear loafers or other slip-ons.

Shop the right time. If possible, try on shoes in the afternoon or evening: Your feet will be a little swollen from the day's use, and you won't wind up with a tighter fit.

Other Foot Issues

Even if your shoes fit right, it doesn't mean that nothing will go wrong with your feet. Eight out of ten of us are plagued by foot and ankle problems, according to the American College of Foot and Ankle Surgeons. The obvious way to soothe foot and heel pain is with a good massage—experts recommend using moisturizing lotion to make the rubbing easier. Here are some other ways to stay one step ahead of what's ailing you below the ankle.

Get soaked. When your dogs hurt because they're tired—burning, itchy and aching—one of the best treatments is a nightly foot-soaking alternating between hot and cold water, says Terry Spilken, D.P.M., a podiatrist and adjunct faculty member at the New York College of Podiatric Medicine in New York City. His advice: Place your feet in cold water for five minutes, then immediately soak in hot water for five minutes, and so forth. This has a "massaging" effect that invigorates feet by opening and closing blood vessels.

Stretch your calf. Heel pain can be caused by inflammation in the bottom of the foot or by bone growths called heel spurs. Stretching your heel cord or Achilles tendon at the back of your foot can reduce or relieve heel pain, says Michael Steinbaum, D.P.M., a podiatrist practicing with the Buenaventura Medical Clinic in Ventura, California. To stretch, stand about three feet from a wall and place your hands on the wall. Then lean toward the wall, bringing one leg forward and bending at your elbows. Your back leg should remain straight, with the heel on the floor. Hold for 20 to 30 seconds. You should feel a gentle stretch in the calf muscle of your back leg. Then switch legs.

Wear arch supports. A lesser-known cause of foot and heel pain stems from the fact that your belly isn't the only part of your body subject to middle-age spread. Fallen arches occur as the ligaments that support your arches give out, causing feet

FAST FACTS

How common: At least 80 percent of men experience foot and heel pain, at least occasionally.

Risk factors: Improperly fitting shoes lead the list, but age, poor hygiene and heredity are also factors.

Age group affected: All, but some types of pain—like that caused by fallen arches—are more common in those over age 40.

Gender gap: Men and women are equally prone to foot problems, but men experience foot problems far more often—largely because they roundly ignore their feet. Men neglect hygiene, buy ill-fitting shoes and are more apt to flock to a Tupperware party than see a doctor.

Who to see: Podiatrist.

to flatten out and spread—usually around age 40. But for less than $10 you can buy some arch support insoles at most drugstores and many shoe stores that provide much-needed support to fallen arches, says Judith Smith, M.D., assistant professor of orthopedic surgery at Emory University School of Medicine in Atlanta.

Don't touch a nerve. Foot pain between the third and fourth toe could be a malady known as Morton's toe or Morton's neuroma. This comes from pressure on the foot bones called metatarsals, which irritate the nerve between them. The culprit here is often tight, pointy shoes. Buy wider shoes, and consider using metatarsal arch supports, which are available at drugstores. If your case is severe, talk to your doctor about a cortisone injection or surgery.

Try patchwork. Some people have a bulging joint in the big toe called a bunion. The close confines of a shoe can rub it the wrong way, causing pain. To reduce the friction, try covering it in a bunion shield, which is available at drugstores.

Change your shoes often. Another cause of foot pain is plantar warts, which are caused by a virus that invades the skin through microscopic cuts or abrasions on the soles of your feet—and grow inward, causing pain as though you're walking on a tack. The virus that breeds plantar warts thrives in warm, moist environments, like the insides of your shoes.

"Wearing the same pair of shoes every day accumulates moisture in the shoe," says Douglas Richie, D.P.M., a Seal Beach, California, sports podiatrist in private practice. "Rotating your shoes greatly improves the health of the skin of the feet." And for the same reason, you should change your socks frequently, preferably twice a day.

See also Athlete's Foot, Blisters, Corns and Calluses, Nail Problems

Foreskin Problems

Keeping Infection at Bay

What's the big flap over foreskins? In a word, circumcision, whose opponents would make it the next battleground in the civil rights movement. "The rest of the world looks upon us as barbarians!" declares Marilyn Milos, R.N., founder of NoCirc, an anti-circumcision group in California. Foreskin problems should be dealt with medically, she says, not "amputation."

For most of us it's a moot point. Roughly 75 percent of American men don't have foreskin problems because they don't have foreskins.

Those who've managed to retain that little flap of skin (the prepuce) over the glans may have the gratification of knowing they're walking around the way nature intended, but they also have some concerns that other guys don't have. There is, for instance, an array of infections known as balanitis, which can cause inflammation and soreness to the head of the penis. It's usually caused by bacterial or fungal infections growing in the moist, warm shelter of the foreskin. Since men with diabetes are said to be particularly susceptible to balanitis, men with recurrent bouts of balanitis should probably get checked out for diabetes as well

Phimosis is another problem that can afflict the uncircumcised. That's when the opening of the foreskin is so small that the foreskin can't be retracted over the glans. Phimosis is usually a congenital problem. Some boys grow out of it as their foreskins grow larger. If they don't, phimosis can make it hard to urinate and difficult to clean the secretions, known as smegma, from under the foreskin.

"In addition, drops of urine get mixed with the smegma, and that combination is highly carcinogenic," says Marc Goldstein, M.D., professor of urology and director of the Center for Male Reproductive Medicine and Microsurgery at the New York Hospital-Cornell Medical Center in New York City. "So there's a significant increase in penile cancer in men with phimosis."

A related problem is paraphimosis, in which the foreskin is so tight that once retracted it can't return to its original position. Essentially what happens is that the foreskin strangles the penis, causing the head of the penis to swell and turn dark blue. "It becomes excruciatingly painful," reports Michael J. Maloney, a dermatologist in private practice in Denver, and must be treated at once, lest gangrene develop.

FAST FACTS

How common: Perhaps 10 percent of uncircumcised men develop problems such as infections.

Risk factors: Poor hygiene, multiple sex partners, unprotected sex.

Age group affected: Usually older men or young children. But thirtysomething guys who don't clean themselves regularly get their share.

Gender gap: Actually, women have foreskins, too, protecting the clitoris. But that's a whole other thing.

Who to see: Urologist.

Other research suggests that uncircumcised men are more likely to contract syphilis and gonorrhea. The bacteria for both can grow beneath the foreskin and find its way into the body, syphilis through the skin, gonorrhea through the urethra. No fun.

There's also evidence of a greater risk of urinary tract infections (UTIs), with the accompanying burning feeling and frequent need to urinate. Infections can appear in the urethra (urethritis), in the bladder (cystitis), or in the kidneys (pyelonephritis). And they can be serious, cautions Dr. Maloney. "You can get a kidney infection and lose kidney function." Some research even suggests that uncircumcised men run a greater risk of HIV infection, which can lead to AIDS.

Clean Up Your Act

Gangrene? Cancer of the penis? AIDS? If this dire list makes you want to run right down to your neighborhood urologist for a circumcision, keep in mind that you probably won't get any of these ailments. Most uncircumcised men, says Dr. Maloney, "don't have any problems." Penile cancer, for instance, usually attacks older men and is quite rare—maybe 1,100 or 1,200 cases out of an estimated 632,000 male cancers a year. The trouble is that almost all of these cases occur in uncircumcised men.

Urinary tract infections are also uncommon among young, sexually active men. Babies and older men are the main male targets. Again the rub: Uncircumcised boys appear to be 10 to 20 times more likely to develop UTIs than circumcised ones. This proclivity to UTIs seems to diminish with the approach of manhood.

There is some logic to the greater susceptibility of uncircumcised men to gonorrhea, syphilis and even HIV diseases since the foreskin provides a hothouse environment where bacteria and other nasties can grow. But with a bit of caution, there's no need to catch any of these diseases.

Wear a latex condom. This simple precaution should prevent syphilis and gonococcal bacteria, as well as HIV, from getting under the foreskin in the first place.

Clean carefully. Dr. Goldstein says he's sometimes "shocked by the poor hygiene in people who otherwise are very clean. Even executives!" If you don't have foreskin problems, don't wait until you do. Keep the penis clean. "Often," says Dr. Maloney, "just cleaning the area and letting it dry out will get rid of an overgrowth of bacteria or yeast."

If you already suffer from a mild form of balanitis, continue to clean gently under the foreskin, but be sure you consult a dermatologist or urologist to find out what's causing the irritation. Dr. Maloney recommends that men with balanitis retract the foreskin and wash the end of the penis with plenty of water—"maybe mild soap and a fingertip, but nothing more aggressive, like a washrag."

He says to keep the foreskin retracted while drying the area off with a hair dryer set on low or letting it air dry in front of a fan. Then apply medicine—perhaps an antiyeast, antibacterial or antifungal cream. The final step: "Take a piece of gauze and make a miniscarf out of it and wrap it around the penis while the foreskin remains retracted."

This may not be the way you'd choose to dress for a night at the opera, but you should start feeling better soon.

Don't rule out circumcision. If balanitis occurs in conjunction with phimosis, you have a much more serious problem, one which frequently calls for a circumcision. Mild cases may be treated with topical steroids. Paraphimosis, of course, is a surgical emergency that almost always requires circumcision, or at least a dorsal slit—an incision in the foreskin that permits it to move over the head of the penis, relieving the constriction. Dr. Goldstein prefers doing a complete circumcision, for cosmetic reasons. "The dorsal slit looks a little funny. It looks like dog ears. It's not a normal-looking penis."

And all we need is for our partner to look at our penis, cock her head to the side, and say, "Woof, woof."

Frostbite

Preventing the Freeze

Oh, what fun—sledding, skiing, ice fishing, one-horse open sleighs. It's easy to forget there's a grim side to winter recreation. When your mind's on jingle bells, it can miss the alarms of freezing skin.

"I have skied for 38 years, so I've seen my share of frostbite out on the slopes," says David C. Novicki, D.P.M., president of the American College of Foot and Ankle Surgeons in Park Ridge, Illinois, and a foot and ankle surgeon in Milford, Connecticut. "Anytime I see someone with what looks like white, frozen skin, I tell them that they must act on this immediately, because sometimes they're unaware of it."

Doctors gauge frostbite by the amount of damage it does. With first-degree frostbite, the mildest sort, the skin turns waxy white and is cold to the touch but not yet blistering. Getting inside and warming the skin will usually prevent serious damage, but you might still need to see a doctor.

In the most serious cases, fourth degree, deep damage occurs. The flesh hardens and turns gray or blue, and eventually all feeling is lost in the affected area. Such patients require hospitalization and often lose body parts to amputation, says Dr. Novicki.

Frostbite commonly strikes the ears, nose, hands, feet and toes. It most commonly occurs when people spend 6 to 12 hours in temperatures of -4° to 10°F. But damage can come much more rapidly. Wind makes the effects of cold worse—the greater the wind speed, the greater the loss of body heat.

Getting wet is a factor, too, because cold water pulls heat from the body 25 times faster than cold air. Touching bare skin to cold metal also can cause frostbite quickly.

A study that followed 812 frostbite patients for up to 18 years after injury found that 82 percent had heightened sensitivity to cold, 73 percent had discolored skin and 58 percent experienced profuse sweating. Other long-term effects can include burning pain, cool extremities, numbness, skin discoloration, joint problems and sensitivity to cold.

People who have had frostbite in the past are more vulnerable to getting it again. Elderly people and people who have been drinking alcohol are more susceptible to frostbite.

Keeping Toasty

If you can't resist that sledding hill, take these precautions to save your skin.

Bundle up. In extreme cold, cover all of your body parts with a hat, scarf, face mask and gloves. Keep your torso well-covered, too. When you're cold, blood tends to leave your extremities and collect in the main body. So warming your torso will warm your toes, too.

See your tailor. Make sure your winter clothes fit. If they're too tight or loose, your chances of damage from the cold are increased. And tight shoes will reduce blood flow to your feet, increasing the likelihood of frostbite.

Dress in layers. "Layered clothing is extremely helpful," says Dr. Novicki. "Many people wear silk liners under their gloves, or a silk long underwear outfit and then a good long pair of pants. A blanket of air builds up between the clothing, and that helps to insulate you."

Keep a lid on it. "People have all of this macho baloney about not wearing hats," says Dr. Novicki. "There's an enormous amount of heat lost from the head. Certainly you want, in cold weather, to keep your head covered."

Boots should breathe. Leather boots are best in the cold because they breathe, says Dr. Novicki. "With leather footgear you will have a tendency to perspire a lot less than with the all-plastic type," he says. "And we recommend layers of socks—a silk liner and a wool or cotton sock."

Don't drink. In cold weather alcohol may feel like it's warming you up, but it's actually having the opposite effect—it causes greater heat loss from the body. And as you might know, alcohol has been known to make people stupid, which you can scarcely afford in an emergency.

When Frostbite Strikes

If Jack Frost does rear his head and bites, here's what to do to minimize the damage.

Get inside immediately. If you have frostbite, get out of the cold. If your hands are affected, warm them in your armpits. Other affected skin can be warmed against dry, gloved hands. Don't rub frostbitten skin—you can cause further damage. If your feet are frostbitten, don't walk on them. If you feel tingling and burning after 20 minutes, then your circulation is returning. If numbness remains, get medical help.

Warm up in water. For minor frostbite warm the skin gradually by immersion in progressively warmer tubs of water, five minutes at a time. Start with water at 60°F and increase the temperature about 10 degrees each time until you reach

FAST FACTS

How common: Increasingly so. The rising popularity of winter sports is a contributing factor.

Risk factors: Bare skin exposed to freezing cold, wind and wetness. The elderly and those who recently consumed alcohol might be at a greater risk than others.

Age group affected: All ages are affected. Elderly people with circulatory problems are more susceptible.

Gender gap: Both sexes are equally vulnerable, although macho behavior such as foregoing hats—you know who you are—increases risk of exposure.

Who to see: Family doctor or emergency room doctor.

105°F. In severe cases involving frozen skin, the warming is done more rapidly in the warmer water, Dr. Novicki says. Such patients need a doctor.

Forego the fire. Don't try thawing your skin by a fire. Your frostbitten nerves won't be able to warn you if you start to roast.

Refreezing is worse. Before you warm up your frostbitten skin, make sure you aren't going to have to head out into the cold again soon. Refreezing your skin will cause much more damage than the original frostbite.

Nix nicotine. Don't smoke when you're suffering from frostbite. The nicotine will limit your circulation, which your skin can't afford.

Genital Herpes

How to Avoid a Touchy Subject

A virus doesn't have to be fatal, crippling or even painful to cause a lot of grief. Case in point: genital herpes.

Most people never know that the genital herpes virus is in their body. And only a minority get short-lived sores from time to time. Still, because the disease is sexually transmitted, can recur and gets lots of hysterical publicity, herpes can take a big emotional toll.

While many guys take herpes in stride—after all, there are a lot more vicious viruses to worry about these days—emotional fallout can range from social awkwardness (when to share the news with a prospective bed partner) to depression, according to Ted A. Grossbart, Ph.D., an instructor in psychology at Harvard Medical School and co-author of *Skin Deep: A Mind-Body Program for Healthy Skin*. "The impact on self-esteem . . . the unwarranted sense of being damaged and unloveable, can be severe," he says. "Some people just avoid relationships."

A Very Common Virus

Everybody knows that herpes isn't rare, but you may find it hard to believe just how common it is: Experts estimate as many as 40 percent of American adults have been exposed to the virus. More surprising, maybe three out of four folks who carry the virus don't know it. Even the initial infection, usually the worst, can be without symptoms, according to Lawrence R. Stanberry, M.D., director of infectious disease at Children's Hospital at the University of Cincinnati.

The virus behind genital herpes is the same one that causes cold sores: herpes simplex. It's transmitted by direct contact, one set of genitals to another, but isn't terribly contagious. A man who has sex for a year with a woman who has herpes has less than a 5 percent chance of catching the disease.

The first episode can be nasty: tingling and itching, followed by a crop of painful blisters, which break to leave an ulcerated sore. It may take three to four weeks for the sore to crust over and disappear. You may have a fever.

When herpes is over, though, it isn't all over. The virus doesn't die, but slinks into hiding in nearby nerve cells. From whence it may return at any time to cause recurrent sores (almost always less painful and shorter-lived than the first ones).

For reasons that aren't well-understood, about one-third of people who have been infected with herpes have virtually no recurrences. Another third have a few—about three per year—and the rest have more. According to Dr. Stanberry, the strain of virus and the amount you were exposed to probably makes the difference, as does the immune system you were born with.

Self-Protection Basics

Since there's no cure for herpes—once it gets under your skin, it has no intention of leaving—the best thing to do is to not get it.

Use a condom. It used to be thought that herpes was only contagious when the virus came out of hiding to cause a visible sore, or the few days before or after. It's become clear, however, that many people shed the virus even when soreless. One study suggested that nearly three times out of four, herpes is in fact transmitted without symptoms.

"The risk of transmission per exposure is highest when the lesions are there," says Gregory Mertz, M.D., section chief for infectious disease at the University of New Mexico in Albuquerque, "and it's important to avoid skin-to-skin contact at this time. But the cumulative risk is higher during the asymptom periods."

So the message is clear, according to the Centers for Disease Control and Prevention (CDC) in Atlanta: Always use a latex condom during sex. The virus can't pass through it.

If you know your partner has ever had herpes, Dr. Mertz points out, you should use a condom every time—not just when the sores recur—given the risk of asymptomatic transmission.

A condom doesn't keep you 100 percent safe, though. It only protects what it covers—the penis itself. If the herpes virus comes in contact with the rest of your pubic area, you could catch it that way.

Limit your sex life. The CDC offers the standard advice for lowering the risk of all sexually transmitted diseases—be selective in your sex partners. The more you have, the greater your risk of exposure.

Be wary of oral sex. "Herpes can also be transmitted from mouth to genitals," Dr. Mertz points out. Like magic, oral sex can transform your girlfriend's cold sore into your genital herpes.

Shun the sun. Ultraviolet exposure at the site of infection is the only factor known to trigger recurrences. This is more often an issue with oral herpes. But if you're a hard core naturist, be warned.

De-stress. Many insist that stress can trigger herpes recurrences, but the data doesn't support it. Still, no one ever says it would hurt to cut back on stress.

Be well-nourished. Lysine (an amino acid) and other nutrients have their partisans, but there's no firm data that they reduce recurrences or make them heal faster, Dr. Stanberry says. But in general, "people in good nutritional shape do heal more quickly."

The Right Medicine

While nothing known can expel the herpes virus once it takes up residence, science has found the next best thing—a drug that shortens episodes and all but eliminates recurrences. That drug, acyclovir (Zovirax), apparently stops the virus from reproducing. If you start taking acyclovir promptly, it can markedly shorten the discomfort from the first herpes episode, and get the sores to heal sooner. Taking the drug at the first sign of an imminent recurrence (often an itching, tingling sensation in the area) can shorten these, too.

Even better for people who've been plagued by frequently returning herpes sores is the ability of acyclovir to keep the nasty virus from acting up. A study at the Baylor College of Medicine in Houston followed a group of people with genital herpes for nine years. When the study started, they were having very frequent recurrences—an average of 12 each year.

After five years of acyclovir therapy the participants were having, on average, less than one attack per year. And 20 percent have had none since starting treatment.

What's more, acyclovir has the potential of reducing the risk of passing the virus between episodes. A study at the University of Washington in Seattle found that less asymptomatic viral shedding occurred when people took the drug twice daily. Viral shedding is what makes it possible for a person to transmit a virus.

Other Treatments

If you're having a severe herpes outbreak, there's a lot you can do to make yourself more comfortable until it goes away.

Bathe often. During an initial outbreak, take a warm shower or bath, two or three times a day. Gently pat (don't rub) the infected area dry. Vigorous rubbing could irritate the area and spread the infection, says Dr. Stanberry.

Dry it out. Apply a drying agent, like zinc oxide or calamine lotion, directly to the sores.

Try cold and heat. An ice pack, an infrared heat lamp or a hair dryer set on a cool or warm setting can relieve pain. But don't overdo it—back off at the slightest feeling of irritation.

Hang loose. Wear loose-fitting cotton underwear: Circulating air avoids irritation and speeds healing.

Don't glop. Avoid gooey ointments with bases like petroleum jelly. "They keep the lesions from drying, so they last longer and shed the virus for longer," says Dr. Stanberry. Over-the-counter topical agents containing zinc may have some antiviral effects, but they haven't been shown to be effective in clinical trials. Still, they may help and probably won't hurt, Dr. Stanberry says.

Scrub thy nails. Wash hands thoroughly with soap whenever you touch the infected area. The virus can live on skin for 30 minutes and can easily spread by contact to other parts of your body, especially your face.

Seek emotional help. If you're suffering emotional distress, consider counseling or a support group. "Sometimes, just meeting and talking to someone who's had more time to adjust to the problem is very helpful," Dr. Grossbart says.

The Herpes Resource Center can provide useful information and help you find a support group. Write to the American Social Health Association, P.O. Box 13827, Research Triangle Park, NC 27709, and include a self-addressed, stamped envelope. Or call the National Herpes Hotline at (919) 361-8488.

See also Cold and Canker Sores, Sexually Transmitted Diseases

Gum Disease

Building a Good Foundation

Most of us think our mouths are in pretty good shape. Most of us are mistaken.

A poll by the Roper Organization found that 80 percent of Americans don't think they have gum disease. In fact, three out of four adults have some form of it.

The Roper poll also found that 78 percent of those who admit to having at least one symptom of gum disease continue to insist they've never had it.

Are we all in denial, or are we just dumb?

Neither, really. The problem with gum disease is that it can develop for years with virtually no symptoms: No pain, no signs that even a dentist can spot with the naked eye. "We make the assumption that if there isn't pain, everything must be okay," says Christine Dumas, D.D.S., who practices in Los Angeles and is an adviser to the American Dental Association (ADA). "Unfortunately, by the time you feel gum disease, it may be too late."

It doesn't help that men don't come in for dental checkups nearly as much as women, Dr. Dumas says. Plus, adults are often confused when visible symptoms finally emerge. Gums that bleed during brushing or flossing are a sign of bacterial infections and that a dentist needs to clean things out. Instead, men think bleeding gums are just a normal part of aging. Or they think that it means they're brushing or flossing too hard, says Joel M. Boriskin, D.D.S., a dentist in Oakland, California, and adviser to the ADA. In that case, men back off doing exactly what they need to be doing more of—brushing and flossing. So the problem gets worse.

Dr. Dumas, however, has found that once men learn they might have gum disease, they get inspired to do battle with it, using any and all of the various mechanical devices available to do so, from floss to irrigators. "I think it becomes a tool thing with guys," she says.

The Plaque Attack

Certain bacteria have been implicated in causing gum disease. Heredity may be one of many factors that determines susceptibility to the bacteria that cause periodontal disease.

FAST FACTS

How common: Three out of four adults have some form of gum disease.

Risk factors: Heredity, poor oral hygiene, smoking.

Age group affected: Neglect your teeth and you can get gum disease, no matter what age you are.

Gender gap: Men and women have equal susceptibility to gum disease. But men see dentists far less than women, meaning their problems often don't get caught early on.

Who to see: Dentist.

As bacteria eat, reproduce and die, these microscopic freeloaders contribute to a filmy substance called plaque (pronounced plak) on our teeth. Over time plaque builds up and may harden into a rocky deposit called tartar. That's the stuff the hygienist takes a pickax to while your fingers are digging grooves into the arms of the dental chair.

Your pink, healthy gums get irritated by the plaque and tartar, at which point you have an early stage of gum disease called gingivitis. If you don't get the plaque out of there, it starts building up between the gums and the teeth, gradually burrowing deeper and deeper beneath the gum line. That's a cozy haven for bacteria to thrive in, and eventually they'll work their way into the very bone to which your teeth are anchored. This advanced stage of gum disease (by now it's actually a bone disease, to be strictly accurate) is called periodontitis. If left untreated, periodontitis will undermine a tooth's support structure so completely that the tooth will get wobbly and finally drop out. Bring on the mashed potatoes.

Waging War

As common as gum disease is, it's one of the easiest maladies in the world to combat, at least in its early stages. Once it becomes more advanced, oral surgery may be required to reshape the gums so that they can once again get a grip on your teeth. But there's no need to let it get that far. This is one shooting war where the firepower is on your side.

Your toothbrush and dental floss are your first lines of defense against gum disease. The third fundamental tool is your dental hygienist: Twice-yearly cleanings to get rid of the plaque you're missing at home are a must. Don't make the mistake of thinking that those checkups alone will keep gum disease at bay, though. Plaque-forming bacteria start recolonizing in your mouth within 18 to 72 hours after you leave the dentist's office, which means it's up to you to keep them on the run between cleanings. For more information on the basics of oral hygiene, see Dental Problems on page 150.

Here are some other tips to help you practice efficient bacterial management.

Starve 'em out. Your mom was right: Sugary foods are bad for your teeth. What your mom may not have known is that sugar hides in some surprising places. Mark E. Jensen, D.D.S., Ph.D., a dentist in private practice in North Oaks, Minnesota, who has done extensive research on diet and gum disease, points out that most starchy foods such as cereals, crackers and breads turn into sugar as soon as we put them in our mouths. Dr. Jensen also points out that sticky foods—peanut butter, dates and raisins, for example—are a bacterium's dream because they coat the teeth and gums, providing a steady source of sugary sustenance for hours.

The solution is not so much to avoid eating starches and sweets (although cutting back on the frequency a bit wouldn't hurt), but to clean your teeth thoroughly after you eat them. And don't snack between meals, says Richard Price, D.M.D., clinical professor of dentistry at Boston University School of Dentistry and an advisor to the ADA. "That way you can have your cake and eat it, too," he says.

Say cheese. Research has shown that cheese eaten at the end of a meal helps fight the formation of the bacteria that cause plaque, according to Dr. Jensen. Virtually any cheese will do the trick, he says, except for goat cheeses, which are higher in bacteria-feeding lactose. Other dairy products, including plain yogurt, 2 percent milk and whole milk, have been shown to have similar, though weaker, plaque-fighting effects. Raw fruits and vegetables also fight plaque because their fibers clean your teeth as you eat them.

Stimulate your spit. When it comes to gum disease, consider saliva a friend: It helps keep the mouth clean of plaque-building bacteria. Dr. Price recommends chewing a piece of sugarless gum after meals to help get those cleansing fluids flowing.

Rinse with fluoride. Nighttime is party time for the bacteria in your mouth because you don't salivate in your sleep. Therefore, it's a good idea, according to Ralph Burgess, D.D.S., former head of preventive dentistry at the University of Toronto Dental School, to gargle with a fluoride rinse before you hit the sack.

"We tend to rinse our mouths out with water after we brush," he says, "so we're rinsing away a lot of the fluoride toothpaste." If you want to save money on the fluoride rinse, he says, just spit the excess toothpaste out of your mouth after you brush and don't rinse with water.

Talk to your dentist. When you visit your dentist, be sure to ask for a comprehensive periodontal exam, which involves measuring with a tiny probe any pockets that have formed between the gum and the tooth. The procedure only takes a few minutes, according to Dr. Dumas.

Inspect your medicine chest. Also be sure to tell your dentist of any prescription drugs you might be taking. George Kivowitz, D.D.S., a dentist in private practice in Holland, Pennsylvania, says that many medications can contribute to gum disease, especially those prescribed for blood pressure problems and for seizures. Dilantin in particular causes extreme sensitivity in the gums, according to Dr. Kivowitz, which can drive anyone with gingivitis up the wall.

Think of your genes. If either or both of your parents lost their teeth, take that as a warning that you need to exercise particular caution. "Several studies have implicated heredity and periodontal disease," says Linda M. Weinfield, D.D.S., a periodontist in private practice in Oak Lawn, Illinois.

Count your Cs. The gums, like the rest of your body, benefit from general good nutrition. "If the body is healthy, the mouth can be healthy as well," Dr. Weinfield says. A healthy diet and good oral hygiene can prevent the occurrence of gum disease, she adds.

Quit smoking. The bacteria in your mouth love cigarette smoke, according to Dr. Kivowitz. The tar and nicotine are toxins that irritate the gum tissues, and hot cigarette smoke lowers blood circulation to the area, impeding the healing process.

Consider your friends. If the possibility of losing your teeth doesn't spur you to flossing and brushing with vigor, perhaps vanity will. One of the later symptoms of gum disease is persistent bad breath.

Hair Problems

Taming the Lion's Mane

Envy the balding man—he no longer has a problem with how greasy, unruly or just plain stupid his hair looks. Freed from the mane concerns of life, he never again has to worry about looking like Alfalfa or suffering the cowlick from hell or having what his wife would call a "bad hair day."

As for the rest of us with some mop still on the top, we face the moment-by-moment hassle of getting our hair to look right. Many of us don't even bother trying.

"Most men, unfortunately, neglect their hair—in fact, they don't really pay much attention to it until it starts falling out," says Gregory Miller, head of the styling department for Vidal Sassoon in New York City. But men can't help it—they know they're never going to look like those guys in the shampoo commercials. Their hair's either too oily, too brittle, too wavy, too straight or some improbable combination of the above. And the things they put in their hair to correct one problem seem to cause another.

Becoming Hair-Brained

That said, you can still have better-looking, or at least more manageable, hair and you won't have to work yourself into a coiffure fury to get it. But first, you need to understand why your hair is the way it is.

"Most hair characteristics, texture, color and so forth, are genetic," says Victor D. Newcomer, M.D., clinical professor of medicine/dermatology at the University of California, Los Angeles, School of Medicine. "You can't do much to change it, so you just have to learn to live with it."

And you can, but it means initially making some conscious decisions about the way you treat your hair. "That's the big obstacle you have to get around," says Miller. "Men don't want to spend any time on their hair. But it's like any other part of your body—you have to spend a little time on it if you want it to be healthy and look good." But Miller adds that once you figure out why your hair's misbehaving, you'll be able to help control the problem in about the time it takes you to lather up with shampoo.

FAST FACTS

How common: Every man has or has had some type of problem with his hair. It's part of your dues for being alive.

Risk factors: Although the root of most hair problems is genetic, men who dye their own hair, wash it too frequently with harsh ingredients or expose it to sun and heat are just asking for a bad hair day.

Age group affected: If you have hair, you're fair game for hair problems. As guys approach their fifties and their hair gets thinner, they're less likely to suffer oily hair—but it's more likely to get dry or brittle.

Gender gap: To hear women tell it, they have far more problems with their hair than men. Overall, though, women take far better care of their hair and are less likely to do to their hair the sort of inadvertent harm that men cause themselves.

Who to see: Barber, hair stylist.

Changing the Oil

Right after baldness and dandruff, oily, greasy, stringy hair ranks as man's chief coiffure complaint. Ironically, our hair needs that oil.

"There are glands in the scalp that secrete oil for each of the hair follicles. This oil actually allows the hair to slide through the scalp, and then protects the hair from the elements," explains Jerome Shupack, M.D., professor of clinical dermatology at New York University School of Medicine in New York City.

But some men have overactive glands, causing them to secrete excess oil. The result: These Oil-Can Harrys tend to feel like they've parted their hair with a dipstick instead of a comb. "It doesn't happen forever. As you get older, those glands get less active," adds Dr. Newcomer. In the meantime you can't shut down those glands, but you can minimize their oil spills.

Get a shampoo and a rinse. Most guys try to impose an oil embargo by washing their hair as often as they can—at least twice a day. Miller says that's fine, but go easy on the actual shampooing.

"When you shampoo, you massage the scalp. That washes the oil off the scalp and massages the glands underneath," he points out. Either of these two occurrences is enough to jump-start those glands, creating more of the problem you were trying to stop. "Instead of shampooing two or three times a day, shampoo the hair once and just rinse it the other times," Miller says. That should keep your hair from looking dull and flat without washing too much of the oil off your scalp.

Can the conditioners. Be especially cautious using hair conditioners or shampoos that contain conditioners. They make hair softer and more manageable, but if you have oily hair, you're compounding the problem.

"One of the main ingredients of most conditioners is dimethicone, a type of silicone, which can make your hair greasier," says Miller. If you can't live without a conditioner, use a lightweight one and be judicious in applying it. "Don't get it anywhere near your scalp," Miller admonishes.

Hands off your hair. Of course, the problem may not be overactive glands at all, but your own nervous habits. "Running your fingers through your hair, holding your head in your hands, scratching your head—some of these things will massage the glands, plus you transfer some oil from your hands to your hair and that gives it a flat appearance," says Miller.

Making Ends Split

Meanwhile, if you don't produce enough oil, or you're exposing your hair to particularly harsh treatment, you can end up with brittle hair.

"When that layer of oil is broken down, the moisture trapped below it evaporates. Then the hair dries out and is more susceptible to damage," says Dr. Shupack. Shortly, you end up with dry, unmanageable thatches with enough split ends and broken shafts to make your head look like a haystack. Luckily, experts say, men can easily protect naturally dry hair or spot habits that might be drying their hair out.

Turn on the hair conditioner. While conditioning is not usually recommended for oily hair, it does plenty of good for dry, brittle hair. A conditioner or shampoo with conditioner coats hair, trapping moisture and protecting it from drying elements.

Spare the sunlight. And speaking of drying elements, few are hotter or more damaging to hair than our own sun.

"As experts we are always telling people to wear a hat in the sun to protect their scalp and hair," says Miller. You can also buy spray-on sunscreens in most drugstores. Although they're designed more for scalp protection, they may also keep your hair from withering.

Watch your water sports. You'd think swimming would be a good, moisturizing sport for your hair. But if you swim regularly in a chlorinated pool, you're doing more harm than good.

"If you have a pair of jeans and you wash them in bleach regularly, what do you think they'll look like?" says Miller. "The chlorine in pools has just the same effect on hair—it's absolutely lethal, especially if you follow that up by going out in the

the male file

The average human head has 100,000 hairs on top that grow an average of 0.01 inches a day. Each day, the average person loses 25 to 125 hairs, which are replaced by new ones, unless you're balding.

sun." Miller suggests shampooing your hair after every dip in the pool. Not only will you save your hair, you may even save yourself from embarrassment. "If it stays on your hair long enough, it's not uncommon for the chlorine to give it a nice greenish tint, too," Miller says.

And even in unchlorinated water, towel your hair off as much as possible when you get out.

"If you walk around in the sun with wet hair, the heat of the sun is going to be magnified by the water droplets and that's going to damage hair, too," says Dr. Shupack.

Don't blow hot air. If you blow-dry your hair, keep the dryer on a low or "cool" setting. "And don't get the dryer too close to the hair—that really dries it out too much," says Miller. Keep the dryer at least a foot from your head.

And if you towel off, pat your hair dry—rubbing it with the towel will only make it more brittle.

Dye in, dry out. By the time we hit middle age, our body's supply of certain pigments starts to decrease—and our hair starts losing its color. Once those few gray hairs start sprouting, more than a few of us come up with the colorful solution of dyeing our hair back to its more youthful hues. Think twice before you cast those dyes. Some commercial hair dyes have a metallic base that builds up on hair, making it brittle. Ask your hair stylist about the base before using the dye.

"Plus, coloring your own hair is a bit like being your own dentist. I mean, you can't really see what you're doing," says Miller. If you want to heed vanity's call, heed it all the way and get it colored by a professional. "The ingredients we use tend to be less of a quick fix than these at-home jobs, and they're not going to be as harsh," Miller adds.

Breaking the Wave

And then there are the hair phenomena that no one understands fully—for example, why our hair develops a sudden kink or wave seconds after we get out of the shower.

"Some of this can't really be controlled. Our hair grows in certain patterns," says Miller. "That's why a hair part falls a certain way, or why some men seem to be stuck with a perpetual cowlick." Most of us just hope for the best, but if you're willing to invest a little extra time and money, you can make your hair more agreeable—possibly even stylish.

Get slick. In addition to whatever shampoo you use, consider adding a styling gel or mousse to your hair. Gel keeps straight hair straight and prevents cantankerous locks from sticking out. Meanwhile, if your hair's wavy or curly in a flattering way, mousse will help keep that wave or curl in place. Finally, a light conditioner keeps hair more manageable.

Don't take any static. In the winter static electricity can make combing your hair look like an impromptu science experiment, with your static-charged appearance being the hideous result. To avoid a shock when you look in the mirror, wet your comb first and pass it slowly through your hair.

Hit the showers. When all else fails, you can always start from scratch. Go back to the shower and wet your hair again. "This time, don't let it dry on its own. Take some time to blow-dry it into the shape that you want," says Miller.

Befriend your barber. Finally, if you ever have any questions about your hair, ask the person who's no stranger to your parts—the barber or stylist who cuts your hair regularly. If you don't have a regular one, get one. And remember: You don't always have to get a haircut to get hair advice. "Most good professionals will be happy to give you a free consultation," says Miller, who recommends seeing your barber about once a month. He or she can be a valuable ally in your quest for style—and keep you from tearing your hair out in frustration.

Hangover

Easing the Morning After

Inebriated man can be a wonder to behold. By night he is charming, witty, glib, fun hog supreme, magnet to gorgeous women, master of his universe—at least in his own mind. By morning this once debonair personage is buffing the underside of the toilet rim with the back of his head.

Actually—as you may well know—dinner revisiting is but one of the many symptoms of a hangover. Fatigue, jittery nerves, depression and a head that has ballooned to accommodate the Stanford marching band can all result from an evening's excess.

We all know what havoc too much drinking can wreak, but no one can tell you precisely what elicits all this carnage.

"Nobody knows what causes a hangover," says Donald Goodwin, M.D., professor of psychiatry at the University of Kansas Medical Center in Kansas City, who has researched the topic extensively. "Hangover is really a catchall for a multitude of symptoms, and it's not well-understood."

No matter. To the man who has overimbibed a cure is of far more concern than a cause. Unfortunately, here again there is plenty of mystery. Why are there so many mixed messages about hangover cures, even from the experts?

"Because no one really knows what works," says John Brick, Ph.D., a biological psychologist in private practice in Yardley, Pennsylvania, specializing in alcohol and drug pharmacology and toxicology. "What works for one person doesn't necessarily work for another. A lot of the hangover recipes are just incredibly anecdotal."

The Night Before . . .

The best way to avoid a hangover is not to drink, a practical option but one few men heed, explaining why a man who has never experienced a hangover is rarer than Christmas specials in July. If you choose not to abstain, a little forethought may help ease your pain the next day.

Watch what you drink. There's still plenty of debate on this, but many experts believe the darker-colored alcohols—whiskey, rum, brandy and the like—tend to wreak more havoc. Why? Because the darker liquors are chock full of congeners, chemicals that add flavor and color. These substances may also magnify a hangover.

Experts agree that red wine can often be a problem, too. Red wine contains tyramine, a chemical that can produce a headache that will stand your hair on end. "If you're prone to headaches, it's definitely true that red wine is most likely to cause them, especially the cheaper brands," says Anne Simons, M.D., assistant clinical professor of family and community medicine at the University of California, San Francisco, and a clinical physician at the Department of Public Health, also in San Francisco.

Slug water before you go to bed. "One part of the hangover is actually caused by cellular dehydration in the brain," says Dr. Brick. "You can minimize that by drinking water before you go to bed. A 12-ounce glass of water will help rehydrate the system. It seems to work for a lot of people."

Dr. Simons advises also downing a few glasses of water while you're imbibing—it will help keep you hydrated and possibly reduce the next day's discomfort.

Eat a big meal. "Drinking on an empty stomach is just going to increase the toxic effects of the alcohol," says Dr. Simons. "Your blood alcohol level will get higher faster, and you'll likely suffer more the next day."

Food slows the absorption of alcohol. Still, a healthy repast is not a license to lie on your back under the keg.

The Morning After . . .

You've ignored all the preceding advice, drowning it in a sea of alcohol. You awake shaky and pained, with the mental acuity of a cantaloupe. Here are a few things you might want to try.

Sleep in. Experts agree this is one of the best things you can do for a hangover, if for no other reason than that it cuts down on the time you have to spend conscious. Be aware that even if you get a solid eight hours, that may still not be enough.

"Alcohol disrupts your sleep cycle," says Dr. Simons. "Even if you sleep for a long time, it may not be good quality sleep. You really need a lot more sleep to make up for having poor quality sleep. If you can plan it so you can stay in bed longer the morning after, that can really help."

Reach for drinks, preferably water. Alcohol dehydrates, no secret to anyone who has woken up the next morning sure that Lawrence of Arabia had been filmed in his mouth. Your body's cells need fluid. Your bloodstream needs fluid. Your tongue has sprouted hair.

What to drink? Advice here runs the gamut. Everyone has his own personal concoction guaranteed to cure. The truth is orange juice or any other fruit juice that contains fructose (a form of sugar) may help your body burn alcohol faster, and

FAST FACTS

How common: Right up there with colds and puberty.

Risk factors: Alcohol—too much.

Age group affected: All ages—from too young to know to old enough to know better.

Gender gap: Men and women are equally as likely to wake up feeling as if they've been hit by a truck. Men may enjoy this experience more often because they often drink more.

Who to see: Sorry, you'll have to face the music yourself.

sports drinks like Gatorade that replace both fluids and electrolytes may come in handy if you've been tossing up the night's excesses. But in most cases, all you really need is plain old water.

"If your bartender or your uncle from Kalamazoo says you should drink a mix of cranberry and tomato juice with a spritz of orange juice, well that's fine," says Dr. Brick. If it helps you, it's simply because you're drinking fluids, he says. Water would accomplish the same thing.

Take aspirin. A mild painkiller like aspirin will help relieve the headache and general achiness of a hangover. Aspirin, however, may irritate your stomach, so you might want to eat something light first, or try an aspirin substitute like acetaminophen.

Will taking aspirin before your binge help? Sorry, old wives' tale, says Dr. Goodwin.

Have a few bananas. No kidding. Drinking depletes the body of serotonin, a chemical compound produced in the brain with the help of certain nutrients found in bananas, says Dr. Goodwin. He allows that he doesn't know if replenishing serotonin will make you feel better, and he admits he knows of no hard scientific evidence to support his claim. But since that's the case with all hangover remedies, this one's as good as any.

Apply ice. "Use a bag of ice either on the forehead, both temples or the nape of the neck," advises Alan M. Rapoport, M.D., a neurologist and co-director of the New England Center for Headache in Stamford, Connecticut. It can help dull headache pain.

Eat . . . delicately. Chosen properly, food may help quell your roiling stomach. Though a cheesesteak hoagie with extra cheese may sound good, you need to steer clear of fatty foods and lean toward high-carbohydrate foods such as cereals, breads and fruits, says Dr. Simons. "You want to eat things that are easy to digest."

Careful with the coffee. There's no scientific evidence that caffeine helps a hangover in any way—and since it's a diuretic it will dry you up even more. Plus, coffee is a powerful stimulant, not the sort of thing you need when you're already jumpier than an amphetamine addict grasping an electric wire.

"Some people have something very much like anxiety attacks with a hangover," says Dr. Goodwin. "If you're feeling jittery and nervous and anxious, coffee is going to make you feel more jittery and nervous and anxious."

But regular coffee drinkers depend on caffeine. When they skip their morning cup they often get a headache—making their hangover worse. "Coffee is a double-edged sword," says Dr. Brick. "You'll have to experiment to see what works best for you."

A Final Warning

Hangovers, for the most part, are a humorous affair, especially if you aren't the one with the hangover. But there are two serious points you need to consider.

First, studies have shown that the effects of a hangover can hang on, and impair performance, for a surprisingly long time. In one study, airline pilots who consumed roughly four drinks were still impaired in their ability to land aircraft (using a flight simulator) 14 hours after their blood alcohol level returned to zero.

"If you're hungover, you may be at a higher risk for accident or error," says Dr. Brick. "Plan on avoiding anything that could get you in trouble."

And though it may seem a blessing, there's cause for concern if you drink and never get hangovers.

"That's a sign of certain types of alcoholism," says Eric J. Devor, Ph.D., professor of psychiatry at the University of Iowa Hospitals and Clinics in Iowa City. "If you drink large amounts of alcohol and don't get a hangover, that's something you might want to have a professional look into."

Headache

Declare Independence from Pain

Thomas Jefferson suffered from debilitating headaches throughout his life. In his Pulitzer Prize-winning biography, *Jefferson and His Time*, author Dumas Malone recounted one episode that delayed Jefferson's return to his beloved Monticello following Congress's adjournment in 1807. "Though somewhat less severe than others he had endured, this lasted about three weeks, keeping him in a darkened room nearly all day when at its worst and, as he complained, leaving him only an hour or two for work."

Jefferson was no slacker. And neither are the millions of Americans who miss work each month because of headache pain. A national survey conducted for Anacin showed that in one month seven million Americans missed one or more days of work because of headaches. Annualized, that would mean an estimated $8 billion in lost productivity for U.S. companies.

The fact that headaches are so common—about 90 percent of the population has them at least occasionally—yet are still considered mostly a women's problem may result in a lot of unnecessary suffering for males.

A study of 2,479 people who get migraine headaches found that men are far less likely than women to seek a doctor's help or to be properly diagnosed if they do. "While it's true migraine is three times more common in women, it still affects 6 percent of U.S. men. This often goes unrecognized," says Richard B. Lipton, M.D., associate professor of neurology at the Albert Einstein College of Medicine in New York City. "The way gender bias works in migraine strikes me as very ironic because women with migraines get stigmatized as having some trivial problem that may not be worth the doctor's attention, and then men with migraines get missed because of that same myth."

The Three Main Pains

There are more than 300 different causes of headaches, ranging from carbon monoxide intoxication to thyroid disease to brain tumors. Some men even get headaches at the point of orgasm during sex—not exactly the kind of throbbing they had in mind. "You're supposed to be feeling good and all at once you get hit over the head with this headache," says George H. Sands, M.D., assistant professor of neurology at Mount Sinai Medical Center in New York City.

But the overwhelming majority—more than 90 percent—of headaches among men fall into three categories. They are:

Tension. The most common by far, tension headaches account for nearly 70 percent of all headaches. This is what most of us would consider as the "Take two aspirin and call me in the morning" variety. It is brought on, as the name implies, primarily by stress or fatigue, although other factors—including caffeine, poor posture and inadequate lighting—can trigger an attack. The pain, generally characterized as mild to moderate, strikes both sides of the head. It is more of a steady pain than pounding or throbbing, and can last anywhere from 15 minutes to a week.

Migraine. This one can send you cowering to a darkened room, much like Thomas Jefferson. Close to a quarter of headaches fall into the migraine category. Migraines typically cause intense, pulsating pain, usually in just one side of the head, and are often accompanied by nausea, vomiting and sensitivity to light, sound and movement. A migraine can last as short as four hours and as long as three days. And it is believed to be largely genetic. "Almost 70 percent of people with migraines have a family history of headaches," says Ninan T. Mathew, M.D., director of the Houston Headache Clinic and clinical professor of restorative neurology at Baylor College of Medicine in Houston.

Cluster. In *Saturday Night Live*'s early days the late Michael O'Donoghue performed a series of hilariously sick celebrity impersonations. With a straight face he would introduce his portrayal of Mike Douglas—or whoever was the target that night—with a sharp needle in his eye. Then, he would writhe on the stage in fake excruciating pain, screaming in agony while covering his eyes. Anyone who saw these warped routines has a good idea what cluster headaches are like. Only there's nothing funny about them. "They're so painful that people commit suicide over them," says Marvin Hoffert, M.D., director of Headache Associates in Boston.

Unlike migraines, cluster headaches occur mainly in men. They got their name because they tend to come in clusters. "Cluster headaches are strictly and always on one side and in a very special location," Dr. Hoffert says. "It's kind of behind the eye and in from the temple. Everybody points to exactly the same spot with cluster headaches. They are overwhelmingly severe. You can't do anything else when you have a cluster headache." They last between 15 minutes and three hours, and can strike anywhere from eight times a day to once every other day.

More than 80 percent of people with cluster headaches have blue or hazel eyes, says Joel Saper, M.D., neurologist and director of the Michigan Head Pain and Neurological Institute in Ann Arbor. More than 90 percent smoke cigarettes and more

FAST FACTS

How common: At least 90 percent of Americans have a headache sometime in a year.

Risk factors: Stress, family history, food sensitivities, disrupted sleeping or eating patterns.

Age group affected: While everyone is subject to headaches, they occur most frequently between the ages of 35 and 45.

Gender gap: Women are three times more likely than men to get migraines, and have a higher overall rate of headaches. Men are equally as likely as women to suffer from tension headaches, but are much more likely to get cluster headaches—for every woman suffering from a cluster headache, there are eight men. Studies show that 99 percent of women and 93 percent of men will have headaches at some time during their lives.

Who to see: If headaches are getting in the way of your everyday life, consult your family doctor. You might be referred to an internist, neurologist or a doctor who specializes in headaches or pain medicine.

than 70 percent drink regularly, he says. What that all means is uncertain. "If the cluster headache patient stops drinking and stops smoking, the headaches don't go away," Dr. Saper says. "They'll be easier to treat, but they won't go away."

Butting Heads over Headaches

There is considerable disagreement within the medical community regarding what causes headaches. The traditional view, espoused by Dr. Mathew, is that headaches usually stem from arteries in the brain constricting and then expanding, pressing against nearby nerve fibers.

Others, including Dr. Hoffert, believe that tension headaches are "head pain, pure and simple," with little to do with arteries. Rather, they are caused directly by muscle tension or soreness, emotional distress or a combination of the two.

As for migraines, this school of doctors believes they stem from an abnormality in the brain's neuron circuits "in which the head pain is really just a side effect," Dr. Hoffert says. The neuron theory accounts for symptoms such as vomiting, sensitivity to light, sound and movement, and clumsiness or confusion, he says.

Then there are those like Dr. Saper, who believe that tension-type headaches and migraines are not two distinct disorders, but the ends of the same spectrum.

"A migraine is more than just pain. It's a constellation of painful symptoms and, in some people, a large array of vague to dramatic nervous-system dysfunctions," Dr. Saper says. "Many people with tension-type headaches have those vague dysfunctions, but they don't reach the threshold to diagnose it as a migraine. It's a very arbitrary line that separates tension-type and migraine headaches."

While doctors may disagree on what causes headaches, there are several things they agree can be done to help prevent or ease the pain.

Heading Off Head Pain

The quickest way, of course, is to take a pain reliever such as aspirin, acetaminophen or ibuprofen as soon as the pain strikes. And migraine sufferers can get relief from a prescription drug called sumatriptan or a powerful class of drugs called ergotamines. Sumatriptan is about 75 percent effective in reversing migraine pain, Dr. Saper says, but warns that it is not a "miracle cure," as some have hailed it. The drug, marketed as Imitrex, poses cardiovascular risks in some patients. It also is short-acting, meaning migraine pain returns within nine hours for about half of the drug's users, Dr. Hoffert says.

Additionally, studies show that men who frequently take painkillers for headaches will need ever larger doses to get the same effects. There's also the risk of "rebound" headaches, in which the drugs themselves cause more headaches to occur, says Bradley S. Galer, M.D., assistant professor of neurology and anesthesiology and medical director of the headache clinic at the University of Washington in Seattle. Here are some other ways to deal with or head off headaches.

Don't take it sitting down. Any kind of vigorous exercise—running, swimming or even walking briskly—not only can help prevent headaches before they begin, but also short-circuit tension headache pain when it does arrive, perhaps by boosting the body's production of painkilling endorphins, says Dr. Sands. "I get headaches sometimes, and when I go for a swim they will usually get better." To get the endorphins going, you probably need at least 20 minutes of intense exercise.

Whoa, Trigger. A study of 494 people with migraines found that certain things served as triggers for attacks. Number one with a bullet was stress. Among men in the study 54 percent said their migraines kicked in during stress. And 22 percent said their headaches started after the stress was over. So it makes sense that stress reduction and relaxation techniques would help reduce the frequency and severity of migraines. Muscle tenseness, as well as emotional stress, can set your head throbbing. Take a few minutes during the day to stretch and relax.

"If it's a headache caused by areas of contracting muscles, called trigger points, I generally counsel my patients to take a hot shower in the morning and stretch those muscles to reduce the contraction," adds Dr. Sands. A massage or a good soak in a hot tub also may ease your aching head, says Dr. Hoffert. Biofeedback—a method of consciously influencing body functions you don't ordinarily control, such as blood flow and heart rate—has proven successful in helping reduce migraine intensity, duration and frequency in many. But biofeedback takes training and time; consult your doctor about it first. Other stress reduction techniques, including meditation, imagery and yoga, may help as well. "Clinical psychologists are available that specialize in teaching these tools to headache sufferers," says Dr. Huffert.

Don't be a caffeine fiend. "For tension-type headaches the most common food problem would be caffeine, because caffeine is a stimulant, both to the psyche and to the muscles," says Dr. Hoffert. "Caffeine will make tight muscles tighter and anxious minds more anxious. So reducing caffeine use will help."

Watch what you eat. Foods were a trigger among 28 percent of men with migraines from the study. And certain foods seem to especially trigger attacks, says Dr. Mathew. Chocolate is a common offender, as is a class of chemical additives called nitrites, often found in processed meats such as sausage and ham. Many men get headaches after consuming artificial sweeteners, or foods laced with monosodium glutamate, a flavor enhancer often used in potato chips and Chinese food.

Don't see red. Red wine may go well with steak, but it also accompanies migraines in some. Check if you're one of them by monitoring whether your headaches start when you drink wine or other alcoholic beverages.

Don't smoke. Yet another reason not to smoke cigarettes—or even be around those who do. "It raises carbon monoxide levels and potentially provokes headaches in predisposed people," Dr. Saper says.

Keep normal hours. "Too much sleep and too little sleep can induce a headache," says Dr. Mathew. "If you need six hours of sleep, then you should sleep six hours every night." The same rule of regularity applies to eating habits, Dr. Saper says.

Be like Thomas Jefferson. Go into a dark room. "Your eyes are sensitive to light, so it feels better," Dr. Saper says.

Let the ice man cometh. If you suspect your headache was caused by muscle trauma to the neck or shoulders, give it the deep freeze, suggests Dr. Sands. Many men get quick relief from this type of headache with cold compresses, adds Dr. Sands. Wrap a bag of frozen vegetables or ice in a towel and keep it where you're hurting for ten minutes, and then remove it for ten minutes and so forth.

Use this cluster buster. Keeping a portable oxygen tank nearby may be a breath of life if you suffer from cluster headaches. Inhaling eight liters of oxygen per minute for ten minutes using a mask knocks down cluster headaches in about 70 percent of people. Talk to your doctor about whether you would benefit by such a setup. Because cluster headaches are so short in duration, drugs aren't much help once you get one. But there are some prescription medications that can help prevent cluster headaches.

When to See a Doctor

For most men it's a matter of personal choice. You should consult with your physician, Dr. Hoffert advises, "when your quality of life is being affected by the headaches. If it's not important to you, then just put up with it." Dr. Lipton agrees. "It is not my view that everyone with a migraine needs to see a doctor. It's a matter of how people are affected."

One thing doctors agree on is that there are several headache alarm bells that should alert you to see your physician. They are: If your headaches are getting worse; if they are less likely to go away with standard treatment than they once did; if they are accompanied by neurological symptoms such as numbness, tingling, weakness, dizziness, visual impairment or difficulty walking; if you run a fever with a headache; if you have a stiff neck; if you have explosive vomiting; and if you develop a new type of headache after age 55. In those cases, your headaches may be a sign that something more serious is wrong.

Hearing Loss

Hear Today, Hear Tomorrow

Whatʼs that? Your wifeʼs accusing you of not paying attention? Everyoneʼs mumbling? Listen up, fella, itʼs your ears.

Sure, hearing loss is something that happens to elderly people. About 30 percent of those over age 65 have experienced some decline; the percentage rises to 40 percent for those over age 75. But the process can begin decades earlier. Hearing specialists say itʼs happening at younger and younger ages.

Why? The incessant din of modern society is taking a toll on our ears, especially the ears of men. While both sexes don earphones and attend live concerts, far more men are exposed to construction and factory clamor, not to mention gunshots, chain saws, jet engines, lawn mowers and leaf blowers. Even the sounds of heavy traffic can rise above the 85 decibel limit that experts consider safe.

Above 85 decibels, noise overstimulates the delicate cells in your inner ears that conduct sound to the auditory nerves. The cells will recover if their exposure to the racket is brief. But prolonged exposure to loud noise destroys these cells. Because the effects are cumulative, repeated noise exposure can lead to permanent decline, says James Lankford, Ph.D., professor of audiology at Northern Illinois University in Dekalb. Men with both loud jobs and loud hobbies multiply their risk.

The Sounds of Silence

Noise is not the only cause of hearing loss, of course. Age, heredity, head trauma, recurring infections and certain medications can even dim the hearing of a cloistered monk. But, while you canʼt get insurance against aging or trade in your genes, you *can* combat the biggest threat of all by simply reining in the decibels.

Turn it down. Get used to lower volumes when you listen to the stereo or television. And donʼt blast away with earphones on or sit too close to the speakers.

Wear ear protectors. Foam plugs inserted into the ear canal or protectors that cover the ears like muffs can blunt sound by 15 to 30 decibels—enough to bring most ambient noise into the safety zone. Which is better, muffs or plugs? "The best kind of protector is the one thatʼs worn," says Dr. Lankford. So the choice is yours—just make sure they fit both ears properly.

245

Tinnitus: How to End Ringing in the Ear

Perpetual ringing in the ears, or tinnitus, is a particularly bothersome problem because there is no cure. Sufferers—and there are a lot—are forced to carry on hearing noise that no one else can hear.

The noise in your head is real, although the exact mechanism is unknown, and when it's loud and persistent, it can drive you to distraction. Indeed, it is sufficiently distracting to account for 12 million doctor visits a year.

What triggers tinnitus? Mostly, it's exposure to loud sounds. Because they are exposed to more noise, men get tinnitus twice as often as women. Plus, just about any ear condition—impacted wax, a tumor and everything in-between—can trigger the personal noise. "Tinnitus is to the ear what pain is to the rest of the body," says Jack Vernon, Ph.D., director of the Oregon Hearing Research Center in Portland. "It's a sign that something is wrong in the auditory system."

There are ways to diminish the perpetual internal noise of tinnitus. Continual exposure to machinery, car horns, rock concerts and other clamor can make tinnitus a constant companion, so avoid loud sounds at all costs. That means getting used to lower volume on the TV, stereo and car radio.

A great many tinnitus victims are told there is no treatment for the condition and all they can do is get used to it. That's not true, say the experts.

Get evaluated. "Have it examined by an otologist or otolaryngologist to be sure it's not a treatable medical condition," says Dr. Vernon. It could be something as serious as a tumor on the hearing nerve, he says. You should rule out that and other disorders. It's also advisable to get a hearing test. Many people with tinnitus have hearing loss without realizing it.

Become a masked man. The treatment of choice, says Dr. Vernon, is a tinnitus masker. It fits into the ear and creates a masking sound that is more pleasant than the sound of tinnitus. Other devices, called tinnitus instruments, combine the functions of a hearing aid and masker. There are also bedside maskers if your head noise makes it difficult to sleep.

Take your medicine. "If masking doesn't work, speak to your doctor about Xanax," says Dr. Vernon. In one study, 76 percent had relief with it, as compared to 5 percent on a placebo. An anti-anxiety prescription drug, Xanax, generically known as alprazolam, doesn't always work, and it can be habit forming.

If your tinnitus is ongoing, Dr. Vernon recommends contacting the American Tinnitus Association. It publishes a magazine, sponsors research and provides referrals. Write to the association at P.O. Box 5, Portland, OR 97207.

FAST FACTS

How common: Approximately 10 percent of Americans suffer permanent hearing loss at some point in their lives.

Risk factors: The main factor is noise. Also, heredity, head trauma, recurring infections, certain medications and exposure to certain chemicals.

Age group affected: Gradual loss of high-pitched sounds may begin in the thirties or forties and extends to lower frequencies by age 50 to 60. By age 75, 40 percent of men have significant hearing loss.

Gender gap: The ears of men and women are built the same, so both sexes are equally susceptible. Men, however, have greater exposure to noise and head traumas, so they tend to have more hearing problems.

Who to see: Audiologist for a hearing test. For medical treatment an otologist or otolaryngologist.

Don't worry about muffling the sounds you need to hear. Protectors neutralize background noise and can enhance the understanding of ordinary speech, says Michael K. Wynne, Ph.D., associate professor in the Department of Otolaryngology at the Indiana University School of Medicine in Indianapolis. "At a concert or a club," he adds, "protectors actually improve the quality of sound, and you can hear the lyrics better." For a hundred bucks or so, you can even purchase the kind of high-fidelity earplugs favored by musicians.

When should you wear ear protectors? If, after you leave a loud place, all sounds appear to be muffled, you've been exposed to too much noise, says Laurence Fechter, Ph.D., professor of toxicology at the University of Oklahoma Health Sciences Center in Oklahoma City. Dr. Wynne's rule of thumb: "If you have to raise your voice to be heard, it's too loud for your ears." But even more moderate levels of noise exposure may have a cumulative effect on hearing, says Dr. Fechter. He suggests wearing ear protectors whenever you use power tools or listen to loud music.

Get away from it all. The longer you're exposed to noise, the greater the damage. Take a break and rest your ears. Give your ears a chance to recover.

Added Protection

Noise is not the only threat. Here are more ways to protect your ears.

Don't stick things in there. Wax is not a waste product. Wax is good. It helps prevent infections. Ordinary washing will take care of any excess, so don't go shoving cotton swabs in your ears in a misguided attempt to clean them. It can push the wax farther into the ear canal and plug it up, says Ronald Amedee, M.D., associate professor of otolaryngology at Tulane University Medical Center in New Orleans. Many a hearing loss has been cured by a professional de-waxing from an ear specialist.

Keep them dry. Water that remains in the ear can alter the acidity level, leading to infections. If you swim a lot, protect yourself. Whether or not you use swim plugs, Dr. Amedee recommends prophylactic drops (Star-Otic Ear Solution). You can purchase a solution at a drugstore, or make your own. "Mix a pint of white table vinegar and a pint of clear rubbing alcohol," he says. "Put four or five drops in each ear when you leave the pool. It helps to restore the proper pH."

Stay in shape. "Eat properly and exercise appropriately," Dr. Wynne advises, "and avoid caffeine and nicotine." All of which will help prevent blood vessel damage. "Hearing can be affected if blood flow to the capillaries is restricted."

When the Ears Fail You

If you find yourself straining to hear or if you have to ask people to repeat themselves a lot, don't play denial games. Have your hearing checked.

Act quickly. "The longer you wait, the more difficult it is to treat and the greater the chance it can get worse," says Dr. Wynne. Getting help quickly is especially important if the hearing loss is sudden, if it's accompanied by dizziness or a relentless ringing in the ears or if it develops in one ear only.

Get a hearing test. The best way to determine the nature and extent of a hearing loss is to have it evaluated by a certified audiologist. They have can be found in large hospitals, medical schools and speech and hearing clinics.

Have a medical evaluation. Dr. Lankford recommends having an otologist or otolaryngologist examine you for underlying medical conditions. Anything from wax buildup to infections to tumors could result in hearing loss.

Make it louder. If medical treatment can't restore your hearing, a specialist might recommend hearing aids. "There has been a renaissance in hearing amplification in the last few years," says Dr. Amedee. Hearing aids are smaller and better; the more powerful ones fit snugly behind the ear, but some fit into the ear canal itself.

If you do decide to buy aids, see a licensed hearing aid professional and insist on a trial period. It takes time to evaluate these devices and adjust to them. And establish a good relationship with the dispenser; the instruments might need to be modified from time to time.

Other amplification devices can be used in addition to or instead of hearing aids. There are wireless systems that transmit sound from a microphone to a set of earphones, and systems that carry infrared signals to a personal receiver that converts the information to sound.

Heart Attack
How to Beat the Clock

It was hardly what you'd expect: An interview with a rock star in which the major focus was not the star's latest album, tour or political cause. The topic: his first heart attack.

The star was John Mellencamp, who described being hit by what he took to be the flu after a concert. "I didn't have pain in the chest or any of the classic symptoms," he told *Rolling Stone* magazine, "so I went out and did 20 more shows."

It was only after that "crazy" feeling in his chest persisted that he went to a doctor and learned the truth: What he'd thought was the flu had been a heart attack that had reduced his heart capacity by something like 12 percent. His reaction was anger, mainly at himself. "The moral of my story," he said, "is that 80 cigarettes a day and a cholesterol level of 300 is like a loaded gun."

Indeed, if ever there's a wake-up call to change your habits, a heart attack is it. What makes the whole topic so scary is that men who don't even know they are at risk drop dead from heart attacks. And not just a few: According to the American Heart Association, about 250,000 people a year die of heart failure suddenly and unexpectedly.

If you want to avoid such an abrupt ending, read on.

Assessing Your Risk

Two out of three people who have heart attacks survive them. The best way to ensure you're among that majority is to make sure you know what a heart attack feels like and what to do if you're having one.

John Mellencamp was not alone in mistaking his heart attack for the flu. According to Jeffrey Anderson, M.D., professor of cardiology at the University of Utah School of Medicine in Salt Lake City, up to a quarter of all heart attacks aren't discovered at the time, either because they're "silent" or because the symptoms are misconstrued as something else.

The fact is that heart attacks usually are not the sledgehammer to the chest many of us assume them to be. Joseph Alpert, M.D., a cardiologist at the University of Arizona, Tucson, and author of *The Heart Attack Handbook*, says that for most people a heart attack is uncomfortable, rather than painful.

He describes the typical symptoms as a heaviness, burning, squeezing, tightening or pressurelike sensation in the middle of the chest, usually behind the breastbone. Sometimes these sensations spread to both arms, especially to the wrists, and up into the neck, jaw or back—any one or all of these places may be involved. Sweating, nausea or shortness of breath may occur. The discomfort can last for several hours, which is why a heart attack can so easily be mistaken for the flu, heartburn or indigestion.

What causes a heart attack? The vast majority—about 85 percent—occur when an artery that feeds the heart, already clogged by cholesterol deposits, gets blocked off entirely by a blood clot. Lacking blood and oxygen, the area of the heart supplied by that blocked artery begins to die. Often the stress of a heart attack causes the rhythm of the heartbeat to be thrown off, and it is this abnormal rhythm that can lead to cardiac arrest and death.

The best way to lessen your risk of having a heart attack is to avoid narrowed arteries and other forms of heart disease by controlling the risk factors that are within your control. For details on how to do that, we've devoted entire chapters to heart disease, high blood pressure and high cholesterol. In the meantime here are some pointers specifically related to heart attacks, especially for those who are collecting risk factors the way some people collect parking tickets.

Couch potatoes beware. If you're out of shape, sudden bursts of activity—shoveling snow is a classic example—can bring on a heart attack, says Scott W. Sharkey, M.D., director of the Cardiac Care Unit at Hennepin County Medical Center in Minneapolis. One study found that the chance of a sedentary person suffering a heart attack during or just after heavy exertion is nearly 50 times that of people who exercise five or more times a week. That's why couch potatoes who plan to start a new program of physical fitness are encouraged to check with their doctors first.

Don't throw the snow. One reason so many men have heart attacks shoveling snow is that cold air causes blood vessels in the heart to constrict. If you must shovel, Dr. Sharkey says, wear a mask or scarf over your mouth that will help warm up the air you breathe.

Don't powder your nose. Another type of snow that's dangerous for your heart, Dr. Sharkey says, is cocaine. Remember the college basketball star Len Bias? He proved that even the best-conditioned of us can die suddenly by shoveling that sort of powder.

Run on. Athletes who don't have risk factors for heart attack but are still concerned about dropping dead in midworkout should relax. Research has shown that

FAST FACTS

How common: Each year at least 1.5 million Americans will have a heart attack. A third of them will die, making heart attack America's single largest killer.

Risk factors: Age, heredity, being male, being overweight, smoking, high cholesterol, high blood pressure, lack of exercise, diabetes, stress.

Age group affected: The average guy is more at risk for heart attack as he gets into his fifties because the bad habits of a lifetime start to catch up with him in middle age. Five percent of all heart attacks occur in people under the age of 40, while 45 percent occur in people under the age of 65. About four out of five people who die of heart attacks are age 65 or older.

Gender gap: Men have more heart attacks than women until women pass the age of menopause. It's thought that women's higher estrogen levels protect them from heart disease during childbearing years.

Who to see: Your family doctor can evaluate your risk of heart disease; a cardiologist will treat you if you have it. If you think you might be having a heart attack, call your local emergency medical service or 911 for immediate help.

people who exercise consistently are "extraordinarily safe" from heart attack, according to John J. Duncan, Ph.D., chief of clinical applications at the Cooper Institute for Aerobics Research in Dallas.

Dr. Duncan cites one study that tracked nearly 200,000 runners who had participated in two major marathons over a 30-year period. Only four sudden cardiac deaths occurred among them, he says, and when autopsied, each of those four showed symptoms of underlying heart disease.

Cool it. Several major studies have shown that anger, stress and severe anxiety can help set the stage for heart attacks. If you're plagued by those emotions, you owe it to your heart to learn how to manage them. "Everyone has stress," says Stephen Hargarten, M.D., interim chair of the Department of Emergency Medicine at the Medical College of Wisconsin in Milwaukee. "It's the *management* of stress that's the issue." Try learning some relaxation techniques, practice meditation, get a hobby, find some counseling or, in severe cases, ask your doctor about medication. And, Dr. Hargarten adds, don't forget to laugh.

Make your mornings mellow. If stress is bad for your heart, stress in the morning is worse. Heart attacks have been shown to occur most often during the early morning hours, Dr. Sharkey says, especially on Monday mornings. The blood is more prone to clotting in the morning, and the body, as it shifts gears from groggy to harried, may undergo hormonal changes that can kick off an attack.

Consider getting tested. Men over age 40 may want to ask their doctors about the possibility of having a stress test to look for signs of heart disease, says Dr. Duncan. A stress test involves walking or jogging on a treadmill while hooked up to an electrocardiogram. Be forewarned, however, that narrowed spots on arteries that are too small to be discovered on stress tests can still cause heart attacks, according to Dr. Sharkey. That means good health habits are still your best defense.

No Time to Waste Time

If you think you're having a heart attack, get to a hospital. *Fast.* "When the heart attack starts, every minute counts," says Paul Ridker, M.D., associate physician at the Brigham and Women's Hospital, Harvard Medical School. "Every single minute, heart cells are dying. Most doctors will tell you that if they had the option, they'd have a heart attack in the hospital so that they could be treated immediately."

In reality, according to a study Dr. Ridker conducted, most doctors who have heart attacks arrive at hospitals within 80 minutes. That's far faster than the average Joe, who waits between five and six hours. Why do people hesitate? Andreas Wielgosz, M.D., head of the Division of Cardiology at the Ottawa General Hospital in Canada, conducted a study of that question. It found, not surprisingly, that confusion over symptoms is among the most common reasons. Many people lengthen the delay when they try to treat themselves for what they think is their problem, taking an antacid, for example, on the assumption they're experiencing heartburn.

Finally, there's the old demon, denial: A lot of people simply refuse to admit to themselves that they might be having a heart attack.

Here's a checklist of what you should do if heart attack symptoms set in.

Talk about it. Dr. Wielgosz's study found that people who told someone else that they feared they were experiencing a heart attack ultimately received treatment earlier. That's because whoever you tell is not as likely to succumb to denial as you are, and thus may be in a better position to decide whether a trip to the hospital is in order. "The decision making should be shared," Dr. Wielgosz says.

Plug into the system. If you're uncomfortable for more than a few minutes, call your local emergency medical service or dial 911. That will put you in touch with knowledgeable people who can advise you and send help if needed. Or, if you can't get through, get your personal doctor on the phone.

Get to a hospital. Don't worry too much about choosing a hospital. According to Dr. Wielgosz, any hospital that provides emergency care will do. "Proximity is by far the most important criteria," he says. And don't be shy about going to the emergency room just because you're not sure you're really having a heart attack. "Don't be embarrassed," Dr. Wielgosz says. "The health profession would much rather assure you that everything is fine than deal with you as a statistic."

Depending on how severe your symptoms are, you may have to make a judgment call between being driven to the hospital—never drive yourself—or asking for an ambulance. The deciding factor, according to Harlan Krumholz, M.D., assistant professor and cardiologist at Yale School of Medicine in New Haven, Connecticut, should simply be which one will get you treatment fastest. Don't forget that ambulance crews can start working on you as soon as they arrive.

Take an aspirin. Aspirin helps reduce the blood's tendency to clot, which can reduce your chance of dying from a heart attack by 20 percent. Dr. Krumholz recommends swallowing two adult chewable aspirin or one adult aspirin.

Relax. As weird as that might sound, anything you can do to allay feelings of panic while you wait for treatment will help your heart. As already noted, stress is a risk factor for heart attacks, in part because our ancient fight-or-flight response mechanism causes adrenaline to be released into the bloodstream. According to Dr. Alpert, adrenaline increases blood pressure and causes the blood to clot more easily. That can be a good thing if your body is preparing for a battle that might cause a wound, but if you're having a heart attack, it definitely makes things worse. Try to sit quietly and think peaceful thoughts.

The Clot-Busting Miracle

The best thing about getting treatment for a heart attack quickly is that doctors now have drugs that can stop the attack cold. That can have a direct impact on the quality of your life for the rest of your life, because tissue damaged during a heart attack is damaged irreversibly. The implications of that are great: Damaged heart tissue means the heart's efficiency as a pump is reduced. Also, your overall stamina will decline—how much depends on how much tissue has died—while the likelihood of succumbing to a second heart attack is increased.

The clot-buster drugs, as they're called, dissolve the clot that's blocking your coronary artery, restoring the lifesaving flow of blood to your heart. According to Dr. Ridker, these drugs can reduce deaths from heart attack by 25 to 30 percent if they're administered in less than six hours from the time the heart attack begins. Administered within an hour of when a heart attack begins, clot-busters increase your chance of surviving by almost 50 percent. Those are definitely odds worth rushing for.

See also Heart Disease, High Blood Pressure, High Cholesterol

Heartburn

Surefire Ways to Extinguish the Flames

You load so much turkey onto your plate that it makes a Dagwood sandwich look thin. You follow that up with apple pie, ice cream and three cups of coffee. By the time dinner's done you feel like a beach ball with legs. Worse, your chest has burst into painful flames. Holiday heartburn strikes again.

Not that heartburn waits for holidays to set your insides on fire. It can occur anytime, although it's most common when you've just stuffed yourself with a rich, multicourse meal. And despite the name, heartburn affects not the heart but the esophagus, the tube leading from the mouth to the stomach.

Also known as dyspepsia or acid indigestion, heartburn occurs when powerful acids inside the stomach (which is well-protected by a tough inner lining) surge upward into the esophagus (which isn't as well-protected). After prolonged contact with the acids, the tender tissues get scorched. "It's analogous to moving your finger very quickly through a flame," says Arthur J. DeCross, M.D., a gastroenterologist in private practice in Rochester, New York. "You can do it 100 times very quickly and you're not going to get burned. But if you stick your finger in a flame and leave it there, you're going to get burned."

Banish the Burn

Stomach acids are normally kept in place by a tough little ring of muscle called the lower esophageal sphincter. But sometimes this protective muscle doesn't do its job properly, says Dr. DeCross, with the result that acids splash upward into the esophagus.

Here are some of the things you can do to help your sphincter keep stomach acids where they belong.

Don't be a pig. Overeating is the number one cause of heartburn, experts say. The more food you stuff into your stomach, the greater the volume of acids secreted, making it more likely to splash into the esophagus, says Dr. DeCross. Eating less—and eating more slowly—are the best ways to stop the burn from igniting.

Watch out for food foes. Many foods and drinks can cause the protective sphincter to temporarily weaken. Chocolate, mints, alcohol and fatty foods all are

Heartburn or Heart Attack?

Yow! You've just stretched out on the sofa when this dull ache starts smoldering in your lower chest. So you struggle with the chest pain dilemma: Do you call 911, only to have an irritated paramedic hand you an antacid? Or do you suffer stoically—and possibly drop dead from a heart attack?

Experts agree that it can be difficult to distinguish the pain caused by heartburn from that caused by a heart attack. One helpful clue is to ask yourself what you were just doing: Were you jogging, for example, or scarfing hot dogs?

"Most people get heartburn at night, or lying down after they eat," says Duane T. Smoot, M.D., a gastroenterologist and professor of medicine at Howard University in Washington, D.C. "Most people get heart pain when they're exercising."

You can also tell a lot by the kind of pain you're having. Heartburn usually causes a burning or dull ache in the lower chest. Heart attack pain, on the other hand, is "a heaviness in the chest," says Dr. Smoot.

To be safe, however, you should consider any sudden and severe chest pain to be a medical emergency, experts say. This is particularly true if the pain radiates from the chest to the shoulders, neck, arms or jaw, or if you're also experiencing dizziness, fainting, sweating, shortness of breath or nausea.

prime offenders, says Larry I. Good, M.D., chief of the Division of Gastroenterology at South Nassau Hospital in Oceanside, New York, and assistant professor of clinical medicine at the State University of New York at Stony Brook. Tea, colas and juices also can cause problems.

Everyone's different, of course. Some guys can eat chocolate all day without pain, while others ignite after a single bite. By paying attention to when heartburn occurs, you'll learn which foods to avoid in the future, says Dr. Good.

Skip the coffee. Both decaf and regular will cause the stomach to secrete more acids, says Dr. Good. At the same time, coffee weakens the protective lining inside the esophagus, making it more vulnerable to acid assaults.

Stay on your feet. When you've just indulged in an epic holiday gorge, the lure of the couch can be nearly irresistible. When you lie down, however, acids come up. To help gravity work to your advantage, stay on your feet—or at least stay sitting up—for a few hours after eating, doctors advise.

Lean left. If you must hit the sack after a large meal, try lying on your left side. In one study 15 healthy volunteers at Jefferson Medical College in Philadelphia were asked to lie down after a high-fat meal. Researchers found that those who laid on their left sides had significantly less acid backup than those who laid on their right.

Keep your head up. To prevent the nighttime burn, try elevating the head of your bed four to six inches by putting blocks under the legs of the headboard, says Daniel A. Norman, M.D., director of the Department of Gastroenterology at Barton Memorial Hospital in South Lake Tahoe, California, and assistant clinical professor of medicine at the University of Nevada School of Medicine in Reno. Sleeping on a slant will help keep stomach acids down, he says.

Banish the butts. Smoking fans the flames in two ways: It reduces the holding power of the protective sphincter, and at the same time, it makes it more difficult for the body to remove acids already present in the esophagus. So if you haven't already quit smoking, now would be a good time to give it up.

Time your workouts. Running right after a meal can cause acids to splash into the esophagus, says Donald Castell, M.D., chairman of the Department of Medicine at Graduate Hospital in Philadelphia. To prevent this, wait at least a half-hour to an hour after eating a light snack and two to three hours after a small meal before hitting the pavement, he says.

Enjoy spicy foods. While men have traditionally blamed today's heartburn on last night's enchiladas, there's little evidence that spicy foods cause anything more than an exciting culinary adventure. After all, stomach acids are naturally more powerful than anything you'll ever put on your plate. Of course, some people are more sensitive than others, adds Dr. Good. So if those hot peppers seem to be causing more "Oy vays" than "Olés," you may want to switch to milder fare.

Stay slim. Some studies have shown that carrying around excessive weight can reduce the holding power of the esophageal sphincter and at the same time increase the upward pressure of stomach acids.

Sure Ways to Douse the Flames

If, despite your best efforts, you still get heartburn, the first thing to do is reach for an antacid. You won't have to reach far: Pharmacies and supermarkets stock dozens of varieties, all of which can cool the heat in a hurry, says Dr. Good. While liquid antacids are less convenient than tablets, they're generally more effective, he adds.

There are four primary ingredients in antacids: sodium bicarbonate, calcium carbonate, aluminum salts and magnesium salts. In addition, some antacids include another ingredient, alginic acid, which lays down a foamy layer on top of the acid

FAST FACTS

How common: Anyone can get heartburn, and most guys occasionally do. Roughly 44 percent of us experience heartburn monthly.

Risk factors: Overeating (particularly fatty foods), smoking, being overweight.

Age group affected: Most common between ages 60 and 70.

Gender gap: Pregnant women are the top candidates for heartburn. Among society's nonpregnant, however, heartburn occurs equally in men and women. Men should be alert to symptoms of heart attack.

Who to see: Most cases don't require a doctor. But if pain is great or prolonged, consult your family doctor. You might be referred to an internist or gastroenterologist.

pool inside your stomach. The weight of the foam—combined with the buffering power of the antacid—helps keep the painful acids safely in place.

While all antacids can be equally effective, the various compounds cause a variety of side effects. Magnesium salts, for example, may cause diarrhea, whereas calcium carbonate may result in constipation. (The two are often combined in one product so their side effects will cancel each other out.) Ask your doctor or pharmacist which antacid may work best for you.

While antacids are considered safe for short-term relief, they may cause a variety of complications—mineral imbalances, for example, or making other medications you may be taking less effective—when taken for long-term relief. So if you've been taking them for more than three weeks, talk to your doctor.

If heartburn hits you more than once or twice a month, your doctor may recommend that you take powerful prescription medications called H_2 blockers. The H stands for histamine, a chemical that stimulates production of gastric acids. Unlike antacids, which neutralize acids, the H_2 blockers actually reduce the amount of acids that are produced. Drugs such as cimetidine (Tagamet), famotidine (Pepcid), nizatidine (Axid) and ranitidine (Zantac) are all commonly used H_2 blockers.

In people who produce too much stomach acid, H_2 blockers will cut production by as much as 95 percent, says Douglas Drossman, M.D., professor of medicine and psychiatry in the Division of Digestive Diseases at the University of North Carolina in Chapel Hill.

When H_2 blockers aren't enough, your doctor may recommend a drug called omeprazole (Prilosec). This medication—doctors call it a proton pump inhibitor—

shuts down an enzyme that the body needs for acid production. After antacids and H_2 blockers, "it's kind of like the third level of treatment," Dr. Drossman says. Omeprazole has been found to reduce acid production by 99 percent.

Another avenue of treatment, says Dr. Good, is cisapride (Propulsid), a drug that will tighten the esophageal sphincter.

When medications don't work, your doctor may consider surgery. Generally, this is considered an option only when one of the following applies: Your entire life seems to revolve around the pain; you wake up choking; you have precancerous changes of the esophagus; there is recurrent bleeding from an injured esophagus; or you suffer from Barrett's esophagus, a peptic ulcer of the lower esophagus.

The surgery typically involves a procedure called fundoplication. This increases pressure on the lower esophagus by wrapping part of the stomach around the lower end, which in turn helps to keep stomach acids out. In nine out of ten cases surgery will significantly help reduce heartburn pain.

Heart Disease

Avoiding America's Top Killer

Okay, guys, this is the big one, numero uno, the killer of killers. Heart disease is the leading cause of death for men in the United States, killing roughly half a million of us each year. Almost twice as many men die from heart disease as from cancer, the number two killer. You're eight times as likely to die from heart disease as you are from an accident.

The message should be clear: If you're serious about your health, start taking care of your heart.

Although it's true that heart disease hits the elderly hardest, that doesn't mean you don't need to think about it until you're retired and standing on the golf course. Autopsies performed on young men have shown that hardening of the arteries—by far the major cause of heart disease—is often underway by the time we're in our teens, notes Robert Rosenson, M.D., director of the Preventive Cardiology Center at Rush-Presbyterian-St. Luke's Medical Center in Chicago.

It's also a cop-out to assume heart disease is a matter of genetics, and therefore something you can't do much about. Yes, heredity does play a role in the development of heart disease. But to what extent is a matter of debate. Thomas Kottke, M.D., a preventive cardiologist at the Mayo Clinic in Rochester, Minnesota, suspects that what is being passed on in families with a history of heart disease are bad habits as much as bad genes. "You learn your eating habits from your mom," Dr. Kottke says. "And she's the same one who cooks for your dad. And who teaches the kids to smoke in a family? Mom or dad, usually."

There's no question that when it comes to your heart, bad habits can kill. One major study found that men who smoked and who had high cholesterol were more than twice as likely to have a heart attack as those who didn't. Adding high blood pressure to that list more than tripled the likelihood of an attack.

What's wonderful about the heart is that the opposite is also true: Good health habits can add years to your life. Heart disease has declined in this country by an astonishing 50 percent during the past 25 years, according to Dr. Kottke, a decline he attributes in large part to healthier diets, more exercise and less smoking. "What people are doing in their daily lives is having an effect," he says.

A Heart Primer

Your heart is the central engine for a power system that delivers fuel that your body's cells need to function—mainly oxygen, proteins and sugars. Blood, which carries these ingredients, is pumped from the heart to the rest of the body in tubes called arteries. Separate tubes called veins bring the resource-depleted blood back to the heart, where it is sent to the lungs to pick up more oxygen. The blood goes back to the heart and the cycle resumes.

But your heart not only pumps blood, it needs blood. After all, it, too, is made up of cells, which need nutrients and oxygen that the blood supplies. The main tubes carrying the blood that nourishes the heart muscles are called coronary arteries. If arteries clog up with deposits of fat and other debris, the blood flow through them gets restricted. This buildup of debris, called plaque, also causes arteries to become less flexible, or hardened—a condition known as atherosclerosis.

A hardened artery is also more prone to cracking. Paul Thompson, M.D., director of preventive cardiology at the University of Pittsburgh Medical Center, compares the effect to a garden hose that's been left out in the sun too long. When a crack in an artery wall occurs, a blood clot can form. If the artery is already clogged by plaque, the clot can get wedged inside the artery like a cork in a bottle. By far the most dangerous clot occurs in a coronary artery. When that happens, the blood flow to the heart is shut off and—boom!—you have yourself a heart attack. In fact, the vast majority of heart attacks are caused by blockages in the coronary arteries.

Besides setting off a heart attack, atherosclerosis can cause high blood pressure. As the width and pliability of your arteries decrease, your heart works harder than it should to push the blood through those narrower, less flexible pipes. The tougher it is for blood to flow, the more your heart has to work to do its job, and the sooner it wears out.

Heart disease is a sneaky killer—you won't feel the gunk accumulating on your arterial walls. If you're lucky, you might get a warning, which comes in the form of an angina attack. Some luck: If you're having an angina attack, you'll feel pain or pressure in your chest, sometimes radiating down the left arm or into the neck, jaw or shoulder. Physical stress or excitement kicks off angina because your heart is asking for more blood during those moments, blood your clogged arteries can't deliver. You ignore angina at your peril: 90 percent of the people who die suddenly of a heart attack have been found to have had two or more narrowed arteries.

The Basics for a Sound Heart

Since heart disease is such a monster health problem, it gets plenty of attention from medical researchers, so there's a great deal of information about its causes and

FAST FACTS

How common: Heart disease causes nearly half of all American male deaths every year. You're far more likely to die from heart disease than from anything else.

Risk factors: Heredity, poor diet, lack of exercise, excess weight, smoking, diabetes.

Age group affected: The risks of dying from heart disease increase dramatically with age—about four out of five people who die from heart attacks are 65 or older.

Gender gap: Men are at greater risk than women of having heart attacks earlier in life. Exactly why isn't known, but it's thought that women's levels of the hormone estrogen may help keep their cholesterol down and their arterial walls more flexible. In any event, after middle age (and menopause) the statistics even out.

Who to see: Family doctor, cardiologist.

how to prevent it. Here's an overview of the fundamentals. Follow these recommendations and your chances of developing heart disease can be substantially reduced.

Control your diet. What we put in our mouths has a lot to do with what ends up on the walls of our arteries. You've heard of cholesterol—it's the soft, fatlike substance that is the principal component of the plaque that blocks arteries. It's also an essential building block that our body produces to strengthen cells and build hormones. We can't live without it, but we can die from too much of it.

The best way to keep excessive cholesterol amounts out of your system is to eat less animal fat. Foods that are particularly high in saturated fats include meat, whole-milk dairy products and fried foods. You also want to avoid eating too many egg yolks or organ meats, like liver. Both are packed with fat and cholesterol.

Salt, too, is something to stay away from, since it constricts the blood vessels, contributing to high blood pressure.

Foods that are good for your heart are the same ones you've been hearing about for years: fruits, vegetables and grains. Fish is good in moderation because it contains an oil called omega-3 that helps prevent blood clots from forming.

Those are the essential elements of the heart-saving menu that a chorus of famous diet doctors has been talking about for years, and for good reason: It works. "Everybody is finally singing the same song with slight variations," says Robert Rosati, M.D., a cardiologist at Duke University Medical Center and director of the

Kempner Rice Clinic, both in Durham, North Carolina, where one of the early low-fat diets was born.

Lose weight. Being overweight is a heart disease double whammy, according to Charles Hennekens, M.D., chief of the Division of Preventive Medicine at Brigham and Women's Hospital in Boston and the principal investigator of the Physician's Health Study. Those extra pounds are a sign that you're indulging in heart-hurting habits, like not exercising or eating too much fat. Plus, being overweight is a risk all by itself, making you more prone to high blood pressure, a high cholesterol level and diabetes.

Despite the dramatic reductions we've achieved in heart disease, more men than ever are overweight. The problem is that even the health-conscious among us tend to gorge ourselves on low-fat foods, forgetting that calories are calories, whether we get them from one cheeseburger or several bowls of oat bran cereal, says Robert Nicolosi, M.D., director of the Center for Cardiovascular Disease Control at the University of Massachusetts in Lowell and a member of the American Heart Association's Nutrition Advisory Committee.

Another way we kid ourselves, he says, is by combining high-fat foods with low-fat foods (pouring gallons of oily dressing over a salad is the classic example), which doesn't help our fat intake one bit. "The idea is substitution, not supplementation," he says. "You want to substitute unsaturated-fat foods for the saturated-fat foods in your diet."

Exercise moderately. The evidence is overwhelming that men who exercise regularly have lower blood pressures, lower cholesterol levels and less tendency to develop blood clots than those who don't exercise regularly. The good news for couch potatoes is that you don't have to kill yourself in the gym to get those results.

Several studies have found that even the tamest forms of exercise, from walking to gardening, can provide all the benefits of more intense exercise, so long as you exercise regularly. "It's just like the pills the doctor prescribes: They work, but if you stop taking them, you don't get the benefit," says John J. Duncan, Ph.D., chief of clinical applications at the Cooper Institute for Aerobics Research in Dallas.

If you can manage it, Dr. Duncan recommends a regimen of 20 to 30 minutes of light to moderate exercise a day—five days a week. Try to go every other day at least. Men who exercise more intensively can get away with exercising less often, he says.

Drink moderately. You've heard the reports that drinking a glass of wine or two a day may actually help prevent heart disease? They're true. "A large body of evidence from various studies shows that a modest amount of alcohol intake is associated with a lower risk of heart disease than having no alcohol at all," says Ronald

Krauss, M.D., a senior scientist at the Lawrence Berkeley Laboratory of the University of California at Berkeley and a member of the American Heart Association's Nutrition Advisory Committee. Exactly why isn't clear, he says. There is evidence that moderate alcohol consumption raises the level of "good" cholesterol in the blood.

But don't take this as a license to get loaded: Once you get past two drinks or so a day, you start adding to your risk of high blood pressure and stroke, according to Virgil Brown, M.D., professor of medicine and director of the Division of Arteriosclerosis and Lipid Metabolism at Emory University School of Medicine in Atlanta, and former president of the American Heart Association.

Mellow thyself. Studies have found considerable evidence that hostility, cynicism, pessimism and stress can increase your risk of heart disease. According to Redford Williams, M.D., director of the Behavioral Medicine Research Center at Duke University and co-author of the book *Anger Kills*, if you're habitually suspicious, controlling or isolated, your emotions may be affecting your health. A more obvious cue would be frequent bouts of belligerent behavior. "If you're the kind of guy who's known for giving ulcers rather than getting them, don't be so cocky," he says. You may be giving yourself a heart attack.

Plenty of techniques are available that can teach you how to lower your negativity quotient, from meditation and yoga to therapy, self-help books, support groups and prayer. Whatever route you choose, the goal is to avoid negativity binges as conscientiously as you avoid gorging on pizza: Both are indulgences that can damage your heart over time.

Quit smoking. Smoking causes blood vessels to contract, makes them more rigid, raises cholesterol and makes blood clot more easily. You couldn't ask for a better setup for heart disease—no wonder smokers are two to four times more likely than nonsmokers to die suddenly from a heart attack or stroke. "Smoking is probably the number one behavior that you can change or modify that would have the greatest impact on reducing heart disease," Dr. Duncan says.

Inhaling the smoke exhaled by others also poses a substantial risk to your heart. According to the American Heart Association, your risk of death from heart disease is about 30 percent higher if you're exposed to tobacco smoke at home—and it could be even higher if you're also exposed at work.

When You Need Treatment

Okay, so you've been too indulgent for too long or you got an unlucky draw from the gene pool and now you have heart disease. Is there anything you can do about it?

The answer is yes, within limits. Thanks to dramatic advances in diagnostic technology and in medications, physicians are catching heart disease earlier and treating it more effectively than ever, prolonging millions of lives in the process.

Perhaps the most exciting breakthrough, in the opinion of many cardiologists, is a new class of cholesterol-reducing drugs called reductase inhibitors. Several studies have shown that these drugs can safely lower a heart patient's cholesterol level by 30 percent or more, which reduces the risk of subsequent heart attacks and slows the development of atherosclerosis.

Whatever drugs your doctor prescribes, he will almost certainly recommend you begin taking a daily dose of aspirin as well. Aspirin causes blood to become less sticky, thereby keeping clots from forming. Geoffrey Tofler, M.D., co-director of the Institute for the Prevention of Cardiovascular Disease at the New England Deaconess Hospital in Boston, says that aspirin reduces the chances of having a second heart attack by about 30 percent. But talk to your own doctor about aspirin first rather than self-prescribing it.

As vital as drugs often are to preventing the progression of plaque development, they usually can't unclog arteries. According to Donald Smith, M.D., director of the Lipid Unit at the Mount Sinai Medical Center's Cardiovascular Institute in New York City, only 10 to 30 percent of heart disease patients actually manage to shrink the plaque on their arterial walls and usually by only a small amount. "People are always hoping for regression," he says, "but that's rare, no matter how low your cholesterol goes."

When a blockage is severe enough, you may need surgery to remove it. Three basic types of procedures are available. With angioplasty, a tiny balloon is inserted into the blocked artery and then inflated to push the blockage aside. A newer variation on this approach uses a laser to literally vaporize the plaque. The second procedure is called atherectomy. Here a tiny drill is inserted into the artery to shave plaque away from the arterial wall.

Finally, there's bypass surgery, an operation in which a blood vessel is taken from another part of the body and used to construct a detour around the blocked artery.

The main limitation of these procedures is that new blockages can always form. That's why most physicians prescribe rigorous lifestyle changes as an integral part of any treatment for heart disease.

Dean Ornish, M.D., helped pioneer that approach at his Preventive Medicine Research Institute in Sausalito, California. Dr. Ornish's regimen includes a super-low-fat vegetarian diet (10 percent fat, as compared to the 30 percent fat recommended for healthy adults by the American Heart Association), regular exercise and

the male file

The human heart beats 2.8 billion times by the time you're age 70.

a stress management program that combines yoga and meditation with group therapy sessions.

According to Lee Lipsenthal, M.D., the Institute's medical director, 82 percent of patients who faithfully adhere to this program have achieved some reversal of arterial blockages. The progress is small—the arteries are about 6 percent more open on average during the first year and about 9 percent after four years, Dr. Lipsenthal says. But if it improves your ability to live life, then that's progress you can take to heart.

See also Heart Attack, High Cholesterol

Heart Palpitations
How to Finish the Race

You can live a whole lot of life and rarely be reminded that your heart is pumping, second after second, year after year. Sure, exercise or excitement will quicken its pace. But even then your heart is in synch with the rest of your body. It all feels right.

But every now and then can come a scarier moment, when you're doing little if anything and suddenly your heart will race as if you are sprinting. Or, just as suddenly, you'll feel as if your heart's stopped for an instant.

That's called arrhythmia, and what you're feeling are heart palpitations. Your chances of having palpitations double every ten years you live, and men are 1½ times as likely to have them as women, according to a study of 4,731 adults.

A variety of causes for arrhythmia exists. In fact, palpitations are normal, many people get them, and if you're healthy, they're usually nothing to worry about. You should only be concerned if you have a heart condition already.

A Hop, Skip and a Jump

The human heart has its own electrical system. A built-in pacemaker called the sinus node sends out electrical signals and the four chambers of the heart follow, causing the well-orchestrated contractions that we know as heartbeats.

But on occasion the signal gets momentarily out of line. The signal might not originate in the sinus node. Or the sinus node changes its signal rate. Or there might even be a blockage of the signal. If any of these occur, the heartbeat rhythm changes and you feel the palpitations. Usually, the arrhythmia lasts only a few seconds and you experience a fluttering sensation in the chest. You might also feel dizzy, faint, out of breath, and there could be some chest discomfort.

"Why the electrical signal changes is a mystery to us still," says Michael Brodsky, M.D., professor of cardiology at the University of California, Irvine, Medical Center. "We can point to alcohol, nicotine, caffeine and cold medicines and say they can bring on arrhythmias. But we don't know exactly why these things bring them on."

Stress can do it, too. Common events such as anticipating a new date, fighting

266

FAST FACTS

How common: Many people experience heart palpitations now and then, but less than 3 percent of men are in any danger from arrhythmia.

Risk factors: Stress, smoking, alcohol, too little magnesium, caffeine, cold medicines, previous heart condition.

Age group affected: Palpitations start in childhood, but the chances of experiencing one doubles every ten years.

Gender gap: Men are 1½ times more susceptible to heart palpitations than women, though doctors aren't sure why.

Who to see: Family doctor or cardiologist.

with the boss or worrying over finances can lead to anxiety-triggered heart palpitations. In fact, almost 50 percent of the people with heart palpitations severe enough for a doctor to order an electrocardiogram (ECG) turn out to have an anxiety or depressive disorder. These arrhythmias are commonly caused by alterations in the nervous systems with increased levels of adrenaline.

In rare instances, arrhythmias can be the result of more sinister causes. Sustained rapid heartbeat—exceeding 120 beats per minute for two or more minutes—can indicate that the heart's electrical system is misfiring, causing the heart to beat erratically.

"If the random fast beating goes on too long, this may indicate that the patient may have underlying heart disease," says Dr. Brodsky.

Bear in mind, however, that death during arrhythmia is exceedingly rare and is virtually always from heart disease, not the arrhythmia itself.

Making Sure the Beat Goes On

It's always good to see your doctor if you're at all worried that your palpitations are more than stress related. Even if arrhythmia is caused by stress, the reassurance that your health is fine can aid in reducing the number of palpitation episodes. Also, if you're suffering severe anxiety and trying to ignore it, it can become disabling. Your doctor, in eliminating all physical causes of your palpitations, can then go on to recommend that you seek psychological counseling.

Of course, the palpitations can harbor the remote possibility that you're suffering from heart disease. That being the case, the sooner it's caught the better.

The principal test your doctor likely will use is a version of the ECG. There are a few versions of the ECG test.

Resting. You lie down and disks attached to you record your heartbeats as wave patterns.

Exercise. You walk on a treadmill or ride a stationary bike while the ECG disks monitor whether exercise aggravates arrhythmia. This test also indirectly measures your blood flow from the heart.

24 hour. You wear disks attached to a small portable tape recorder that records heart activity as you go about your business for a full day.

Transtelephonic monitoring. You carry a monitor and if you experience arrhythmia, you can telephone a central monitoring system, which will then record those particular heartbeat waves.

What Becomes of the Broken Hearted

In the vast majority of ventricular arrhythmia cases drugs are not prescribed for treatment, notes Abdul Hakim Khan, M.D., associate professor of medicine at Brown University School of Medicine in Providence, Rhode Island. "Only in the presence of persistent or symptomatic arrhythmia caused by heart disease or arrhythmia occurring in people resuscitating from cardiac arrest is drug therapy advisable," he adds. "Even then, we remember to try to weigh the benefits of treatment against the risks of drug side effects."

Magnesium has been found to be crucial to cardiovascular health, and therefore, Dr. Brodsky recommends that you maintain a diet rich in magnesium, with plenty of vegetables, grains and dairy products. Other tips for avoiding heart palpitations include:

Quit smoking. Doctors note that smoking is particularly dangerous if you have cardiac arrhythmia.

Ease in and out. Warm up before exercising and cool down afterward, ten minutes each.

Ease up. If you're not too happy with your palpitations, keep away from such heart-racing activities as rock climbing and paragliding. You might even wish to drop competitive sports. Competition not only pushes the body hard but generates lots of stress.

Breathe deeply. And take life as it comes. Those who hold their breath when they're upset or scared face upsetting their natural heart functions.

Just say no. As with so many medical problems too much caffeine and alcohol makes things worse.

Heat Injuries

Throwing Ice on the Summer Slammer

His body burns. The end zone down the field seems wrapped in a gray mist; the young running back keeps blinking his eyes, trying to focus through sweat and fatigue that is making the football feel like a rock instead of leather filled with air.

He staggers a little as he takes his place in the backfield and waits for the call: "Gotta do this, gotta do this," he tells himself, shaking his head to try to clear it. The snap comes, he takes the handoff, runs.

And then it all goes black.

"Heatstroke is a truly horrible thing," says James Knochel, M.D., a nationally recognized expert on heat-related illness and chairman of the Department of Medicine at Presbyterian Hospital in Dallas.

Heatstroke can whack your thermostat in a matter of hours—a single wicked game of rugby, for example, or a hot summer run through the fields. A man suffering from heatstroke has been so badly hammered that immediate, major medical intervention is needed.

"Heatstroke victims usually die if they don't get the correct care quickly," Dr. Knochel says. "And by quick I mean you have maybe five to ten minutes to start doing something about it."

That care—the right care—may not be available at your local macho-sweatbox, un-air-conditioned weight room, or during that long training run in the country. So what to do?

Step one: Keep reading.

Hot Time Health

"The more an athlete knows about heat illness, the less likely he is to get whacked by it," Dr. Knochel says. "It is absolutely preventable if he knows what he's doing."

So what do you need to know? Start with the basic spectrum of heat illnesses—knowing what happens when goes a long way toward making sure the summer sun doesn't lay you out on the road during your next triathlon.

269

Heat illness, phase one, in an otherwise healthy man: heat cramps. If you have heat cramps, usually in the large muscles of your legs, then you know two things: One, you're drinking adequate water but you're not getting enough salt, because that's what causes them; and two, you are not in significant trouble at this point but you're on your way.

Heat illness, phase two: heat exhaustion. At this point, you've really pushed it. You're experiencing, well, exhaustion obviously, but the list also could include severe thirst, headache, nausea, vomiting, even diarrhea. If you've reached this point on the chart, you know two things again: One, you're in trouble; and two, you may be in serious trouble.

"It's generally not life-threatening," Dr. Knochel says, "but if you try to push through this—and men are a lot more likely to keep hammering than women—chances are pretty good you'll end up with heatstroke."

Heat illness, phase three: heatstroke. At this point, you're not just in trouble—you're probably going to die unless you get help, and quickly.

Symptoms beyond those in phase two include not sweating but skin that is hot and flushed. The sufferer could be delirious, hysterical, convulsing or hallucinating.

That's all happening for a reason: You're body temperature is so high, anywhere from 103° to 112°F, that you're in the grips of what the medical community likes to call severe central nervous system dysfunction.

Translation: Your brain's fried, and you're going with it. If you do not receive proper medical care in very short order, you're going to die.

"These people pretty much have to be in a hospital environment if they're going to pull through," Dr. Knochel says.

Medical intervention at this point generally involves moving the victim to the shadiest, coolest location available, keeping the airway clear, checking for cardiac arrest and shock and perhaps most importantly, doing whatever can be done to cool the patient: removing his clothing, splashing him with whatever cool fluid is available, putting him in front of a fan or air conditioner and icing him down.

the male file

The human body can withstand extreme external conditions. In a 1960 experiment conducted by the U.S. Air Force, naked men could withstand a dry air temperature of 400°F. In heavy clothing, they could endure 500°F. Comparatively, it takes a heat of only 325°F to cook a steak; the average sauna is 284°F.

FAST FACTS

How common: Heat injuries occur frequently in the summer, but exact numbers are not known.

Risk factors: High heat and humidity lead the pack, followed by overexertion, poor fitness, obesity, age (seniors frequently have aging-compromised cooling systems, and children don't sweat as easily) and illness (which for obvious reasons can affect your body's cooling mechanisms). Those who take diuretics for high blood pressure or nasal decongestants (which slow sweating) or those with viral illnesses are also at risk.

Age group affected: Elderly and children.

Gender gap: In theory women may have a slightly elevated risk since their cooling systems rely more on circulation of blood than sweating; but in general men appear to suffer heat injuries more frequently than women.

Who to see: Nearest available emergency medical provider for heatstroke; nearest provider of shade, fluids, rest and coolants for heat exhaustion.

Generally, if you get the right sort of care in the right time frame, you'll be okay. But there are no guarantees.

"Men who've developed heatstroke once seem more susceptible to recurrences," Dr. Knochel says. "And brain damage is one possible consequence." Unpredictable results may also include vision problems, speech problems, uncoordination and numbness, all of which are of uncertain duration.

Keeping Cool

But it's all preventable if you follow the tips outlined here.

Don't overdo it. This is the single most important tip for avoiding heat injuries. When it's hot out, watch your activity level; if you notice any of the symptoms of approaching heat injury, such as dizziness or major fatigue, do the smart thing: Back off. In this arena pain doesn't mean progress, it means peril.

"Women seem much less likely to go through any of this," Dr. Knochel says. "I think that's chiefly because they're smarter than we are about recognizing their limits. They'll stop when a guy might decide to push it just a little further."

Start off slowly. It's important to plan ahead if you intend to avoid heat injuries in the summertime—and by planning, the medical community means making time for acclimation. Dr. Knochel says, "By sequentially increasing the period of work in the heat over a period of seven to ten days, we become acclimated. This means we can get away with a level of work in the heat that two weeks previously might have killed us. When you're fully acclimated, you should be able to match or come close to your normal performance level."

Drink a lot. "Thirst is a very poor indicator of your need for fluids," says Richard Keller, M.D., assistant managing partner and director of occupational medicine at Northern Illinois Emergency Physicians in Waukegan, Illinois.

"You need to stay hydrated during hot weather, which basically means making a point of taking fluids during activity whether you feel like it or not."

"Pound down the Gatorade," Dr. Knochel says. "Before, during and after exercise, take fluids—water, Gatorade, whatever, it doesn't really matter, as long as you keep your intake elevated."

The reason: Your body can sweat off two to three liters of fluid per hour during hot weather exercise. Dehydration is a real risk, and a dehydrated sportsman is a sportsman in danger for the simple reason that you need that fluid to operate your primary cooling system—sweating.

Avoid caffeine, alcohol and salt tablets. Coffee, a lot of soft drinks and tea all contain caffeine, an alkaloid that can improve your physical performance in some ways but which, in summer, could end up impairing you more. The reason: Caffeine is a diuretic that will accelerate the loss of fluid from your body tissues, increasing your risk of heat injury.

Alcohol and salt tablets will also accelerate fluid loss: In both cases, your body will pull water from your tissues in order to dilute the concentration of either and flush them from your system. Alcohol you don't need at all, and salt, which you do, is better and more effectively replaced through ordinary means or by drinking any one of the popular drinks available containing electrolytes.

Change your workout schedule. Take that routine lunchtime run and switch it to early morning or late afternoon. Both times are cooler periods of the day when heat, and therefore risk, is less.

"Even professional athletes do this," Dr. Knochel says. "It's not something to hang your pride on."

Go easy. This makes sense for anybody, acclimated or not. If you don't have to push it—to get ready for that road race, or whatever—then don't.

"High performance means high heat," Dr. Knochel says. "Slowing things down is a sensible way to keep your body heat under control."

Wear the right clothes. Loose hats, like the old Vietnam jungle caps or ventilated baseball caps—anything that lets air circulate and keeps the sun off—are a good idea for summertime athletes who want to stay cool. Loose clothing that lets sweat evaporate and air circulate is highly recommended, hat or no hat; natural fibers and newer synthetics, like Coolmax, that wick moisture are advisable.

Watch the weather. If the humidity's above 70 percent on a hot day, it does not matter how much you sweat. None of it's going to evaporate, and if it doesn't evaporate, it doesn't cool your body.

"The Midwest is the prime region for heatstroke and related heat injuries," Dr. Knochel says. Not, as you might expect, the extremely hot but dry Southwest.

"The chief reason for that is the weather there. That particular combination of high heat and high humidity. You may be sweating a lot but you're not getting much cooling at all."

So when the heat's on and humidity is high, consider bagging it, before they bag you.

Hemorrhoids

Relief for Down Under

They lurk in the dark like betrayals from the primeval past—anatomical proof that human beings, from the anal point of view, weren't designed to stand on two legs.

After all, dogs and cats don't get hemorrhoids. Neither did we when walking on all fours was the only way to travel. But when man stood up, blood rushed down—right into the anal veins, says Daniel A. Norman, M.D., director of the Department of Gastroenterology at Barton Memorial Hospital in South Lake Tahoe, California, and assistant clinical professor of medicine at the University of Nevada School of Medicine in Reno. One theory is that the veins, like water balloons, began to stretch and swell. They turned into hemorrhoids.

There's another theory. "Cushions" filled with blood help keep you continent and support the anal lining during poops. Elastic tissue is supposed to hold these cushions in place. But aging, hard stools and years of downward pressure make the supportive tissue lose elasticity. That allows the cushion to sag: hence, hemorrhoids.

Hidden Inside

Whether they're swollen veins, sagging cushions or both, everyone has hemorrhoids. But because they're usually tucked away inside the anus, we're not aware of them, says Juan Nogueras, M.D., a colon and rectal specialist at Cleveland Clinic in Fort Lauderdale, Florida. There are two things, however, that can suddenly heighten our awareness: Hemorrhoids can bleed, or they can pop outside.

Hemorrhoids that bleed are rarely serious and will usually clear up on their own. In some cases, however, anal bleeding can be caused by something else, such as cancer. Even if you're creative with mirrors, this is one condition you can't diagnose yourself. A checkup is strongly recommended, says Dr. Nogueras.

Hemorrhoids that appear outside the anus can also bleed. More often, they're simply quite tender. Sometimes, however, a blood clot forms inside the hemorrhoid—a condition doctors refer to as thrombosis—and the pain can be excruciating. "I can spot men with thrombosed hemorrhoids down the hallway from my office," says Dr. Nogueras. "They have a characteristic shuffle."

FAST FACTS

How common: More than 50 percent of Americans will have problems with hemorrhoids at some point in their lives.

Risk factors: Being overweight, lifting heavy weights, straining to have a bowel movement, sitting or standing for long periods of time.

Age group affected: Most common after age 40.

Gender gap: Men and women are equally likely to have hemorrhoids.

Who to see: Proctologist.

Safe Passages

Given time, even the most painful hemorrhoid may disappear on its own. There are, however, many things you can do to help prevent them from forming. Here's what the experts recommend.

Start with fiber. Straining to have a bowel movement puts enormous pressure on the anal veins, making straining the most common cause of hemorrhoids, says Dr. Norman. It's also the easiest to prevent. By eating several servings a day of fruits, vegetables, whole grains and other high-fiber foods, you will make your stools softer and easier to pass. Less strain, experts say, means less pain.

Wash it down with water. Just as your car's pistons will grind to a halt without oil, so will your insides lock up if you don't keep them well-lubricated with water. Drinking at least eight eight-ounce glasses of fluids a day will help keep things moving with a minimum of friction, experts say.

Don't be pushy. As men, we don't like taking "no" for an answer. We'll stay on the court all day to get the perfect shot, or turn every screw under the hood until the engine feels just right. The same goes for our bowels: If they don't move on command, then by gosh, we'll sit there until they do. The result, of course, is less likely to be satisfaction than a bumper crop of new hemorrhoids. You can't rush nature's call, warns Dr. Nogueras. If you've finished an entire issue of *Car and Driver* and you're still stuck in neutral, take a break until your insides are ready to shift into drive.

Lift with care. When you're pumping at the gym, do you punctuate each lift with an explosive oomph? Those grunts may impress the guys on machines, but they also generate huge amounts of internal pressure, says Dr. Nogueras. "I see a lot of thrombosed hemorrhoids in guys who say they've done some heavy lifts that day." If you can't breathe normally, you're probably hefting too much, he says.

Lighten your load. Lugging around a huge belly can also put unwanted pressure down below. Try to slim down to help prevent or treat hemorrhoid problems.

Stopping the Pain

Step into the "hemorrhoid" aisle of your local drugstore and you'll find a re-markable array of products with ingredients ranging from petroleum jelly and shark-liver oil to local anesthetics. All can be somewhat helpful, but don't expect miracles. "Most over-the-counter products work because they help lubricate the anal canal or because they have some soothing properties," explains Dr. Nogueras. "But will they help the hemorrhoids shrink or heal more quickly? Probably not."

A less-expensive—and probably equally effective—option is to lie in a warm bath for half an hour several times a day, says Dr. Norman. It won't make hemor-rhoids disappear, but the soothing warmth will temporarily relieve some of the swelling and discomfort, he says.

If your hemorrhoids are simply too large or painful to endure, your doctor may recommend that you have them removed. This may be done with a simple tech-nique called banding, in which a rubber band is snapped around the base of the he-morrhoid, cutting off its blood supply. Within a week the hemorrhoid will drop off, passing out of the body in the stool, says Dr. Nogueras. "I had one patient who got very concerned because he wasn't sure how he was going to put the rubber bands on," said Dr. Nogueras. "I had to explain to him that I put them on."

A quicker, if somewhat scarier (for the patient, not the doctor), approach is to open up the hemorrhoid with a scalpel and remove the clot that's causing all the pain. The procedure is a simple one, requiring just a few minutes and a local anes-thetic, says Dr. Nogueras. Best of all, the relief is nearly instantaneous.

For the most severe cases, your doctor may recommend having the entire hem-orrhoid removed, a procedure called hemorrhoidectomy. This is done under gen-eral or spinal anesthetic, and you can expect to spend several days in the hospital. While the procedure can be quite uncomfortable, it has one major advantage: Once a hemorrhoid is removed, says Dr. Nogueras, it never comes back.

Hepatitis

Know Your ABCs

Dr. Jack Kevorkian is certainly not the only person to contract hepatitis through a blood transfusion. But chances are the controversial physician sometimes called Dr. Death is the only one to get it while conducting experiments on cadavers.

According to news reports, Dr. Kevorkian—who would later earn notoriety for assisting terminally ill patients commit suicide—contracted hepatitis in 1964 when he injected himself with blood from a blood bank. Kevorkian and two assistants were acting as "controls" while they gave other patients blood from corpses. The idea was to see if blood from cadavers could be used for transfusions. While those who got the cadaver blood reported no ill effects, Kevorkian reportedly wound up with hepatitis C from a tainted blood bank sample.

Because of better screening, the risk of contracting hepatitis today through a blood transfusion has been significantly reduced, notes James Spivey, M.D., assistant professor of medicine and senior associate consultant at the Mayo Clinic in Jacksonville, Florida. But that doesn't mean the disease has gone away; tens of thousands of Americans still get hepatitis each year.

In most people hepatitis typically produces symptoms resembling the flu, and they get over it. But in rare cases (2 to 3 percent), liver failure occurs, and the patient may die. And in others (percentages vary depending on the virus), chronic hepatitis sometimes progresses to cirrhosis, often a precursor of liver cancer.

"Hepatitis simply means inflammation of the liver, and a lot of different things can cause it," says William B. Ruderman, M.D., chairman of the Department of Gastroenterology at the Cleveland Clinic Florida in Fort Lauderdale.

The main culprits are viruses imaginatively labeled hepatitis A, B and C, which together account for about 90 percent of all cases. Also mixed into the viral alphabet soup, although in far smaller portions, are hepatitis D and E. Disorders that attack the whole body, like lupus, can cause hepatitis. So can alcohol, mononucleosis, even heat injury—as well as at least 30 different viruses.

There is a vaccine for hepatitis B, and more recently, researchers have developed a vaccine for hepatitis A, but it is only partially protective and given mostly to children. No vaccines have been developed for the other hepatitis viruses.

Alphabet Soup

It helps to know your ABCs, especially if you want to prevent contracting hepatitis.

Hepatitis A causes about 30 percent of all cases in the United States. It is passed along primarily through fecal contamination of water or food, although sexual contamination also is possible. It typically produces symptoms resembling the flu—fatigue or low-grade fever, for example—and clears up in days or weeks without significant medical intervention.

Hepatitis B is the most common strain, responsible for about 40 percent of cases in the United States. It's generally spread through blood and blood products, and the flulike symptoms resolve themselves within six months. Healthcare workers who are exposed to other's blood are at some risk, but the disease is more common among intravenous drug abusers and homosexuals. The good news about hepatitis B is that 95 percent of those infected get over it without lasting consequences. But 2 to 3 percent develop the chronic form of hepatitis B, which could lead to liver disease, cirrhosis and, ultimately, liver cancer.

The best news about hepatitis B is that it is completely preventable through the use of commercially available vaccines.

Hepatitis C is responsible for about 20 percent of the cases in the United States. According to Dr. Ruderman, half of the patients infected with hepatitis C, which is transmitted mainly by blood and blood products, develop chronic hepatitis. "And probably up to 50 percent of patients with chronic hepatitis C infection will ultimately develop cirrhosis," Dr. Spivey adds.

Although chronic hepatitis can eventually cause death, those infected can still have a relatively normal life span with the right medical care. "Hepatitis C may be present for decades before complications such as cirrhosis or cancer develop," Dr. Spivey says.

The other half of hepatitis C sufferers usually get over it in six months or so. But it remains the leading cause of fatalities caused by hepatitis.

Treatment of chronic hepatitis chiefly revolves around symptom control, since very few effective antiviral medications are available. The message is clear: Prevention is essential.

Staying Out of Harm's Way

Hepatitis prevention is mostly a matter of common sense—at least for those who don't use drugs, engage in homosexual sex or routinely travel in high-risk

FAST FACTS

How common: Roughly 170,000 new cases of hepatitis C are reported each year in the United States, although the actual number of cases is thought to be much higher.

Risk factors: For type A, consuming traces of feces, including water or shellfish that is contaminated by sewage; to a lesser extent, it can be spread through sex; For type B, any activity that results in exchange of blood products (includes tattooing with unsterile needles and drug use) or sex with a virus carrier; For type C, shared needle use or tainted blood.

Age group affected: All. Higher risk attaches to healthcare workers, drug abusers, homosexuals and those who travel in high-risk areas. Children born to mothers infected with hepatitis B have a higher risk of contracting the disease.

Gender gap: Generally none.

Who to see: Any physician specializing in diseases of the liver—typically, a gastroenterologist.

Third World regions. It boils down to one thing: Stay out of harm's way.

Get vaccinated. Healthcare workers and anyone else exposed to needles and the exchange of blood products should get the hepatitis B vaccine to prevent the disease. All children of school age should be vaccinated against hepatitis B, says Dr. Spivey.

Don't eat raw shellfish. You may think the world's your oyster, but before you slurp it down, you'd better think again. Hepatitis A is commonly spread by shellfish from contaminated waters.

Practice safe sex. Hepatitis B and, to a lesser extent, hepatitis A can be spread through sex. Wear a condom if you have any doubts about your partner or yourself.

Take your best shot. If you think you've been exposed to hepatitis A, talk to your doctor about getting a shot of gamma globulin. This blood product boosts immunity and helps exposed individuals stay uninfected.

Store your own blood. If you're going to need blood for elective surgery, consider storing your own. In the past, about 5 to 10 percent of all those receiving blood transfusions developed hepatitis C. The risk is much lower today, however, as a result of effective testing. "There's never been a safer time to receive a transfusion in the United States," Dr. Spivey says.

Hernias

Win the Battle of the Bulge

You twist hard to get away from your touch football opponent and bang—burning in the groin.

You reach down to grab that whole stack of two-by-fours and bang—burning in the groin.

That burning might be an indicator of that ancient bane of manhood—the hernia, the medical community's term for when an organ or tissue protrudes through the structure containing it. In the groin area the muscles of your abdominal wall weaken or rip, and an organ or tissue covered by the inner lining of your abdomen gets pushed through the opening. The term itself derives from the Latin meaning of rupture.

The most common types of hernia are the inguinal, umbilical and incisional. Inguinal hernias occur in the groin, umbilical hernias come through the navel and incisional hernias develop along surgical incisions. Men and women are susceptible to all, but inguinal hernias are more common in men.

In fact, inguinal hernias account for the vast majority of all problem bulges—about 600,000 to 700,000 each year, according to Parviz K. Amid, M.D., co-director of the Lichtenstein Hernia Institute in Los Angeles.

While a strenuous physical activity might be the final trigger for a hernia, it is not the sole cause, and exercising your abdominal muscles will not reduce your risk.

"Your physical fitness isn't a critical factor, and in fact, there isn't much you can do to prevent them since most hernias occur because of collagen deterioration in the groin—a weakening of connective tissue there," Dr. Amid says. "No one's precisely sure why this problem occurs, but it is the root cause of a typical hernia and may be hereditary."

The triggering event for most hernias: Anything that produces a sudden surge in abdominal pressure sufficient to tear that weakened tissue. Physical exertion is a common cause—those two-by-fours again—but lots of men have had that sudden, unwelcome bulge pop out after laughing hard or even just coughing.

Most of the time, a hernia is not something to get terribly upset about: The typical case is not a life-threatening emergency.

FAST FACTS

How common: Very common, with increasing incidence with age. About 600,000 hernia operations are performed each year in the United States.

Risk factors: Primarily age; to a much lesser extent, surgery, being overweight and genetics.

Age group affected: Tends to strike men in their fifties or older, but can strike from childhood on.

Gender gap: More common in men, though women are not immune.

Who to see: Family doctor is fine for initial diagnosis; a hernia specialist is recommended for the actual repair, since they routinely post much lower rates of recurrence than nonspecialist surgeons.

"A good general practitioner can make the diagnosis in 98 percent of the cases," Dr. Amid says. "Typically, he'll then refer you to a surgeon for the repair itself."

But on occasion, a hernia can pose an immediate risk to your health sufficient to warrant immediate medical intervention.

"Many hernias can be reduced by the patient himself—pushed back in through the opening," says Robert Bendavid, M.D., a surgeon at Shouldice Hospital near Toronto.

"Others can be reduced by a physician, generally because we have a better idea of where and what we are pushing. A hernia that can't be reduced is called incarcerated, and is something that needs to be treated immediately because a patient with an incarcerated hernia runs the risk of the hernia strangulating," says Dr. Bendavid.

A strangulated hernia is a hernia with its blood supply cut off or significantly reduced. The result is usually necrosis—death of the protruding portion of bowel or tissue—if left untreated. In 2 to 5 percent of such cases, death also results.

The important point in this discussion is simple: Any hernia may eventually strangulate. This explains the medical community's standard advice: Get it fixed surgically, and the sooner the better.

Fixing It Right

The key indicator of a freshly arrived hernia is a burning or stinging sensation in the groin, accompanied by a brand-new bulge. But pain in the groin doesn't necessarily mean a hernia, and you can have a hernia without pain.

"A lot of things can masquerade as a hernia," Dr. Amid says. "A pulled groin muscle is a common one—kind of like tennis elbow but in the groin. The only way to definitively determine what's causing it is to get a medical examination."

There are three principal surgical approaches to repairing a hernia. Under the conventional approach, refined over the past century from the first procedures for hernia repair, the hernia is reduced and the opening in the abdominal wall closed by stitching together the proper muscular layers. This well-established operation has a very low recurrence rate, and most surgeons that specialize in hernia repair are proficient at it. Dr. Bendavid, an expert in this method, says recovery time is about four to five days, a vast improvement over its previous weeks-long convalescence period.

An approach that began to spread in the mid-1980s involves inserting a synthetic mesh across the opening where the hernia protrudes. The mesh, anchored between the patient's tissues, serves to replace the weakened or torn tissue and keeps the internal organs where they belong. It is frequently referred to as a tension-free repair because the margins of the opening aren't pulled together and stitched. Dr. Amid, who helped develop this technique, reports same-day discharges are common with a recovery time of two to three days.

The newest approach involves inserting a small hollow tube with a camera on one end into the abdomen, a process known as laparoscopy. This permits surgeons to make a much smaller incision to perform the operation with less effect on the abdominal muscles and, according to its advocates, full recovery often in about three days. "It's an advancement of surgical technique that allows surgeons to see and repair hernias on both sides through the same incision without entering the abdominal cavity, thus avoiding a lot of the controversy over this type of repair," says Charles B. Itzig, Jr., M.D., a general surgeon in private practice in Shreveport, Louisiana, who specializes in this method.

What controversy? Boiled down, it's that some surgeons believe the newest method isn't as safe as the other methods because of a reportedly higher risk of complications and that it is still in an experimental phase. The new method also calls for a general anesthetic rather than a local, another argument against it.

Which approach is best for you? Ask your surgeon (or ask two surgeons) to explain the good and the bad points of each and make the decision together.

High Blood Pressure

How to Mellow the Flow

Kidney stones burn your gut like a blowtorch. The flu can lay you out for days. And a broken leg? Hey, that hip-to-toe cast isn't there to make some sort of fashion statement.

You can complain all you want about health problems like these. But at least you know you have them, and that they'll be getting fixed. High blood pressure is different: Not only is it silent, it's far more dangerous. You can have it for *years* and never even know. You don't feel any different, look any different or notice any symptoms. Yet all that time, high blood pressure can quietly be setting you up for heart attacks, strokes and even kidney failure.

"It would be nice if high blood pressure announced itself a little more clearly," says Robert Toto, M.D., associate professor of internal medicine at the University of Texas Southwestern Medical Center at Dallas. "But unless you somehow find out about it, a lot of damage can be done."

Men have an especially rough time with high blood pressure, also known as hypertension. One out of every three white American males ages 18 to 74 has high blood pressure. Among black men, the figure is even higher at 38 percent. Men have a significantly greater chance than women of developing high blood pressure before age 55—probably because we don't get the heart-saving benefits of the female hormone estrogen.

The worst part is that nearly half the men in America with high blood pressure don't even know it. Which brings us to an important rule: Get your blood pressure checked every year. "You couldn't even imagine how many lives would be saved if people had their blood pressure measured," Dr. Toto says. It's simple. It's painless. And it could add years to your life.

Know Your Numbers

Your heart has it rough enough already, pumping blood second after second, minute after minute, day after day. Quite frankly, it doesn't need the extra pressure. When blood pressure rises, it puts stress on arteries and veins, Dr. Toto says. This can leave nicks and scratches on the linings of blood vessels, creating snags

283

where plaque can gather. This narrows the openings in the arteries—creating even more high blood pressure as your heart tries to pump blood through smaller tubes.

When doctors measure your blood pressure, they take two readings. The first, called the systolic, measures how hard your heart must beat to pump blood through your veins and arteries. The second, the diastolic, measures the resistance your blood vessels exert when blood flows back to the heart.

A reading of about 120/80 is considered optimal. When blood pressure readings creep toward 140/90, doctors begin to get concerned. That's considered borderline high blood pressure, the point at which serious health problems can start. Men with high blood pressure are 10 to 12 times more likely to have a stroke, and 5 to 6 times more likely to suffer a heart attack. High blood pressure also can lower the flow of blood to organs and tissue, depriving them of precious oxygen and nutrients. That's why high blood pressure can lead to kidney disease or even complete kidney failure, especially among black men, Dr. Toto says.

Some experts believe that decreased blood flow also can cause brain damage. Researchers took magnetic resonance images of 35 men ages 51 to 80 and found that those with high blood pressure showed significant deadening of brain tissue on the left side and greater fluid buildup on both sides of the brain. This could be a sign that their brains had actually shrunk in size—perhaps because high blood pressure prevented small vessels from delivering enough blood and nutrients to the brain cells, according to Declan Murphy, M.D., senior lecturer and consultant psychiatrist with the Institute of Psychiatry in London.

High blood pressure can even affect your sex life. Men being treated for high blood pressure are up to four times more likely to become completely impotent in later life, according to Kenneth Goldberg, M.D., director of the Male Health Center in Dallas and author of *How Men Can Live as Long as Women*.

Unsolved Mysteries

We know what it is, and we know what it does. But what *causes* high blood pressure? "That's the $64,000 question," Dr. Toto says. Because in more than 95 percent of high blood pressure cases, doctors can't pinpoint the cause.

Two factors are probably at play, says Carlos Ferrario, M.D., director of the Hypertension Center at the Bowman Gray/Baptist Hospital Medical Center in Winston-Salem, North Carolina. The first is genetics. If your family has a history of high blood pressure, you're probably at much greater risk of developing it. Dr. Ferrario says researchers are getting closer to identifying the specific genes linked to high blood pressure. That would allow doctors to test whether you're in danger. Until

No Low Is Too Low

Ever stand up from a chair and suddenly feel like you're on the Whirl-a-Wretch ride at the state fair? The room is spinning, your feet are unsteady, your head is lighter than helium for a few seconds—and then everything's okay again.

That unsettling sensation has a scientific name: orthostatic hypotension. It's caused by a temporary drop in blood pressure, and it's usually nothing to worry about. The only time you should be concerned, experts say, is if you have this experience more than a couple of times a year or if you have ever fainted from it.

In fact, most of the time blood pressure readings are like the limbo—the lower you go, the better you are. "Generally speaking, as long as you feel well and have no symptoms, there's little concern about how low your blood pressure is," says Robert Toto, M.D., associate professor of internal medicine at the University of Texas Southwestern Medical Center at Dallas. "In fact, people with lower-than-average blood pressure readings tend to live longer, healthier lives."

Some British research shows that people with very low systolic blood pressure readings—consistently below 100—may have problems with tiredness and occasional dizziness (systolic is the first number in a blood pressure reading and measures pressure going away from the heart). But doctors don't recommend trying to raise blood pressure levels in these cases, since the overall death rate is lower among people in this group.

Ironically, about the only time you may need to worry about low blood pressure is if you're being treated for high blood pressure. Some evidence shows that dropping your diastolic level (the second number in a reading, measuring pressure as blood returns to the heart) below 85 may increase the risk of heart problems. Talk to your doctor about this if you're taking blood pressure medication.

then, he suggests you shake your family tree a little. If you find an uncle, aunt, sister, brother, parent or grandparent with high blood pressure, be sure to get regular blood pressure checks.

Even if you have heredity working against you, you may not get high blood pressure. "Very much depends on your lifestyle," Dr. Ferrario says. Being over-weight, not getting enough exercise, smoking, high-fat, high-salt diets and stress all may contribute to high blood pressure. "When you start combining those factors—such as being overweight and smoking—the risk really begins to increase," Dr. Ferrario says.

If you already have high blood pressure, doctors may need to prescribe medication to bring it under control. There are four main classes of drugs. Diuretics, which help the body excrete extra fluids to lower blood pressure, are usually tried first. Beta-blockers are designed to slow the heart rate and reduce the amount of blood the heart pumps. ACE inhibitors help reduce the chemicals that cause your blood vessels to constrict. And calcium channel blockers also help to relax and widen blood vessels.

Depressurizers

Drugs should be your last option, however. They all have side effects, ranging from fatigue to headaches to depression. Besides, there's a lot you can do to help lower blood pressure on your own. And keep in mind that every little bit helps. For each point you drop in the diastolic measure, for example, Dr. Goldberg says you cut your risk of heart attack by 2 to 3 percent. And a massive study of approximately 350,000 American men found that life expectancy in the United States would jump by 1.5 years if the average systolic blood pressure reading fell just 10 points, from 130 to 120.

Here's how to do your part for America.

Get measured. Get your blood pressure checked by a trained professional. "In many cases, it's the only way you'll ever find out that you have high blood pressure," Dr. Toto says. Once a year is enough unless your doctor says otherwise.

Those do-it-yourself machines you see in pharmacies and supermarkets can give you a rough idea of your blood pressure. But pressure rises and falls through-out the day, and the machines may not give accurate readings. So be sure to visit the doctor—or take advantage of free screenings that hospitals sometimes offer in shopping malls and other places.

Drop 20 to drop 10. Losing weight can have a significant effect on your blood pressure. One study of 301 overweight people found that losing about 20 pounds can shave ten points off your systolic reading and eight points off the diastolic reading. "Weight loss remains one of the most important ways to lower blood pressure without medication," says Norman Kaplan, M.D., professor of internal medicine and chief of the Hypertension Division at the University of Texas Southwestern Medical Center at Dallas.

FAST FACTS

How common: Roughly one in four American men over the age of 20 have high blood pressure.

Risk factors: Family history of high blood pressure, plus being overweight, high stress levels, smoking and a diet low in potassium all may contribute to high blood pressure. Black men are at greater risk.

Age group affected: Blood pressure rises with age. Men between the ages of 65 and 74 are most likely to have high blood pressure.

Gender gap: Men have a significantly higher risk before age 55. While the increase in risk for women is greater than that for men after age 60 or so, as a whole, men continue to suffer more from high blood pressure.

Who to see: Family doctor.

A bonus: If you're already taking blood pressure medication, studies show that losing weight makes the drugs significantly more effective.

Walk it down. Exercise is another key to lower blood pressure. Reports from the American College of Sports Medicine show that even moderate exercise—like walking 20 to 30 minutes a day, three to five times a week—can help lower pressure by as much as ten points on both the systolic and diastolic readings in people with mild hypertension. If you have high blood pressure, see your doctor before beginning an exercise routine.

Avoid the shakes. Sodium doesn't affect everyone's blood pressure. But there's no test out there to tell who's at risk. And most of us eat way too much sodium anyway, in the form of salt.

"It's good across-the-board advice to cut back on sodium," Dr. Kaplan says. This holds doubly true if you already have high blood pressure—and triply true for African American men, who may be more sensitive to the effects of sodium than white men.

Experts recommend limiting sodium intake to 2,400 milligrams daily; the typical American, however, ingests 3,000 to 6,000 milligrams a day. The best way to reduce sodium intake is to cut back on salt. For starters, avoid fast food. A fancy burger and fries could give you up to half the recommended daily limit. Fill up instead on fresh or frozen fruits and vegetables. Beware of canned: They often are high in salt. In fact, read the labels of all processed foods. Products labeled "low sodium" must have no more than 140 milligrams of sodium per serving, so they're a good place to start.

Eat rocks and live. Three minerals known as electrolytes—potassium, calcium and magnesium—have shown varying amounts of promise in battling blood pressure. Of the three, potassium appears to have the strongest link, Dr. Toto says. That's because it appears to counteract the effects of excess sodium in the body. Experts haven't settled on the ideal amount you need to do the trick—but it certainly wouldn't hurt to pump up your potassium intake. The National Resource Council recommends about 3,500 milligrams of potassium per day. Big potassium sources include baked potatoes (610 milligrams each), orange juice (496 milligrams per cup), bananas (451 milligrams each), spinach (312 milligrams per cup) and broccoli (286 milligrams per cup). Dr. Toto warns not to take potassium supplements without first seeing a doctor, since too much potassium can cause kidney problems.

Calcium's role continues to baffle researchers. Some studies show that large doses of 1,500 milligrams per day, nearly twice the recommended daily allowance, may reduce blood pressure in people with high blood pressure. Other studies show just the opposite. Dr. Toto says the best advice for now is to get the Recommended Dietary Allowance (RDA) of 800 milligrams. Good sources include low-fat plain yogurt (415 milligrams per eight-ounce container), skim milk (302 milligrams per cup) and canned salmon (181 milligrams per three-ounce serving). As with potassium, don't take supplements until you talk to your doctor. Too much calcium can cause kidney stones in some people.

Magnesium seems to be fading as a high blood pressure fighter, Dr. Toto says. But just in case, he says it's still a good idea to take the RDA of 350 milligrams. Good sources include dried pumpkin seeds (152 milligrams per ounce), halibut (91 milligrams per three-ounce serving), almonds (87 milligrams per ounce), lima beans (50 milligrams per ounce) and fortified cereals (varies).

Do the chill thing. Relax. Vegetate. Unwind. "Stress reduction can certainly play a role in blood pressure," Dr. Toto says. So take whatever steps you can to reduce the chaos in your life. Find a relaxing hobby. Lounge on the hammock. Better yet, get some exercise. And if you're one of those workaholic types, try taking a day off once in a while. Studies show that a man's blood pressure is significantly higher in the office than it is at home.

Butt out. Smoking may not cause high blood pressure but it can worsen the effects by damaging veins and arteries. "You should stop smoking under any circumstances. But if you have high blood pressure, it's very important to quit," Dr. Kaplan says.

Grin and beer it. Here's some good news. Moderate drinking isn't likely to raise

High Blood Pressure Self-Test: Give It a Whorl

Are you at risk for high blood pressure? The answer may be right at your fingertips.

A study published in Britain concludes that there may be a link between the pattern of your fingerprints and your risk of developing high blood pressure. Men who had three or more fingers with whorl patterns tended to have significantly higher blood pressure than men with arches or loops.

A whorl pattern looks like a bull's-eye. The center of the print contains a series of complete circles within complete circles. This differs from the arch pattern, which is a series of wavy lines, and the loop pattern, in which the lines form ovals but don't connect into closed circles.

Researchers discovered that the link between whorls and blood pressure was especially strong on the right hand. They speculate that the whorls could be caused by high fetal blood pressure between the 13th and 19th weeks of pregnancy.

If you notice whorl fingerprints, experts recommend having your blood pressure checked by a doctor. And be sure to tell him about your fingerprints. They could be just the clue he's looking for.

your blood pressure. But remember the key word here: moderate. Some research shows that 3 ounces of alcohol a week is about as much as you should drink. You get about 1 ounce of alcohol in a 12-ounce beer or a mixed drink containing one shot (1½ ounces) of liquor.

Evidence is growing that wine, both red and white, may actually help lower blood pressure, say Dr. Ferrario. He says that may be because grapes contain phytoestrogens, a plant-based form of estrogen. But until the evidence becomes stronger, he suggests no more than one or two five-ounce glasses of wine per day.

High Cholesterol

Unplugging the Fuel Lines

If you owned a Porsche, would you pour syrup into the gas tank? No way. Yet many of us perpetrate the same sacrilege on the delicate machinery of our bodies when we stuff cheeseburgers, french fries, candy bars and a zillion other cholesterol-laden foods down our gullets on a regular basis.

Heart and blood vessel diseases are by far the leading cause of death for men in the United States, and high cholesterol is one of the leading causes of heart disease. The cholesterol level of the average American male rises steadily between early adulthood and middle age, increasing in tandem his risk of heart attack, stroke and assorted other unpleasantries.

It isn't necessary, of course. Although some men have a tendency to develop higher levels of cholesterol than others, a large majority of us can significantly lower the amount of this dangerous gunk in our arteries if we practice some basic rules of good health.

The Good, the Bad, the Ugly

Cholesterol is a soft, fatlike substance transported in the blood. It's important stuff—we couldn't live without it. Cholesterol is the raw material our bodies need to make certain hormones, as well as bile, which is essential for food digestion. Thing is, the body makes all the cholesterol we need; many of us, however, tend to consume too much of the foods that cause cholesterol production, and that's where our problems start.

"Cholesterol is like water," says Manfred Kroger, Ph.D., professor of food science at Pennsylvania State University in University Park. "You need water but if you get too much of it, you drown."

Excess cholesterol builds up on the walls of our arteries. If the arteries supplying blood to our hearts and our brains get clogged enough, we can have heart attacks or strokes. Cholesterol can also block arteries leading to the legs, and it's a major cause of gallstones as well.

The body makes two types of cholesterol: low-density lipoprotein (LDL) cholesterol and high-density lipoprotein (HDL) cholesterol. LDL cholesterol is the "bad" cholesterol that clogs your arteries; think of the L as standing for "lousy." HDL is the "good" cholesterol; it actually helps clear your arteries by flushing the bad cholesterol out of your system. Think of the H in HDL as standing for "helpful."

One other cholesterol term you may hear tossed around is triglyceride. Triglyceride is another form of fat in the blood and as such, it is another signpost doctors use to gauge whether your bloodstream has more fat in it than it should. If you have a high level of triglycerides, you're likely to have a high level of LDL cholesterol and a low level of HDL cholesterol. All indicate that your fuel system is running dangerously rich.

How to Get a Reading

There's a simple way to find out whether or not you have a cholesterol problem: Get a blood test. Any man over the age of 21 should be tested. In many cases doctors will just test for total cholesterol and possibly HDL cholesterol. But if a doctor senses a reason to test more fully, a full profile will measure total cholesterol, LDL cholesterol, HDL cholesterol and triglycerides. Then you'll be stuck with a lot of numbers that won't make sense.

Here's a quick decoder: The American Heart Association defines a "desirable" total cholesterol level as anything under 200. Readings between 200 and 239 are classified "borderline high"; by the time we reach our fifties, more than 70 percent of us will be in or above that range. Your risk of heart attack in that category is twice as high as it is for men in the "desirable" range. If you have a reading above 240—between 20 and 30 percent of men will fall into this range by the time they hit middle age—your doctor will most likely suggest substantial changes in your eating and exercise habits. He may even prescribe cholesterol-lowering drugs.

The Cholesterol Busters

One of the great success stories in American health history has been the huge decline in the rate of deaths from heart attacks over the past 40 years, a decline of more than 50 percent.

The decline is in good part attributable to a decline in the number of smokers, not to mention improved medical care and a clearer understanding of the problem.

But it's also no coincidence, says Basil Rifkind, M.D., a senior scientific adviser in the Division of Heart and Vascular Diseases for the National Heart, Lung and Blood Institute in Bethesda, Maryland, that our average cholesterol levels have dropped significantly during that same period. Here's how you can cut your cholesterol levels, too.

Cut the fat. The American Heart Association claims that by consuming a diet that is 30 percent fat, we can significantly reduce our cholesterol levels and our risk of developing heart disease.

In particular, what you want to reduce in your diet is saturated fats, which generally generate a high cholesterol level in the body. These fats occur most plentifully in meat and dairy products.

Here are ten food fundamentals from the American Heart Association that can go a long way toward helping you keep both your fat and dietary cholesterol in check.

1. Eat no more than six ounces a day of lean meat, fish and skinless poultry. The leaner the cut, the better.

2. Try making main dishes that are primarily pasta, rice, beans or vegetables.

3. Try to limit the amount of oil you consume in a given day to between five and eight teaspoons. That would include the oil used in cooking and baking, and also the oil in salad dressings and spreads. Use vegetable oils sparingly. Choose monounsaturated oils (olive and canola) first, polyunsaturated oils (corn, sunflower and safflower) second.

4. Cook the low-fat way: broil, boil, bake, roast, poach, steam, stir-fry or microwave. Don't fry. Sauté only with no-stick sprays, broths or fruit juices, not oils.

5. Trim off the visible fat before cooking meat and poultry, and don't eat the skin. Drain off the fat after browning meats. Chill soups and stews after cooking them and remove the hardened layer of fat from the top.

6. Limit the amount of egg yolks you eat in a week to three or four. That includes the eggs used in baked goods.

7. Say no to organ meats—liver, brains, kidneys and the like. Like eggs, they're packed with cholesterol.

8. Use skim or 1-percent-fat milk and nonfat or low-fat yogurt and cheeses. Choose soft margarine over stick margarine—the hardening process produces saturated fat. Avoid butter.

9. Eat five or more servings of fruits or vegetables each day.

10. Eat six or more servings of breads, cereals or grains each day.

Stay trim. If you're substantially overweight, your body is producing more cholesterol, and it's pushing that cholesterol into your bloodstream more rapidly than if you were slimmer, says Donald McNamara, Ph.D., professor of nutritional sci-

FAST FACTS

How common: More than half of all American men—between 40 and 50 million—have high cholesterol, a number that helps explain why the United States has one of the world's higher rates of death from cardiovascular disease.

Risk factors: Heredity, fatty diet, lack of exercise, smoking, obesity.

Age group affected: The amount of cholesterol in men's blood tends to rise gradually from their twenties into their fifties. At that point, it usually levels off for a decade or so and then declines. Research suggests that high cholesterol ceases to be a risk factor for heart disease once we get into our seventies.

Gender gap: For most of their adult lives, men have higher cholesterol levels than women on average. It's thought that the female hormone estrogen combats low-density lipoprotein cholesterol and causes high-density lipoprotein cholesterol to rise; after menopause, however, when their estrogen levels drop, women's cholesterol levels tend to exceed men's.

Who to see: Family doctor for a cholesterol test. If your levels are high, you might be referred to a cardiologist or a dietitian.

ences at the University of Arizona in Tucson. Most likely, your triglyceride level is also too high, while your level of HDL cholesterol is probably too low. That's a prescription for heart disease.

One of the main reasons men's cholesterol levels tend to rise from their twenties to their late fifties is that their waistlines expand during those years, at the rate of about a half-pound a year, says William Hazzard, M.D., chairman of the Department of Internal Medicine at the Bowman Gray School of Medicine of Wake Forest University in Winston-Salem, North Carolina. Dr. Hazzard adds that a potbelly usually means you risk having high triglyceride levels, since the gut is where triglycerides tend to collect. That's why the American Heart Association recommends that a man's waist measurement should not exceed his hip measurement.

Work it out. People who exercise regularly have lower levels of LDL cholesterol. Exactly why that's so is not understood, according to David Spodick, M.D., professor of medicine at the University of Massachusetts Medical School in Worcester. Part of the reason may be that the type of men who work out regularly also tend to watch their diets and their waistlines.

Either way, exercising is one of the few ways you can raise your level of HDL cholesterol. You don't need to run a marathon, either. John J. Duncan, Ph.D., chief of clinical applications at the Cooper Institute for Aerobics Research in Dallas, says a regimen of 20 to 30 minutes of low-intensity exercise—anything from walking to gardening to dancing—is perfectly adequate, as long as you do it several times a week.

Don't smoke, drink a little. Besides exercising, there are two other ways to raise your HDL cholesterol. The most important is to quit smoking. Tobacco smoke suppresses good cholesterol and also damages your heart and arteries in other ways.

Meanwhile, if you drink, only drink a moderate amount of alcohol. A moderate amount, according to Virgil Brown, M.D., professor of medicine and director of the Division of Arteriosclerosis and Lipid Metabolism at Emory University School of Medicine in Atlanta and a former president of the American Heart Association, is two drinks a day. Any more than that, he warns, and you may well increase rather than decrease your risk of blood vessel disease.

When You Need Assistance

Help is available when it comes to battling high cholesterol. If controlling your bad habits hasn't brought your levels down, your doctor can prescribe a number of cholesterol-lowering drugs that are effective and, for most men, safe.

One group of drugs in particular, called reductase inhibitors, or statins, has proved to be remarkably successful. According to Dr. Rifkind, statins can lower bad cholesterol counts by 20 to 30 percent in most patients, and if used in combination with other drugs, by as much as 50 percent.

As impressive as those results are, don't count on drugs to bail you out of cholesterol problems if you don't have to. For one thing, you could be one of the rare few to develop significant side effects.

Second, drugs aren't often prescribed until you already have a problem—heart disease, in other words. And even with successful drug treatments, advanced heart disease is almost impossible to reverse. It's far better to avoid getting it in the first place by taking care of yourself over the course of a lifetime.

Impotence

Up from Erection Problems

We take our bodies for granted. When we want to shoot hoops, we expect our arms and legs to listen. When we want to tinker with our cars, we expect our fingers to comply. And when we want to make love, we expect our equipment to stand tall like a young Marine recruit.

Unfortunately, our penis doesn't always get the picture. Instead of standing tall, it sometimes plays dead. And instead of being our pride and joy, it becomes our biggest source of embarrassment.

The problem is called impotence, and 10 million American men regularly suffer from it. Impotence is defined as the inability to achieve or maintain an erection sufficient for satisfactory intercourse.

The causes of impotence fall into two categories: psychological and organic. Psychological causes, such as performance anxiety, depression or stress, were once believed to be the root of all impotence. But in the majority of cases in men over age 50, it's organic problems at work. Organic causes are when body mechanisms don't work right, and include poor blood flow, injury or a drug reaction. Even younger men can be impotent for organic reasons.

The Ins and Outs of Impotence

Most men have had a bout of temporary impotence at one time or another. A familiar scenario plays out sometime after the last call at the bar, when our minds (and imaginations) tell us we're a hunka hunka burning love, while our lethargic penises prove the deflated contrary.

Tension and fatigue also can cause temporary impotence, says Irving J. Fishman, M.D., associate professor of urology at Baylor University School of Medicine in Houston. But when we're talking chronic impotence—the kind that doesn't go away when you sober up—the scenario changes.

The most common cause for chronic impotence—especially in men over age 50—stems from circulation problems in the penis, says Harin Padma-Nathan, M.D., assistant professor of urology and director of the Center for Sexual Function at the University of Southern California Medical Center in Los Angeles.

Normally, blood fills the arteries and the spongy tissue in the penis, making it erect. With age these arteries become clogged from fatty deposits that accumulate over the years. Clogged penile arteries mean less blood, and less blood results in a weaker erection—or none at all.

Other causes for chronic impotence include endocrine disorders such as diabetes or thyroid problems; neurological conditions, like stroke or multiple sclerosis; and reactions to medications, most commonly thiazide diuretics (Naturetin, Hydrex, Diuril and Thalitone), blood pressure medication or tranquilizers.

Although psychologically caused impotence occurs within any age group, it is most commonly seen in younger men and is caused by the most powerful sex organ of all: the brain.

"Psychological erection problems can be caused by problems at work or in a relationship," says C. Steven Manley, Ph.D., staff psychologist at The Male Health Center in Dallas. "They can also be caused by anger, depression or a suppressed fear of failure."

Depression, for example, increases certain body chemicals that can result in lowered potency. Performance anxiety is another erection stopper. With performance anxiety you worry excessively about your sexual performance, Dr. Fishman says. The more you worry about performance, the harder it is to get hard. The harder it is to get hard, the more you worry about performance. It's a vicious cycle.

The good news is that impotence is a hands-down winner when it comes to easily treated sexual dysfunctions. "It's not a difficult situation to overcome at all," Dr. Manley says.

Mind over Matter

Before trying to put the "erect" back in your erection, make sure you really have a problem. If you can't get it up once in a blue moon—or it takes you longer to get a full erection—it's probably part of growing older. After all, by nature we take longer to get a full, strong erection as we age. (The flip side of this is we have better ejaculatory control and fewer problems with premature ejaculation.)

But if you're unable to get an erection for a few weeks in a row—or about 75 percent of the time you attempt sex—then it's time to take action.

Don't hesitate to ask for help. This is our best advice: Don't be shy about seeing a specialist. You're not alone.

"It takes a lot of courage for a man to get to the point of seeing someone, but it's worth it," says Dr. Fishman. "Many of my patients have said, 'Gee, I wish I knew about this before.'"

Seeing a specialist will help determine the cause of your impotence, be it psy-

FAST FACTS

How common: About one in every nine American adult males suffer chronic impotence.

Risk factors: Vascular diseases (hardening of the arteries); endocrine disorders (thyroid problems, diabetes); neurological conditions (stroke, multiple sclerosis); psychological factors (depression, stress, performance anxiety); medications (certain diuretics, blood pressure medications, tranquilizers); smoking; excessive drinking and alcoholism; and groin injuries.

Age group affected: Men of all ages, but most commonly seen in men over age 50.

Gender gap: Men only.

Who to see: Endocrinologist, psychologist, sex therapist and urologist.

chological or organic. Since some diseases, like diabetes, can cause impotence, it's important to find what's causing your problem as soon as you can.

Cut the fat. Even if you're not impotent now, prepare for the future by keeping to a low-fat diet. Just as fat can help clog the blood flow through your heart, it can staunch the flow through your penis.

Sound dietary strategies: Limit red meat, eggs and whole milk—opt instead for chicken, fish, egg whites and skim or low-fat milk. Limit junk food and fatty foods. Instead, eat lots of fresh fruits, whole grains and vegetables.

Ax impotence with aerobic exercise. You know aerobic exercise is good for a healthy heart, but did you know it's also good for a healthy erection? Aerobic exercise increases blood flow, and good blood flow is important for a strong erection. To get your heart pumping—and help keep your manhood firm—get about 30 minutes of exercise at least three times a week.

Don't let your erection go up in smoke. Smoking causes blood vessels throughout your entire body to constrict, reducing the amount of blood that can fuel an erection. Even smoking just two cigarettes can inhibit an erection. "If you measure the blood flow in a man's penis and then have him smoke a cigarette, you'll see a dramatic fall," says Dr. Fishman.

Your best bet is to kick the butts for good. If that's out of the question, avoid smoking for several hours before sex. That should help keep your machinery primed and ready.

Take some R and R. If you're living a six-day workweek, keeping tight deadlines and enduring bumper-to-bumper commutes, your mental health probably isn't the only casualty.

"Stress is probably one of the most common causes of impotence today," Dr. Fishman says. Therefore, it's critical to cut yourself some slack *before* you go to bed, he adds.

Need a suggestion? Take a fast walk or listen to soothing music. Exercise or unwind by reading a book or magazine. The emotional energy you recoup will be well-spent when it's time to rise to the occasion.

Think success. One sure way to scare away an erection is to worry about it. Like we mentioned before, the more you worry, the more you'll have to worry about. In time, rather than looking forward to sex, you'll begin to fear it. Doctors call this performance anxiety, and it's a difficult cycle to break, Dr. Manley says.

It's critical, he adds, for a man to focus on a positive attitude. So the next time you find the "what ifs" creeping into your thoughts, identify exactly what's tripping you up and mentally change it.

"You can usually identify the point at which you've lost mental control and have begun to worry," says Dr. Manley. By identifying negative thoughts, you can replace them with positive ones, thus stopping a self-defeating cycle before it starts.

Here's an example: Rather than focusing on past failures, think about how you'll soon be enjoying sex the way you used to. Picture every pleasurable detail of your next encounter, and see yourself working at peak performance.

Fantasize for fun. Arousing fantasies can be your gateway to Erection City. By relaxing and concentrating on what really arouses you—even if it seems perverse—you'll open up erection opportunities.

"When you fantasize about a situation, you substitute a positive outcome in the fantasy for a negative one," says Dr. Manley. "As you practice this, you'll develop a sense of relaxation and that's very important, too."

Remember that there's a difference between fantasizing to supplement arousal and actually acting out the fantasy. And there's nothing wrong with a fantasy that turns you on as long as it doesn't become an obsession.

Put intercourse on hold. One of the best ways to ease performance anxiety is to stop performing for a while. Explain to your partner that you'd like to delay intercourse until you're a little more confident about getting and keeping an erection.

This doesn't mean avoiding sex. Quite the contrary. Have all the sex you want, but avoid penetration. Try an arousing 20-minute full-body rub without touching the genitals. Use your mouth, your hands and, best of all, your imagination.

Medical "Firmups"

Even if your impotence is caused by an irreversible disease, such as diabetes, it doesn't necessarily mean a life sentence of flaccidity. Today there are more successful impotence treatments than ever to choose from. Here are some of the common ones.

Injection erection. A natural and highly effective treatment is self-injection therapy. However disturbing this may sound, it is easier done than said. It involves injecting one or more drugs into the penis. These drugs—prostaglandin E_1 and papaverine, sometimes along with phentolamine—will cause a hard, long-lasting, natural erection in 15 to 30 minutes.

While these shots are nearly painless, most men are understandably squeamish and look to other forms of therapy. The good news: A new delivery system in which a small pellet is inserted, not injected, into the tip of the penis is undergoing clinical studies.

Penis pump. A drug-free alternative is the penis pump, a specialized vacuum that draws blood into the penis. Slipping a tight ring around the base of the penis traps blood and sustains an erection. When properly used, this device is safe and usually effective, although some men report discomfort and trouble ejaculating.

Penile prosthesis. The most drastic and permanent solution to impotence is the penile implant, an artificial rod or pump surgically placed inside the penis. With a rod version, the penis remains constantly semirigid; with the pump, as the name implies, you pump it up when desired.

Prostheses are considered the "gold standard" of impotence treatments when the causes of the problem are organic. The semirigid models are less costly. The more expensive inflatable models may be more practical, but 50 percent malfunction within five years.

Medicinal solutions, Dr. Padma-Nathan argues, are beginning to eclipse prostheses as the preferred solution to organic impotency. Not only are drugs being developed that are more effective, he says, but they might possibly cure, not just deal with, impotence.

Inflammatory Bowel Disease

When a Swell Time Isn't

When a guy gets a gut feeling about something, he usually can use it to his advantage. That's why we often heed the age-old advice to "go with our gut."

But some gut feelings defy that wisdom, particularly when it comes to inflammatory bowel disease (IBD). Maybe you're alternating between diarrhea and constipation. Could be you've noticed some rectal bleeding. Worst of all, you might have significant pain in your lower abdomen—your gut feels wrenched, your colon seems more like an exclamation point.

If you've experienced any of these symptoms, chances are you're also getting a different gut feeling—one that's telling you to see your doctor.

Punctuated with Pain

The different medical problems that fall under the name IBD are a mysterious lot. Doctors know that the main ones are ulcerative colitis and Crohn's disease, and that the symptoms can flare up for weeks then disappear for months or years. But experts have no clear idea how men get them in the first place.

"There are a lot of theories out there—and they vary from problems with the immune system to some sort of slow viral infection, but the fact is we don't know for sure," says Bernard Schuman, M.D., professor of medicine at the Medical College of Georgia in Augusta. Most experts think that IBD can start as some kind of infection. There's also evidence that some men have a genetic tendency toward the disease—about 20 percent of IBD sufferers have family members with the same malady.

If you're having occasional bouts of diarrhea or stomach pains, don't immediately assume it must be IBD. Roughly one million men may suffer from IBD, but that's a small fraction of the number of men in the United States. On the other hand, everyone gets diarrhea and vague intestinal distress now and again. As a rule, if you suffer these symptoms on a regular basis or you have bouts that last longer than a few days, it's smart to see a doctor. Pain and diarrhea are symptoms of many health problems that men are more likely to develop, such as stress-related condi-

FAST FACTS

How common: Roughly one million men suffer from some type of inflammatory bowel disease (IBD).

Risk factors: Doctors aren't sure what causes IBD. They do know, however, that men who have a family history of IBD are more likely to develop it.

Age group affected: For reasons as yet unknown, men between the ages of 20 and 40 are most likely to get IBD.

Gender gap: Overall, men and women suffer from IBDs equally. Men, however, are somewhat more likely to develop ulcerative colitis, while women tend to develop Crohn's disease.

Who to see: Family doctor, gastroenterologist.

tions like irritable bowel syndrome. The bottom line is you shouldn't mistake a case of the runs for IBD.

Its origins may be uncertain, but the symptoms of IBD are distinct. With ulcerative colitis microscopic sores develop in the colon, resulting in diarrhea, abdominal pain and rectal bleeding. Ulcerative colitis is more common among men than Crohn's disease.

With Crohn's disease the entire digestive system, from the esophagus to the colon, can be affected, although the bowel is the most common target. Unlike ulcerative colitis, Crohn's is somewhat more common in women. During flare-ups the affected part of your digestive system becomes inflamed, causing pain and either diarrhea or constipation. Sometimes Crohn's disease is so severe that the bowel narrows. This can lead to a bowel obstruction, a serious complication that requires immediate attention. Other symptoms include fever, weight loss and skin irritations.

There is almost no way to predict your susceptibility to IBD. Nor could you prevent it even if you could detect that tendency. By the time you notice the symptoms, you have the disease. And IBD is chronic—once you have it, you likely have it for life. But you can learn to live with it—and you should. Left untreated, IBD could lead to more serious health problems such as cancer or even death. Fortunately for the men who suffer the burden of this problem, there are a number of ways to treat IBD effectively, avoid flare-ups and live normal and active lives.

Tabulate trouble foods. Eating generally won't cause a flare-up of your IBD, but certain foods could make your symptoms worse during flare-ups, or create new problems. Milk products are an example, since they all contain the sugar lactose.

"A lot of people with IBD problems tend to be lactose intolerant," explains Bret

Lashner, M.D., director of the Center for Inflammatory Bowel Disease at the Cleveland Clinic Foundation in Ohio. Dr. Lashner suggests consulting with your doctor and a dietitian to determine what foods your system can and can't tolerate.

Other classic foods to avoid include snack foods, like nuts, seeds or popcorn. "If you have Crohn's disease, where there's a possibility of strictures or blockages, nuts and seeds are more likely to get caught in the narrow segment of the bowel and cause obstruction," warns Dr. Lashner.

Stop smoking. Here's one more reason to kick the habit: Researchers have found that Crohn's disease sufferers make their symptoms worse by smoking. On the other hand, many doctors have found that treating colitis sufferers with transdermal nicotine patches or nicotine gum actually relieves symptoms during flare-ups. "No one is recommending smoking as a way to control IBD," stresses Dr. Lashner. "But nicotine—when used for defined periods of time as directed by your doctor—does seem to alleviate ulcerative colitis symptoms."

Bulk up, bulk down. Fiber is an important part of any diet, but IBD sufferers should be judicious about what type of fiber they eat and when they eat it.

"During any flare-up you should avoid high-fiber or roughage-type foods," says Dr. Schuman. These foods could irritate the intestine or even get caught in the digestive passages. For patients with colitis some doctors suggest soluble fiber such as pectin, which is found in apples. Just don't eat hard-to-digest seeds or skin. Psyllium, found in products like Metamucil, is also a good source of soluble fiber.

Scratch spice. Rich or spicy foods tend to be frequent offenders in inflammatory bowel disease patients, says Dr. Lashner. "Patients need to avoid foods that may irritate the gastrointestinal tract such as spicy, greasy or fried foods," he adds.

Say no to NSAIDs. Ironically, many common anti-inflammatory drugs such as aspirin can do more harm than good to people with inflammatory diseases.

"Nonsteroidal anti-inflammatory drugs may be harmful for some people with inflammatory bowel disease," says Arnold Wald, M.D., associate chief of the Division of Gastroenterology at the University of Pittsburgh Medical Center. "In fact, they have been known to cause flare-ups." This class of drugs includes over-the-counter pain relievers, like aspirin and ibuprofen. If you're taking anti-inflammatories for problems like arthritis, talk to your doctor about other options. Otherwise, for basic pain relief stick with products that contain acetaminophen.

Find folic acid. Many of the prescription drugs used to treat IBD have an odd side effect insofar as they limit your body's ability to absorb certain vitamins and minerals. The most important one is folic acid, a B vitamin.

"Lack of folic acid may contribute to anemia," a fatiguing condition that results from a lack of red blood cells in the body, according to Arvey Rogers, M.D., chief of gastroenterology at the Veterans Administration Medical Center in Miami. Unfortunately, major sources of folic acid include high-fiber fruits and vegetables—the ones you're supposed to avoid during flare-ups. Dr. Rogers suggests taking a daily multivitamin that contains folic acid.

Take it easy. Stress can cause flare-ups, too, according to Stephen Hanauer, M.D., professor of medicine and clinical pharmacology at the University of Chicago Medical Center. "It's usually your major stresses—divorce or death of a loved one—that can contribute to a flare-up," he says. But if you feel that day-to-day stress affects your symptoms, it's a good idea to try to minimize it, possibly through meditation, scheduling rest periods during the day or exercising regularly.

Medically Managing Your IBD

If all else fails, some IBD sufferers may benefit from surgery.

"It's always an option, but it's really a last resort, especially for Crohn's disease," says Dr. Wald. Because Crohn's disease can attack anywhere along the digestive system, surgically removing one part of that system is no guarantee of stopping the disease. In fact, half of all Crohn's patients who undergo surgery suffer recurring symptoms within five years.

In contrast, surgery is the only definite cure for ulcerative colitis. "But of course, it's a drastic measure," says Dr. Wald. Only about 15 percent of colitis sufferers eventually need surgery.

Experts say some patients want surgery just to avoid the pain and misery of their bowel disease, but men should think twice before they go under the knife.

"Surgery may cut nerves and muscles in various areas of the rectum," says Dr. Lashner. For men, that translates into concerns about impotence. "The surgery can be very effective for treating an inflammatory bowel disease, but there are definite impotence risks," he says.

Fortunately, there are a number of prescription medications for IBD which, if used properly, can be a better option than surgery. The main weapon in the arsenal against IBD is the prescription drug sulfasalazine (Azulfidine). But this powerful sulfa drug does have side effects—the chief one being infertility.

"It only lasts as long as you're taking the drug, but while you're taking it, the sulfasalazine will reduce sperm counts," says Dr. Lashner.

"There are newer medications available that don't have the sulfa component, so they're easier to tolerate. Best of all, patients can take them as a regular form of control for their diseases," says Dr. Hanauer.

Inhibited Sexual Desire

Getting Out of Low Gear

Ah, youth. Back in those desirous days when it wasn't a question of *if* you wanted to have sex—the answer was always yes—but where, when and how often. But these days? If you're like a lot of guys, it's gone from "more" to "chore" . . . or even "snore."

Sure, it's natural for a man's desires to downshift at various times in his life. But if it seems as though your sex drive lately has been stuck in "Park"—as occurs, at least occasionally, for nearly half of all men in America—then you could be suffering from inhibited sexual desire.

ISD, as it is called, is not the same as impotence. In most cases, the equipment works fine but the desire isn't there to fuel it. So even though a man is able to get an erection and have sex, he doesn't want to—or doesn't become very aroused when he does.

Problems with Mind and Body

"There are a huge number of things that can inhibit men from wanting sex: Stress at work, stress with the children or being with a partner who does not stimulate you the way she used to," says Jay Hollander, M.D., associate director of Beaumont Center for Male Sexual Function at William Beaumont Hospital in Royal Oak, Michigan. "Problems with the penis can't be divorced from psychological problems."

Even if the problem isn't in your head, you may still have trouble down below: Just try to juggle a hectic 50-hour workweek with weekend soccer games and home repairs and still have enough time and energy for quality consummation. Even a sudden change in your life can effect change in your sexual frequency. "Any major change—the birth of a child, the death of a loved one or a serious illness—has the potential to cause some type of sexual impairment," says C. Steven Manley, Ph.D., staff psychologist at The Male Health Center in Dallas.

And then there are physical factors: Certain prescription drugs, disease, even low testosterone levels can shoot down a man's libido quicker than an overzealous Marine.

FAST FACTS

How common: Up to 48 percent of men in the United States have inhibited sexual desire (ISD) to some extent.

Risk factors: Stress, anger, boredom, performance anxiety and other emotional issues are common causes, as are physical factors, like low testosterone levels, diabetes and depression, and even some prescription medications.

Age group affected: ISD is most common in men over age 40.

Gender gap: While therapists once believed that ISD was far more common among women, research suggests that it's probably equally common in both sexes.

Who to see: Start with your family doctor. You might get referred to an endocrinologist, psychologist, sex therapist or urologist.

Top Sexual Complaint

Whatever the reasons—and there are plenty—ISD is America's number one sexual complaint, affecting to some degree anywhere from 11 to 48 percent of men in the United States. Of course, the definition of exactly what constitutes an "inhibited" sexual desire isn't so well-defined. "There was a man in my office yesterday who thought that if he and his wife didn't have sex every day, then there was a really serious problem," says Dr. Manley. "Other men don't feel like anything's seriously out of line until they go a month or so. There's a pretty wide spectrum of what's 'normal.'"

His advice: If both you and your partner are satisfied with the amount and quality of sex you're having (however much or little it is), then there's no problem. But if one of you is unhappy in the quality or quantity of your love life, something is going on, which may or may not be inhibited sexual desire.

So what should you do about it? A good first step is to talk about it. This isn't the time to feel guilty or place blame, says Dr. Manley. Instead, try to understand how you and your partner are feeling, and share your insights into when the change in relationship occurred—and why. And don't forget about those feelings *outside* the bedroom. Nothing extinguishes passion more quickly than pent-up anger and frustration, says Peter A. Wish, Ph.D., a psychologist and co-director of the Sarasota Consulting Group in Sarasota, Florida. "You have to find out what there is about the relationship that is tripping those defenses." Meanwhile, here's some other advice on how to rekindle those fires.

Get a physical. Any number of health conditions can cause your libido to go into hibernation. "ISD is one of the symptoms of either clinical depression or low testosterone levels," says Dr. Manley. Other desire-reducing problems include diabetes, hormone imbalances and even severe stress. Some medications—those used for high blood pressure or antidepressants, for example—can also cause erectile difficulties or a drop in libido, so get a checkup and discuss this with your doctor.

And get physical. Sexually speaking, a regular trip to the gym is not an exercise in futility. In one study men who got a good workout three or four times a week reported more (and better) sex than guys whose only exercise was walking slowly. Experts believe that vigorous exercise boosts testosterone levels and may improve blood flow to all parts of the body—including the genitals. Of course, working out will also make you look and feel better—powerful aphrodisiacs in their own right.

Take five to revive. When you're working ten-hour days six days a week, there's not much energy (or even time) left over for intimacy. "Stress can be a major problem," says Dr. Wish. Obviously, you can't quit your job and hang out on the beach all day in order to have good sex . . . although it's certainly an idea worth pondering. But you can take a few minutes every few hours to relax and unwind. Read the newspaper. Listen to some music. Take a walk or talk with a friend. By scheduling these brief "fun" breaks for 5 to 15 minutes every so often, Dr. Wish says, you'll be amazed at the energy you'll save that can be put to better use come bedtime.

Eat lean and mean. If you are what you eat and you eat a lot of junk food, what does that say about your sex life? Plenty, says Wayne A. Meikle, M.D., professor of medicine in the Division of Endocrinology and Metabolism at the University of Utah in Salt Lake City. A steady diet of fatty foods may curb the production of testosterone—so if you're a steak and 'taters kind of guy, eating leaner may help bring back that loving feeling.

Shake things up. In sex, as in life, doing the same old things day after day can only lead to boredom—and you know what that means between the sheets. "As a couple, you need to recognize the value of bringing novelty into your relationship," says Robert W. Birch, Ph.D., a psychologist and marital and sex therapist in private practice in Columbus, Ohio. That doesn't mean using whoopee cushions or Groucho faces as marital aids. Instead, he advocates a "more creative" approach to lovemaking: Take a long shower together or share massages with sensual oils. Try some new positions or reveal some secret fantasies.

Get into the light. Believe it or not, research shows that exposure to the sun can be sexually stimulating and that people who get a lot of sunlight have stronger sex

Museum Strategy and Marketing

Museum Strategy and Marketing

Designing Missions
Building Audiences
Generating Revenue and Resources

Neil Kotler and Philip Kotler

JOSSEY-BASS
A Wiley Imprint
www.josseybass.com

Published by Jossey-Bass
A Wiley Imprint
989 Market Street, San Francisco, CA 94103-1741   www.josseybass.com

Jossey-Bass books and products are available through most bookstores. To contact Jossey-Bass directly call our Customer Care Department within the U.S. at 800-956-7739, outside the U.S. at 317-572-3986 or fax 317-572-4002.

Jossey-Bass also publishes its books in a variety of electronic formats. Some content that appears in print may not be available in electronic books.

Credits are on p. 396.

Library of Congress Cataloging-in-Publication Data

Kotler, Neil G., date.
Museum strategy and marketing : designing missions, building audiences, generating revenue and resources / by Neil Kotler and Philip Kotler.
p. cm. — (The Jossey-Bass nonprofit and public management series)
Includes bibliographical references and index.
ISBN 0-7879-0912-2 (acid-free paper)
1. Museums—Planning. 2. Museums—Marketing. 3. Museum attendance. 4. Museum finance. I. Kotler, Philip. II. Title. III. Series.
AM5 .K68 1998
069—ddc21
                                                                98-8964

Printed in the United States of America
FIRST EDITION
HB Printing   10 9 8 7 6

The Jossey-Bass
Nonprofit and Public Management Series

CONTENTS

ix

TABLES, FIGURES, AND EXHIBITS

TABLES

FIGURES

EXHIBITS

MODEL MUSEUM PRACTICES

To our mother, Betty Kotler, and to Nancy, Wendy, Jena, Jessica, Melissa, and Amy, our national living treasures, we dedicate this book.

PREFACE

*The Museum can reach only those whom it can attract. This fact alone is enough
to compel it to be convenient to all, wide in its scope, varied in its activities,
hospitable, . . . eager to follow any lead the humblest inquirer may give.*
—John Cotton Dana, founding director, The Newark Museum (1917)

Inside the entrance of the Walker Art Center in Minneapolis, Minnesota,
youngsters are milling around or are seated at tables, working with art materials, fabrics, and collectibles. Elsewhere in the museum, high school students are serving as docents, taking visitors on a tour of a photography exhibit.
The upper-story galleries are filled with Willem de Kooning paintings—large
canvases of lyrical lines and pastel hues forming a continuous ribbon of color
weaving through luminous galleries. A musical performance is just winding
down in the auditorium; a storytelling workshop, using museum collections, is
taking place down the hall; and in a nearby studio teenagers are rehearsing a
play. It is Free First Saturday at the museum, a monthly event in which the
Walker hosts a day of family-oriented activities devoted to creative expression.

This illustrates a trend: museums are broadening their image, audience, programming, and support. Like bandwidths in the digital and broadcasting
worlds, museums can be thought of as ranged along a continuum, from "nar-
rowband" museums at one end to "broadband" museums at the other. The former are museums that take a narrow view of their missions, programs, and
audiences. The latter are museums that have a broad sense of mission, an ex-
pansive image to communicate, a variety of programs, and a large, diverse audience to serve. Just as bandwidths in the digital world vary according to the
extent of information they can channel in a given time frame, so too "bandwidths" in museums differ in terms of the range of programs, experiences, and
services they offer their audiences.

Museums, to be sure, are as different from one another as a Picasso painting is different from the beaverskin top hat Abraham Lincoln wore the night of his assassination—a precious object the Smithsonian Institution displayed in its 150th anniversary exhibition that toured several U.S. cities beginning in 1996. Indeed, the appeal of a museum lies in its individuality and distinctiveness. Yet regardless of their particular qualities, museums increasingly recognize that they have to compete for audiences, support, and resources; offer quality programs; communicate their distinctiveness; build long-term relationships with their communities; and find the means to sustain themselves financially, as once-reliable public-sector funding dwindles.

The most successful museums offer a range of experiences that appeal to different audience segments and reflect the varying needs of individual visitors. Research has shown that museum visitors seek experiences that cross the boundaries of learning, doing, and relishing. They are quite capable in the space of a single day of absorbing thrills and excitement, relaxing, and finding delight in aesthetic pleasures as well as cerebral discoveries. To the extent possible, successful museums provide multiple experiences: aesthetic and emotional delight, celebration and learning, recreation and sociability.

The trend toward broader offerings, wider audiences, and market-oriented programs carries some costs as well as benefits, although we believe that the benefits outweigh the costs in the long run. The broadband museum has encountered criticism and resistance in parts of the museum community. The criticism is rooted in differing conceptions of the museum mission and identity.

Four varieties of museums illustrate these differences in mission and identity: the traditional object-oriented museum, the modified traditional museum, the community-oriented museum, and the storytelling, experience-oriented museum. The differences reflect on important issues that will be examined throughout this book: whether fine and rare museum objects can stand by themselves or require extended interpretive texts, contexts, and meanings; whether museums should limit their audiences to provide a contemplative, focused setting or make their offerings available to the largest number of people, even at the expense of crowds and congestion; whether ancillary programs such as community events, continuing education, and concerts weaken or interfere with core activities and, if not, what is the right balance with core activities; and whether museums should become market-oriented entities, catering to audience and community preferences, or should preserve their identity as primarily scholarly, educational, or esoteric organizations. (These issues are discussed further in Chapter Two.)

Museums are also finding that they can use the tools of strategic planning and marketing to reach their goals without compromising their missions and their integrity. Indeed, high-quality planning and marketing are instruments rather than ends; they are adapted to the purposes and the objectives that museum managers define. In a competitive world, museums are being measured by the experiences, benefits, and outcomes they generate as much as by the collections and other resources they possess. Strategic planning and marketing are instruments for shaping, communicating, and distributing quality experiences and programs and reaching the broadest possible audience.

PURPOSE

This book offers the museum community a philosophical and methodological framework for examining a museum's resources, mission, opportunities, and challenges. Solid self-assessment and research become the basis for setting goals and implementing strategies.

Museum Strategy and Marketing is the first comprehensive and systematic book devoted to the uses of strategic planning and marketing in museums. It covers all phases of planning and marketing and offers a set of detailed auditing and review tools. It is the first book to examine the full range of marketing skills relevant to museums: existing product marketing, new product marketing, channel and distribution marketing, service marketing, sales and promotion marketing, price marketing, donor marketing, and image and brand marketing.

This book gives focus to the concept of the "museum experience" as a key outcome of museum visits—specifically, a range of experiences including learning and celebration, recreation and sociability, aesthetic pleasure, and enchantment. The book examines the evolving concept and role of the museum: from the collection and conservation of material culture to information and education to providing experience and meaning.

Museum Strategy and Marketing highlights three critical features of museum management: distribution, added value, and museum alliances and partnerships. Museums are increasingly making objects and exhibitions, educational offerings, and services available beyond the halls of the main museum building. Digital and electronic media and geographically dispersed satellites and facilities provide additional distribution channels. Like other organizations, museums are finding ways to add value to their offerings. They are supplementing collections and exhibitions with interactive and multimedia technologies, are expanding their gift shops and restaurants, and upgrading services they provide to visitors. Museums, in addition, are building partnerships with other museums and with outside cultural and educational organizations as a means to raise visibility, assemble greater resources, and elevate programming quality. Museums have also organized joint marketing programs and joint purchasing co-ops to reduce costs.

Museum alliances and partnerships are appropriate responses to another type of challenge: the competitive inroads of information, entertainment, and media conglomerates that have far greater resources, more elaborate distribution channels, and more extensive product lines. In today's world, museums compete for audiences with the electronic media (and stay-at-home habits); with the recreational alternatives offered by movies, theme parks, and sports competitions; and with "edutainment" organizations such as Disney and themed "destination" shopping malls and restaurants. Can museums, through partnerships, raise their visibility, assemble resources, and upgrade offerings to compete with conglomerates bent on capturing and dominating consumers' time, minds, and spending? One promising response is aggregating several museums in cultural districts that are compelling destinations for tourists and local residents and significant generators of local economic development.

This book is filled with illustrations of sound museum practices and models of museum problem solving.

AUDIENCE

Museum Strategy and Marketing is written for museum professionals who deal daily with challenges, choices, and decisions. Museum staff in all areas and specializations can benefit from the concepts, tools, and techniques presented. So, too, can members of museum boards; professionals in the arts, cultural, and educational sectors; and supporters of museums among foundation, corporate, and public-sector organizations. This book is also a text for museum studies and training programs as well as professional development programs in arts and cultural resources management and administration. The strategic planning and marketing concepts also have relevance to professionals in the travel and hospitality industries, insofar as tourism is a growing source of museum audiences.

OVERVIEW OF THE CONTENTS

Museum Strategy and Marketing is distinctive for its range of examples and illustrations of museum practices, programs, problem solving, and organizational behavior. Museum examples appear in every chapter and illustrate every major concept and theme. Eight museums, in addition, are highlighted in features headed "Model Museum Practices," extended discussions that appear toward the end of most chapters. The model museums illustrate topics and themes covered in the chapter. Yet the museums identified in this book constitute only a small sample of exemplary museums and museum practices. The museum world is filled with a great many admirable organizations and approaches; given the individuality and the scope of museums, generalizations are necessarily difficult. Thus the examples in this book should be regarded as illustrative only; it is our hope that their behaviors and practices will inspire adaptation to other settings and situations.

Part One (Chapters One and Two) of this book explores the challenges and the opportunities that museums are facing as the twenty-first century approaches. Chapter One looks at museums' variety, historical origins, and development, at how museums differ and what they have in common. Chapter Two examines three contemporary challenges: formulating a distinctive, engaging, and appropriate mission; building community support and larger, wider audiences; and acquiring needed revenues and resources.

Part Two (Chapters Three through Five) provides the framework of strategic planning and marketing that is developed throughout the book. No single marketing and planning formula is applicable to all museums, but every museum can benefit from one or another facet of planning and marketing. Chapter Three analyzes a museum's external and internal environments; the processes in formulating a mission, set of objectives, and strategy; and the possible effect of strategies on existing organizational design and systems. This chapter is essential to designing a strategic planning and marketing system.

Visitor studies confirm the importance of understanding museum audiences. Chapter Four looks at audiences, their characteristics and subgroups, and the ways individuals choose among recreational and leisure alternatives, including museum-going. Chapter Five applies marketing principles to audiences: segmentation, targeting, and positioning the museum and its offerings.

Part Three (Chapters Six through Twelve) presents the specific tactics, tools, and applications that transform marketing knowledge into implementable systems. Chapter Six describes the uses of marketing and museum research and information-gathering techniques. Chapter Seven focuses on strategic development of the museum's offerings (exhibitions, programs, services)—how to design and upgrade museum offerings to make them attractive to various types of visitors. Museums are also distributing their offerings more widely than ever; Chapter Eight considers various distribution channels (traveling exhibits, branch sites, electronic media, and other innovations) for making museum offerings more available.

Museums seeking to raise their visibility, project appealing images, and create effective promotion and communication programs will find Chapter Nine useful. It explores image building and brand identity, advertising, public relations, direct marketing, and sales promotion. Museums are also paying increased attention to pricing and revenue-raising strategies. In the past, most museums charged no admission or seriously underpriced their offerings. Chapter Ten examines pricing strategies and techniques, covering admissions, special exhibitions, sales in gift shops, memberships, and rental of museum facilities.

Chapter Eleven examines how museums can attract new resources and increase existing resources—for example, by converting infrequent visitors into regular ones, visitors into members and volunteers, and small gift-givers into larger gift-givers. The chapter covers membership, corporate contributions and sponsorships, foundation grants, and public-sector support. It probes fundraising concepts, tactics, and practices. Chapter Twelve rounds out the discussion of strategies and tactics, providing a broad view of the museum as a marketing system and organization. It describes how museum managers can best use plans, budgets, and controls to achieve objectives and strategies. The Marketing Audit Guide, at the end of the chapter, takes museums through a full assessment of their environments, objectives, resources, and organizational designs.

In the concluding chapter, we consider the range of factors and conditions that can help museums secure their future in the twenty-first century. The chapter provides a summary of the findings and recommendations presented throughout the book. In the Appendix, Stephen Weil's essay "Twenty-One Ways to Buy Art" is a fitting finale. It brings readers full circle, back to the first task of a museum: to create and care for a collection. Weil, one of the museum community's most fecund thinkers, guides the reader in the realm of acquiring objects and building collections.

In the final analysis, museums provide a unique and distinctive offering: rich, sensory, multidimensional experiences with authentic and tangible objects in scholarly, informational, and interpretative contexts. We offer this book to all people to whom museums matter; our intent is to help them build and manage successful museums and to meet the challenges museums will face in the twenty-first century.

February 1998

Neil Kotler
Arlington, Virginia

Philip Kotler
Evanston, Illinois

ACKNOWLEDGMENTS

We wish to acknowledge individuals who have contributed to our research and ideas and two institutions that have helped shape excellence in the museum world.

The Smithsonian Institution, one of the world's great museum and research institutions, is a national meeting place, where people raise their sights, celebrate history, deepen their learning, stretch their imagination, and enjoy incomparable museum-going experiences. Four Smithsonian colleagues, in particular, helped make this book possible: Ruth Selig, Marc Pachter, Stephen Weil, and Barbara Schneider.

We also acknowledge the J. Paul Getty Trust, which has sponsored since 1979 the Getty Leadership Institute for Museum Management, where top-level museum professionals have received important training in museum leadership. We want to thank the following members and staff of the Getty Leadership Institute Advisory Committee for conversations and exchanges about the museum world: Ellsworth Brown (president, The Carnegie, Pittsburgh), Amina Dickerson (distinguished visitor, John D. and Catherine T. MacArthur Foundation), Alberta Sebolt George (president and CEO, Old Sturbridge Village), Katharine C. Lee (CEO and director, Virginia Museum of Fine Arts), Gregory R. Long (president, New York Botanical Garden), Raymond E. Miles (professor emeritus, Haas School of Business, University of California, Berkeley), George P. Moynihan (executive director, Pacific Science Center), Philip Nowlen (academic director, Getty Leadership Institute), Maureen Rolla (administrative director, Getty Leadership Institute),

John W. Rosenblum (dean, Jepson School of Leadership Studies, University of Richmond), Serena Rattazzi (director, American Federation of Arts), Stephen E. Weil (senior scholar emeritus, Center for Museum Studies, Smithsonian Institution), and Harold Williams (president and CEO, J. Paul Getty Trust).

We also owe a debt of gratitude to the museum leaders who so graciously offered us opportunities to learn about their museums and explore a range of museum ideas, practices, and challenges.

—N. K. and P. K.

THE AUTHORS

Neil Kotler is a program specialist at the Smithsonian Institution in Washington, D.C., where he has worked since 1986. He received a B.A. degree (1962) from Brandeis University, an M.A. degree (1963) from the University of Wisconsin, Madison, and a Ph.D. degree in political science (1974) from the University of Chicago. He is a former legislative director in the U.S. House of Representatives; professor at Georgetown University, the University of Texas at Austin, Dartmouth College, and De Paul University; and a Peace Corps volunteer and secondary school teacher in Ethiopia. He is the editor of several publications at the Smithsonian Institute Press, including *The Statue of Liberty Revisited: Making a Universal Symbol; Sharing Innovation: Global Perspectives on Food, Agriculture, and Rural Development*; and *Completing the Food Chain: Strategies for Combating Hunger and Malnutrition*. He has co-produced two educational videos: *Democracy and Rights: One Citizen's Challenge* and *Citizen Stories: Democracy and Responsibility in American Life*.

Philip Kotler is the S. C. Johnson Distinguished Professor of International Marketing at the J. L. Kellogg Graduate School of Management, Northwestern University. He has been honored as one of the world's leading marketing thinkers. He received his M.A. degree (1953) from the University of Chicago and his Ph.D. degree in economics (1956) from the Massachusetts Institute of Technology and has received honorary degrees from the University of Zurich, Athens University of Economics and Business, and De Paul University. He is author of over one hundred articles and seventeen books, including *Standing Room Only: Strategies for Marketing the Performing Arts, Marketing for Hospitality and Tourism, Marketing Management, Strategic Marketing for Nonprofit Organizations, Social Marketing, Marketing Places, The Marketing of Nations,* and *The New Competition.* He has been a consultant to IBM, General Electric, AT&T, Bank of America, Merck, Motorola, Ford, and other organizations. He is a member of the board of governors of The School of the Art Institute of Chicago and a member of the advisory committee of the Getty Leadership Institute for Museum Management.

Museum Strategy and Marketing

PART ONE

MUSEUMS FACE
THE TWENTY-FIRST CENTURY

CHAPTER ONE

The Diverse World of Museums

An overcrowded museum is a healthy museum.
—S. Dillon Ripley

Museums are solemn spaces.
—Otto Mayr

The Art Institute of Chicago's blockbuster exhibition of the works of Claude Monet drew 960,000 visitors during a nineteen-week period in 1995. The Monet show generated substantial increases in museum membership, gifts, corporate relationships, museum shop earnings, and rental fees; its impact on Chicago's economy in revenues and jobs was estimated to be nearly $300 million. The 1996 Cézanne exhibition at the Philadelphia Museum of Art drew 550,000 visitors during a thirteen-week period, generating ten thousand room-nights for the city's hotels and an estimated $86.5 million in added income for the city. A city-commissioned report concluded the museum is a prime tourist attraction and the city awarded the museum a substantial grant to promote its programs. Museums in the closing decade of the twentieth century are drawing larger audiences and offering a greater variety of exhibitions, programs, and services than ever before. If the number of new museums and museum additions is any indicator, the museum world is reaching wider audiences and acquiring a visibility in some cases rivaling that enjoyed by popular culture and the mass media. Let us examine the distinctive qualities of today's museums.

THE MUSEUM EXPERIENCE

Museums offer experiences, ideas, and satisfactions not found in other places. These derive from authentic objects of nature, history, science, and the arts that museums collect and display; the sensory experiences with three-dimensional

3

objects that museums present and interpret; and the research, scholarship, and interpretation that support museum collections and exhibitions.

A visit to the Philadelphia Museum of Art's Grand Salon from the Hôtel le Tellier in Paris or to its Indian Buddhist temple or its Japanese teahouse offers a one-of-a-kind experience of being transported back in time and being immersed in a complete environment of great beauty and enchantment. The experience of remembrance and bonding with the history and glory of the United States was a palpable part of visits to *America's Smithsonian,* a traveling exhibition celebrating the 150th anniversary of the Smithsonian Institution's founding in 1846. The exhibition was filled with great objects of the American past, including the famous 1853 Rembrandt Peale portrait of George Washington, a sword worn by Washington in the Revolutionary War, gowns worn by the wives of U.S. presidents, objects of U.S. technological history such as the Apollo 14 space capsule, and the top hat that President Abraham Lincoln was believed to be wearing the night he was assassinated in 1865. Visitors stood in awe of these objects. One said: "I feel like somebody sprayed me with gold. That's how beautiful and fortunate I feel." Another said: "The longer I stay, the more intense it gets. To see the things that Abe Lincoln wrote, to be so close to something that is woven into the fabric of our history—it goes beyond words." Standing before the painting of Washington, yet another visitor said: "He looks so noble. Serene. It's holy" (Waxman, 1996, p. C6).

A visitor to the Smithsonian's Museum of Natural History in the winter and early spring of 1996 could view *Landscape Kimonos,* a once-in-a-lifetime exhibition of Japanese kimonos handwoven and hand-painted by Itchiku Kubota. Kubota, a seventy-nine-year-old Japanese artist, re-created a sixteenth-century technique and tradition of fabric dyeing, transforming it into a unique art form of the twentieth century. Visitors encountered in a large oblong gallery a series of thirty-five silk kimonos, hanging side by side. Each depicted a fragmentary moment of seasonal change reflected in the landscape. Moving from the left side of the room to the right, the visitor viewed through color, line, form, and texture the passage of seasons from autumn to winter, a changing landscape of mountains, fields, lakes, and skies in the varying light and shadows cast by sunshine, rainfall, cloud cover, and snowfall. Visitors expressed a sense of being transfixed by an artistic vision of the natural world that allowed them to see nature in a wholly different light.

A visit to the vast and rich Paul Gauguin retrospective exhibition at the National Gallery of Art in Washington, D.C., in the late 1980s produced a transformative experience for one of the authors. For several days following the show he would step outside the front door of his house in the early morning to fetch the newspaper and peer out on the world as if he were viewing it through Gauguin's eyes, imagining the luminous colors of Gauguin's Tahiti transposed to the midst of Arlington, Virginia.

Science and natural history museums offer biological specimens, ecological settings, scientific instruments, and objects of engineering and technology that can arouse curiosity, illuminate patterns, and lead to important discoveries. Maxine Singer, a biochemist and president of the Carnegie Institution of Washington, can recount memorable experiences as a youngster visiting New York City's American Museum of Natural History. Freeman Dyson, a physicist and scholar at the Institute for Advanced Study in Princeton, New Jersey, can relate visits as a youth to London's British Museum and the Museum of Natural History, experiences that shaped his love and pursuit of science. Museum collections and exhibitions are often a springboard to scientific vocations.

Great museum exhibitions offer visitors transcendent experiences that take them outside the routines of everyday life and transport them into new and wonderful worlds of beauty, thought, and remembrance. The psychologist Abraham Maslow termed these "peak experiences," experiences that are totally absorbing and at the same time transforming of perceptions and understanding. At their best, museums elevate the spirit, enlarge thought and feeling, stretch the imagination, and offer enchanting experience.

Museums are engaging in greater self-assessment as a means to improve their offerings and organizations—examining opportunities and obstacles in the larger environment and planning tools with which to adapt to changing circumstances. Some museums are reinventing themselves. The Detroit Historical Museum, for example, a venerable seventy-year-old city-run institution, facing substantial cuts in state funding and a 40 percent staff reduction in the first half of the 1990s, undertook a significant and transforming reorganization. According to museum director Maud Lyon (interviewed Mar. 12, 1996), the changes, along with a greater commitment from the board of directors, led to a major refocusing on community involvement, participation, and support. The museum organized a new permanent exhibition, *The Motor City,* which increased visitorship by 60 percent over three years. Every significant group in the city involved in automotive history participated in conceptualizing and designing the exhibit. For example, in discussions with the labor unions, museum staff realized that the exhibit should highlight the role of labor unions in advancing the position of industrial workers. Community mobilization led to growth in donations, volunteers, donated services, and other resources. A television station established a partnership with the museum to produce public service announcements highlighting Detroit's history. The city of Detroit is making plans to commemorate its 300th anniversary in the year 2001 and has asked the museum to play a major role in organizing this tricentennial celebration.

In this chapter we will examine what a museum is, what museums have in common, and how they are different. We will also view museums historically to trace their evolution and development.

WHAT IS A MUSEUM?

According to a 1989 survey, there are an estimated 8,200 freestanding, independent museums in the United States. If museum branches and the historic homes and sites are included, this number exceeds 15,000 museum sites (American Association of Museums, 1994, pp. 23, 27). Of U.S. museums, 55 percent are historical museums and historic sites; 15 percent, art museums; and 14 percent, nature and science-and-technology-oriented museums, including zoos and botanical gardens. The Institute of Museum and Library Services, a U.S. federal agency, estimates the total number of independent U.S. museums in 1992 at 8,934 (Danvers, 1992, p. 21). Great Britain has an estimated 2,000 museums. Numbers fluctuate, of course, as museums start up or shut down.

The American Association of Museums (AAM) defines a museum as an institution that is "organized as a public or private nonprofit institution, existing on a permanent basis for essentially educational and aesthetic purposes," that "cares for and owns or uses tangible objects, whether animate or inanimate, and exhibits these on a regular basis," that "has at least one professional staff member or the full-time equivalent," and "is open to the general public on a regular basis . . . at least 120 days per year" (1994, pp. 18–19).

Even given this very broad definition, it is sometimes difficult to know what is a museum and what is not. Indeed, some people visiting Venice, Italy, have concluded the entire city is a museum, not just the particular buildings that promote themselves as museums, such as the Museo Archeologico and the Museo Orientale. The same thought arises when visiting Hampton Court or Warwick Castle in England. Do they not contain great collections of fine and decorative arts and represent history as well as or better than some "history museums"?

Is Atlanta's Cyclorama a museum? The Cyclorama tells the story of the Civil War Battle of Atlanta (July 22, 1864). Its centerpiece is the world's largest painting, a canvas in the round weighing nine thousand pounds and measuring 358 feet by 42 feet—longer than a football field. Extending thirty feet out from the painting is a diorama-like foreground containing hundreds of three-dimensional figures and objects (wagons, munitions, and natural landscape). Audiences view the painting from a moving platform with theater-like seating. In another part of the building are cases filled with Civil War uniforms, guns, and memorabilia. The battle scene for the most part depicts a historical narrative. Yet the guide points out that one slain figure in the foreground is the likeness of Clark Gable, who starred in the movie *Gone With the Wind,* set during the Civil War. Gable visited the Cyclorama in the late 1930s and expressed his enjoyment but also his dismay that his own image was missing from the painting; the owners subsequently added the Gable figure. Further, the guide explains, the painting was inspired by a Confederate general, John B. Hood, and was commissioned twenty years after the Battle of Atlanta. Parts of the painting glorify Hood's role in the battle. Do advocacy and the fictive elements diminish the standing of the Atlanta Cyclorama as a museum?

How Museums Differ

Museums vary in extent of collections, size of staff, endowments, revenues and expenses, physical plants, and hours of operations.

Collections. Ninety-three percent of U.S. museums, it is estimated, own collections; yet children's museums, science and technology centers, and history centers often possess negligible collections or no collections at all. The Museum for African Art in New York City organizes on-site and traveling exhibitions of objects borrowed from private collectors and other museums. The Contemporary, in Baltimore, is a museum without walls, an organization of museum professionals who bring together interpretative work and expertise, objects and collections borrowed from other places and create exhibitions for the public at different sites in the city.

Collections that embody a record of history, art, nature, or science contain objects that are of value in and of themselves. However, science and technology centers often contain tools, props, interactive machines, and materials with which to demonstrate science and technology. These objects are tools rather than rare, authentic pieces.

Museums are in the business of caring for, interpreting, and showing authentic objects. However, the Museo del Falso (Museum of Forgeries and Counterfeits), in Salerno, Italy, which opened in 1991, is dedicated to the collecting, study, and viewing of faked objects. Its earliest exhibitions were devoted to counterfeit foods, detergents, and precious metals.

Most museums are organized around a specialized collection or else multiple collections specific to a particular field. However, the South Carolina State Museum, located in Columbia and publicly funded through the state legislature, is five museums in one, featuring regional and contemporary art collections, regional historical collections, technology and engineering collections, natural history collections, and a science center that help it fulfill its core mission of educating young people. Many museums that are acquiring objects are likely to deaccession and sell off or exchange objects to make room for others. Yet the Isabella Stewart Gardner Museum, in Boston, has a distinguished collection of more than twenty-five hundred objects of Western art that cannot be sold or added to, according to the founding charter. In addition, the installations and interior design of the building cannot be altered in any significant way. The vast majority of U.S. museums are nonprofit organizations. However, some museums, such as the New Jersey Children's Museum, in Paramus, are organized as for-profit businesses.

Most museums ask their visitors not to touch objects. The Atlanta History Museum's 1997 exhibition, *Metropolitan Frontiers: Atlanta, 1835–2000,* had signs posted in several areas urging visitors to touch certain objects. The Shotgun House, situated at the exhibition's center, is a reconstructed nineteenth-century working-class dwelling. A sign at the porch entrance read: "Please feel free to touch all objects in the Shotgun House." Virtually all museums are secular and research-minded in their assumptions about objects, evidence, and authenticity. The Living Bible Museum, in Mansfield, Ohio, however, is an institution preserving and presenting a belief system (Christianity rooted in the Old Testament). It advertises itself as nonsectarian, but it is located within the Diamond Hill Cathedral in Mansfield.

Ownership. An estimated 59 percent of all U.S. museums are privately governed and 41 percent are government run (7.3 percent by the federal government and 27 percent by states and municipalities). In France, by comparison, approximately 80 percent of the museums are run by the national government. Museums in Great Britain vary from national museums, such as the British Museum, that are substantially maintained by the government to small local museums and museum services that are supported by a combination of local government grants and private contributions.

Size and resources. Small museums, defined by the Institute of Museum and Library Services as having "five or fewer full-time paid or unpaid staff, or an annual operating budget of under $250,000," account for 75 percent of all U.S. museums. The average smaller museum is open 221 days in the year and serves 16,000 visitors annually. It has two full-time staff and an annual operating budget under $90,000 (Danvers, 1992, pp. 9–10). For example, the Maryland Ornithological Museum and Clyburn Nature Center and Arboretum, located in Baltimore, together occupy a large nature preserve. In the mid-1990s the museums were managed by an all-volunteer staff; the director was a city official working at a distance from the museums and lacking museum training. A typical small, rural U.S. museum is the Morrow County Museum, in Heppner, Oregon. This thirty-two-year-old museum has a mission to chronicle the history of the local agricultural area, from the pioneering period in 1890 to the early settlement in 1920. Community members donated most of the collection's five thousand pieces. Only in recent years has the museum adopted acquisition, collection management, and conservation policies. The director works full time but is paid at three-quarters time; there are no other paid staff. The museum lacks storage facilities and conservation materials, and virtually all of the collection is shown in the galleries (Danvers, 1992, pp. 18–20).

In contrast, the largest museums, such as the Metropolitan Museum of Art, in New York City, and the Smithsonian Institution, have several thousand employees and budgets in the hundreds of millions of dollars. A few U.S. museums have endowment funds reaching one billion dollars or more. The J. Paul Getty Museum in Malibu and Los Angeles, California, is a subsidiary of the

Getty Trust, a U.S. charitable foundation that has in excess of $4 billion in assets. At the other extreme, the Waterloo Area Farm Museum, in Stockbridge, Michigan, has an annual operating budget in the neighborhood of $15,000 and an all-volunteer staff. In the late 1980s, the total value of U.S. museum endowments was $14 billion; 93 percent was accounted for by large museums and 76 percent by art museums (American Association of Museums, 1994, pp. 87–88).

Hours of operation. Some museums are open to the public only a fraction of the year, and others, like the Smithsonian Institution, are open eight hours each day, every day of the year except Christmas. Sixty percent of U.S. museums are open every week of the year, and fewer than 1 percent are open only by special arrangement or appointment. One-third are open less than thirty hours a week, 44 percent between thirty-one and fifty hours per week, and one-quarter in excess of fifty hours per week.

In addition to all these operational differences, of course, museums vary by their subject matter: there are aquariums, planetariums, botanical gardens, and zoos; science and technology centers, art museums, and children's museums; nature centers and natural history and ethnographic museums; historical museums, and many small specialty museums with narrowly defined collections (see "Types of Museums" at the end of this chapter).

The range and diversity of museums in the United States have given rise to dozens of specialized museum associations, organized in different regions, states, and fields of collecting. Given the heterogeneity and variability of museums, the American Association of Museums in 1970 established a museum accreditation process, with procedures and standards that verify that a museum has "achieved and continues to meet generally understood standards of professional performance." By the mid-1990s, approximately 730 of the estimated 8,200 U.S. museums had achieved accreditation status.

What Museums Have in Common

What, then, can be said about most if not all museums? Virtually all museums are organized around collections of art, material culture, or specimens of nature. They share the goals of acquiring and conserving their collections and of interpreting and exhibiting this human and natural heritage to public audiences. They are expected to care for and preserve their collections as a public trust for future generations. The Grand Hall of the Canadian Museum of Civilization in Hull, Quebec, as shown in the photograph on p. 10, exemplifies the distinctive character of museums.

Museums are normally invested in missions that serve the public, and these missions are educational, aesthetic, scientific, or historical. The great majority of museums in the Untied States are organized as private, nonprofit organizations or as agencies of state and local governments. As nonprofit educational organizations, these museums receive certain privileges and exemptions under

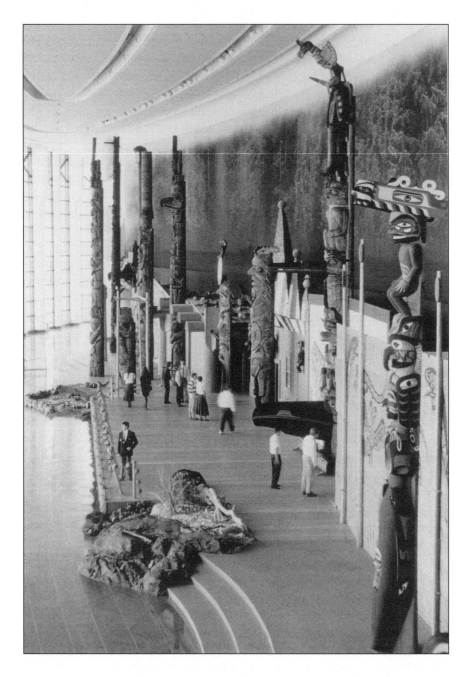

Canadian Museum of Civilization/Musée Canadien des Civilisations, Hull, Quebec. The Grand Hall, shaped to symbolize Raven's Canoe, is a "villagescape" representing Native cultures from Canada's Pacific Coast.

Photo by Harry Foster.

U.S. laws and tax regulations, in return for which they are expected to function as publicly minded educational and public service–oriented organizations.

MUSEUMS EVOLVE

Museums originated among the ancient Greeks prior to the Christian era as scholarly, religious, spiritual, and creative centers, engaging a small number of participants and far removed from everyday life. Our word *museum* comes from the Greek *mouseion*, a temple of the muses—in Greek mythology, goddesses of inspiration and learning and patrons of the arts. One of the earliest museums was built in Alexandria, Egypt, in the third century B.C., by Ptolemy II Philadelphus, the most accomplished of the Ptolemaic kings following Alexander the Great. Alexandria was then the preeminent city of learning in the Mediterranean world, and this Ptolemaic museum functioned as a scholar's library, a research center, and a contemplative retreat.

In ancient Rome during the second century B.C., museums became associated with the storage and display of collections acquired in colonial and military campaigns. The instinct for collecting evident throughout human history was elevated by the Romans into a major art form and a systematic enterprise. After imperial wars and conquests, Roman generals returned to Rome, as Fulvius did in 189 B.C., for example, with thousands of bronze and marble statues and gold and silver pieces, the plunder of military campaigns. The center of Rome itself became a museum, filled with objects from subdued nations (Ripley, 1978; Alexander, 1979).

During the medieval period in the West, the Roman Catholic Church became a preeminent intellectual center and patron of the arts. A significant art collection, overseen by Pope Sixtus IV, had been amassed in Rome by the end of fifteenth century. The period of the Renaissance in Italy, beginning in the late fourteenth century, marked the rise of humanism and secularism as leading ideas in society. Renaissance thought reflected strong interest in the study of nature and in inventiveness and artistry. By the sixteenth century, Italy was home to great private collections and museum-like buildings that housed botanical and zoological specimens, historical artifacts, skeletal remains, curios, shells, coins, bronzes, sculptures, and paintings. Collections depicting the range of world habitats and cultures were also highly sought after, becoming known in the eighteenth century as *cabinets of curiosities*. The term applied to the collections as well as to the spaces and furniture in which they were housed (Ripley, 1978). Far-ranging, encyclopedic collections developed out of these earlier collections, and today they are found in great international museums such as the Louvre, the British Museum, the Hermitage, and the Prado.

Collections in modern Europe and in England were assembled by kings and nobility, by the established churches, and later by wealthy merchants. Housed in palaces and grand private residences, they were open to highly selective audiences. Science and natural history collections were available to scholars but off-limits to most people. The first university museum was Oxford University's Ashmolean Museum, opened in 1683. The museum's literature identifies it as "the oldest surviving purpose-built museum building in the world" and the earliest museum open to public visitors as well as scholars.

The public museum, open to people regardless of rank or class, arose first in London in the eighteenth century. Sir Ashton Lever, a country gentleman and graduate of Oxford, collected live birds and, later, shells, fossils, stuffed birds, costumes of native peoples, weapons, and every variety of exotic object. Having outgrown the space of his ancestral home, he opened a public museum in London in 1774. An admission fee was charged to cover costs and to regulate the number and manner of visitors. Lever's experience with visitors, however, was adverse, and he eventually put this notice in a London newspaper: "This is to inform the Publick that being tired out with the insolence of the common People . . . I am now come to the resolution of refusing admittance to the lower class except they come provided with a ticket from some Gentleman or Lady of my acquaintance" (Ripley, 1978, p. 32).

The tension in museums between serving scholars, connoisseurs, and savants on the one hand and encouraging public learning on the other grew in the eighteenth and nineteenth centuries. Nevertheless, museums gradually evolved into broader, public-minded institutions. In the transition stage, museums often set aside special hours or times of the year for ordinary people to visit. The British Museum, for example, opened its doors to the public in 1759, at least to visitors with proper identification, between the hours of 11 A.M. and noon. The Louvre in 1793, following the French Revolution, opened its doors to the public three days each week.

Museum Development in the United States

The pattern of museum development in the United States differed from the pattern characteristic of museums in Europe. Although there are exceptions on both continents, many European museums were created as instruments of ruling classes and governments to celebrate and glorify the national culture and the state. The great majority of U.S. museums, by contrast, were created by individuals, families, and communities to celebrate and commemorate local and regional traditions and practices and to enlighten and entertain people in local communities. The earliest American museums emerged in the latter part of the eighteenth century in places like Charleston, South Carolina; Salem, Massachusetts; and Philadelphia.

U.S. museum development was influenced by the ideas of leaders such as Charles Willson Peale in the late 1780s in Philadelphia; George Brown Goode at the Smithsonian in Washington, D.C., in the late nineteenth century; and

John Cotton Dana in Newark, New Jersey, in the early twentieth century. Others like Philip Youtz, director of the Brooklyn Museum; Francis Henry Taylor, director of the Metropolitan Museum of Art; Henry Watson Kent, the Metropolitan's supervisor of instruction; and Theodore Low, the Metropolitan's head of education, also exerted major influence.

Charles Willson Peale, the celebrated early American painter and portraitist, opened an art and natural history museum in Philadelphia between 1782 and 1786. Its explicit purpose was to instruct and engage ordinary citizens who lacked formal education (Brigham, 1995). Peale's museum was open certain evenings of the week in order to reach working people. He advertised that the extended evening hours were "to accommodate those who may not have leisure during the day light to enjoy the rational amusement which the various subjects of the Museum afford." Burgiss Allison, a supporter of Peale's museum, explained this mingling of reason, education, and entertainment: "With regard to amusements . . . it must be evident to every person of the least reflection . . . that if we can contrive to amuse whilst we instruct, the progress will be more rapid and the impression much deeper" (Brigham, 1995, pp. 19–20; see also pp. 1–5).

The Metropolitan Museum of Art offered lectures for adults beginning in 1872, two years after its founding. Boston's Museum of Fine Arts inaugurated adult education classes in 1876. George Brown Goode, director of the Smithsonian's earliest national museum, advanced the view that museums should serve the broad public and have clear educational purposes. He wrote: "The museums of the future in this democratic land should be adapted to the needs of the mechanic, the factory operator, the day laborer, the salesman and the clerk, as much as to those of the professional man and the man of leisure. . . . No museum can grow and be respected that does not each year give additional proofs of its claims to be considered a center of learning" (Boyer, 1993, p. 18). Goode pioneered in making museums accessible by creating the first explicitly educational exhibitions, with labels and texts to enlighten the public.

John Cotton Dana, founder of The Newark Museum, continued in Goode's path and became the leading proponent in the early twentieth century of audience-, community-, and education-centered museums. He wrote: "We believe that it will pay any community to add to its educational apparatus a group of persons which shall form the staff of a local institution of visual instruction. . . . [And museums] will transform themselves slowly into living organisms, with an abundance of teachers, with ample workshops, classrooms and spaces for handling the outgoing and incoming of objects" (Dana, [1917] 1988, pp. 7–8). His "new museum" made special efforts to attract young people.

Some urban American museums in the late nineteenth and early twentieth centuries had missions to help train workers in the arts and in design and engineering skills that were needed in the industrial era. In Ohio, the Toledo

Museum of Art and the Cleveland Museum of Art established training programs. The charter of the Cleveland Museum of Art in 1913 stated, among its objectives, to "maintain an industrial training school" (Newsom and Silver, 1978, p. 14; see also pp. 13–26). This also reflected the nation's growing interest, converging with the new philosophy of progressive education, in self-improvement, self-teaching activities, and informal and supplementary adult education practices.

America's industrial and mercantile leaders in the late nineteenth and early twentieth century—Andrew Carnegie in New York City and Marshall Field and Julius Rosenwald in Chicago, among others—founded museums and libraries in the spirit of noblesse oblige for the explicit purpose of reaching lower-income and working-class people and immigrants who lacked formal education and strong acculturating influences. In Chicago, Field, Rosenwald, and other municipal leaders conceived a series of museums that were situated in the city's public parks. Both the museums and the parks were intended to be *people's parks*, reaching the majority of citizens who were unschooled or out of school; combining recreation, education, and nature study and offering wholesome, all-encompassing leisure-time activities.

Many U.S. history museums and historic sites developed from the bottom up, as a result of community initiative that sought ways to memorialize a community's history and celebrate its traditions and achievements. No list of influences shaping U.S. museums would be complete without mention of the showman P. T. Barnum (1810–1891), founder of the jumbo-scale circus. Barnum was in the museum business as well, opening museums in New York State and in the Midwest. He combined entertainment, adventure, and exotic experiences with an appeal to natural curiosity, if not enlightenment. Rubens Peale, son of Charles Willson Peale and manager of the Peale Museum in Baltimore between 1822 and 1837, was one of the first museum leaders to raise concerns about competitors. The family's archives preserve a comment he wrote in 1822: "Since the opening of the circus, I have been completely deserted" (Peale family papers, Peale Museum, Baltimore, Maryland).

Changes in Museum Design and Presentation

The design of early museum galleries and exhibitions reflected the learning of the people who enjoyed access. As long as museums embraced mainly scholars, connoisseurs, savants, and the wealthy, their collections and exhibitions required little explanation or interpretation. A typical nineteenth-century natural history museum, for example, was filled with cabinets and cases containing artifacts and art, ethnographic objects, specimens, and other natural objects, mixed together in a seemingly haphazard arrangement. Nineteenth-century museums provided little or no historical or contextual information; they held esoteric collections for the initiated. The absence of descriptive, contextual, and interpretive materials posed no great hindrance to this narrow band of visitors.

This did not mean, however, that museums lacked a point of view. Nineteenth-century natural history museums in London, New York, and elsewhere embodied a concept of history—history seen as moving along a providential path. The collections were regarded as records of human and moral progress, evolution from the primitive to the civilized—a notion clearly reflecting the ideas of the Enlightenment.

Museums evolved in other respects as well. The earliest history museums collected objects that reflected aristocratic or elite ideas, symbols, and culture. History museums typically collected and exhibited busts and paintings of heroes and famous historical figures and artifacts and specimens depicting great battles and historical events. Their purpose was to inspire by example as well as to enlighten. The Smithsonian's National Museum of American History (named the National Museum of History and Technology until 1980) was one of the first history museums to collect and show objects depicting everyday life and to interpret history from the point of view of ordinary citizens. Its exhibits of eighteenth- and nineteenth-century America featured the implements and objects of everyday life, ordinary dwellings, common religious practices, and letters and documents recounting the daily lives of citizens. In similar fashion, history museums in the United States in the late twentieth century have evolved along one further path: collecting artifacts, artworks, and records reflecting on different cultures and ethnic communities, particularly "minority" and newly emerging communities.

Museum presentations today feature a variety of new elements—electronic and interactive media (videos, CD-ROMS, computer interactives, the Internet); hands-on tools and demonstrations; and storytelling, theatrical, dance, and musical performances. These interactive and multimedia museum presentations reflect recently developed educational concepts emphasizing multiple intelligences, divers learning styles, and a range of culturally defined learning modalities.

Historically, museums were seen as authoritative custodians and interpreters of culture and knowledge. The presumptive authority of museums resided in their rare and authentic collections and in the curator's and scholar's expertise in interpreting the collections. By the latter decades of the twentieth century museums have for the most part evolved along egalitarian, democratic, culturally diverse, and popular lines. Collections, always the core of museums, now coexist with narratives and educational programs as prime museum values. Exhibitions increasingly offer multiple perspectives. The evolution of central museum concepts—from collections to information and education and from learning to experiences—has reflected a gradual shift from control by experts (curators, educators, scholars) to control by audiences. Museums traditionally controlled their collections and interpretations thereof, whereas audiences control their own experiences. Hence marketing, with its focus on the museum experience from the point of view of visitors and consumers, reflects the latest stage in museum evolution. As museums evolve further, new ways of balancing disparate and sometimes conflicting elements and aims must be found.

SUMMARY

Museums offer distinctive things not found in other places, notably the enjoyment of rare and authentic objects, the sensory experience of encountering items of beauty and interest, and knowledge deriving from the research and scholarship behind collections and exhibitions. Although the presence of tangible objects characterizes virtually all museums, in many other respects museums can be as different from one another as they are collectively from movie houses, theme parks, and sports arenas. Museums differ in size and in resources, in numbers of staff and hours of operation. Museums also differ in architecture, facilities, and collections, exhibitions, and services. Historically, museums have evolved from elite organizations accessible only by the nobility to broader-based public institutions. Museums have also redefined their raison d'être along more egalitarian, democratic, and consumer-oriented lines. Museums, for much of their history, were valued primarily for the care and preservation of their rare collections as keepsakes for future generations. Because collections were the dominant focus, museum offerings and the museum-going experience were controlled by museum keepers and experts. But by the early twentieth century, the focus of museums had shifted toward informational and educational resources, programs, and purposes. An even more evolved view is that a museum's main function is to provide appealing and memorable museum experiences. The move from information and learning toward an experience in a distinctive environment is also a move toward giving museum "consumers" a much greater voice in defining museum quality and service.

○

TYPES OF MUSEUMS: A SURVEY

Museums are organizations with different collections, missions, and objectives. Here we review the major types of museums, their historical developments, their characteristics, and the issues faced in each group.

Art Museums

Art museums have evolved into broad, public institutions more slowly than have science and history museums. Aesthetic norms, connoisseurship, taste, and restrictions on entry worked to limit participation, but art museums are evolving toward openness and inclusivity, with education receiving increasing emphasis. So-called blockbuster exhibitions have generally proved to be means of attracting large audiences and raising the visibility of art, artworks, and artists.

Art museums, it can be argued, have two audiences to deal with. The first consists of the patrons, collectors, and donors who contribute the artworks and other resources that sustain the museums. The high prices of works of art reinforce patrons' and collectors' status so that a high level of involvement in art museums symbolizes or even confers high social status. The second audience consists of visitors, members, and the general public. Correspondingly, art museums evidence a division of labor between patrons' and visitors' needs and interests; for example, art museums typically have extensive programs catering to donors and patrons. Art museums are building collections that go beyond the traditional emphasis on the fine arts—paintings, sculptures, drawings, and prints. Increasingly, they are collecting decorative arts and crafts, design materials, architecture, and photography.

Art museums have the challenge of acquiring artworks that are costly and precious. They compete in this with other museums and with corporations and wealthy private collectors. They also compete with one another for gifts and donations. Art museums also have active culling and deaccessioning policies and use the funds obtained from sale or transfer to reshape their collections. In some museums, purchasing a costly work of art is viewed as trading off conservation, education, and museum services. The alternative uses of an art museum's budget can become a highly charged issue.

Art museums face a particular challenge in attracting visitors. The public is less likely to identify with the arts than with other areas of knowledge such as science. Art history, studio arts, and art education are experiencing cutbacks. The absence of awareness among young people in the value of the fine arts can lead to inattention later in life. Museums therefore have an added role in education. An excellent example of museum education in the arts is the Visual Learning Center at the High Museum of Art in Atlanta. It has computer-interactive screens with information about the paintings, drawings, and prints that hang on the surrounding walls. At one screen a visitor can learn about the element of line in works of art; at another screen, color; at a third, light; and at a fourth, composition. Thus the interactive learning is integrated with and reinforces the visual encounter with the works of art in the gallery.

Art museums can provoke controversy and confusion. Some forms of contemporary art are unfamiliar to broad segments of the public and are distasteful to some people. The creation of art is often associated with individuals who harbor "avant-garde" and sometimes antisocial ideas. The very impulse among artists to push the boundaries of the customary can be interpreted as signs of radicalism, decadence, or disreputability.

Many art museums are entering the electronic information age with great vigor. They view the electronic information highway as a premium distribution channel for reaching large audiences and especially as a link to young people, who are acclimated to computer and video technology. Even small art museums can maintain Web sites on the Internet, thanks to the relatively low cost and the relative abundance in most communities of computer whizzes willing to donate their services. There are risks in the electronic environment, however. Viewing art on a computer screen should not be a substitute for seeing art in museums. Digital images vary in quality and can be manipulated. Museums that put art on the Internet lose control of those images, with repercussions for copyrights and standards. Nevertheless, art images on videotape, film, and CD-ROM are now as widely disseminated as art images in books, and both forms can be of great aesthetic and educational value.

History Museums, History Centers, and Historic Houses and Sites

A survey of public interest in history museums and sites reveals two contrary tendencies—a great potential for public interest and yet level or declining visitorship. "In developed countries," Victor Middleton (1994) observes, "there has been an extraordinary period of growth of interest in heritage. In part this reflects public interest and demand, in part the interests of supplying organizations dedicated to the conservation ideals. . . . The growth is a manifestation of relatively mature, educated and wealthy societies, able and willing to forgo some part of potential present consumption of resources for the sake of posterity" (p. 6). Kevin Britz (1995) refers to *community memory* in his chronicle of the rise of small-town historical societies and museums. He notes the upsurge in communities' interest in honoring, recording, and interpreting their past and transmitting local values to future generations. Public interest in history and history museums is reinforced by holidays and commemorative events such as the 1976 U.S. Bicentennial celebration, which sparked the rise of many new history sites and museums.

A major issue for history museums is presentation. Books on a particular historical topic can claim to be comprehensive, and they usually include extensive bibliographies. Lectures are formats for learning a great deal about a particular subject of limited scope, and they often allow the audience to comment or ask questions. Museum exhibitions, however, are necessarily more selective and compressed than books and often less responsive to audience inquiries than lectures with a question-and-answer period. The need to compress a large amount of information and interpretation into a historical exhibition that is limited in size and space can lead to charges that the exhibition is biased, excludes certain perspectives, or favors certain groups over others. History museums are increasingly searching for ways to present multiple perspectives, particularly when controversial topics are involved. They are also investing in surveying group and community perspectives on important historical topics and providing supplementary resources that visitors can consult for expanded treatment.

As American society and culture become more variegated and splintered, museum curators and historians face pressure to incorporate an ever-greater range of ethnic, cultural, and class perspectives. Inclusiveness is sometimes limited by gaps in museum collections, especially with respect to newcomer or emergent ethnic communities, or a tendency to reflect the views of a particular generation or gender. Thus history museums are being called on to record and represent a common heritage in a given community as well as the singular threads of ethnical, cultural, and generational groups and their degree of integration with or separation from the mainstream. Similarly, history museums are being challenged to deal with relative views, truths, and perspectives and eschew absolute ideas and claims to authority that characterized traditional museums. Community perspectives are being combined with curatorial perspectives. History museums are expected to be celebratory in portions of their exhibitions but are also expected to provide critical perspectives on other (or even the same) topics. Historical interpretation is itself subject to continuous rethinking and reanalysis; such "revisionism" is frequently a source of controversy among tradition-minded groups. Historians point out that scholars in other fields like biology, medicine, and economics are expected routinely to revise and upgrade their knowledge, yet historians are expected to stick to conventional interpretations, no matter how outdated by subsequent findings they may be. History museums in particular can be challenged by stakeholder groups who see their role as guardians of tradition and convention.

Two new directions in history museums have had a major impact. History museums, especially history centers, are engaging in the study and interpretation of contemporary issues and their effect on families, communities, cities, and society as a whole. They are employing their historical resources to illuminate contemporary conditions—and in some cases they are creating exhibitions and public programs that point the way to solving problems. History museums and centers are also experimenting with new presentation methods. One aim is to connect visitors with historical experience by linking broad historical processes and events to historical forces within their own communities and families. Museums are using personal as well as narrative elements to make history more current and engaging. An example is the Lower East Side Tenement Museum in New York City. Visitors view several restored rooms with the original furnishings, photographs, and letters and diaries.

Science Museums and Science and Technology Centers

Science museums and science and technology centers are experiencing high rates of increase in museum visitorship. There are several reasons for this. Communities, school districts, and corporations have supported science museums as education centers and as training grounds for skill building among young people. Science museums can supplement the limited science resources available in schools. They offer, to a greater extent than other museums, hands-on, interactive tools and exhibits of particular appeal to young people. Science museums and centers are process oriented rather than object oriented; this gives them greater contact with visitors and more audience involvement than most other types of museums.

Science museums and centers are experimenting with techniques and approaches for communicating science to a broad-based public. They have led the way in building IMAX and Omnimax theaters. San Francisco's Exploratorium pioneered in the use of interactive exhibitions, hands-on tools, and demonstrations of scientific inquiry and methods. The Carnegie Science Center, in Pittsburgh, offers science programs targeted to different age groups. The Maryland Science Center and the Shedd Aquarium offer unusual experiences with science and nature, including overnights and science camps. Science and technology centers have excelled in designing environments that are dynamic looking, colorful, and visually and aurally inviting. Science centers are relatively free of the obligation to maintain large collections (although many have collections); their objects are typically instruments and tools for doing science. Because they demonstrate so many things in so many ways, science museums and centers use more volunteers and staff, which requires training and quality control. Science museum and center managers say that one of the thorniest problems is maintaining interactive and computer equipment in working order. Active use by young people and also inadequacies in design and engineering result in frequent breakdown of the hands-on and interactive equipment.

Natural History, Anthropological, and Ethnographic Museums

Natural history museums are perhaps the most museum-like of museums. They tend to have enormous collections requiring a great deal of attention, care, and conservation—meaning large staffs and high operating costs. Nearly 60 percent of objects and specimens in permanent museum collections are accounted for by natural history museums. In contrast, science and technology museums account for only 2 percent of total permanent collections; art museums, just under 2 percent; and historical museums, approximately 12 percent (American Association of Museums, 1994, pp. 55–57).

Because the largest natural history museums originated as research organizations, employing scientists and scholars, their missions have emphasized research as well as exhibitions and programs for the public. The result has often been tension in allocating resources; balancing scholarly, curatorial, and public service roles; and integrating professional loyalties with museum loyalties.

Exhibitions at natural history museums tend to be longer lasting than those at art and science museums. Because these museums are generally older, their facilities tend to be less modernized, giving some natural history museums a quaint, old-fashioned feel. Natural history museums were among the first, however, to create designed environments as contexts for objects, collections, and exhibitions. In recent years the cases filled with disconnected specimens and objects have given way to dioramas with realistic settings for ethnographic objects and animal and plant species. Old-time cabinet-of-curiosities-style galleries are being replaced by themed rooms, exhibitions with narratives, videos, and interactive tools. Larger natural history museums have built IMAX and Omnimax theaters and are attracting large audiences.

Natural history museums with significant anthropological and ethnographic collections are facing the issue of repatriating portions of their collections to groups that claim traditional ownership. Some natural history collections were acquired from people in colonized societies. Increasingly, these people are questioning why their cultural patrimony has been turned over to outsiders. New U.S. policies and programs for the repatriation of Native American specimens and artifacts were established in the late 1980s and early 1990s.

Natural history museums are being challenged to devote a greater portion of their resources to representing and interpreting critical contemporary issues such as environmental degradation, ecological sustainability, and protection of the natural world's biodiversity. These museums, once windows onto the past, are more and more becoming windows of the future. Environmental conservation and education are major programs at natural history museums, with a focus on research, policy, and instruction. Herein lies a great opportunity for natural history museums to reach larger audiences.

Zoological Parks and Botanical Gardens

Zoos and botanical gardens are the most frequently visited types of museums in the world. They also are visited by a broader cross section of their communities than other museums are. Median attendance at U.S. zoos in the early 1990s was 482,000, compared to median attendance of 22,000 at history museums, 60,000 at art museums, and 94,000 at science museums. In terms of children who visit as part of a school group, median attendance at U.S. zoos was 47,000, compared to 14,500 at art museums, 16,000 at history museums, and 14,000 at science museums. Zoos are among the most costly museums to operate. For this reason it is not surprising that 67 percent of U.S. zoos are government run or supported, compared to 34 percent of U.S. science museums and 31 percent of U.S. art museums (American Association of Museums, 1994, pp. 40–53, 65).

Zoos first developed as private menageries and collections maintained by kings and nobility in Egypt (approximately, 1500 B.C.) and in China and the Middle East (approximately 1000 B.C.). The first modern zoo opened in Vienna in 1752, although it was closed to the general public for its first thirteen years. The earliest U.S. zoo is the Philadelphia Zoo, opened in 1854. Zoos have evolved in their missions. William Hornaday, the first director of the New York Zoological Society stated that his zoo's mission was "to collect and exhibit fine and rare animals" and enable "the greatest possible number of people to see them with comfort and satisfaction" (Alexander, 1979, p. 113). Today, zoos are in the forefront of worldwide efforts to save endangered animal species, protect ecological systems, and train people in the challenges of preserving biodiversity and the environment. Large research-oriented zoos are engaged in cutting-edge research in the fields of genetics, reproductive physiology, veterinary medicine, and wildlife conservation. Zoos worldwide have developed highly intensive electronic information systems through which they can collaborate in protecting endangered species and aiding their reproduction in captivity. Computerized databases enable a zoo in, say, Africa to find out almost instantaneously the animal stock available for breeding in U.S., Asian, and European zoos.

A new direction in zoos is to integrate and develop holistically the animal collections, the plantings and botanical species, and the ecological systems in which they all exist. The National Zoological Park, for example, is transforming itself from a zoological park into a *biopark*. Zoo Atlanta has designed highly innovative ecological settings featuring combinations of animals found together in the wild. Its Masai Mara habitat includes zebras, giraffes, gazelles, black rhinos, cranes, and ostriches. Zoos are also playing a leading role in designing educational programs focusing on environmental conservation. The National Zoological Park, for example, has satellite- and computer-based education programs that reach school classrooms in the Washington metropolitan area, bringing together zoo scientists and educators in digital workshops with teachers. In recent years zoos have developed extensive sponsorships and partnerships with business corporations that have resulted in sizable financial support to renovate habitats, construct new facilities, and sustain educational and public outreach programs (Maple and Archibald, 1993).

Children's and Youth Museums

Children's and youth museums are one of the fasting-growing segments of the museum world. The great majority of U.S., British, and European children's museums have developed in the last twenty years. The Brooklyn Children's Museum, founded in 1899, was the first U.S. museum dedicated exclusively to young people. This museum and others that followed reflected developments in educational philosophy and psychology associated with Jean Piaget, Maria Montessori, and John Dewey, early-twentieth-century pioneers who created models of progressive education with hands-on, experiential learning. The growth in children's museums has accompanied the growing emphasis on preschooling and early childhood learning. Considerable evidence indicates that early childhood learning is enhanced by multisensory stimulation, tactile and kinesthetic experiences, and designed environments that foster youngsters' curiosity, imagination, and active participation. Children's museums have become important adjuncts to formal education. Educated parents are increasingly turning away from television and mass media and seeking nonmediated forms of learning, experience, and participation.

Some children's museums have been criticized for being little more than playlots. Yet these museums vary considerably in their programs, goals, and methods. Some, like the Please Touch Museum in Philadelphia, offer extensive children's play activities, exhibits, and equipment that encourage children to be active. Others, like the Children's Museum of Manhattan, use material objects, collections, and exhibitions, in addition to play equipment, to engage children. The Capital Children's Museum, in Washington, D.C., makes extensive use of artworks, stage settings, and designed environments that depict various world cultures and offer cross-cultural experiences. The Habitot gallery of the Minnesota Children's Museum is devoted to infants and toddlers six months to four years of age. The highly celebrated Children's Museum of Indianapolis and the Children's Museum in Boston are large enough to offer a full range of learning and entertaining experiences for young people. A growing issue for children's and youth museums is finding ways to reach children of minority ethnic groups and children at risk.

Community and Ethnic Museums

Large U.S. urban centers with sizable immigrant and minority ethnic communities have witnessed the growth of community museums devoted to the representation and interpretation of local ethnic cultures. Chicago, for example, has a Polish museum, a Lithuanian museum, a Ukrainian museum, a Mexican American museum, a Jewish museum, a Swedish museum, and an African American museum, among others. Community museums represent their local cultures in positive ways, first, to members of the cultural group represented in the museum and, second, to members of the larger society. Community museums seek to solidify community ties by furnishing through artifacts and artworks the ideas and symbols that strengthen cultural identities.

A problem arises, however, when ethnic and community museums appeal almost exclusively to members of their own communities and fail to reach out to other groups and disseminate their cultural ideas to the broader society. Community museum staff tend to be involved in ongoing community issues and concerns, deflecting resources and energies away from research and interpreting museum collections. Chicago's Ukrainian Institute of Modern Art has attempted to reach a wider local audience through exhibits of works by contemporary Ukrainian and Ukrainian American artists and performances of contemporary music written by Ukrainian composers. The Mexican Fine Arts Center Museum, also in Chicago, has established a range of programs to communicate and promote the cultural traditions of the city's Mexican American community. At the same time, it engages a wider audience by sponsoring public artworks in the neighborhoods, art classes for children, and teacher workshops that meld museum resources with formal schooling.

Specialty Museums

Museums collect every type of specimen, artifact, and object. Not surprisingly, Great Britain, an island nation and major maritime power, has nearly two hundred naval and maritime museums. The Time Museum in Rockford, Illinois, is dedicated to collecting time pieces from all over the world. The Samuel D. Harris National Museum of Dentistry, in Baltimore, focuses on human teeth and advances in dentistry and oral hygiene. The museum's star attraction is George Washington's lower dentures. Museums are devoted to famous personalities (for example, Elvis Presley's Graceland), historical eras (Richmond's Museum of the Confederacy), human records of achievement or statistical anomaly (Copenhagen's Guinness World Records Museum), and public institutions (New York's Museum of American Financial History). A growing number of specialty museums are halls of fame devoted to a sport, a type of music or literature, or some other specific field. The International Tennis Hall of Fame and Tennis Museum, in Newport, Rhode Island, not only houses collections but is also situated, according to its brochure, adjacent to "the only lawn tennis courts in the country that are open to the public."

Businesses and industries have established museums to record their commercial accomplishments and celebrate the products they have made famous. Jim Beam's American Outpost, located in Clermont, Kentucky, celebrates a firm that is Kentucky's oldest continuing business. The Pennsylvania Anthracite Heritage Museum, in Scranton, records the life and times of the region's coal industry. The Mushroom Museum at Phillips Place, in Kennett Square, Pennsylvania, lies in the heart of the U.S. mushroom-growing industry and is owned by one of the largest mushroom-producing companies. One of the world's most unusual museums opened in 1994 in a suburb of New Delhi, India. Dedicated to the history of latrines, waste disposal systems, and human hygiene beginning in 2500 B.C., the Sulabh International Museum of Toilets was created by the founder of the Sulabh International Social Service Organization, a corporation that generates fuel from human excrement and that owns and manages 650,000 public pay toilets in India's cities and along its roads.

General Museums

Some of the finest museums house collections involving diverse fields of knowledge and human activity. The Ashmolean Museum at Oxford University in England, for example, contains collections of the fine arts and decorative arts; ethnographic, archeological, and anthropological collections from nations once part of the British Empire; natural science collections; and collections of tools, technologies, and scientific equipment. Museums that embrace two or more distinctive collection areas are known as *general museums.* The Reading Public Museum, in Pennsylvania, contains 250,000 objects drawn from the decorative and fine arts, anthropology, and archaeology and includes one of the largest and most distinguished butterfly collections in the United States. Another example of the general museum is the Niagara Falls Museum, in Ontario, Canada. The museum was founded in the early nineteenth century in Canada, moved to the United States in 1888, and moved back again to Canada in 1958. Its collections are an assemblage of Egyptian mummies and taxidermy specimens, dinosaur and whale bones, rocks and minerals, Oriental art, Native American artifacts, medieval weaponry, and oddities and freaks of nature. The museum's Daredevil Hall of Fame features objects and stories of people who had adventures at the falls, including a woman who in 1901 went over the falls in a barrel and lived to tell about it. It has been argued that one of the great values of general museums is the variety of objects placed together, the juxtaposition of highly dissimilar objects and thus the opportunity to explore differences, make comparisons, and probe patterns in nature and in art. The hodgepodge of objects that general museums house provoke curiosity and wonderment, especially among children.

Encyclopedic Museums

Great art museums with collections that incorporate art from many different cultures, civilizations, and historical periods and include the fine arts, decorative arts, and craft arts, are known as *encyclopedic museums.* Examples are the Louvre in Paris and the Metropolitan Museum of Art in New York City. Encyclopedic museums of natural science, natural history, archaeology, ethnography, and anthropology also exist: European examples are the British Museum and the Deutsches Museum; U.S. examples are the American Museum of Natural History, the Field Museum, and the Smithsonian Institution's National Museum of Natural History.

Small Museums

Three out of four museums in the United States are defined as small museums. Many report resource deficits alongside rising levels of demand for services. The Institute of Museum and Library Services indicated in 1992 that 97 percent of small U.S. museums reported a need for additional funding, 94 percent needed more staff, 94 percent needed better equipment, and 87 percent needed staff training.

Small museums face a series of challenges. They tend to be located in small, rural communities that have experienced population loss. They are not usually tourist destinations. And they have difficulty obtaining traveling exhibitions or acquiring loans from other museums.

Mary Kay Ingenthron, a consultant to small museums (interviewed on Jan. 22, 1996), observes that a major concern of smaller museums is their lack of access to and resources for professional training and development. By their very nature, many of these museums are rooted in traditional and informal community practices that stand in the way of adapting to new situations and forces. Yet small museums, with a great many things to offer the public, can benefit from new concepts and techniques of museum management. For example, small museums are often in reach of professional resources in their own communities yet may not be familiar with ways to enlist these resources. Professionals in public relations, marketing, and accounting may be willing to join their boards if approached properly. Many small museums are building community support. An example is the Racine County Historical Society and Heritage Museum, in Racine, Wisconsin. The museum has two full-time, three half-time, and one quarter-time paid staff members and 180 volunteers. It has a budget of $250,000 and receives support from the city's business community. In the mid-1990s, it revised its mission to focus on the inventiveness, product development, and entrepreneurial skills that characterize the region.

Small museums are discovering the value of special events to build memberships and raise revenues. Maria Holperin, former director of two small museums and now a museum consultant (interviewed on Oct. 15, 1996), points to the variety of special events that are appropriate for small museums: community picnics, membership dinners, award ceremonies, charity breakfasts, and auctions. An usual museum event occurred in the mid-1990s in Springfield, Missouri, when the History Museum for Springfield/Greene County and the Springfield Little Theatre collaborated in producing a series of "murder mystery" dinner theater events. Volunteer actors, trained in improvisation and audience interaction, staged a series of theater pieces that required the audience's locating objects in the museum collections in their quest to solve the mysteries. Each performance was preceded by cocktails and dinner. Special events of all kinds have proved highly popular with local residents.

Small museums in rural areas can take advantage of trends toward metropolitan dispersal. Computers and telecommunications are making it possible for increasing numbers of individuals to work at home or in the local community. It is important for small museums to monitor demographic changes in their communities, areas of growth, and new groups of residents. Newcomers can bring skills and energies and are potential museum visitors and supporters of a community's cultural life.

A major challenge is for small museums to raise their visibility and attract the audiences and patrons they need for self-support. Small museums are prime candidates for collaborations and partnerships. They can build public relations, promotional, and marketing partnerships with other small museums in their area. They can band together and promote themselves to local and state tourist agencies and the travel and hospitality industry. They can encourage companies to support a cluster of museums in a given area to form a framework for cultural activities. Local and regional museums contribute to the quality of life of residents and employees, advantages that businesses are likely to appreciate and support.

Small museums in the United States have established a marketing, communications, and development voice in the Small Museums Administrators' Committee (SMAC), a professional standing committee of the American Association of Museums. SMAC's newsletter reports on best practices in small museums and profiles successful institutions. Collaboration among small museums in the United States has spurred development of membership directories and better communications, inventories of collections, and regional partnerships for promotion and marketing.

CHAPTER TWO

Strategic Museum Challenges

Mission, Audience, and Funding

*People want to step away from the routine of everyday life, stretch the mind
and imagination, and nourish the spirit. They use their leisure time to
achieve this. Education and entertainment may be two poles, but they
interpenetrate. A question for museums is how best to organize the
museum-going experience so as to offer a deeper level of meaning than
theme parks yet also make it inviting, orienting, and comfortable.*
—Marc Pachter

A growing number of museums today are reinventing themselves—adapting to changing expectations and conditions and responding with new
forms of organization, exhibition design, programming, and services. The
changes museums are making can be seen as responses to what museum managers and professionals view as challenges that lie ahead, challenges in many
areas. This chapter examines three of these challenges: defining a distinctive,
engaging mission and striking a workable balance between the mission and demands from outside; building a solid audience and community support; and
generating sufficient funds and reserves to sustain a museum over the long run.

One cautionary note is appropriate here. Some museums are finding that
their responses to changes are ill adapted to the challenges they face. They produce piecemeal and incremental responses rather than timely, well-thought-out
plans for long-term solutions. Policies and plans may lack coherency, a long-
range perspective, a dispassionate assessment of mission and resources, and a
strategic planning and marketing framework.

CHALLENGE ONE: MUSEUM MISSION AND IDENTITY

Museums are complex organizations with multiple purposes, functions, and
roles to perform. Their multifaceted programs and operations make defining a
mission and identity a challenging task. Multiple purposes and competing expectations require striking a balance.

Museums are called on to show and interpret their collections and exhibitions and make them accessible, yet they are also obliged not to risk the deterioration of objects and collections from heavy use, which would make it impossible for future generations to enjoy them. Museums seek to maximize audiences (within the limits of public safety, comfort, and convenience) and at the same time provide high-quality visual, aesthetic, and learning experiences for those audiences—two goals that sometimes conflict. Some blockbuster exhibitions, for example, boost visibility, visitation, and revenues, but their very success at drawing large crowds can result in an unsatisfactory museum-going experience marked by congestion and noisiness. Museums large enough to support research staff are also expected to provide labor-intensive services to the public.

Considering the multiplicity of goals and constituencies that museums have to satisfy, the challenge is to create a coherent mission and identity around which the museum's values and resources can be effectively organized, communicated, and deployed. Its mission determines the functions, roles, and purposes it serves and its distinctive offerings, services, and operations.

A Museum Chooses Its Mission

A museum's fundamental mission, regardless of its particular characteristics, is to collect objects and interpret them, show them and educate the public about them, and inspire people to support the museum. Without support, a museum cannot last. The core, it can be argued, is a museum's collection, and the best statement we have seen regarding the mission of a museum and the purpose of collections was offered by William W. Moss, retiring after ten years as director of the Smithsonian Institution Archives, in the archives' 1993 annual report:

> Archives, museums, and libraries are institutions intentionally created by people to preserve material things we believe are of lasting value. . . . We know that nothing material is permanent. . . . We also know that in the modern world, information is plentiful. . . . In such a world, why do we need archives, libraries, and museums? . . . The answer is "so we may not be misled by fakes." . . . It is socially necessary and probably psychologically essential that we prevent others from fooling us about the past. If all history is inevitably interpretation, it is best that we have the most reliable and most durable interpretation available. . . . We need durable evidence, evidence that survives over time, through changes in interpretation, to give us confidence in the information we use so freely. . . . [These] are places . . . for a "reality check" in a world of plentiful, competing, and sometimes contradictory information.

Museum missions should be distinctive, yet there is wide latitude in framing a mission. A museum's mission can direct the museum to be predominantly research oriented and to offer limited public services. Or the mission may be broader in scope and direct the museum to present offerings that are both educational and entertaining and to provide a wide array of services. Thinking about museum missions often involves tensions among a museum's multiple and sometimes contrary goals. This is inherent in any mission-driven organization. The root of the word *mission* means "to send off," as to fulfill a calling or to convert others to a cause. A contemporary art museum, for example, is likely to be devoted to advancing awareness and enjoyment of contemporary art and at the same time persuading people that such artworks, often unfamiliar or even confusing, are objects of beauty and imagination that capture important human experiences and meanings.

Though all museum offerings derive from objects, collections, and exhibitions, museum professionals disagree along two dimensions. One is the extent to which a museum should focus on its collections and the unique knowledge residing therein and consequently appeal to the relatively limited audience that is likely to find that collection appealing; or else augment objects and collections with rich interpretive materials, supplementary programs, pleasing amenities, and consciously created experiences designed to attract a broader, larger audience. The second dimension involves who or what agency defines and determines a museum's offerings: museum professionals or audiences and the marketplace—or a combination of the two. These disagreements are heard more frequently in art museums than in history or science museums.

The museum world, with its great variety and scope, offers considerable latitude for different museum concepts and missions. The following reflections by distinguished museum leaders, past and present, illustrate a range of views of what museums should be and should do. Alan Fern, director of the National Portrait Gallery at the Smithsonian Institution, argues for a relatively traditional view. He observes: "The core business of the museum . . . is to allow people to experience the qualities of fine and rare objects that would otherwise be unavailable to them, thereby enriching their knowledge and experience . . . [in] an appropriate and dignified setting in which visitors and artworks can meet one another" (letter, Sept. 2, 1997).

Sherman Lee, director of the Cleveland Museum of Art in the 1960s and 1970s, affirmed the missionary character of museums with an emphasis on the need for art museums to shield themselves from public ignorance or disfavor. The context for his remarks was the trend in art museums toward blockbuster exhibitions. "It's part of the gradual businessization or PR-ization of art museums. Americans have never been happy with art, so they want to try to turn it into business, which they understand better. If you put hype around the visual arts and 'market' them, you fundamentally change the nature of what you're working with. Art is being sucked into a world of which it should not be a part" (1979, pp. 8–9).

Paul Perrot, who served in the 1970s and early 1980s as an assistant secretary for museum programs at the Smithsonian Institution and is a former director at the Corning Glass Museum in New York State and the Virginia Museum of Fine Arts, while not opposed to broadening the scope of museum offerings and services, argues for the distinctive mission of a museum to instruct the public. He wrote in the early 1970s: "Giving the visitor what he wants is not necessarily advisable: the purpose of an educational institution is to channel the client so that he will want the *best*. Therefore, it should present to him increasingly higher standards, while at the same time making sure that these standards are intelligible—that they are not a 'narcissistic' demonstration of the staff's own brilliance" (1972, p. 2).

A broader view of a museum's mission and objectives, with an emphasis on audience-centeredness, is offered by Harold Skramstad, former president of the Henry Ford Museum & Greenfield Village. Skramstad observes: "It has been a tradition in the museum and arts community to think that if somebody doesn't like us or support us or understand us, it's their problem. No, it is our problem. . . . Adding value is the critical issue. Not value added according to us, and our standard, but according to the community's standards" (Garfield, 1995, pp. 46–47). In another context, Skramstad advanced the view that a museum's "specialness will result from the experiences it provides" (Museums for the New Millenium, 1997, p. 38).

Julian Spalding, director of the Glasgow Museums and Art Galleries in Scotland, also takes a broad view of a museum's mission and objectives, with a particular emphasis on the need for community support. He writes: "Museums in Glasgow get talked about a lot—the best marketing is by word of mouth. People in Glasgow talk about our museums and support us and it is that swell of public opinion that ultimately can be turned into cash. . . . I think our main challenge is to . . . establish a real body of support within the public and show that it is well spread throughout all levels and communities" (1991, pp. 79, 86).

Stephen E. Weil, former deputy director of the Hirshhorn Museum and Sculpture Garden and a luminary in the museum field, has observed that museums, in most cases, are mission-driven organizations and that an inherent tension exists between a museum's mission and its environment, in particular public demands and in some cases the marketing strategies that some museums have adopted. Yet Weil argues that despite the parameters, museums should broaden their aims and offerings and should communicate more readily with audiences and with the surrounding communities. He writes: "The traditional concept of the art museum as a temple in which to celebrate the human genius of the few must be expanded into a view of the art museum as a place in which to celebrate the human accomplishment of the many, a place where the visitor may come to gain a better appreciation of that uniquely human capacity for creative transformation" (1995, p. 108).

Bran Ferren, executive vice president for creative technology, research, and development at Walt Disney Imagineering, highlighted before a 1996 professional museum audience the importance of storytelling, context, and meaning in supplementing the viewing of objects and collections. His view focuses on the transition in museum roles from offering information to offering experiences:

> A big part of your [museum] job is contextualizing the objects in your collections for your visitors. Storytelling is the most powerful technology at our disposal with which to accomplish this. . . . Establishing context is an essential part of making people believe that they are getting a valuable museum experience. Sometimes, it's been done for you—like Dorothy's red shoes. Other objects require more exposition. If I present to you an old piece of wood and say, "This is an old rotting piece of wood," you will say, "Yes, please get if off my desk." If, however, I can present the case with some degree of authority that it is, in fact, a piece of the original cross, it will take on a whole new meaning. . . . Why do people come back [to a museum]? I would say it is about content (the collection plus its context) and trust [*Museums for the New Millennium*, 1997, pp. 128–135].

The museum world's diversity makes generalizations risky, but it may be helpful to suggest a fourfold typology that depicts the main directions museums have taken in recent years:

Traditional museums (for example, the Ashmolean Museum, Oxford University)

Modified traditional museums (for example, the Art Institute of Chicago)

Process-oriented experiential museums (for example, the Minnesota Historical Society)

Community-centered museums (for example, the Corcoran Gallery of Art, Washington, D.C.)

This typology is neither exhaustive nor methodologically rigorous. The different characteristics of museums will dispose them to one side or another of any given category. But in general, art museums are more likely to be traditional and object centered and science centers are more likely to be process oriented and experiential.

Museums Acquire a Broader Image, Broader Offerings, and a Broader Audience

Museums in the United States have been encouraged since the late 1960s to adopt broader missions and identities. In 1967, President Lyndon Johnson asked for a study of the condition of museums, their unmet needs, their relationships to schools and universities, and their particular needs for funding. The resulting influential report, *America's Museums: The Belmont Report* (American Association of Museums, 1969), helped expand federal government support. It urged museums not only to take care of their collections but also to become more committed to public service, to design more educational programs, and to create "a lively place" where audiences can find "pleasure and delight" (pp. 1, 23). It also sparked dissent. Charles Parkhurst, then director of the Baltimore

Museum of Art and a member of the panel that drafted the report, pondered in another publication: "Are museums developing their own form of separatism, polarized as activity centers to serve as cultural dance halls as opposed to museums dedicated to preserve, display, and elucidate manifestations of man's essential tendencies of mind, and nature's varied resources?" (1969, p. 12).

A later stage in the broadening of museum missions and identities occurred with the 1992 report of the American Association of Museums (AAM), titled *Excellence and Equity: Education and the Public Dimension of Museums.* The report stated that education is "central to every museum's activities" and called on museums to "reflect the diversity of our society." The report stated: "Museums can no longer confine themselves simply to preservation, scholarship, and exhibition independent of the social context in which they exist" (p. 8). A further influence on U.S. museums to broaden their offerings occurred with the 1995 AAM publication of *New Visions: Tools for Change in Museums.* This report urged museums to improve their organizations, render their internal cultures more congenial to the public and consumers, and build more mechanisms for serving the public, providing education, and reaching diverse communities.

Stephen Weil, who currently serves as senior scholar emeritus at the Smithsonian Institution's Center for Museum Studies, has written widely on the relationship of museum missions to museum outcomes and accountability. Noting that museums are under increasing pressure from public-sector agencies for funding and to provide public-oriented benefits that are not available elsewhere, Weil (1994) advises museums to ask themselves a series of hard questions (and act accordingly):

> What outcomes does the museum aim to accomplish, and what results are in fact achieved?
>
> Does the museum have ways to measure outcomes and performance?
>
> Are the museum's mission and goals realistic and achievable, given its resources?
>
> Does the museum accomplish its mission effectively and efficiently, with better results at a lower cost than other organizations can accomplish?
>
> What does the museum offer that is distinctive and of special value in its community that other organizations do not offer?

Weil argues that the public view of the value that museums offer has evolved in recent years from a focus on "inputs" (collections, staff, and other resources) to a focus on "outputs" (frequency and scope of exhibitions, educational programs, and other offerings) and finally to a focus on "outcomes" (the effects of museum offerings on visitors, on learning, and on the experiences audiences take away).

Museums are indeed capable of broad missions and identities without compromising their core functions and values. It is also true that museums with too many offerings and facets can easily exhaust their resources. Emphases and priorities have to be articulated. Museum missions are significant anchors and must not be too vague, yet they should not be overly confining or narrow. One conceptual and methodological principle is worth reiterating here. Research has shown that different types of visitors focus on different kinds of experiences and that most museum visitors are seeking a *range* of experiences. People are quite able to absorb a variety of experiences and nuances during a visit to a single museum. They can welcome excitement, amusement, and diversion at one point and in another moment be reflective or relish the aesthetic pleasure of viewing a rare work of art. Visitors can oscillate between sociable experiences, celebrative and learning experiences, and enchanting and transcendent experiences. Exhibit 2.1 offers another way of viewing the scope of museum-going experiences and describes the six main varieties. Museums should strive (within their resources) to offer an array of experiences to their visitors to ensure enriching and satisfying visits.

Museums Reconcile Research, Education, and Entertainment

Museum professionals in the 1970s and 1980s began to examine the multiplicity of roles museums have been expected to perform, particularly larger museums that view themselves as research, educational, and popular institutions wrapped into one. Museum professionals (curators, researchers, and scholars in particular) view their role as building knowledge and finding truth wherever it may lie. They are highly trained individuals; they work in fields incorporating principles and methodologies not readily understood by the general public; their work is guided by standards of inquiry. Thus museum professionals sometimes regard popular views, community standards, and marketing norms as hindrances to their professionalism. A large number of museum professionals view their work as similar to that done by university professors and researchers. Yet there is an important difference: museum offerings are created specifically for a public audience, whereas academic work is usually oriented toward professional peers.

Tensions exist among the disparate museum roles. They arise, for example, when stakeholders or a community group seeks to censor exhibitions on grounds that they are "indecent" or "unpatriotic." One of the central tenets of any professional community is giving professionals the widest possible intellectual freedom and trusting in their training, expertise, and authority in their field. Pressure to curb the ability of curators to present exhibitions as they see fit—indeed, censorship in any form—runs contrary to professional norms and expectations, as well as intellectual freedom.

The concerns of a mission-driven museum's drive to protect its mission and its independence have in recent years come up against pressures to become more public and visitor oriented, taking more account of audience interests and needs and the demands of the marketplace generally. The issue many museums

○○○○○

Exhibit 2.1. Six Types of Museum-Going Experiences.

Recreation

Enjoyment of free, relaxed, unstructured time and activity . . . playful and diversion-ary activity . . . activity that can refresh body and spirit (walking around carefree, visiting different galleries, trying out interactive devices, sitting down for a meal, shopping in a gift shop)

Sociability

Meeting with or participating with others . . . looking at and being together with others . . . taking part in shared, public activity (visiting an exhibition in a group, meeting someone over lunch, looking at other visitors)

Learning Experience

Gathering and acquiring information . . . perceiving new things and new patterns . . . exer-cising curiosity and a sense of discovery . . . trying to understand things . . . contem-plating and reflecting . . . practicing cognitive skills (doing a science experiment, viewing new art forms, reading labels and texts for context and meaning)

Aesthetic Experience

Engaging in sensory perceptions, especially visual and tactile . . . seeing objects with a view toward their beauty, rather than what is moral or useful . . . comparing things and finding patterns . . . engaging in an intensive, focused activity (comparing paint-ings by the same artist to assess their qualities, similarities, and differences; enjoy-ing multimedia presentations that engage different senses)

Celebrative Experience

Observing and honoring a leader, event, group, or organization . . . sharing in histori-cal achievements . . . extolling something . . . connecting with the past, the historic record, the chain of causes and effects, changes in materials, and continuity through history and time . . . encounting high standards that refine sensibility, enlarge thought, and shape aspiration (view rockets and technologies in a science museum with a sense of achievement, view an icon with reverence and respect)

Enchanting Experience

Encountering things that uplift the mind, imagination, and spirit . . . finding magic, de-light, fascination, and rapture in things and places . . . lifting oneself from the routine of everyday life (view an art exhibition with a sense of enchantment or an exhibit of sci-ence and technology with a sense of awe)

○○○○○

face is that by virtue of the very evolution of the museum role and identity, museum professionals have lost varying degrees of independence and control over museum offerings. Once museums ceased to be regarded exclusively as collection-driven repositories and came to be viewed as information and educational centers, museum professionals lost part of their justification as collection experts and authorities in particular fields. And then when museums became experience centered, museum employees gave up some more of their initiative to their audiences, for visitors define their own experiences. Marketing is resisted precisely because it focuses on museums from the point of view of visitors, members, and other consumers.

Although there are no easy answers to mission tensions, museum professionals are discovering that these tensions are not inescapable; they often relate more to methods than to ends and are sometimes reconcilable with a little effort. Curators developing exhibitions are teaming up more and more with designers, educators, and communication and marketing specialists, recognizing the advantage of a division of labor. Thus certain decisions are primarily curatorial, others are primarily market driven, and still others warrant joint involvement. Furthermore, professionals recognize that serious topics can be given lively presentations and that entertainment can be an adjunct to exhibition quality. Museum managers also recognize differences in the quality of outside communications, public relations, and marketing resources they use. Marketing, for example, is primarily a set of concepts, tools, and methods; done right, a marketing plan furthers the museum's objectives and purposes in a targeted manner. Marketing does have a point of view, but its greater utility lies in the practical applications to reaching audiences and solving problems.

Museum Missions and Controversies

As museums have broadened their image, offerings, and audiences, they have become more visible in the public eye. Consequently, they are more susceptible to public, stakeholder, and community pressures. And the growing tendency of museums to situate their missions locally, provide community services, seek community support, and become part of community life is laudable from a variety of perspectives. But there is a potential negative effect. Museums in the past were largely self-contained and not dependent on the community or on large and diverse audiences. Their boards and patrons shielded them from outside pressures. However, as museums move closer to their communities, they risk becoming lightning rods. As community symbols, museums—especially those that have become tourist destinations and generate substantial revenues for the community—can be sources of local pride and honor or else risk becoming the focus of controversy and ill-will.

Museum controversies can be traced back to a variety of conditions and factors. They have arisen for decades, although they seem to be more frequent and more highly publicized nowadays. Many museum controversies involve a conflict between community (or stakeholder) standards and professional standards. That was the case for a 1996 exhibition at the Phoenix Art Museum titled *Old Glory: The American Flag in Contemporary Art,* which alienated veterans groups, politicians, and other people. Intended by the curators as a survey of the flag's image in U.S. history and in modern social movements, the exhibition featured certain works that showed the flag in ways that some visitors perceived as irreverent and insulting. A 1990 exhibition of Robert Mapplethorpe photographs at the Contemporary Art Centre, in Cincinnati, Ohio, led to community conflicts extreme enough to call out the police; the exhibition ultimately went on as scheduled. A planned exhibition at the Smithsonian Institution's National Museum of American History, re-creating a California sweatshop, was attacked in 1997 by U.S. clothing industry groups, charging that it would be unfair to the apparel trade and biased toward workers and against owners and managers. The greater an institution's visibility, the greater the chances that exhibitions that involve contested perspectives will arouse controversy or attract notoriety.

That was the case with the plans at the National Air and Space Museum to create an exhibition in 1995 to coincide with observance of the fiftieth anniversary of the end of World War II in the Pacific and the dropping of the first atomic bomb over Hiroshima, Japan. The initial script sought to tell the story of the bomb and its aftermath in terms of the public anxiety and superpower conflict that marked the atomic age. Part of the script dealt with estimates of the number of U.S. soldiers who might have been killed had Japan been invaded on land instead—long cited as a justification for dropping the bomb. One early exhibit script contested the claim that an invasion would have involved a great loss of American lives. This generated significant opposition from veterans groups, military associations, industrial firms working in the defense industry, and members of Congress—illustrating the influence of stakeholder groups, particularly in history museums. The controversy led the Smithsonian's secretary to abandon the initial plan and transform the exhibition into a chronicle of the *Enola Gay,* the airplane from which the bomb was dropped, its crew, and the Smithsonian's efforts to restore the plane.

In some places, museum controversies have had a chilling effect on professional staffs and their willingness to develop exhibitions. Ordinarily, controversies must be dealt with and settled on a case-by-case basis, confronting the particular conflicts and groups involved. Yet from the standpoint of public relations and marketing, museums that enjoy high visibility, deal with potentially controversial objects and topics, and have strong stakeholder groups can take steps to avert or minimize controversies. One step is to set up a thorough review process. Another is to make the lines of authority absolutely clear. A third step is to train museum staff to anticipate and deal with controversies. Yet another is to undertake research far in advance of an exhibition's design to gauge public and stakeholder attitudes.

CHALLENGE TWO: BUILDING AN AUDIENCE

Arnold L. Lehman is director of the Brooklyn Museum and previously director of the Miami Art Museum and of the Baltimore Museum of Art. Before taking on the directorship at each of these institutions, Lehman walked around the museum and asked the question, "What makes a museum friendly to people who don't know it?" (Martin, 1997, p. B1). The question Lehman poses may seem simple at first glance, yet it holds a key to museum success. Museum leaders and staff in past years, and sometimes today, have failed to ask that question.

The Museums & Galleries Commission, the British government's principal advisory body on museums, reports that "studies have shown that, if persuaded across the threshold of a museum, most people find something to interest them and make a visit worthwhile. The challenge is not only to provide a good experience for those who do visit, but to improve marketing techniques in order to attract those who do not" (1992, p. 33). Harold Williams, the recently retired president of the Getty Trust, concurs: "We have got to get people into the museum. And that is going to require marketing in all kinds of ways" (Feldstein, 1991, p. 122).

Diverse Audiences, Multiple Constituencies

Museums serve diverse audiences, multiple constituencies, and visitors who have disparate interests, intentions, and expectations. Museums are expected to give special attention to young people, although older adults often form the core of their support. In addition to their visitors, museums have boards of directors, patrons, donors, and members, all of whom have a greater than average stake in what museums are doing and how well they are doing it. Museums that receive public-sector funding have to maintain good relations with governmental constituencies. Many museums also depend on corporate and business support to fund exhibitions and other programs—yet another constituency. Yet if a museum fails to reach and attract sufficient audiences, it is not likely to survive.

Attracting, building, and retaining an audience are leading objectives of museums. In their simplest form, these objectives boil down to three tasks: first, winning over people, many of whom have never been to a museum, by making the museum visible, familiar, and inviting; second, persuading people to visit again and again and designing and delivering engaging offerings and satisfying experiences that will dispose them to become regular visitors or even members; and third, competing successfully with other providers of leisure-time activities, which occupy the bulk of most people's free time. These three tasks can be expanded into several specific challenges:

- Finding ways to reach and attract nonvisitors (in most communities the great majority of residents)
- Diversifying the audience and reaching newcomers and emerging ethnic communities (see Chapter Eight's Model Museum Practice)
- Encouraging occasional visitors to visit more regularly and persuading regular visitors to increase their involvement as members, volunteers, or patrons (see Chapter Eleven)
- Creating programs and services that result in an enjoyable and rewarding museum-going experience (see Chapter Seven)
- Becoming a tourist destination and building partnerships with the travel and hospitality industries and with local and regional governments (see the Conclusion)

We discuss audience building, particularly competing with other providers of leisure activities, in Chapter Four. Here we focus on some of the main issues in dealing with visitors and audiences.

Attracting Audiences in the Face of Competition

Building museum audiences, as suggested earlier, involves having to face competition from four different types of alternative leisure activities. The first competitor to museum-going is stay-at-home behaviors, such as watching television, listening to music, reading, using the computer, playing electronic games, gardening, and entertaining friends. The second form of competition is activities such as going to shopping malls, dining in restaurants, going to the movies, taking nature hikes, attending professional sports events, and visiting theme parks. The third competitor is participation in cultural and educational activities other than going to museums, such as taking adult education courses, attending the theater or concerts, going to libraries, and visiting commercial art galleries and art fairs. The fourth type of competition museums face is other museums. And all of these options are proliferating as never before.

Making museums more familiar and inviting is a primary task. The National Endowment for the Arts examined audience size at art museums in the early 1990s and reported that 73 percent of the American people fail to visit an art gallery or museum in any given year (Anderson, 1994, p. 37). The Atlanta History Center commissioned a mail survey of citizens in the Atlanta metropolitan area to find out how they spent their leisure time during the year. The sample was weighted toward people who expressed an interest in cultural activities, although the questionnaire covered the full range of their leisure-time interests. Nearly 40 percent indicated that they had very little time for leisure activities of any kind. Respondents were asked what they do, sometimes or often, in their spare time. Ninety-one percent of the respondents indicated that they sometimes or often watched television or listened to music at home; 65 percent gardened; 83 percent entertained at home. Outside the home, 93 percent went shopping; 73 percent went the movies; 70 percent attended sports events; 73 percent went to parks or on hikes outdoors; 42 percent went to the theater or concerts; and only 31 percent, sometimes or often, went to art museums and 38 percent to history museums. One conclusion of the study is that "getting people off the couch and outside the home offers the greatest challenge" (*Positioning for the Future*, 1994, p. III-4).

Another way to view the competition for audiences is to compare the rates of participation of audiences in museums with the rates in a variety of other leisure activity settings. A 1995 Smithsonian report titled *Who Attends Our Cultural Organizations* estimated participation in various museums in 1994: a total of 28 million adults (eighteen years of age and older) made at least one visit to a natural history museum (15 percent of the adult population); 41 million (22 percent) made at least one visit to a science and technology center; 44 million (24 percent) went to an art museum; 69 million (37 percent) went to a history museum or historic site; and 85 million (46 percent) made at least one visit to a zoo or an aquarium (Doering, 1995, pp. 1–9).

The Census Bureau of the U.S. Department of Commerce in Washington, D.C., has collected statistics on attendance and participation rates for various leisure activities. The last complete series is for 1992, and the survey was commissioned by the U.S. National Endowment for the Arts for its report *Arts Participation in America, 1982–1992*. The report estimates the percentage of adults attending or participating at least once in the activity during the twelve months prior to the survey. Here are some of the results: 3 percent of the adult population attended an opera performance, 27 percent went to a museum, 35 percent visited a "historic park," 59 percent went to a movie, 37 percent attended a sports event, and 50 percent went to an amusement park.

Competitive pressures on museums also reflect the findings that more and more people enjoy less and less leisure time. One study found that people are working harder for a given paycheck; more people are working; more people are working longer hours; the proportion of single-parent households has grown significantly; two spouses in more families are employed; and greater population dispersal means more time is spent commuting (Schor, 1991). Another study found that leisure time declined by 37 percent between 1973 and 1987—from 26.2 hours per week to 16.6 hours (Kotler and Scheff, 1997, p. 9).

Given diminishing leisure time and the overwork and stress in contemporary life, an argument can be made that the museums, cultural organizations, and other providers of leisure activities that can best organize and structure the limited free time people have will be the ones that succeed in overtaking the competition. This means that museums have to lower the psychic, physical, and time costs involved in visiting them. Museums have to raise their visibility through image building and promotion and should devote resources to building brand identities—images, messages, and cues that lead people to place their trust in the organization and to form a long-lasting relationship with the organization and its products. Brand images dispose consumers to make choices among a few selected organizations and products, thereby reducing their decision time.

Retaining Audiences

Charles Parkhurst, director of the Baltimore Museum of Art in the late 1960s, expressed concern that museums were becoming social and community centers. "In this brave new museum world, the center replaces the museum, and the new institution becomes a constellation of events instead of being a constellation of objects" (1969, p. 11). Parkhurst may have overlooked the complementarity between drawing visitors and members into museums on the basis of events, on the one hand, and supporting a museum's collections and overall operations, on the other. He also failed to take into account the social and interpersonal benefits of museum-going that many visitors value. Museums working to retain audiences understand this complementarity and these benefits.

Marketing professionals have long distinguished between the *tangible* and *intangible* benefits of goods and services, a differentiation that can be useful in the museum context. The tangible benefits of being a museum member, for example, would include acknowledgment in the annual report, invitations to special events, discounts on adult education classes and gift shop purchases, and other gifts. Intangible benefits might include meeting new people at museum events or through volunteer work, hosting the museum visit of an out-of-town friend, forming a sense of community, and taking satisfaction in supporting a worthy cause. Similarly, museum members enrolled in continuing education classes are not just receiving an education but are engaging in social and potentially companionable activities.

Museums are well advised to look at their missions and their offerings in the broadest possible ways while holding firm to their core mission and offerings. Individuals seek to fill their free time with a variety of activities and experiences. Likewise, visitors to museums generally enjoy multilayered experiences. To keep visitors and members satisfied, museums can change their offerings periodically, present a variety of activities, and aim to provide the widest possible range of experiences. This variety of offerings will augment rather than detract from the core mission of the museum.

Johan Huizinga, the early-twentieth-century Dutch intellectual historian, wrote a classic treatise on the central role of play and playfulness in human life. Tracing the "play element" in history and culture, Huizinga (1949) concluded that play was a universal need and embraced learning and leisure, education and entertainment. Museums must recognize that the difference between education and entertainment is less important that the difference between attentiveness or engagement and inattentiveness or disengagement.

The Corcoran Gallery of Art in Washington, D.C., exemplifies the strategy of augmenting and diversifying offerings as a way to build and retain audiences. Janet Solinger, director of the Smithsonian Institution's Resident Associate Program in the 1980s, built it into one of the most successful membership programs in the nation before directing her skills in the late 1990s to the Corcoran in the position of director of public programs. At both institutions, Solinger set out a wide assortment of benefits, attractions, and experiences that people could enjoy. These included in-house concerts, theatrical performances, poetry readings, lectures by famous personalities, continuing education, study tours, book signings, food-tasting events, and social receptions. Solinger also created novel events using the unique opportunities the nation's capital offers—for example, open houses and tours at embassies that ambassadors are encouraged to sponsor. At the Corcoran, Solinger built membership and patronage by orchestrating distinctive and sought-after social events. Solinger succeeded by defining the needs, interests, and satisfactions (often interpersonal, social, and bonding needs) sought by museum members and then offering them one-of-a-kind, high-satisfaction experiences.

Building Quality Visitor Experiences

Beverly Serrell is a student of the museum-going experience. She has watched visitors at hundreds of exhibitions in dozens of museums as they look at objects, stroll around exhibits, and navigate gallery spaces. She has calculated that three-quarters of the visitors she has observed spent less than twenty minutes at a given exhibition (1993, p. 49). Serrell concluded that many shows are underutilized because they fail to engage the visitors' attention and interest.

At the same time, studies indicate that typical museum visitors spend significant time browsing in museum gift shops, dining in the restaurants, and making use of rest room facilities. This suggests that museums should also provide a high quality of services. Museum managers recognize that museum visits have built-in difficulties. Visitors have to stand for extended periods of time and tend to walk about a lot. They complain about having too much rather than too little sensory experience in museums, bordering on sensory overload. Visitors with children must attend to the children's needs. Museums in the past were known for their chilly treatment of visitors. They offered little or no orientation, assigned few employees to welcome and assist visitors, and made no effort to gain a meaningful place in the minds of visitors. This situation has changed in a growing number of museums. Museums today research public perceptions and attitudes, the characteristics of visitors and nonvisitors, and visitor comments on their experiences. The results help museum managers redesign their programs and redeploy their resources to achieve a higher level of satisfaction among visitors. Managers must come to appreciate the fact that the quality of the museum-going experience will in large part determine whether visitors will visit again or will recommend the museum to other potential visitors.

Three particular challenges in attracting and satisfying audiences are being tackled by museum managers: visitor demand, visit length, and cost.

Visitor Demand. The economic concept of demand is of major interest to museums. Museums are typically open year round, yet many go begging for visitors at various times and for extended periods. Conversely, art museums that organize blockbuster shows face the challenge of accommodating great demand at specific times and in a limited time frame. Under these circumstances, influencing visitor demand for museum programs and services becomes a strategic consideration.

In most cases, museums do not know what the size of their audience will be at any given time, day, or season, other than by extrapolating patterns and trends from past audience behavior. The exceptions are the special exhibits or social events for which tickets purchased in advance are required; group tours and visits by school groups booked ahead of time; and the summer, vacation, and tourist seasons, during which time museums in urban centers in particular can anticipate larger-than-normal audiences.

Forecasting total demand over the course of a year is one issue; another is trying to even out lumpiness in demand across the seasons and among different audience segments. Museums can control heavy demand by ticket sales and timed entry, by allowing visitors to stand in long lines, thereby discouraging others, or by closing the doors for varying periods to allow the crowds inside to lessen. Museums that charge an admission fee can influence demand by giving discounts for particular groups and by canceling fees on slow days. Creating events and programs during weekday evening hours has proved to be an effective means of attracting visitor segments such as young professionals who might not otherwise have time or inclination to visit.

Extending the Length of Museum Visits. The length of a museum visit is related to the scope and quality of a museum's offerings, the depth of a visitor's experience, and behavioral characteristics such as an individual's propensity to dine in restaurants, browse in gift shops, and relax in pleasant surroundings. Extending the time a visitor spends is a way to enrich and deepen the visitor experience and at the same time add to the museum's revenues. Studies show that typical visitors spend about ten minutes in a museum gallery and a total of about an hour in all galleries combined. They spend about an equivalent amount of time in gift shops and restaurants when such amenities are available. How do museums get visitors to spend more time?

Some museums are redesigning the spaces in their halls and galleries to slow a visitor's passage and capture more attention. The Reptile Discovery Center at the National Zoological Park, in Washington, D.C., has reconfigured its galleries so that visitors must move in zigzags rather than in straight paths. Texts and labels are more prominent when visitors have to move toward them and then around them. A combination of unusual animal exhibits and environments, texts, photographs, posters, demonstrations, and behind-the-scenes activities such as animal feeding and care encourage the visitor to spend more time than was typical before the redesign.

An increasing number of larger museums are setting up a variety of small gift shops and commercial kiosks instead of having a single large gift shop. Dispersed around a museum, these kiosks encourage visitors to take breaks from the galleries and spend time and dollars in the shops. The National Air and Space Museum has experimented successfully with a range of smaller shops, sometimes connected to special exhibits, that feature special merchandise built around particular themes.

Orientation films at the start of a museum visit provoke interest and increase awareness. Research has shown that visitors who obtain orientation and wayfinding information tend to spend a longer time in a museum than visitors who do not (Lankford, Bitgood, and Cota, 1995).

Reducing the Costs of Museum-Going. In marketing analysis, a consumer is viewed as likely to purchase or adopt a thing when convinced the benefits will outweigh the costs. An individual who decides to visit a museum likewise faces various costs and sacrifices. Museum visits take time—not merely the time spent in the galleries but also the time required to travel to the museum, find a parking space, purchase tickets, stand in line to view a special exhibition, and gain entrance to the museum restaurant. A museum visit can involve financial costs for parking, food, and gift shop purchases. Another cost can be thought of as stress—the fear of feeling uncomfortable in strange surroundings or not knowing what to make of what one is seeing. The fact that many people never step inside a museum and that only a minority of residents in most communities actively visit museums suggest that many people perceive a museum visit as involving relatively more costs than benefits.

Museums are taking a variety of actions to reduce their perceived costs: providing parking lots and lighting on walkways, offering better orientation and information services, making more staff available to welcome visitors and answer their questions, and furnishing better transportation options for reaching museums and better directions once inside them. The Museum of Science &

Industry in Chicago is building underground parking to allow visitors to move comfortably and securely between their cars and the museum in all seasons. The National Museum of American History is undertaking a major redesign of its entrances to furnish greater orientation and information and provide adequate and comfortable seating and rest areas.

CHALLENGE THREE: ATTRACTING FINANCIAL RESOURCES

A third challenge is finding the resources to pay for the varied and costly activities of running museums. At the close of the twentieth century, museums are confronting several major challenges with financial consequences:

- Responding to a rising level of demand for museum services and programs, which consequently require bigger staffs and sometimes larger facilities

- Reaching broader audiences, underserved groups, and minority ethnic and cultural communities, an objective that can be costly and time consuming

- Expanding their educational roles, in particular by investing in costly electronic information, computer, hardware, software, interactive, and digital technologies to supplement museum offerings and to reinforce learning

- Playing a larger role in the community

In 1984, the Commission on Museums for a New Century reported that "the economic conditions at the beginning of this decade have forced a fundamental shift in the outlook of museums toward their future financial stability. Times *are* hard, and money for museums *is* scarce" (p. 110). These findings have been confirmed by subsequent events.

The U.S. economic recessions in the 1980s had a considerable impact on museums. Museum managers found their government funding reduced at all levels (federal, state, and local) as a result of shifts to social spending and pressures to curb deficits. They also found it harder to raise support from corporations as the latter were subjected to a greater variety and extent of demands for support from a greater number of nonprofits and charities. Museums with substantial endowments found themselves reaching deeper into that income to cover costs of operating and of building new and larger facilities. Art museums were facing the special burden of rising prices for works of art; at the same time, potential donors were encountering reduced tax advantages for making donations and gifts. Some museums had to close down galleries and entire wings, cut staff, reduce hours, or shut down periodically. Art and history museums, particularly in economically hard hit urban centers, encountered serious difficulties. Cutbacks in museum funding also occurred in Great Britain and Continental Europe.

Creative America, a report prepared by the President's Committee on the Arts and Humanities (1997), echoed the findings in the 1980s: "For the past decade there have been disturbing signs of a weakening philanthropic spirit. . . . [P]rivate contributions to the arts and the humanities, when adjusted for inflation, remained at essentially the same level. . . . Recent reductions in the budgets of the two National Endowments and the Institute of Museum and Library Services are already having adverse effects on the nation's cultural infrastructure" (pp. 18, 28). The report also pointed out that among cultural organizations, museums are most dependent on government funding and least generative of earned-income revenues. The report urges the federal government to maintain the existing public-private partnership pattern of cultural support and calls for the creation of a second federally sponsored revenue source in addition to the existing federally sponsored National Endowments for the Arts and the Humanities.

Some museum leaders view museum finances as cyclical, directly related to broader business and economic cycles. Others have reached the conclusion that the financial woes besetting museums have become structural and endemic. "Unfortunately, there are no easy solutions," Thomas W. Leavitt, a former museum director, wrote in 1991, "[museums] are, with few exceptions, chronically undercapitalized, underbuilt, and understaffed. There is simply no easy way out" (pp. 58–59).

Varieties in Museum Financing

Museums finance themselves in a variety of ways, varying in their financial pictures just as they vary in all other characteristics. In France, the major national museums are financed largely by the central government in Paris. Long regarded as symbols of national greatness, museums such as the Louvre are generously and carefully maintained in their physical plants, operations, collections, and programs. Elsewhere in Europe, museums are typically funded by a combination of national and local government support along with private gifts and earnings. An example is the Deutsches Museum, in Munich, one of the world's leading science and technology museums. In the Netherlands, a number of government-funded national museums were privatized in the late 1980s and early 1990s, although the Dutch government, as trustee of the collections, will continue its support.

Allocation of government funding to British museums is determined by a museum's status as a national, regional, or local museum. The majority of British museums are funded and supervised by local government councils. National museums, primarily located in London, are supported by parliamentary appropriations. The British Museum, for example, received 81 percent of its funding in 1993–94 from government grants, another 9 percent from indirect support provided by local and national government sources, and 10 percent from private gifts and donations and earned income. In recent years, however, the share of government revenues going to British museums has declined, and these museums increasingly have turned to patrons and private-sector sources, including corporations, for the support of programs. A major addition to cultural funding in Great Britain was the establishment of a national lottery. Lottery funds support capital investments and infrastructure and conservation needs of cultural and educational institutions, including museums. Lottery support in the 1990s grew into one of the most significant sources of nongovernment funding for these organizations (Museums & Galleries Commission, 1992).

The museum-funding picture in the United States is typically multilayered, combining private- and public-sector support, and includes appropriations, grants, and tax receipts; individual, foundation, and corporate gifts and grants; and earned income (admission and exhibition charges, gift shop and catalogue earnings, restaurant and food service revenues, membership and event dues, product licensing fees, publication sales, facility rental fees, and revenues deriving from loans and traveling exhibitions).

Increasingly typical of large science museums and science and technology centers is the financial profile of the Pacific Science Center in Seattle, Washington: 89 percent of its operating budget derives from earned income (including 14 percent of earned revenues from membership, 8 percent from traveling exhibitions and loans, and 30 percent from admission and other charges). Conner Prairie, a major living history museum and historical site in Fishers, Indiana, identified its 1993 revenue sources as gifts and memberships, 9 percent; gift shop and restaurant income, 23 percent; endowment, 35 percent; and earned income, specifically admission and special event fees and rental fees, 33 percent. Conner Prairie is a leading example of the new entrepreneurial and business directions taken by museums. The Art Institute of Chicago, for the year ending June 30, 1995, had an annual budget of $66.5 million, and reported the following revenue sources: 13 percent from endowment; 13 percent from state and local grants and appropriations; 17 percent from private giving, including memberships and gifts; 13 percent from earned income; and 44 percent from tuition and fees from the School of the Art Institute, one of the major art schools in the United States.

Public-sector museum support in the United States is variegated. St. Louis, Missouri, and the counties surrounding it allocate a fixed portion of personal property and real estate taxes to local cultural institutions, including museums and the St. Louis Zoo, using the financing means of a *cultural tax district* (Costello, 1985). The Detroit Historical Society (overseeing the Detroit Historical Museum) operates as an agency of the municipal government (staff are employees of the city government, and operating costs are covered by city appropriations), and at the same time, the society has a private nonprofit arm responsible for private support. The museum's director is responsible to two boards of directors, a municipally appointed board and a private board of patrons and community leaders. A majority of U.S. state governments set aside annual appropriations dedicated to support of the arts and cultural life, including museums. Funds are channeled to organizations through state arts councils and in some cases to local arts councils.

Four Financing Challenges

Museum finances have been affected by four trends and conditions: a decline in public funds, flat or falling levels of private giving, a rise in operating costs, and pressures to cut or eliminate tax privileges and other subsidies enjoyed by museums. Let us examine each of these developments in more detail.

Cutbacks in Public Funds. Although new museums start up virtually every day, a number of existing museums have been forced to close down, substantially scale down staff and operations, or curb their missions, all as the result of financial pressures. For example, in the early part of 1993, the 188-year-old New York Historical Society, unable to meet payments on a nearly $6 million annual budget, closed its galleries to the public, announced it was close to bankruptcy, and made plans to downsize, redesign its mission, and sell and transfer parts of its three-million-piece collection. The museum subsequently reopened with a scaled-down operation and a transformed mission.

The Detroit Institute of Arts (DIA) in the early 1990s experienced significant city funding reductions. When Detroit's economy declined, budgets were cut across a range of programs, and $7 million was cut from DIA's $26 million budget. The museum, with internationally renowned collections, had to release 140 employees, reduce its weekly hours from 48½ to 25, and close half its halls and galleries. DIA's financial woes have continued, but not as a result of poor management or of public disapproval of its mission. A variety of circumstances have led to the funding cuts, but the common thread was the pervasive pressure on governments at all levels in the United States to reduce aggregate spending, shift resources to urban and social services, and find ways to balance their budgets. In short, the cuts reflect a shift in public priorities.

Increasing Competition for Private Support. As public-sector funding for museums has declined, museums are under pressure to expand their private-sector funding. As they endeavor to increase their corporate, foundation, and individual support, they are encountering increasing competition from other cultural and educational institutions and from social service agencies, all of which are reaching for a relatively fixed amount of support.

U.S. business corporations, despite several years of high earnings, have only recently been increasing their charitable contributions. Corporate giving (measured in constant dollars) declined from 1986 to 1991. It began to increase after that, to $8.5 billion in 1996, a rise of 4.8 percent (in constant dollars) over the 1995 level (Gray, 1997, pp. 40–41). The problem for museums, which are basically local institutions, is that the business sector is increasingly conglomerated and internationalized. Fewer local business elites—traditionally, supporters of local cultural institutions—remain. In their place are franchises or branch offices that are more likely to offer support, if at all, for marketing reasons than for reasons of affinity and loyalty. Indeed, much corporate support has shifted from philanthropic giving to arrangements that promote corporate images and products. Corporations are demanding a far higher price for their support of museums: large audiences, reliable audience data, discretion in communicating corporate products.

Individual charitable giving, which provides 80 percent of all charitable contributions in the United States, amounted to $119.9 billion in 1996, a 4.12 percent rise (in constant dollars) over the 1995 level. In recent years, Americans have not increased the share of income that goes to charity by much. Furthermore, half of all charitable giving is received by religious organizations. Contributions to the arts (in constant dollars) have remained relatively flat during the 1990s. In the twenty-year period from 1976 to 1996, charitable giving to arts organizations in the United States increased from $7.02 billion to $10.92 billion, a far lower rate of increase than that experienced by religious and educational organizations (Gray, 1997). In both corporate and individual giving, private support flowing to cultural organizations and museums has not kept pace with increases in costs for expanded programs, facilities, and staff.

Museums are becoming more aggressive in building earned-income programs as major means of support. An increasing number are charging admission fees, building membership programs, and expanding museum commerce such as renting out facilities and developing larger and better shops and restaurants. However, as museums move toward earned income, they face greater dependence on the marketplace and the need to meet consumer desires, find and cultivate the right target groups, and invest more in promotion and marketing. To the extent they become perceived as businesses, they also risk jeopardizing their nonprofit status and tax subsidies and face business competition. The single most significant revenue-enhancing area for art museums, and the one closest to their missions, is the organizing of blockbuster exhibitions, which have a track record of attracting audiences and significant revenues. Large-scale, high-visibility exhibitions, however, are increasingly costly to organize, are subject to growing competition among museums worldwide, and if done too frequently, have shown diminishing returns.

Museum leaders are increasingly sensitive to the balancing act between costs and benefits that revenue raising entails. Alan Fern (interviewed Oct. 8, 1996), director of the National Portrait Gallery, points out, for example, that increased visitation levels generally mean greater costs, especially for museums that are publicly supported and free of charge. If it costs a museum $18 to service each visitor (in fixed and variable maintenance, overhead, and staffing costs), it is difficult ordinarily to recover these costs through gift shop and restaurant receipts (unless a museum can regularly organize a series of high-visibility exhibitions). Therefore, museums are examining the direct and hidden costs involved in generating earned income so that they can identify programs that are more rather than less cost effective.

Increasing Operating Costs. Museums have become far more costly to operate than in the past. The last several decades brought an extraordinary expansion of museum facilities, staff, and programs, not only in the United States but also in Germany, Great Britain, and in Japan. Expansion, in turn, results in larger operating budgets. As collections increase, museums require more staff to care for and manage them and need more storage space and maintenance facilities to house and conserve them. As facilities expand, museums require more security guards and other personnel.

Neil Rudenstine has examined thirty- and forty-year trends in art museum spending, sampling several U.S. museums. Between 1950 and 1987, the number of art museums increased from about 100 to 550. During the period from 1950 to 1979, more than 100 existing museums added a total of over ten million square feet of new space to their facilities. The pace of new museum building, including additional facilities, continued in the 1980s and 1990s. During the period from 1980 to 1987, museum staff increased about 25 percent. At the same time, the number of exhibitions grew by about 37 percent and thus the outlays on increased staff, space, and materials. The result was that museums assumed greater and greater fixed operating costs (Feldstein, 1991, pp. 73–86).

Museum operating costs have been rising as a proportion of total museum costs. The Commission on Museums for a New Century (1984) reported that operating costs consumed one-half of most museum budgets in 1970; by 1980, however, the proportion of operating costs to total museum budgets rose to two-thirds. In the 1980s, according to Rudenstine (Feldstein, 1991, p. 78), the operating budgets of a sample of art museums grew by 136 percent (13 percent a year), while operating budgets for a similar sample of private universities rose 103 percent, and for symphony orchestras, 83 percent. As operating costs have escalated, all other museum activities have had to take a reduced budget share (Commission on Museums for a New Century, 1984).

Some museums are having difficulty meeting operating cost deficits as a result of expansion. In the early 1990s, the Oregon Museum of Science and Industry (OMSI), in Portland, built a new $40 million, 210,000-square-foot museum, including a state-of-the-art Omnimax theater. The combination of major cost overruns, increases in operating costs, and flooding on the Willamette River on which the new museum is situated, resulted in more than a $20 million operating deficit, which the museum is attempting to cope with through increased private- and public-sector support.

There are some factors offsetting rising operating costs. First, museums depend heavily on volunteers for managing significant parts of their programs. The American Association of Museums reported in 1994 that nearly 377,000 volunteers were offering their services, 2.5 times the total paid museum staff, full time and part time (American Association of Museums, 1994, p. 81). A second factor is that nearly two-fifths of total U.S. paid museum staff work part time. This pervasive part-time employment pattern reflects in part the existence of seasonal museums, such as outdoor historic sites, nature centers, and parks, and also the employment of college and graduate students on work-study programs and internships. The third factor is that compensation for museum occupations, overall, lags behind compensation scales in other sectors of the nonprofit world such as hospitals and universities and far behind compensation available in the private sector. In addition, the large proportion of part-time employees indicates that many museum employees are going without full compensation and benefit packages. One can conclude that the growth in museum operating costs is less the result of salary hikes and more the result of expanded operations, materials, and staff size.

One last consideration emerges from an analysis of museum operating costs: many museums are lacking in endowments, reserves, and other forms of capital that can not only insulate them from economic downturns and crises but also enable them to expand and improve their programming, marketing, and promotion. A study of museum endowments in the late 1980s indicated that only one-half of U.S. museums have endowments, and these endowments are distributed unevenly: three-quarters of large museums and only 45 percent of small ones have endowments; 93 percent of the $14 billion in total value of U.S. museum endowments is held by large museums; art museums possess 76 percent of the total. Furthermore, the median endowment for all U.S. museums was estimated at $125,000, hardly an ample reserve to draw on (American Association of Museums, 1994, p. 87).

Reduction or Loss of Tax Privileges and Other Subsidies. U.S. museums, along with religious, charitable, and educational organizations, are typically established as nonprofit organizations and thus obligated to fulfill certain educational and public purposes that without nonprofit organizations would presumably go unmet. In return, nonprofits enjoy privileges under the federal tax code: they are normally exempt from property tax levies, are often exempt (given certain conditions) from sales taxes on certain items in museum gift shops, and enjoy lower postal rates for mailings. They can also receive charitable contributions, which carry tax deductions and other incentives for donors.

Not surprisingly, the financial privileges that museums and other nonprofit organizations enjoy have been subject to criticism by certain groups of citizens and by business people who are in competition with museums' commercial operations. Museums face a challenge to their tax-exempt status when they earn income from items and activities that might be considered *unrelated businesses.* Firms such as the Museum Company, which operates stores in dozens of shopping malls across the United States and sells reproductions of museum objects and collections, have challenged the tax privileges museums enjoy. A business lobby, the Coalition for Fair Business Practices, has also challenged nonprofits' privileges. The argument is that because a museum is able to sell its collection-related products without paying taxes on the earnings, it derives a larger profit than the for-profit business selling similar goods and paying taxes. In recent years, as large museums have established satellite stores in shopping malls and expanded shop and catalogue sales, for-profit companies have expanded their legal and tax challenges.

U.S. tax courts are considering these challenges, and congressional committees have held hearings on the tax privileges enjoyed by nonprofit organizations. Museums continually negotiate with taxing agencies. Increasingly, shops in large, urban museums have been taxing themselves on portions of their inventories not closely related to museum collections. This can satisfy the tax agency, avert time-consuming negotiations, head off further protests, and stall unfavorable changes in the tax code (Goedert, 1996). In short, museums face the dilemma that as they increase their sources of earned income to make up for the loss of public-sector support and stagnating private and corporate contributions, they risk jeopardizing their nonprofit status. Furthermore, as museums become more commercial in their orientation, the public's perception is liable to shift toward regarding museums as commercial enterprises and therefore less deserving of subsidies and tax advantages. In Colorado, a citizen initiative in the early 1990s placed on the ballot an amendment to eliminate virtually all local property tax exemptions currently enjoyed by churches and other nonprofit organizations in the state. State officials estimated the amendment would place nearly $3 billion worth of land and buildings on state tax rolls, yielding nearly $70 million in new property tax revenues. Though the amendment failed, public sentiment can easily increase toward reducing or eliminating the privileges enjoyed by nonprofit organizations, especially in revenue-poor communities and in recessionary periods.

Leaner government budgets in the face of increasing demands for public funds have led to a heightened sense of accountability toward nonprofits and recipients of public-sector funding. Museums, too, are increasingly called on to account for their funding, the outcomes of their programs, the benefits they offer individuals and communities, and the ratio between their costs and benefits. An example is the U.S. Internal Revenue Service Form 990. Nonprofit organizations are required to file this form and report their sources of income, assets, expenses, compensation paid to top officers, and information related to program activities. The form consisted of only a few pages in the past; today, it has twelve pages. Citizens today can readily obtain copies whereas restrictions on its use existed in previous years. Misstatements are subject to federal criminal law penalties.

Museum Financing Opportunities

Alongside their serious and sometimes critical funding challenges, museums can take varying advantage of trends and conditions to generate funding opportunities. Some of these are more available to large urban museums than small rural or exurbanite ones, yet at some level these opportunities can be mined by all museums. Here we will briefly highlight the opportunities in financing support.

Tourist Development. Tourism is one of the world's largest and fastest-expanding industries. And increasing numbers of tourists are seeking cultural and heritage tourism and not simply recreational travel. As G. Donald Adams, a pioneer in museum public relations and marketing, has observed, museums "are uniquely positioned to derive greater benefit in the future from the growing number of cultural tourists. . . . [T]he tourism industry will continue to recognize more fully how very important America's museums and other cultural attractions are to the success of their businesses. Acceptance by the tourism industry and growth in the cultural tourism market will combine to position museums . . . as major generators of tourist dollars" (1995, p. 37).

Corporate Marketing Sponsorships and Partnerships. A growing number of firms and business corporations are engaging in partnerships with museums and other nonprofits. Such partnerships, to be sure, have to be carefully researched, selected, and monitored. Business goals are not always consonant with museum goals. Yet these corporate partnerships and sponsorships can yield visibility, promotion, income, and support.

Asset Development. Art museums have long recognized that popular, large-scale, high-visibility exhibitions, such as the 1996 Vermeer exhibition at the National Gallery of Art and the 1996 Cézanne exhibition at the Philadelphia Museum of Art, are considerable revenue-producing assets that attract large audiences and generate corporate, municipal, and hospitality and tourist industry support. Yet they are also learning that building solid collections can also attract audiences and outside support. Museum collections are distinctive assets that draw audiences, particularly when museum buildings, collections, and exhibitions together offer exceptional experiences. Museums that possess objects regarded as treasures or icons have the advantage of premium assets. Museum collections also are assets as electronic information and entertainment products (videos, CD-ROMs, and so forth). Asset building among museums, through collections, traveling exhibitions, and loans, is likely to increase as museums and other cultural organizations continue to build collaborations and partnerships across communities and among different types of organizations.

Marketing Museums. In 1986, G. Donald Adams wrote about museums in a way that not too many years earlier would have been regarded in the museum world as taboo: "What if somebody told you that you were in show business? Your reaction might be somewhere between revulsion and a quizzical look. . . . But the fact is museums are competing for people's leisure time and money. And in that regard they compete in an arena that runs the gamut from VCRs and home entertainment centers to the best that Broadway, Hollywood and Madison Avenue can deliver" (Adams and Boatright, 1986, p. 16). Adams put his finger on a significant facet of the museum world earlier than many of his colleagues. Traditional museums typically invested little or nothing in promotion, advertising, public relations, or marketing. They made few efforts to raise demand for the products and services they offered. Compared to the marketing of commercial entertainment, information, and "edutainment" firms, museums operated in the little league.

This is changing. Museum leaders are finding that investments in image building and brand naming, media advertising and public relations, and marketing and communication can be highly productive in building audiences and revenues and cost effective in generating the ends they seek to accomplish.

Voluntary Contributions. Most museums, even the largest, make appeals for volunteers and voluntary contributions. Small and medium-sized museums, however, vitally depend on volunteers and contributed goods and services. Voluntary support for museums exists in most communities, although it requires cultivation. The work of volunteers in museums, donations of equipment by local companies, in-kind contributions of professional and technical support services and skills, all represent vital contributions to museums that lack adequate financial resources. Small museums are launching a growing number of initiatives that tap community, business, and volunteer support and that raise the resources the museums require.

Consolidations and Mergers. There is a body of opinion in the museum community that museums may have reached a plateau in their funding and that smaller museums in particular will have to consolidate and merge or else lose their viability. There is concern that growth in the numbers of museums may have outstripped the market and the support for their offerings.

Museum consolidations and mergers thus far have been relatively scarce, but there are signs that they will increase. Mergers have combined children's museums and science centers, art museums and historical museums. For example, two major museums in Cincinnati, the Natural History & Science Museum and the Cincinnati Historical Society, merged in the mid-1990s and now occupy a grand site in a renovated historical railroad station. The merger over a several year period of two art museums in Southern California—the Laguna Art Museum and the Newport Harbor Art Museum—finally took place in 1996. Consolidation can also take the form of sharing collections, distributing loans and exhibitions, and organizing other forms of collaboration. Sharing collections is far more widespread than in the past. Marketing and promotional alliances among museums in a local community are also more widespread. Local museums also are joining together in purchasing cooperatives to bring down operating costs. These alliances, partnerships, and collaborations help museums increase their visibility, assemble greater resources, and attract larger audiences.

SUMMARY

Every organization has to cope with changes in its environment and should be watchful for both threats and opportunities. Museums are facing many challenges related to changing conditions. One challenge arises from a financial environment characterized by burgeoning operating costs and lagging income. Another challenge derives from increasing competition for audiences, competition among a growing number of providers of leisure-time activities, all going after a share of individuals' diminishing free time. Yet another challenge arises when museum missions come up against market forces. The audience challenge is particularly critical. Museums compete for audiences against stay-at-home behaviors (watching television, using the computer, reading a book), other leisure activities (shopping, movies, sporting events, hiking), other cultural activities (theater, concerts), and other museums. Museums have to build audiences by attracting new visitors, especially from underserved groups; by retaining existing audiences and encouraging them to become more active; and by providing exhibitions and other offerings of outstanding quality and appeal.

PART TWO

STRATEGIC PLANNING
FOR MUSEUMS

CHAPTER THREE

Museums Turn to Strategic Planning

Market-oriented strategic planning is the managerial process
of developing and maintaining a viable fit between the organization's
objectives, skills, and resources and its changing market opportunities.
—Philip Kotler

This chapter takes museums through the initial stages of thinking about their marketing approaches. The *strategic market planning process* (SMPP) allows museums to shape, plan, and implement their missions, offerings, and the markets to be served. If consumer orientation is the way to think about marketing, SMPP is the way to do marketing. A word about marketing is appropriate before proceeding to strategic planning.

Marketing is at its core an exchange process between those who seek a product or service and those who can supply that product or service. It is formally defined as "a social and managerial process by which individuals and groups obtain what they need and want through creating, offering, and exchanging products of value with others" (Kotler, 1994, p. 6). Marketing begins with the view that each person has an assortment of needs and wants to fulfill (self-esteem, food and shelter, education, sociability, entertainment, a certain standard of living, creative achievement, and so on) and that these are satisfied through a variety of products and services. Marketing takes place when five conditions are met: (1) at least two parties are involved; (2) each party has something of value to offer the other party; (3) each party is capable of delivering on its half of the exchange and of enjoying some benefit or satisfaction from the exchange; (4) each party is free to accept or reject an offering; and (5) each party believes it is appropriate and desirable to deal with the other party.

Marketing professionals work to identify and satisfy consumers' needs by matching these with individuals or organizations that can meet those needs. A corollary of this is that the supplying organization (regardless of whether it is a business producing consumer goods, a law firm offering legal services, or a museum offering exhibitions and programs) should be oriented toward the consumer (or customer or client or user or visitor). From this, two distinctive characteristics of marketing practice follow: first, a reliance on systematic research to learn about one's consumers, the organization's ability to meet their needs, the larger environment in which both the consumers and the organization interact, and the competitors who seek to meet the same consumer needs; and second, experimentation, innovation, trial and error—a search to develop products and services that will succeed in the exchange process, within the framework of an organization's objectives.

Resistance to marketing often reflects misinformed notions about it. Marketing offers every type of organization a set of principles, methods, and tools for advancing the organization's purpose with its consumers or users. Marketing professionals are not expected to impose their goals on organizations; rather, they are expected to probe an organization's objectives and apply their expertise to realizing those objectives. Thus marketing is primarily an instrument to achieve certain *ends,* but it must work in tandem with the professional skills and resources at its disposal and must take account of professional viewpoints and values. Marketing is a discipline with decades of experience behind it; though not a precise science, it is built on extensive experience, sound behavioral principles, and rigorous methodologies. In the hands of competent marketing professionals, it gives effective results of high quality.

We see the SMPP process as embracing three elements, discussed in the following sections: a strategic market planning system, an organizational design that matches the chosen strategy, and systems design for market information, planning, evaluation, and control.

STRATEGIC MARKET PLANNING SYSTEM

Developing a strategic market planning system, the first element of the strategic market planning process, requires four steps: (1) analyzing the environments in which any marketing plan must operate; (2) analyzing internal resources; (3) formulating a mission, objectives, and goals; and (4) formulating strategy (see Figure 3.1).

Environmental Analysis

All organizations are affected by several environments. Museums need to scan their individual environmental conditions, opportunities, and the threats presented and adapt their missions, objectives, and goals accordingly.

Museums operate in five environments:

- *Internal environment*—the organizational life of a museum and its internal publics, such as the museum board, director, staff, advisory board, and volunteers

Figure 3.1. Strategic Market Planning Process.

- *Market environment*—groups and organizations (visitors, members, community residents, stakeholders, activists, media, and so on) with whom the museum works to accomplish its mission

- *Regulatory environment*—groups and organizations (government, regulatory, and accrediting agencies) with an interest in how the museum conforms to laws, rules, and regulations

- *Competitive environment*—groups and organizations that compete with the museum for the attention and loyalty of customers and donors

- *Macroenvironment*—forces and conditions (demographic, economic, technological, political, and social) that shape opportunities and threats but that are largely outside of the museum's control

We examine each of these environments to identify current trends and factors for museums to consider as they analyze their own environmental conditions.

Internal Environment. The museum's internal environment consists of the groups or offices that have primary responsibility for programs and operations and for carrying out museum goals and strategy. The core internal publics are the museum's board of trustees, director, paid staff, and volunteers. At the same time, certain external publics can exercise a strong internal influence. For example, art museums are highly dependent on patrons, collectors, artists, and art dealers in building and maintaining their collections. In many cases, individuals from one or more of these groups sit on boards of directors or else serve as major stakeholders in friends-of-the-museum associations.

Museum boards. Museums operated as nonprofit organizations have boards of trustees as their highest governing body, and the role of these boards has changed. Museum boards are expected to set policy and oversee management. Yet boards function in a variety of ways, depending on the particular characteristics of a given museum, its history, the type of community it serves, its scale, and other factors. Museum board members have traditionally been recruited for their power, prestige, or wealth in the community. Board members at art museums, particularly, have been recruited for their potential giving and their support of the institution's collections. Stories are legion about art museum board members who offered much-needed financial support at critical times.

Museum boards vary in their involvement in a museum. Certain board members and boards are notable for their deference to museum directors. Others are known for a penchant for micromanagement. Relations between boards, directors, and top-level managers are especially critical when boards get involved in management. Because of the respect and influence their board members command, in times of crisis or controversy boards can help deflect pressures from a museum's management and defuse controversies and missteps before they become overwhelming.

However, as Harold Skramstad observes, "the day when most museums could live under the umbrella of their own endowment and their own agenda and their own goals . . . the age of the board getting around the table and divvying up the deficit, are gone" (Garfield, 1995, p. 34). Museums are becoming more institutionalized and formal, more oriented to public audiences, and are giving more emphasis to business skills than in the past. In recent years, board composition has shifted or broadened to include professionals and specialists whose skills can bring substantial advantage to a museum's management.

Board members are being recruited for their management, marketing, public relations, communications, and fundraising skills. They can be called upon to provide in-kind services in specialized areas of need, in addition to their general services on the board (for an excellent discussion of museum boards, see Ullberg, 1981).

Museum directors. As museum boards have been shifting their emphasis from internal to external factors, so, too, are museum directors expected to focus more of their time on audiences, donors, sponsors, balancing the budget, and cultivating an organization's image that will attract more visitors and supporters. "My task on arrival was quite clear," Malcolm Rogers said as he assumed the directorship of Boston's Museum of Fine Arts (MFA) late in 1995. "I had to eliminate the budget deficit, raise public awareness of the museum, and raise the esteem in which the museum is held. I also had to look to the morale of the staff." Rogers's early initiatives to eliminate MFA's budget deficit required museum reorganization and downsizing of staff (Runyard, 1995, p. 21).

Increasingly, directors of large museums are engaged in restructuring their organizations, developing viable, long-range financial strategies, and shifting internal museum cultures, typically inward looking in the past, to outward looking and publicly responsive. When Glenn D. Lowry assumed the directorship of New York's Museum of Modern Art (MOMA) in 1995, for example, he had already shown considerable acumen and leadership in dealing with financial and marketing issues. As director of Toronto's Art Gallery of Ontario, Lowry faced a situation in which provincial and local support for the gallery had been cut in half, construction on a new wing halted, staff reduced by half, and the gallery doors closed for seven months until new funding could be found. Lowry found a funding solution by persuading the Barnes Foundation to include the museum in its highly acclaimed international tour of its collection of modern French paintings (see Exhibit 9.1). Lowry and the board had to raise nearly $4 million to finance the exhibition and persuade local and regional governments that the exhibit cost was a sound investment in generating heightened cultural, tourist, and economic activity. The Barnes traveling exhibit at the Ontario Art Gallery succeeded in reaching the museum's goals, generating sales of more than half a million tickets, earning nearly $3 million in revenues, and raising the museum's image and base of support in the community. During his Toronto tenure, Lowry had raised $58 million for the museum. Upon his arrival in New York, the MOMA board had high expectations that he would accomplish similar things for MOMA. The new director immediately faced the challenges of building a major endowment campaign, cutting museum costs, and at the same time finding ways to keep most of the staff intact, raise salaries, and improve internal morale (D'Arcy, 1995).

Willard Boyd (1995), former president of the Field Museum, has pointed to the increased turnover of museum directors as a sign of the growing complexity of museum leadership and management. He lists four areas of particular importance for museums to consider in hiring a new museum director: (1) the director's intellectual vision, the capacity to develop the mission and push it in significant new and more public directions; (2) the director's ability to build strong programming that will appeal to existing audiences and arouse support among new constituencies; (3) the director's experience and expertise in relation to the museum's distinctive offerings and the targeted markets it has to attract; and (4) the director's ability to enlarge the museum's financial base by engaging in more community relationships, forming more partnerships with corporations and other supporters, and building a broader and larger membership base.

Traditionally, museum directors have been drawn from the ranks of museum curators and researchers and from the academic world. In recent years, however, a growing number are moving to large and medium-sized museums from management roles in corporations and other large private and public organizations. Directors of most museums are now expected to have skills in image building, raising funds, and building audiences and community support.

Museum staff. Museum staff are the paid employees: directors, curators, educators, collection managers, exhibit specialists, marketers, development specialists, secretaries, service workers, and so on. Management builds effective staff members by defining job positions and responsibilities, by recruiting qualified people, and by effectively training, motivating, compensating, and evaluating people after hiring. Employee training is a critical task with significant marketing implications. Those employees who come into direct contact with visitors have to be trained in a *customer service* orientation. Curators, educators, and external relations staff who are cold or indifferent to visitors are likely to create negative feelings and word of mouth, and this can lead to declining attendance.

Motivating staff members takes careful planning. Staff expect several things from the museum: adequate salaries, fair treatment, respect and recognition, and the feeling of being a valued member of a worthwhile museum. Management has to offer incentives and create benefits if it expects staff to deliver, in turn, high morale, solid work, and ongoing support. It is noteworthy that many museum staff are motivated more by professional service motivations and values than by material rewards. Advancing knowledge, pursuing research, safeguarding a mission that is part of a public trust, earning professional recognition and acclaim, educating the public, and doing good work for society are the values and expectations that characterize many who work at museums.

Yet income and material incentives occupy staff to varying degrees. Museums typically have limited income, and their employees receive fewer material incentives and lower wages than private-sector employees with similar backgrounds and skills. Academic pay scales come close to museum pay scales, although at larger universities the highest-paid professors earn considerably more ble working rules, so that during the peak summer season, service staff can give greater emphasis to traditional roles of guarding exhibitions and handling crowds, but in off-peak seasons, their roles can expand to include assisting children, providing information to visitors, interpreting collections, and promoting the museum's services and products (Watson, 1995).

Staff at the Exploratorium, in San Francisco, one of the earliest and most innovative of U.S. science and technology centers, unionized in 1993, following forty months of demoralization, conflict, and negotiation. Under its founder Frank Oppenheimer, the museum functioned as an unusually informal organization, offering staff considerable mobility and role change, access to management, and ease of communication. Staff could sit in on board meetings and, except for the founding director's position, met with little hierarchy in the ranks. By the 1990s, the organization had become more formal. A series of directors and top-level managers had come and gone, the financial situation was trying, and staff dissatisfaction had grown. The precipitating event took place in November 1990, when the leadership, responding to increasing deficits, laid off ten employees and reduced the working time of nine others. The layoffs and the process by which they were arrived at further lowered staff morale. Fifty staff organized an effort to avert the layoffs by calling for across-the-board salary reductions. Working with a sophisticated and supportive union team, the pro-union staff waged a year-and-a-half campaign to unionize, first meeting with management opposition, later being offered an option to establish a staff association, and finally winning board approval for a union. Two years after unionization, the union did provide a framework for expressing grievances, coordinating actions, and improving communication between staff and management (Gurian, 1995).

Museum volunteers. Most museums use volunteers in a variety of areas—as docents who conduct tours, as staffers of information kiosks and orientation services, and as helpers in gift shops. The Field Museum places volunteers as assistants in curatorial, conservation, and research departments.

Some museums employ large numbers of volunteers that sometimes equal or exceed the numbers of full-time paid staff. Science and technology centers tend to use greater numbers of volunteers than art museums. Hands-on tools and machines, interactive exhibitions, discovery rooms and other educational facilities, demonstrations, and laboratories all boost the need for staff and volunteers to communicate and work with visitors. The Oregon Museum of Science and Industry, in Portland, with annual average visitorship of one million, in 1995 employed 158 full-time paid staff, 71 part-time paid staff, and 500 part-time volunteers. The Newark Museum, a leading art and science museum, had 190 part-time volunteers in 1995, compared with 90 full-time and 150 part-time paid staff.

than high-ranked curators and even museum directors. Some
compensation is consistent with nonprofit organizations and
and represents a form of subsidy that museums cannot afford t
lack of material rewards, however, can make the employees'
tion even stronger. After all, if a museum cannot compensate
fashion commensurate with expectations, it certainly can expec
fessionals at least, demands for other satisfactions, including ir
tonomy, and responsibility. For this reason, museums have to
demands for incentives, opportunities, and recognitions that
demic training, achievement, and professional status.

Alongside complaints and low morale in the top and middle
ums are dissatisfactions among service workers, primarily guards, c
tenance workers, and food service workers. Museums for years
as attendants and guards older individuals, often retirees. The ti
job placed limited demands on these employees; they were exp
over the collections and exhibitions and were discouraged from t
offering information to visitors, on the theory that this would de
security role.

However, new types of job recruits and new organizationa
defining even these lower-level jobs. Part of the reason for the
from the fact that new job recruits increasingly are women with
are younger than the traditional guard; some have considerable s
cational backgrounds. Because these new job candidates have h
tions than their predecessors, museums are finding that undema
work is considered boring and leads to low morale and commitn
ing worker attitudes and identifying opportunities for new roles
new ways to make museum work more productive and satisfying
seums are in the forefront of this redefinition. The Doncaster Mus
Gallery, London's Transport Museum, and the Colchester Museur
figuring staff roles and elevating training and professionalism. Th
Museums changed the titles of attendants and security guards to
sistants. Instead of just guarding exhibitions, they play roles in
school groups; providing introductions and orientations to visitors;
itors find their way through the museum; offering information abc
activities and programs and also galleries that visitors might overlo
moting museum services such as the restaurants and gift shops
1995; Falconer, 1995; Seaman, 1995).

Redefining jobs, however, also requires balancing a variety of ir
needs, benefits and costs. Britain's Great Yarmouth Museums, fc
found that in redefining and elevating the roles of service personne
had to adjust upwards compensation and other benefits and to neg
complicated work arrangements. They negotiated with the unions a

Volunteering clearly plays a significant role in museums and is an important part of the internal environment for museums to examine and manage. Many museums could not afford to offer the range of services they do if these services had to be provided by salaried staff. Volunteers typically arise out of the ranks of museum membership and other supporter groups. They can be counted on to offer financial support as well as intense personal involvement.

Market Environment. A museum must deal with a number of external publics who greatly affect its goals and strategies. Some of these publics constitute the museum's market environment: they are the museum's members and visitors, community residents, stakeholders and activists, and the media. (Competitors and regulatory agencies are also part of the market environment and are discussed later in the chapter.) One of a museum's important tasks is to distinguish among the various publics being served and their varying needs and relative priority.

Museum visitors and members. Museums visitors and members represent the museum's primary external public. Museums have to relate to a range of visitors—individuals and families who regularly participate, active members, visitors who visit infrequently, groups on school visits, tourists on organized tours—and serve them all effectively. Yet the interests of one group can conflict with the interest of other groups. Regular visitors have an interest in seeing new museum exhibits and new types of programming. Tourists want to see a blockbuster or the permanent collection and the facilities in a one-time experience. And museum members expect a rich menu of high-quality, diverse programming such as lectures, special tours, continuing education, and social events.

Thus museums face *opportunity costs* insofar as resources invested in one particular activity or audience segment are unavailable for other uses. Museums trying to attract low-income, less-educated groups for the sake of diversity face trade-offs in that resources have to be diverted from satisfying regular visitors who tend to be well-educated and middle- to high-income people. Assessment of such opportunity costs requires thinking about which activities and groups will best enable a particular museum to achieve distinction, gain resources, and be of service to the community.

Community residents. Museums are physically located in geographical areas and come into more than casual contact with neighborhood residents and community organizations. These groups are likely to take an active interest in what a museum does. Residents in close proximity to a museum are likely to have concerns about traffic congestion and parking. A museum should designate one or more staff members to maintain liaison with the community. Responsive organizations do not wait until local issues erupt. They make investments in their community and proactively build goodwill.

Any area's demographic patterns are likely to change over time. Many urban museums, for example, the Philadelphia Museum of Art and the Cleveland Museum of Art, at one time catered to population segments and social classes that no longer reside near these museums. U.S. cities, in particular, have witnessed significant population shifts in the last several decades: a movement out of central cities by European Americans of middle and high income and a movement in of African Americans and Latinos, who tend overall to have lower incomes and differing cultural interests. Large, urban U.S. museums are challenged to respond to the interests and needs of the new groups. The social pressures on these museums to serve all parts of the community are reinforced by the fact that central-city museums are often recipients of local government grants and subsidies and therefore are obligated to serve all groups. (Chapter Four offers an extended discussion of tourists and other audience segments.)

Stakeholders and activists. Museums in recent years have become increasingly aware that they have *stakeholders*—groups with an active interest in museum policies and programs. Art museums, historically, have paid attention to art collectors and patrons, who at times functioned as shadow cabinets alongside management. These stakeholders also have been highly effective in recruiting from their social circles other collectors, donors, and patrons. It is not surprising, therefore, that they have long constituted a principal support and stakeholder group for art museums.

History museums in recent years have also become aware of stakeholder groups that pay critical attention to their collections, exhibits, and other programs. A vivid example is the *Enola Gay* exhibition that the National Air and Space Museum, in Washington, D.C., modified substantially after criticism from veteran and military groups. The actions of these groups also contributed to the removal of the museum director.

Museums would be foolish to ignore stakeholder and activist groups that perceive themselves to be special constituencies. Responsive museums can do two things. First, they can include representatives of stakeholder groups in their decision making or, at a minimum, give voice to these groups in other ways. Representatives of stakeholder groups can be invited to sit on a museum's board of trustees or serve as advisory group members. Second, museums can assign staff responsibility for contact with these groups, to ensure that stakeholder views are communicated to management and management views to stakeholder groups.

Media. The media—television and radio stations, newspapers, magazines, journals—are part of the market environment, conveying news, features, and editorial opinion. Marketing managers should be acutely sensitive to the role the media play in shaping public perceptions. Museums, in particular, rely on the media to publicize their shows, programs, and special events. Media reviews of museum exhibits carry weight similar to film, theater, and performing arts reviews. They can kindle or dampen audience interest. Museums, particularly in urban areas, increasingly are building ongoing, long-range relationships with their local media. As a museum becomes more market- and customer-focused, it seeks to shape an image of its institution that is visible, attractive, and consistent in the public eye, and local media are the principal conduits for communicating this image. Local media can also be museum sponsors and marketing partners.

Regulatory Environment. Regulatory organizations such as federal, state, and local government agencies, professional accreditation associations, and to some degree, educational organizations are external publics that impose rules of conduct on museum organizations. Museums have a keen interest in satisfying these rules in order to attract and maintain a resource base and attract visitors.

U.S. museums have to satisfy the laws that govern charitable organizations and the rules imposed by the Internal Revenue Service (IRS). For example, U.S. museums frequently negotiate with the IRS over rules limiting the types and extent of commercial enterprises museums can operate. Museums that receive grants, subsidies, and other forms of support from government agencies are subject to oversight, if not regulation, in regard to their uses of public funds and their compliance with rules and laws protecting individual rights, such as equal employment and equal opportunity rules. U.S. museums may benefit from accreditation by the American Association of Museums; donors and collectors might be reluctant to contribute to museums that lack accreditation.

Competitive Environment. Competitors, yet another external public, are becoming a significant environmental factor in the recreational, cultural, and educational marketplace of the 1990s. Yet many nonprofit cultural organizations refuse to give competitors the attention they deserve. Competition is too often perceived as an attribute solely of the private sector. Nonprofit organizations would typically rather view nonprofit organizations serving similar needs as sister organizations, and museums have usually not thought of other museums as competitors even though they seek patrons, members, visitors, and volunteers largely from the same pool of potential supporters. Nor have museums recognized other leisure organizations or other leisure activities, such as couch-potato viewing of television sets and videos or active involvement with computers and cyberspace, as competing with museum visits. However, museums do in fact compete with these behaviors as well as with going to theme parks, theaters, sports arenas, and restaurants; taking a drive in the countryside or a hike in a nature reserve; and doing exercise or gardening. And museums face competition from libraries, lecture halls, continuing education centers, colleges and universities, and even the digital information environment. In short, the competitive environment, for nonprofits and businesses alike, has to be viewed broadly, continuously, and strategically.

There is nothing like the specter of competition to give museum directors a jolt. To compete, they have to rethink how their products and services are perceived by the public relative to the products and services offered by similar organizations. They have to view their consumers more carefully to see if there are better ways to meet consumer needs and wants—for example, by additional offsite and electronic and digital programming. They have to consider the need to communicate and promote their offerings more effectively, adjust their pricing, refurbish physical facilities, and expand services. One way in which museums can meet the competition is to use the principles and tools of positioning, developed by marketers. (Positioning is discussed further in Chapter Five.)

Museums should be aware of four major types of competitive pressure and competitors:

- *Desire competitors*—the range of general desires and preferences that potential consumers might have (for example, traveling, reading, watching television)

- *Generic competitors*—the range of ways potential consumers can satisfy a particular need or desire (for example, learning something by attending a lecture instead of visiting a museum)

- *Form competitors*—the range of alternative services that would satisfy the particular type of leisure activity selected (for example, viewing a museum's art collection on the Internet instead of viewing it at the museum)

- *Enterprise competitors*—the range of other types of organizations that can satisfy the needs of potential consumers (for example, visiting a major downtown art museum rather than visiting a smaller neighborhood art museum or going to a theme park or a shopping center for recreation)

The most intense competition in the business world usually is at the enterprise level. However, the most intense competition for museums is likely to be at the desire and generic levels. Each museum has to understand who its competitors are, how people perceive their needs for particular types of services, and what the museum's specific organizational strengths and weaknesses are.

The competitive environment can be illustrated by examining the competitive pressures faced by a large, urban museum. Consider a young professional woman in New York City deciding what to do on a particular evening (see Table 3.1). The young woman realizes she has several desires that can be satisfied—finishing a project at work, engaging in physical fitness exercise, attending to household responsibilities, going after entertainment, or seeking an aesthetic experience. If she determines that she desires an aesthetic experience, she has to consider several generic competitors, including watching television, seeing a movie, going

Table 3.1. Decision Making and the Four Types of Competition.

Desire Competition	Generic Competition	Form Competition	Enterprise Competition
What desire do I want to satisfy?	How do I want to have an aesthetic experience?	What form of art experience do I want to have?	Which museum do I want to go to?
Work	TV at home	Theater	Big downtown
Exercise	Art on video	Symphony	museum
Household chores	Viewing art on	Rock concert	Smaller
Entertainment	the Web	Dance	neighborhood
Learning	Movie	performance	museum
Aesthetic	Experience art in	Museum	University art
experience	a public place	Outdoor art fair	gallery
			Private gallery

Source: Strategic Marketing for Nonprofit Organizations (5th ed.) by Kotler and Andreasen, © 1996. Adapted by permission of Prentice-Hall, Inc., Upper Saddle River, NJ.

to a theatrical or dance performance, or visiting a museum. If she chooses to visit a museum, she has to decide on which one to visit and what exhibits to see. The probability that she will choose a particular museum clearly falls as her perceived options multiply.

Macroenvironment. The macroenvironment consists of forces and conditions that shape opportunities and pose threats to an organization. Examples include demographic shifts, economic and business cycles, cultural value and attitude shifts, political realignments, and government and regulatory program and policy changes. Organizations have to monitor these forces for their effects on both short-range and long-term planning. For example, during an economic recession, corporate contributions are likely to be reduced, thereby requiring a nonprofit organization to seek revenue from alternative sources—or else retrench. Similarly, organizations ought to be sensitive to demographic shifts, targeting youthful cohort groups, for example, so that they are not left serving largely aging audiences.

Threat analysis. Strategic planning involves analyzing potential threats to an organization and major opportunities for the organization. An *environmental threat* is a challenge posed by an unfavorable trend, factor, or condition that can lead, in the absence of deliberate managerial and marketing action, to the stagnation, decline, or demise of an organization or its products and services. Not all threats warrant the same attention or concern. Managers have to assess each threat according to its potential severity (measured by the extent of resources the museum would lose if the threat materialized) and its probability of occurrence.

Suppose a museum director identified the following four threats:

1. The museum anticipates a 10 percent decline next year in visitorship.

2. The museum's cost of operation is likely to rise 15 percent next year.

3. The museum might lose the support of a major foundation that contributed $200,000 in each of the past three years.

4. The museum might lose tax-exempt status for its highly profitable and expanding gift shop.

When each of these threats is evaluated according to potential severity and probability of occurrence, suppose the results are those shown in Figure 3.2. The most serious threats are those that fall in the upper left cell; management should prepare contingency plans for these. The least serious threats fall in the lower right cell; management can safely ignore these. The other two cells contain threats of medium seriousness; management should monitor these. By identifying and classifying threats, management knows which environmental developments to plan for, monitor, or ignore.

Opportunity analysis. Opportunity analysis is also of great importance to an organization. By managing its threats successfully, an organization can stay intact and avert trouble, but it will not necessarily grow. However, by managing its opportunities successfully, an organization can advance its mission or business. A *marketing opportunity* is defined as an attractive arena of appropriate marketing action in which an organization is likely to enjoy superior competitive advantages. Every level of museum management should make an effort to identify the opportunities facing the museum.

Suppose an art museum director perceives the following opportunities:

1. The museum could launch a studio arts program to capitalize on the growing demand for art instruction and continuing education.

2. The museum could open a small satellite museum in a nearby city that has become a place of considerable population influx, with

Figure 3.2. Threat Matrix.

		Probability of Occurrence	
		High	Low
Potential Severity	High	1, 2	3
	Low	4	

Source: Kotler, 1982, p. 86.

middle- and upper-middle-class households. The parent museum caters to a strong tourist public, but the satellite museum would cater to a largely residential public.

3. The museum could open a gift shop in a major suburban shopping mall, one that caters to upscale consumers and offers a promising market for museum products.

4. The museum could develop jazz music and dining programs to attract young professionals, single people, couples, and individuals seeking after-work relaxation and sociability—population segments that have been flocking increasingly to restaurants and clubs in the museum's neighborhood.

Not all opportunities are equally feasible or attractive. An opportunity needs to be assessed on an opportunity matrix with two dimensions: (1) *potential attractiveness,* measured by the amount of revenue and resources or other results that a museum might value; and (2) *success probability,* measured by the museum's ability to develop and capitalize on the opportunity. Possible results for the art museum are shown in Figure 3.3. Launching a studio arts program appears to be the best opportunity because the museum has determined that the program is likely to produce a good revenue stream and a loyal membership and that the museum has a high probability of running a successful studio arts program. However, opening a gift shop in a suburban shopping mall falls in the lower right cell because the museum has analyzed that it would be costly to operate and is not likely to weather the competition. It should be rejected. Opportunities identified in the other two cells may be worth monitoring, although specific planning at this point may not be warranted.

Internal Resources Analysis (Strengths and Weaknesses)

Marketers must assess a museum's external opportunities and threats in relation to its internal resources. A great marketing opportunity is no opportunity at all unless an organization has the necessary resources and capabilities to

Figure 3.3. Opportunity Matrix.

Source: Kotler, 1982, p. 86.

carry it out. It is likely that any museum will have a mixture of strengths and weaknesses. The museum does not have to correct all of its weaknesses. Rather, it may settle on a strategy to rectify certain weaknesses that relate to specific opportunities. A big question for any museum is whether it should limit itself to those environmental opportunities where it currently possesses the required strengths or should consider more beneficial opportunities and acquire or develop the requisite strengths to take advantage of these stronger opportunities.

Museums have to review their internal resources and capabilities in each operational area. A large museum, for example, may have strengths in management but weaknesses in product development. Or it may have strengths in collections and exhibitions but weaknesses in communications and marketing. A small museum often lacks a significant collection that can form the basis of strong exhibits and other programs. A museum should audit its relative strengths and weaknesses, using a form like the one shown in Exhibit 3.1. (A more advanced instrument, the marketing audit, is discussed and a sample audit instrument shown in Chapter Twelve.) Internal audits are a means to take stock of the resources that exist within an organization. They allow an organization to appraise its strengths and weaknesses in relation to one another as well as in relation to a changing environment. An audit is a basis for assigning priorities. It can lead an organization to address its weaknesses by either eliminating or modifying certain programs and operational practices. It can lead to an effort to refocus on existing strengths. Or an audit can lead to adoption of an entirely new strategy.

Seizing an Opportunity to Convert a Weakness into a Strength. A growing number of museums have had to reduce their budgets in response to funding cutbacks by public authorities or other sources. As a result these museums often have to reduce staff and risk a reduction in programs, educational outreach, and visitor services. Yet there are instances in which museums have successfully transformed fiscal crises into opportunities and weaknesses into strengths.

An example is the Detroit Historical Museum (DHM). This museum has operated as a hybrid organization: it is an agency of municipal government, overseen by the mayor and a municipal commission, and having a staff of civil servants; and it also operates as an agency of a private association, the Detroit Historical Society, overseen by a board of the society. Certain of its activities and operations have been publicly financed; others, privately financed. Between 1991 and 1995, DHM was forced to reorganize, from top to bottom, in the face of substantial cutbacks in state and local government support. Its municipal, public-sector budget decreased from $5.1 million (1991) to $2.8 million (1995). A major part of this decline resulted from a more than $2 million cut in state government support, accompanied by smaller reductions in municipal support. The staff was cut from seventy-two to forty-five.

According to Maud Lyon, DHM's director (interview, Mar. 12, 1996), an inventory of the museum's weaknesses, midway through its fiscal crisis, might have looked like this: "DHM paid considerable attention to its collections and little attention to its visitors and the community as a whole. The city's population had changed considerably in terms of ethnic and racial mix, yet the museum made little effort to reach new groups of residents. Visitorship stagnated. While the museum experienced cutbacks in public-sector support, it lacked skills and experience to go after sources of private support."

Yet DHM, like other museums, was surrounded by untapped opportunities and resources that it had overlooked: "DHM's private side (the historical society board, and so on) was relatively inactive," Lyon observed, "although members were available for larger roles and bigger challenges. A variety of leaders and leadership groups were available but were disconnected from the museum. A lot of latent pride in the city and surrounding metropolis existed. Leaders were searching for ways to build and express local pride and self-identity. Detroit in the year 2001 would commemorate its 300th anniversary, marking the time of the first settlement, and presenting a major opportunity for the museum to play a role in Detroit's anniversary celebrations."

DHM took positive steps to reorganize and reorient its mission and roles. Work on a strategic plan began in 1992. Trustees, staff, and community and business leaders were all involved in the planning process. The remarkable transformative behavior of the museum was evident in its efforts to reach out to the community. This began with joint projects with the African American museum two blocks away. The DHM conceived of a series of special museum events celebrating ethnic heritage. It joined forces with local radio and television stations to foster interest in local and regional history, publicize museum activities, and create media programs built around local loyalty and pride. When a television station called on DHM to design a series of thirty-second spots focusing on Detroit's history, the museum furnished unusual stories about local and regional history—and at the same time raised museum visibility. Municipal and suburban officials began to view DHM as a vital institution linking city and suburbs, facilitating communication among parts of the metropolis, and generating a positive image of the whole. The museum also committed itself to playing a prominent role in the plans and programs for Detroit's 300th anniversary celebration.

Building on a Strength as a Future Opportunity. Some museums have untapped strength in their names and reputations. Museums can have strong collections and yet fail to recognize their potential for building strong and popular exhibitions. Museums can overlook the powerful stories and themes embedded in their collections, which resonate with the memories, associations, and interests of visitors. Museums that possess attractive facilities can overlook the use

Exhibit 3.1. Strengths and Weaknesses Analysis.

	Performance					Importance		
	Major Strength	Minor Strength	Neutral	Minor Weakness	Major Weakness	High	Medium	Low
Programs								
1. Museum reputation								
2. Core product quality (exhibits)								
3. Interpretative quality								
4. Orientation quality								
5. Volunteer services quality								
6. New exhibit development								
Audience Development								
1. Visitorship level								
2. Visitorship diversity								
3. Repeat visitorship								
4. Visitor service quality								
5. Membership program quality								
Marketing								
1. Image effectiveness								
2. Public perceptions of accessibility								
3. Promotion effectiveness								
4. Pricing effectiveness								
5. Product mix								

Finance

1. Cost/availability of capital				
2. Cash flow				
3. Financial stability				
4. Fundraising effectiveness				
5. Government support				
6. Earned income support				
7. Corporate support				
8. Individual giving				

Organization

1. Visionary, capable leadership				
2. Dedication of employees				
3. Entrepreneurial orientation				
4. Innovativeness				
5. Staff responsiveness to public service, educational outreach				
6. Flexibility and responsiveness, overall				

Source: Marketing Management (9th ed.) by Kotler, Philip, © 1997, p. 83. Adapted by permission of Prentice-Hall, Inc., Upper Saddle River, NJ.

OOOOO

of their museum as a venue for business or social events or as a place for the community to gather on special occasions.

The Art Institute of Chicago (AIC), one of the world's great art museums, has a variety of strengths in its reputation, collections, educational programs, gift shops and catalogues, and audience development activities. AIC has on the average 1.3 million visitors a year. Yet, by the mid-1990s, the museum recognized that it had to boost its annual visitorship to maintain a requisite level of revenue and programming. Of its several world-class collections, AIC's Impressionist art collection is one of the strongest. The collection is a source of loans to museums throughout the world. AIC's ability to borrow works from other museums is in turn considerable. AIC, in other words, has strong relations with other museums and easy access to other collections.

The AIC has a history of organizing large-scale exhibitions that have won critical and audience acclaim. A recent example was the Monet exhibition, which drew 960,000 visitors. The Art Institute has organized exhibitions through the 1990s by a number of leading impressionist painters. Yet it has been careful to balance its overall schedule, allowing the surpluses generated by these exhibitions to subsidize, in effect, the museum's ability to present works of less familiar artists and cultures, thereby utilizing its strength in one of the most popular areas of Western art to strengthen its mission of bringing a wide range of the world's visual arts to Chicago. AIC recognizes that an overdependence on the most popular aspects of its collections would be shortsighted, even though they constitute an essential strength for its marketing and development efforts.

Using an Internal Audit to Correct a Weakness. The Memorial Art Gallery of the University of Rochester (MAG) has focused its strategic planning on attracting a greater number of young and middle-aged people to the museum as visitors and members. According to museum public relations manager Deborah Rothman (interviewed Oct. 10, 1996), this priority developed from an audit of the museum's strengths and weaknesses and the intent to overcome a weakness. MAG offers an illustration of the uses of internal audits for goal setting and strategy. The museum is situated in downtown Rochester, at a distance from the university that sponsors and supports it. It is perceived as a city museum, though it receives no financial support from the municipal government. It has a distinguished collection of decorative and fine arts, a $2.5 million annual budget, forty-one full-time staff, and an annual audience of three hundred thousand people.

Through its planning process MAG recognized its membership base was aging and declining. Eighty percent of its members were fifty years of age or older. Membership renewals were down. The museum exists in an older northern city that like other U.S. cities has undergone displacement of its industrial base, shrinkage, and decline. Once headquarters to several major national corporations, only a handful remain. Its major industry has lost employment. A growing number of the museum's core supporters have moved south to warmer climes or spend less time residing in the metropolitan area. MAG has taken steps to counteract these trends in the city. A new museum wing was built and new programs were launched that together, over a ten-year period, led to a doubling in visitorship. In 1989, the museum launched a new program to attract young professionals working in the city. Once a month, MAG opens its halls for First Friday, a social event for young professionals. The event has attracted as many as 1,600 people. At times, the crowd cuing up in front of the museum exceeded the number of people who could be accommodated under the fire code. These social gatherings have generated strong support in the community and brought in eight hundred new members, nearly 10 percent of the membership. Planning for these events is in the hands of a volunteer committee of young professionals. These First Friday gatherings have convinced staff that the once-a-month event has not exhausted the demand for such uses of the museum facilities. The value of such museum events, for a significant segment of the community, appears to exceed the supply. Management is considering additional programs to expand the membership, particularly the target group of younger professional people.

Mission, Objective, and Goal Formulation

Any organization can benefit from a SWOT analysis: an analysis of its *strengths* and *weaknesses* in relation to its *opportunities* and *threats*. This analysis of environment and resources provides a background and stimulus for management thinking regarding the museum's basic mission, objectives, and goals.

Every organization at its beginning is fairly clear about its mission and goals. However, as it develops and accomplishes the initial objectives, and as its environment changes and presents new challenges, its management will have to review and reassess its mission and goals. In some organizations a review will convince management that the current mission and goals are clear, appropriate, and effective. In others, management might find that the goals are clear but of diminishing appropriateness in relation to changes in the environment and organizational capabilities. In still others, management will discover that the goals no longer are clear or appropriate; the result then is an organization adrift. The purpose of developing a clear and appropriate mission and set of objectives and goals is to keep the organization from drifting into an uncertain future.

Mission. We need to draw a distinction between three commonly used terms in strategic planning: *mission, vision,* and *values.*

> *Mission* is the answer to the questions: What is the purpose of our organization? What is distinctive in what we do? What do we aim to accomplish (image or niche in the marketplace, quality of products and services, market share)?

Vision is what the organization wants to be or become (the ideal or the best possible form and substance it aspires to) and reflects the organization's priorities.

Values are the core beliefs and norms of the organization, beliefs of what is right, fair, just, or desirable.

For example, the Museum of Modern Art (MOMA) has the *mission* of collecting, interpreting, and displaying the best embodiments of modern art, with a focus on works spanning the Impressionist era through the end of World War II.

Today, the museum is considering whether to adopt an expanded *vision* that includes the active acquisition of works of contemporary art. A vision can embrace views of how large the museum should be in the next decade, whether it should run satellite facilities, how important educational outreach should be, and the organization's emphases and priorities overall.

As for *values*, MOMA staff are committed to studying, collecting, and showing the finest artworks, displaying them in the finest facility, and making the best possible efforts to involve the public in the museum. The museum regularly de-accessions artworks judged to be of inferior quality to help finance acquisition of new works of high quality.

Museums for much of their history did not have to articulate and communicate their missions. Museum leaders had confidence in the traditional purposes and contributions of their organizations. They perceived their primary obligation as collecting, studying, and conserving collections—tasks that few other organizations performed. They operated under the assumption that appropriate visitors would be drawn to view their collections and that there was little need to appeal to a wider public. Museum missions and mission statements assumed larger significance as changes occurred in the environment. Competition from other organizations and an increase in the number of museums forced individual museums to define more carefully their particular roles, functions, and markets. Competition for financial resources and diminishing support from traditional sponsors has led museums to redefine their accountability. Expanded roles compelled museums to husband their limited resources and assign priorities to the roles they could fill effectively. Museums today need to clarify their mission, as Peter Drucker (1974) pointed out years ago. He called on organizations to answer the following questions to clarify their missions:

What is our business?

Who is the customer?

What is value to the customer?

What should our business be?

What will our business be?

Differing views of a museum's mission. The first question, What is our business (or mission)? might sound simple, yet it is the most profound question an organization can ask. A museum, for example, can define its business as research, or education, or caring for a collection, or providing entertainment, and so on. Experts have quite different views on the mission of a museum. As Mihalyi Csikszentmihalyi (1991, pp. 125–126) has noted, "Visitors do not expect intellectual thrills from attending a museum. They are, rather, hoping for surprise and excitement as they escape temporarily the predictable confines of existence in an environment where the constraints of everyday life appear to be suspended." More tradition-minded museum leaders are likely to focus on the objects and materials museums contain. As Sir David M. Wilson, director of London's British Museum, has written, "Museums are about the material they contain. The first duty of the museum curator is to look after that material. . . . His second duty is to make that material available to whoever wants to see it" (1991, p. 11).

A product-centered definition of a museum's mission is different from a market-centered definition. The product-oriented definition emphasizes what the museum produces that it expects consumers to purchase. The market-oriented mission emphasizes the needs of museum consumers—the benefits, values, and satisfactions they seek—irrespective of particular products. There is clearly a difference between an art museum mission that emphasizes the informational and experiential preferences of audiences and one that focuses on collections, research, and the aesthetic qualities of the museum setting.

Multiple markets, multiple missions. Today's museums have to think about how they want to position themselves in different markets and in several possible markets. Each one represents a need, value, or satisfaction that patrons or various types of visitors seek in exchange for a museum visit:

- What place should a museum occupy in the education market, and more particularly in relation to preschools, schools, colleges, and universities?

- How should a museum position itself in the recreation and relaxation market?

- What role should a museum play as a space for interpersonal and social exchanges, where people meet and socialize, and as a center of community life?

- What role should a museum play as a place for celebrating a community's history, heritage, and accomplishments and for building a sense of community pride?

- What role should a museum play in building skills and in transmitting basic concepts (especially for young people) in science, history, or art?

A market orientation encourages museums to define their missions broadly in relation to publics and consumer groups that will be served, customer needs that will be met, and techniques or technologies that will satisfy customer needs. Marketing professor Theodore Levitt has advanced the notion that market definitions of what a business is are superior to product or functional definitions of what a business does. He argues that businesses (or nonprofits) are more effective when they view themselves as "a customer-satisfying process" rather than "a goods-producing process" (Kotler, 1997, p. 38).

The implication of Levitt's argument is that interest in particular products may change over time but basic needs and satisfactions endure. A history museum, instead of focusing merely on historical artifacts, could also focus on communicating a people's heritage. An art museum, instead of centering on blockbuster exhibitions, could also take a broader view on using artworks to interpret and communicate the creative process and the human skills that it taps. A science and technology museum, instead of homing in on famous pieces of technology, could also illuminate scientific concepts and scientific methods. Although museums of sufficient size and resources can operate in multiple markets, there is a danger that a museum with many roles can lose its focus and its distinctive quality. Museums have to identify their core mission and then rank-order the other roles they are able to perform.

Developing a mission statement. A museum's mission is generally shaped by five factors. First, the museum's *prior history* has an influence. In the extreme case, a museum established by a single benefactor could be legally bound by the terms of the founder's will, agreement, and bequest. An example is the Barnes Foundation, in Merion, Pennsylvania; its mission for many years was limited to the founder's vision. Albert Barnes declared in his will that his extraordinary collection of Impressionist, European, American, and African art would not be loaned out to other museums or allowed to travel. Sixty or so years had passed before the museum's director could modify these terms through a court judgment. Museum tradition is also a powerful influence.

Second, the current *preferences* of the museum's management and staff (and in some cases, of the leading patrons and supporters) will play a role.

Third, the *environment* in which the museum operates—economic, financial, regulatory, and so forth—will influence its mission. Because most U.S. museums are established under federal rules as charitable and educational nonprofit organizations, they are required to fulfill certain educational and public service purposes as part of their core missions.

The museum's *resources* are a fourth important factor, because the level of resources will make certain missions feasible and others impractical.

Finally, the museum's distinctive *competencies* must be weighed in shaping a mission. Virtually all museums are collecting institutions. Their missions therefore have to encompass collections acquisition and deaccessioning, care and conservation, display and interpretation.

A museum's mission often takes form during the process of designing a mission statement. The mission statement is an important tool for strategic planning and for engaging management, staff, members of the public, donors, and other stakeholders in the planning process. However, designing a mission is both complex and time consuming. Different publics, inside and outside the museum, will have different views of what the organization is and should be doing. Meetings will have to be organized to build consensus on the core mission.

An organization should strive after a mission that is feasible, motivating, and distinctive. The goal of *feasibility* directs an organization to aim high, but not so high as to create an unachievable mission or engender loss of confidence or credibility among the public. A *motivating* mission allows those working for the organization to feel they are part of a worthwhile organization that has valuable aims and purposes to fulfill. Supporters are inspired by the organization's aims and feel that its mission enriches their lives. A *distinctive* mission defines the competitive domain in which an organization operates. If all museums in a city closely resembled each other, there would be less loyalty shown to any particular museum. People take pride in identifying with an organization that "does things differently" or "does things better." By cultivating a distinctive mission, an organization stands out and is likely to attract a committed base of support.

Examples of museum mission statements. Museum mission statements vary considerably because they reflect a museum world of great diversity in missions, organizations, and purposes. In general, however, museums strive to communicate the distinctiveness of what they do—their collections, their buildings and facilities, their subject matter, the scope of research and interpretation, their public programming, and the services and experiences they provide. Here are some examples.

The National Museum of American History dedicates its collections and scholarship to inspiring a broader understanding of our nation and its many peoples. We create learning opportunities, stimulate imaginations, and present challenging ideas about our country's past.

The mission of the Virginia Museum of Fine Arts is to collect works of art of all types and from all periods of world history and to interpret these through permanent and temporary exhibitions, publications, lectures, seminars, and a variety of outreach programs. The Museum's highest priorities are to develop the art collections through purchases, gifts and loans, to preserve and conserve these collections, and to have the collections used and appreciated by the Museum's audience, which includes all segments of society from the general public to students and scholars locally, nationally, and internationally.

The mission of the Women of the West Museum, a new institution opening in Boulder, Colorado, at the end of the 1990s, is to become the nation's leading institution devoted to tracing and interpreting the multicultural history and contributions of women in the American West. It will also further scholarly research, serve as an archival center, and increase public understanding of the impact of women on all aspects of the western experience.

The current mission of the Sixth Floor Museum is to preserve and protect the former Texas School Book Depository building, Dealey Plaza, and environs for the benefit of all peoples; to provide educational programs which interpret those sites; and to operate a historical museum with a principle focus on the life, times, death, and legacy of President John F. Kennedy.

Changing the museum's mission. Because the environment in which an organization operates is continually changing, a mission that was appropriate at a particular time in the past may no longer be appropriate in the present day. Although an organization's mission should not be revised lightly or frequently, it is worthwhile to reexamine it periodically.

Some mission revisions are made necessary by organizational changes and growth. Other museums have to redirect their missions because of loss of their visitor or funding base. For example, the Parrish Art Museum, in Southampton, New York, was dedicated to its collection of artworks of ancient Greece and Rome, including excellent copies of marble statues and works of European and American artists. Having developed out of a private collection and a strong-willed collector, the museum continued to reflect the founder's wishes until after his death. By the 1950s, however, visitorship had declined, and the management and staff began to reexamine the museum's mission and the highly eclectic and unfocused range of the collection. With a change in leadership, the museum shifted its focus to American art, particularly the art of the region of Long Island where the museum is situated. The redefining of the Parrish Art Museum, the decision to focus on regional artworks and artists, of which there were an abundance, resulted in an expanded audience and a reinvigorated organization (De Salvo, 1993).

The Henry Ford Museum & Greenfield Village (HFM/GV), one of the leading U.S. historical museums and sites, launched a major redefining process in 1991. This was not the result of financial difficulty or a shortage of visitors and members. HFM/GV, for much of its history since 1929, has been a well-endowed, significant, and popular U.S. history museum. Founded by the American automobile magnate Henry Ford, whose collection was vast, eclectic, and idiosyncratic, the museum is a twelve-acre complex with eighty historic structures in addition to the main building. The museum has enjoyed the advantage of the Ford Motor Company's support. The average annual visitorship in the late 1980s and early 1990s was over one million people, and a large proportion were visitors living at a distance of 250 miles or more. HFM/GV's staff consisted in 1994 of 245 full-time and 790 part-time paid employees, along with 643 part-time volunteers. By any measure, the Henry Ford Museum & Greenfield Village is a major U.S. museum complex.

However, museum management had undertaken considerable research into visitor perceptions and preferences, the museum's external relations, and the images the museum communicated. Beginning in 1991, the museum began a process of strategic planning, a major part of which was reexamination of its mission. According to its director at the time, Harold Skramstad:

> We realized we had to focus. . . . In a sense, we're a museum that is about everything. By being about everything, there is no focus. It is hard to use resources effectively. Our collection could continue to grow in every direction, because what's American history? It is everything. That was a direction we couldn't continue to go. We recast our mission statement and market position— to celebrate the spirit of innovation in America. What our collections kept telling us was that our great strengths were those things that relate to the story of change as driven by resourcefulness, ingenuity, and innovation. Our visitors were telling us that, our influentials were telling us that, the founding vision of Henry Ford was telling us that [Garfield, 1995, p. 33].

The long-standing mission of the Henry Ford Museum was broadly conceived as interpreting the American experience, with some emphasis on the relation between technology and social change. At one point, the museum had advertised itself as "A Great American Museum that is Great Fun." By 1994, HFM/GV had adopted this mission statement: "Henry Ford Museum & Greenfield Village provides unique educational experiences based on authentic objects, stories, and lives from America's traditions of ingenuity, resourcefulness, and innovation. Our purpose is to inspire people to learn from these traditions to help share a better future."

HFM/GV has recreated itself as a highly distinctive museum complex, offering unique and distinctive value to its community and the nation. Its current logo says, "Celebrating the Spirit of Innovation in America." So committed is management and staff to the newly defined mission that the museum's new mission statement is printed on the back of every business card carried by every member of the staff. And the first experience visitors have at the museum is to encounter and participate in a game that demonstrates the spirit of innovation. A large gallery is filled with tubes containing different colored balls, and groups of visitors are invited to work together as teams to figure out the best ways to separate the balls by color. The game, which lasts several minutes, introduces visitors to the process of collaboration and the mind-set that generates ingenuity and innovation.

The new orientation and mission at HFM/GV has proved highly successful. Management has even extended the museum theme of teaching innovation beyond museum walls. A new business unit has developed programs for training people in the skills, processes, and values of inventiveness and innovation. The museum unit provides training for corporate and nonprofit organizations, programs that generate museum revenue. In 1996, HFM/GV also formed a partnership with the Ford Motor Company to create a new secondary school in Dearborn, Michigan, devoted to teaching inventiveness and innovation to students. In focusing its mission, repositioning its programs, and marshaling its resources around a distinctive niche of value, experience, and learning, the Henry Ford Museum & Greenfield Village has built a unique public image and organization that distinguishes it from all other museums, cultural, and educational institutions.

Objectives. The mission of an organization suggests more about where the organization is coming from than where it is going. It describes an organization's broad purposes rather than its particular aims and methods. Organizations also have to develop long-range objectives and goals, as well as a set of objectives and goals for each planning period.

For every type of organization, there is usually a potential set of relevant objectives, and the organization's task is to make choices among these objectives. For example, a museum would likely identify these objectives:

- Increase numbers of visitors
- Build membership
- Expand the collections
- Design exhibits and programs that attract a diverse cross section of the community
- Extend educational outreach
- Make improvements in the facilities
- Improve services to visitors
- Increase the endowment
- Eliminate the operating deficit

However, a museum cannot successfully pursue all these objectives at one time; certain objectives are incompatible with others in the short term, and in any case, budget resources are likely to be limited. In any given year an organization will select certain objectives to emphasize and others to defer action on or ignore. A typical museum, for example, might decide that improvements in its physical plant and the services provided to visitors have to take precedence over changes in exhibitions and programs. This might reflect a strategy of improving accessibility and building new audiences as a precondition for diversifying offerings that will, in turn, reach a wider audience and stimulate repeat visits. Therefore an organization's major objectives are likely to vary from year to year, depending on management's perception of the major problems and the phasing of solutions to those problems.

Museum directors and boards have to keep financial and budgetary considerations in mind at all times when analyzing opportunities and setting objectives. They have to ask the questions: Can we afford to do this? Will the added expenditures result in significant gains? What are the opportunity costs of a given choice?

Here is a set of management, financial, and budgetary objectives that organizations, including museums, might pursue:

Surplus maximization. A museum might want to accumulate as much cash surplus as possible in order to build a new wing or renovate existing facilities. In this case all efforts will focus on increasing revenue and reducing costs.

Revenue maximization. A museum might seek to maximize its total revenue, perhaps under the assumption that a high level of revenue communicates a message to donors that the museum is doing important work. Management might think that a large revenue base will facilitate future donations.

Usage maximization. Many nonprofit organizations are primarily interested in maximizing usage of their facilities and services. Granting institutions and other contributors typically look at a museum's visitor level and membership growth as yardsticks for determining funding support.

Capacity targeting. Organizations with fixed service capacities typically set their price and marketing expenditures to produce an audience that can be handled by the existing capacity. For example, a museum that is offering a major exhibition and is experiencing relatively low visitation might consider lowering its admission fees or offering discounts to particular target groups in order to fill the space. However, if the potential number of visitors exceeds capacity, a museum might consider raising fees, rationing tickets, or offering incentives that encourage visits in slack periods.

Full cost recovery. Many nonprofit organizations are primarily interested in breaking even each year. They would like to provide as much service and programming and as many resources as they can as long as their sales revenue, donations, and grants cover their costs. Many museums want to be in the position of spending just short of the amount at which they would have to report a deficit. They also may want to avoid showing too large a surplus, so that granting agencies will not reduce their support.

Partial cost recovery. Other nonprofit organizations operate with a chronic deficit each year. Their aim is to keep this annual deficit from exceeding a certain set amount. Private foundations, corporations, or individual donors often are solicited, on a "crisis" basis, to cover the annual deficit.

Budget maximization. Many organizations act as if they are attempting to maximize the size of the staff, the number of programs offered, and the number of markets reached. These organizations seek program grants and donations without fully considering their ability to use contributed funds effectively. They are reluctant to trim programs or staff, even in the face of evidence that parts of the organization are nonproductive. Trimming operations would of course raise image problems.

Producer satisfaction maximization. Some argue that many nonprofit organizations and their staffs are basically self-serving and primarily oriented toward maximizing their own interests. Self-serving interests exist in all organizations, although it can be argued that not being under the discipline of profit maximization, nonprofit organizations have more room to indulge such interests. In museums, for example, some curators spend much of their time on research and devote relatively little to public service. Museum directors also might pursue their own interests without factoring in the needs of internal and external stakeholder groups.

Example of setting objectives. The Johnson County Museums (JCM), in Shawnee Mission, Kansas, launched a process of self-assessment, objective setting, and strategic planning in the early 1990s. This history museum complex near Kansas City, Missouri, offers a good example of a museum successfully engaged in setting and achieving objectives.

JCM, an agency of the country government, was founded in 1967. The museum complex has a nonprofit arm to raise private support and also receives relatively large county government support. Museums director Janet Bruce Campbell (interviewed Apr. 22, 1996) observes that for much of its history, JCM had had a devoted, albeit narrow, band of supporters but lacked broad community involvement and support. The collections reflected upper-middle- and upper-class households and their histories. In 1987, annual attendance dropped to five thousand visitors a year. The turnaround came with the hiring of the new director, who launched in 1992 a long-range planning process involving all sectors of the community.

A principal objective emerging from this process was to reorient the museums to the local community, providing residents with museums that symbolized a sense of place and communicated both the common and the diverse heritages of the community. This objective required reaching all segments of the community and instilling a sense of participation in the museums. Implementing the objective of community involvement has led to an increase in members, volunteers, and visitors. The JCM friends organization is on its way toward raising a half a million dollars. (JCM is discussed further in the Model Museum Practice at the end of Chapter Five.)

Goals. An organization's chosen objectives have to be restated in the operational and measurable form known as goals. Without goals, anything a museum does or achieves can be considered acceptable; there is no standard or set of standards for planning, choosing among limited resources and marketing opportunities, and measuring or evaluating outcomes.

Thus a museum's objective of increased visitorship has to be turned into a goal (usually with a deadline) of, say, "a 10 percent increase in visitorship in the next twelve months." A statement of goals permits an organization to think concretely about its needed plans, programs, and management controls. A number of questions may then arise: Is a 10 percent increase in visitorship feasible? If so, what strategy should be used? What resources are required to achieve that increase? What activities will have to be carried out? Who will be responsible and accountable? How will the organization monitor and measure progress toward the 10 percent goal? Each question is a critical issue that has to be settled prior to determining whether or not to adopt a proposed goal.

Strategy Formulation

Strategy formulation is the museum's effort to figure out its broad strategy for achieving its goals. There are two basic stages in strategy formulation: (1) the museum examines its current offerings, products, and services to determine which ones it should build, maintain, reduce, or terminate; on this basis, it develops a *product portfolio strategy;* (2) the museum then examines new products and new markets that it can expand into and proceeds to develop a *product and market expansion strategy.*

Product Portfolio Strategy. Most museums are multiproduct and multiservice organizations. A major museum is likely to have, in addition to its core collection and exhibition operations, a program area focusing on children and an area dealing with adult continuing education. Over time, an art museum may add a studio arts continuing education curriculum for its members. A history museum may add courses on creating genealogies, doing oral history, exploring a neighborhood's history, and so on.

A museum's programs will vary in their importance and contribution to the core mission. Some program areas are large; others, small. Some are expanding; others, declining. Some are of high quality; others, low quality. Different programs have to be viewed in terms of their stage in the product *life cycle.* Some offerings and programs might be obsolete or unnecessary, having outlived their relevance to audiences.

Museums find it easier to add new programs than to reform or remove failing ones. Existing programs come to have stakeholders, built-in advocates. In prosperous periods a museum may have sufficient resources to satisfy everyone. However, in periods of slowdown or decline, management is forced to make hard choices.

An increasing number of museums are making such hard-nosed assessments of the programs in their portfolio. A first step in portfolio analysis is to identify the museum's key programs and businesses. A sound working principle is to invest resources in those programs that are high in attractiveness and for which the organization has the relevant strengths. Two approaches to portfolio analysis are described here.

General Electric approach. General Electric (GE) has formulated an approach to portfolio evaluation that is also applicable to nonprofit organizations. Known as the Strategic Business Planning Grid (Figure 3.4), it makes use of two basic dimensions: *market attractiveness* and *organizational strength.* Market attractiveness is a composite index comprising such factors as *market size, market growth rate, revenue and costs, competitive intensity, cyclicality,* and *seasonality.* Organizational strength is a composite index, also, reflecting the museum's *program quality, efficiency, market knowledge,* and *marketing effectiveness.*

The factors making up each dimension are scaled and weighted so that each existing program receives two numbers, one for market attractiveness and one for organizational strength. Each program is plotted on the grid, which is divided into three zones. The first zone consists of the three cells at the upper left and indicates programs located in attractive markets and for which there exists considerable organizational strength. The implication is that the organization should invest in and build up these programs. The second zone consists of the diagonal line of cells stretching from the lower left to the upper right and indicates programs that are medium in combined attractiveness and organizational strength. The organization usually will spend the resources necessary to maintain these programs rather than expand or contract them. They should, however, be monitored frequently for signs of changes. The third zone consists of

Figure 3.4. Strategic Business Planning Grid.

Source: Adapted from Kotler, 1997, p. 75.

the three cells on the lower right and indicates programs low in combined attractiveness and organizational strength. The organization should give serious thought to reducing these programs or eliminating them altogether.

Museum portfolio approach. Nonprofit organizations might seek to build their own portfolio evaluation schemes. Identifying the criteria for judging programs is the major task. A museum might consider the following three criteria for measuring program attractiveness:

- *Centrality*—the degree to which a particular program is central or vital to the museum's mission

- *Quality*—the measure of the quality, image, or reputation that the particular program enjoys

- *Market viability*—the degree to which the market interest in a particular program is sufficient in size and growth

The first two criteria, centrality and quality, can be combined in a grid, as shown in Figure 3.5. Each program is then evaluated as high, medium, or low for each criterion and entered in the appropriate cell. Market viability, the third criterion, is indicated as high, medium, or low in each cell, next to the program name. A major benefit of this type of analysis is to signal opportunities, problems, and possible solutions for each product area and for all the product areas as a whole.

Figure 3.5. Museum Portfolio Approach.

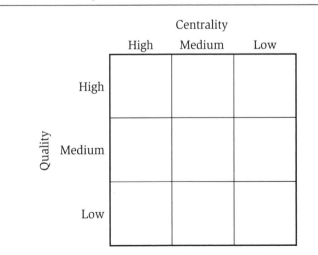

Source: Strategic Marketing for Nonprofit Organizations (5th ed.) by Kotler and Andreasen, © 1996. Adapted by permission of Prentice-Hall, Inc., Upper Saddle River, NJ.

Product and Market Expansion Strategy. Portfolio evaluation is useful for assessing a museum's current programs. But it does not assist the museum manager with two of the most difficult problems that manager will face: (1) how to find promising new offerings, and (2) how to build and convert promising new offerings into stars.

What is needed is a systematic approach to opportunity identification. A useful device is the Product and Market Opportunity Matrix (Figure 3.6). Markets are listed at the left; products, along the top. Management should first consider cell 1, market penetration. This cell asks whether a museum can maintain or expand its visitor base by deepening penetration into its existing markets with its existing programs and offerings. If further market penetration does not look promising, then managers seek solutions as indicated in the other cells.

Cell 2 asks whether the museum can bring its existing offerings to a wider geographical market. An urban museum can open a satellite museum in another part of its city or in a different city. For example, a number of large, urban museums have opened satellite gift shops in urban shopping malls. Cell 3 asks management to consider marketing existing programs to new markets. A large, urban museum, as an example, might make a strong effort to attract first-time visitors among underserved ethnic groups. In cell 4, the museum management considers whether it should modify some programs and offerings to attract more of the existing market. For example, a museum can extend its hours of operation and

Figure 3.6. Product and Market Opportunity Matrix.

	Offerings		
Markets	Existing	Modified	New
Existing	1. Market penetration	4. Modification for existing markets	7. Product innovation
Geographical	2. Geographical expansion	5. Modification for dispersed markets	8. Geographical innovation
New	3. New markets	6. Modification for new markets	9. Total innovation

Source: Strategic Marketing for Nonprofit Organizations (5th ed.) by Kotler and Andreasen, © 1996. Adapted by permission of Prentice-Hall, Inc., Upper Saddle River, NJ.

offer additional programs in new time periods, such as evenings. Cell 5 involves modifying products for geographically dispersed markets. Cell 6 considers modifying products for new markets. To penetrate the senior citizen market, for example, a museum might shorten its standard tour or provide printed brochures that have larger type. Cell 7 directs management to examine product innovation, which can take the form of offering new exhibit tours, new lecture series, and new types of exhibits. Cell 8 relates to geographical innovation, which involves finding new ways to serve new geographical areas. Electronic information technologies using the computer networks of the Internet and the World Wide Web are making it possible for museums to offer their resources to new national and international audiences. Cell 9, the final category, considers total innovation, entirely new products for new markets.

The product and market opportunity matrix gives museum leaders a systematic way to conceive new opportunities. These opportunities are then evaluated, and choices are made. The results of this product and market analysis and of the previous portfolio analysis enable an organization to formulate its strategic plans.

Setting the Marketing Strategy

Once management has completed the first four steps of the strategic marketing planning process—analyzing the environment; analyzing the museum's resources and competencies, its strengths and its weaknesses; determining the mission, objectives, and goals; and formulating the broad strategies—the various functional personnel and managers—curators, conservers, educators, exhibit design staff, marketers, and development staff—can proceed to develop their specific plans. *All these specific plans, including the marketing plan, have to be nested within the larger strategic plan.* Subsequent chapters of this book will discuss elements of marketing strategy, including target markets (Chapter Five), competitive positioning strategies (Chapter Five), and marketing mix strategies (Chapter Seven). (The Model Museum Practice at the end of this chapter provides an extended example of strategic planning at the Museum of Contemporary Art in Chicago.)

ORGANIZATIONAL DESIGN

The purpose of strategy formulation is to develop strategies that will assist the organization to achieve its goals in a changing environment. The existing organization, however, has to be capable of carrying out these strategies. It must have the *structure*, the *people*, the *operating norms and procedures*, and the *organizational culture* that enable successful strategy implementation. An organization might even have to change its structure to permit pursuit of its strategic plan. Thus organizational design is the second key element affecting implementation in the strategic market planning process. For example, if a museum plans to open a satellite museum, it must have staff competence in researching potential new markets, locating real estate, negotiating deals, and developing facilities. Or if a museum seeks to attract a new market, such as an underserved ethnic community, it must ensure that it has the collection and programming resources that are attractive to the new market, staff who are responsive to the new market, and services that make the museum accessible to the new market.

Many organizational theorists insist that *structure should follow strategy.* At the same time, organizational structures are difficult to modify or replace. Vested interests build up over time in any organization. When a new external environment calls for change, management has to develop a plan to market the desired organizational changes to internal staff. If management fails at this, the organization is stuck with its old situation and structure, despite the new environment.

New strategies have to be responsive to an organization's current structure, and yet they may require managers to reconfigure that structure and also the internal organizational culture. Changing an organizational culture is a huge task, but it may be essential if the museum is to survive in the new environment. *Organizational design*, then, is this process of matching an organization's structure, staff, and culture to a new strategic plan.

A good example of the issues involved in strategic planning and organizational design and transformation is found at the Glenbow Museum, in Calgary, Alberta, Canada. The Glenbow is a relatively new museum. It was founded in 1966 by a public law passed by the provincial government of Alberta, Canada. The impetus for the museum was the largest private gift of cultural resources ever made in Canada—the transfer of an enormous collection along with some endowment support from a wealthy oil and gas entrepreneur named Eric Harvie to the people of Alberta. An estimate of the market value of the Harvie gift in the mid-1990s put it at $120 million. The museum today combines military, social, and cultural history and also ethnology and mineralogy; in addition, it includes an art gallery, a library, a large archival center, and a traveling exhibition service. In the early 1990s, the museum complex had to address a major fiscal crisis: nearly a 40 percent reduction in provincial government support, a cut of thirty-one full-time staff, and the shift of eleven other staff from full- to part-time work. Fiscal projections for a five-year period, moreover, had estimated a cumulative deficit of nearly $8 million, which the museum board determined that it could not allow. Some projected bankruptcy by 1998.

Museum leadership responded by adopting a core strategy of building up the private, entrepreneurial side of the museum and stabilizing public-sector support. This involved reconfiguring the organization, transforming its culture, and reducing operating costs. Portions of the collections were offered for sale. Twenty-two departments were consolidated into five units, and management ranks were cut. Teams of curators and other professionals were established to alter the organization's discipline- and research-based orientation. The museum began to collaborate with other nonprofit organizations. It formed business-oriented commercial partnerships, and a new entrepreneurial unit, Glenbow Enterprises, was established to generate product licensing, retail sales, facility rentals, and consulting services in the heritage and museum exhibit fields. The new strategy led to an audience development plan and active collaboration with the corporate sector. Over a seven-year period, the Glenbow Museum went from roughly 65 percent government support and 35 percent private support to 65 percent private support and 35 percent government support.

Once it had built up credible private support, the Glenbow Museum was able to negotiate with the provincial government for support on the basis of a stronger bargaining position. Negotiations were directed toward defining what museum programs and services the provincial government would continue to support, rather than the elimination of support, an earlier aim of provincial officials (Janes, 1995).

Museums are highly individualized and even idiosyncratic organizations, rooted in particular histories, circumstances, and environmental conditions. Their core strategies have to reflect these circumstances. (Strategic planning is discussed further in the Model Museum Practice at the end of this chapter.)

SYSTEMS DESIGN

The final stage in the strategic market planning process is systems design: establishing the systems that enable the museum to develop, carry out, and monitor the set of activities that will implement the new strategy. Without effective implementation, the best strategic planning in the world will come to nothing. The three principal systems for controlling the implementation of a new strategic plan are the marketing information system, the marketing planning system, and the marketing control system. They are introduced briefly here and discussed in more detail in later chapters.

Marketing Information System

The job of effectively running a museum calls for continual monitoring of consumer publics, intermediaries, competitors, and the larger macroenvironmental factors, forces, and trends. This information is obtained from various types of marketing research (see Chapter Six).

Marketing Planning System

Information, to be effectively used, should be incorporated in the planning system. An increasing number of museums are operating formal planning systems in which long-term and short-term goals, strategies, marketing programs, and budgets are developed annually and at other intervals. Successful planning calls for a planning staff, planning resources, and a planning culture. The marketing planning system is the set of procedures for incorporating marketing research and information into planning and development, enabling managers to respond to new factors in the environment (see Chapter Twelve).

Marketing Control System

Once again, plans are useful only when they are implemented. The purpose of a marketing control system is to evaluate performance and measure the ongoing results of implemented plans against the goals and, when necessary, take corrective actions before it is too late. Corrective action may take the form of changing the goals, strategies, plans, or the means of implementation in the light of new circumstances. One of the key control tools used by organizations is the *marketing audit.* It is important that museums from time to time undertake such an audit of their opportunities and performance in order to identify areas needing improvement. (See Chapter Twelve for the marketing audit.)

SUMMARY

The strategic market planning process is the framework by which a museum organization shapes, plans, implements, and controls the mission it has designed; the programs, products, and services it offers; and the outreach to the audience segments it seeks to attract. The process works in three stages: (1) setting up a planning system that analyzes environmental factors, organizational strengths and weaknesses, mission, objectives, and goals and then determines strategies; (2) crafting an organizational design adapted to the chosen strategies; and (3) creating systems to monitor planning implementation and outcomes, specifically market information, planning, and control.

○

MODEL MUSEUM PRACTICE

Strategic Planning at Chicago's Museum of Contemporary Art: Building a New Museum

Chicago's Museum of Contemporary Art (MCA) reopened on June 21, 1996, with an impressive new $46 million museum facility of 220,000 square feet. Situated in one of the most prized areas of the city, one block west of the Lake on Chicago Avenue and one block east of Michigan Avenue, the museum occupies a building nearly five times larger than its old facility. In 1996, the MCA's operating budget was over $10 million, compared to $2.5 million in the late 1980s. At the start of 1997, the MCA projected yearly attendance at 500,000; its attendance at its former facility averaged 100,000. In the early 1990s, the MCA had a membership base of roughly 3,000. Spurred by the excitement of having a new facility and the plans for growth, its membership in October 1996 reached 16,000.

The MCA had occupied for twenty-five years a 33,000-square-foot facility in a cramped building and an inconspicuous location on the city's east side. The old building had limited exhibition space and virtually no space for visitor orientation, members' meetings, or amenities such as a restaurant and shop; it was unable to display significant portions of the museum's world-class collections. How did the MCA accomplish its remarkable growth, and how is it dealing with the challenges that lie ahead?

"The museum couldn't survive into the new millennium without becoming more competitive," observed Kevin E. Consey, the MCA's director and CEO. "We faced the sobering choice of having three options: maintain the status quo at the old facility and remain a 'regional' museum dwarfed by the city's world-class museums; scale down the collections, programs, and operations, eroding the resources and eventually dissolving; or take risks to grow and expand significantly. We needed a signature facility of great prominence in a city that celebrates its architecture; and we needed expanded programs for tourists and residents and a higher level of services and amenities."

With the assistance of a leading business consulting firm, the MCA board in the late 1980s chose the growth option, and a core group put forward a significant commitment of financial support. A new director was hired. A strategic planning process was launched by a newly hired associate director. Planning was further expanded in the early 1990s. The growth option had to be translated into a set of goals: expanding membership, donorship, and community support; achieving ambitious funding goals enabling the expansion and relocation; designing and constructing a new facility of distinction; and achieving "people" goals, primarily through creative and exciting new offerings and services. The John D. and Catherine T. MacArthur Foundation gave the museum a vote of confidence in awarding it a $2 million planning grant to develop education programs.

A critical issue was to find a new museum site. The MCA found an exceptional site on the grounds of an old armory building slated for demolition and owned by the state of Illinois. The museum was able to lease the land for its new facility at $1 per year; in exchange, it offered the state a property the museum owned. At key junctures, the MCA marshaled the support of the Illinois governor and the city's influential corporate community. Project construction for the new facility was funded through tax-exempt borrowing under state auspices. The museum found a leading European architect, Josef Paul Kleihues.

In a later phase, the MCA planned for the new museum's opening and the achievement of its objectives. Four areas of planning were critical:

- *Artistic and educational goals*—setting and maintaining high standards for collections, exhibits, and educational programs

- *Leadership and staffing*—building a management team with expertise in critical areas and a staff and organization that supports the strategic goals, and incorporating board expertise and expanding corporate involvement

- *Fundraising*—successfully completing the endowment campaign and building broader donor support

- *Marketing*—enlarging and diversifying visitorship and membership, identifying key audience segments and the appropriate strategies and tools to reach them, and planning for membership retention

The MCA's strategy for growth depended on several conditions. The MCA's board of trustees had to embrace the growth plan. Management had to convince the board the risks of relocation and expansion were manageable. Planning staff spent considerable time anticipating and analyzing risk factors, calculating risk levels, and generating various scenarios that could arise. MCA board members contributed $36 million toward a fundraising campaign that ultimately exceeded its $55 million goal, with a final total of $72.5 million.

The MCA is not without challenges. It has to capture a large audience and donor share, with yearly visitorship of at least 350,000 to meet its financial goals. The MCA's costs compelled a 30 percent increase in the admission fee ($6.50 a ticket). Having seen its membership quintuple, the MCA has to find ways to maintain a high renewal rate as well as expand its membership further. The MCA has already expanded its endowment from a tiny $3.5 million (in the late 1980s) to $29 million in 1996. Yet this level falls short of what museums of comparable size and cost are advised to have. Finally, like other contemporary art museums, the MCA faces a continuing challenge in raising awareness of the beauty and value of contemporary art, a far more difficult marketing situation than museums that offer Impressionists, Rembrandts, and Vermeers face.

All signs point to promising growth at the Museum of Contemporary Art in Chicago. The MCA has become a symbol of civic pride and a favored destination for tourists. The new museum's opening in July 1996 permitted the offering of significant new programs. "Without careful planning, it's unlikely the MCA could have developed from a small, regional museum into a world-class institution," comments Mary Ittelson, a consulting executive and former associate director at the MCA in charge of planning. "When the expansion plan was first announced, a lot of people thought the vision was audacious, even reckless. Yet the success lay in the planning process—charting, step by step, the paths to take to reach the goals and then executing each step, one at a time. That's the way we achieved what many people thought was impossible."

CHAPTER FOUR

Understanding Museum Audiences

*Museums let adults engage in playful behavior—using their imagination,
exploring, and engaging in interactive games. On the other hand,
museums let children try out adult roles—gathering information,
solving problems, becoming experts.*
—Barbara Franco

*A great escape. [From] when I walked in the door until I left,
it was a different world. I could totally forget everything.*
—First-time visitor to the Art Institute of Chicago

Audience development is a prime objective of museums today. This was not always the case. As a curator at a university art museum remarked in the mid-1990s: "Ten years ago, art museum staff might easily have asked, 'Is an audience necessary?'" However, the museums that once put their collections or their research first are now placing their audiences at the center of their activities: building relationships with their communities, investing resources in attracting larger and more diverse audiences, and applying new concepts and methods to helping audiences derive satisfaction and education from museum offerings.

On any given day, U.S. museums are likely to be filled with a variety of people: school children touring as part of a field experience, families with young children, older adults visiting individually or in couples, extended families, unrelated adults taking a group tour, scholars and connoisseurs, and college-age students. Audiences can be identified along the lines of gender and age, ethnicity and race, social class and educational background. Overall, museums attract primarily adults and a disproportionate number of higher-educated people. Older people, in couples and groups, are the typical visitors in all types of museums in the fall and winter. Zoos attract a mix of visitors that is more representative of the community's social classes and ethnic groups. Science museums and science and technology centers, more than other types of museums, attract greater numbers of young people and families with children. Museum visitors also differ in other aspects: the frequency and the length of their visits;

whether they are local residents or tourists; their motivations, interests, and expectations; and their prior awareness and knowledge of museums. Museums, clearly, have to respond to an extremely heterogeneous population and shape their programs accordingly.

People have different attitudes toward museums. Some never step into a museum, either because its existence is unknown to them or because its image is intimidating. Some visit occasionally but think museums are stuffy and elitist. Some like to visit a few times a year, especially when family and friends from out of town are paying a visit. Some are so stimulated by museums that they visit whenever they can. As museums increasingly try to understand their audiences and to shape their programs and services accordingly, they are learning more about the processes by which people make their choices of leisure-time activities. They are identifying the elements of a visit that contribute to a positive, satisfying experience—perhaps an experience like that of the first-time visitor to the Denver Art Museum who said, "The museum inspired me to want to go back and learn more. It prompted me to ask questions about things I had not previously given thought to" (Walsh, 1991, p. 13). As a result of visitor research, museums are making their facilities more physically accessible and comfortable, creating orientation and information areas, redesigning exhibit halls to make presentations more attractive, and organizing exhibitions that have a broad appeal.

This chapter begins by examining the major characteristics of the museum-going audience, summarizing the results of a number of studies. Next it presents a model of consumer decision making leading to a visit to a museum. It also assesses the influence of such factors as ethnicity, social class, life cycle stages, lifestyles, socialization, and social trends in motivating museum-going.

CHARACTERISTICS OF THE MUSEUM AUDIENCE

Museum audiences are varied. They include people who just wander in and people whose visits are planned in advance. Although most museums are open to the public virtually every day of the year (unlike other suppliers of leisure activity, such as amusement parks and professional baseball and football teams), their audiences still vary with the seasons. Tourists are dominant at large, urban museums during the summer months; local residents form a larger segment in the off-peak seasons such as winter; and older people typically visit museums during the autumn months.

A museum learns about its visitor characteristics through surveys. The National Air and Space Museum (NASM) conducted in 1994 a broad-ranging study of 2,975 visitors. NASM has the distinction of being the most visited museum in the world, attracting nearly nine million visitors a year. This study provided a glimpse of their characteristics (Ziebarth, Smith, Doering, and Pekarik, 1995, pp. iv–vii):

In all seasons, more men than women visited NASM (in a ratio of about three to two).

The NASM audience was 75 to 80 percent Caucasian (varying by season), and more Asians visited than members of other minority groups.

The proportion of local visitors was much higher in winter.

In every season, at least two out of every ten visitors were residents of foreign countries.

In the fall, visitors were more likely to arrive alone or in pairs and less likely to bring children.

Among visitors aged twenty-five and older, 63 to 73 percent (depending on the season) had college degrees.

More than half of all visitors had no specific thing to see.

First-time visitors accounted for half of the audience in summer and fall.

Audiences differ by museum type. John Falk and Lynn Dierking (1992, p. 20), citing visitor studies in England and the United States, report that an estimated 70 percent of visitors at the Natural History Museum in London visit as members of social groups, predominantly family groups. In the United States, families with children are frequently found at zoos, science and technology centers, and children's museums and less often at art, history, and natural history museums (families with children are estimated to comprise 10 percent or less of art museum visitorship). Science and technology centers are more likely than other types of museums to attract older children and teenagers.

The most striking characteristic of the majority of museum visitors is high educational attainment, followed by high income. However, variations in educational level are associated with attendance at different types of museums: visitors to U.S. art museums tend to have the highest educational level, followed by visitors to science and technology centers and history and natural history museums. The majority of visitors to zoos have a high school education or less.

Methods of Counting Museum Audiences

Estimates of the size of museum audiences are often imprecise. People going to concerts, the theater, and sports events have to purchase tickets, and tickets are a reliable measure of audience size. However, perhaps as many as half of the museum-goers in the U.S. visit museums that do not have admission fees, offer free days, or do not use tickets or turnstiles. Only 55 percent of U.S. museums in 1988 charged for entry. In Great Britain in the early 1990s, two-thirds of the museums charged an admission fee (American Association of Museums, 1994, p. 89; Runyard, 1993, p. 4).

Many museums report the *number of museum visits* rather than *number of visitors.* Individual visitors may leave and return several times in one day (to feed a parking meter or step out for a smoke), yet each entry is counted as a separate visit. Thus basing figures on visit counts is likely to inflate audience size. In museums that are free of charge or lack tickets, staff at entrances use mechanical or electronic counters to log visitors, but this method lacks reliability. Staff may not be continuously posted or uniformly attentive. Reliability is also compromised by any failure to distinguish visitors from staff and volunteers. During museums' peak seasons, large crowds make counting difficult for even the most conscientious staff. When museums organize special events geared to holiday celebrations, it can be hard to differentiate visitors attending these events from gallery visitors. Similarly, urban art museums are likely to count the participants at social events (such as evening mixers for young professionals) as museum visitors even though they may not enter a gallery or view an exhibit.

The American Association of Museums (AAM) reports that just two-thirds of museums "arrive at attendance figures through an accurate count; most others estimate the count, but some museums use both methods" (1994, p. 63). An example of the resulting imprecision is reported by Stuart Davies, who examined the range of estimates of visitorship in British museums in 1992. The most commonly used figure that year was 79 million visits to all of Britain's museums and art galleries. Other studies showed widely varying figures: a *Sightseeking* study, 77 million; a *Leisure Futures* study, 120 million; and so on. Davies's reestimate for 1992 is 110 million visits. He observes that "faced with staggering inconsistencies in collecting and reporting, it can only be reluctantly concluded that unless attendance figures are based on ticketed admissions, they should not be regarded in any way as reliable for forecasts, projects or performance criteria" (1994, pp. 9, 49).

Poor counting practices can pose problems for any museum that seeks to understand its audience or justify its community value. Moreover, as corporations increasingly tie their financial support of museums to achieving marketing and public relations returns, they are requiring museums to supply reliable data on audiences: their size, their composition, and even the length of their visits. These potential sponsors are likely to want to ascertain the impacts museum visits have, particularly the attention visitors pay to exhibit sponsors. Therefore visitor counts and visitor research are becoming significant factors as museums raise more and more private support.

Counting the Total Museum Audience

A number of surveys have tried to gauge what proportion of the population visits museums and how often they do so. Visitation figures, as we mentioned, are not always reliable. A Smithsonian Institution study in 1995 estimated that two-thirds of U.S. adults (at least eighteen years of age) attended at least one museum or museum-like facility during the year previous to the study—122 million individuals out of an adult population of 185 million. Visits to all types of museums, from modern art museums to aquariums, were included. An estimated sixty-three million adults did not visit a cultural institution at all during the year previous to the study, and 90 percent of the nonvisitors were found to have a high school education or less (Doering, 1995, p. 2). John Falk (1993, p. 73), on the basis of reviewing museum audience studies, estimates that "regular museum-going" (visiting a museum at least once a year) accounts for probably less than 40 percent of the population and that frequent or active museum-going (four or more visits per year) accounts for about 20 percent of the population. A visitor frequency study in British museums yielded the following estimates: 40 percent of British adults are regular museum visitors (visit at least one museum each year); another 40 percent are occasional visitors (visiting less frequently than once a year but within a three-year period); and 20 percent are people who rarely or never visit a museum (Schuster, 1991, pp. 30–32).

One of the pioneering analyses of the types of museum visitors and the frequency of their visits in the context of leisure choices was done by Marilyn Hood in 1980 and 1981 at the Toledo Museum of Art. Hood divided Toledo's adult population into three groups—*frequent visitors* (who visit the museum at least three times a year), *occasional visitors* (who visit once or twice a year), and *nonparticipants*. Frequent visitors accounted for 14 percent of adults in the Toledo area; occasional visitors, 40 percent; and nonparticipants, 46 percent (Hood, 1983, pp. 54–55).

Hood then interviewed respondents to analyze the factors that shaped their choices of leisure activity and, in particular, their preferences for museum visits. She identified the following six attributes, which may occur singly or in various combinations, that influence leisure choices (p. 51):

- Being with people, or having social interaction
- Doing something worthwhile
- Feeling comfortable and at ease in one's surroundings
- Having a challenge of new experiences
- Having an opportunity to learn
- Participating actively

Some of these attributes describe interpersonal and social behavior; others, cognitive and intrapersonal characteristics. They can also be clustered into these three categories: emotional (for example, "feeling comfortable"), rational (for example, "having an opportunity to learn"), and sensory (for example, "having a challenge of new experiences," "feeling comfortable in one's surroundings"). The frequent visitors in Hood's study valued most highly three attributes: the opportunity to learn, to undertake new experiences, and to do something worthwhile in their leisure time. The occasional visitors were individuals who were social-ized early in life to seek active participation, social interaction, and entertain-ing experiences as the ingredients of their leisure activities. This group tended to seek after relaxing experiences, comfortable settings, and interaction with other people. Family-centered activities were more important for this group than were activities that involved learning new things and being challenged sensorially. The third group, the nonparticipants, tended to value being together with other people, engaging in high levels of activity, and feeling comfortable in their sur-roundings. For the most part they lacked early experiences in museums, and any involvement in cultural activities they had arose later in life. These people viewed museums as inaccessible and unfamiliar places. Hood's study was par-ticularly groundbreaking because it linked visitation, nonvisitation, and fre-quency with motivation, personality, and socialization factors.

One other survey of attendance at U.S. art museums undertaken in the 1980s was noteworthy. The National Endowment for the Arts, the U.S. Bureau of the Census, and the University of Maryland collaborated on a survey in 1982 and again in 1985. Known as the Survey of Public Participation in the Arts (SPPA), it asked respondents whether during the previous twelve months they visited an art museum or an art gallery. The 1985 SPPA survey estimated that 22 per-cent of adult Americans—two out of every nine adults—had visited an art mu-seum or gallery at least one time in the previous year. Comparative data on museum visitorship in Great Britain, France, and Sweden, showed that 29 per-cent of the adult British population were said to have visited an art museum or gallery at least once a year, 30 percent of the adult French population, and 31 percent of the adult Swedish population (Schuster, 1991, pp. 2–18).

The SPPA survey also reported noteworthy data on the education and social class of art museum visitors. Although 4 percent of respondents with some grade school education had visited an art museum in the last twelve months, 45 percent of respondents with a completed college degree and 55 percent of respondents with graduate school education reported such visits. Fifteen per-cent of respondents earning $10,000 to $14,999 reported visiting an art museum at least once; 45 percent of respondents reporting incomes of $50,000 or greater had visited. The survey also reported marked differences between urban and rural respondents. Fourteen percent of rural respondents had visited an art mu-seum at least once compared to 25 percent of respondents from large metro-politan areas (Schuster, 1991, pp. 10–13).

Tourism as a Source of Visitors

Museums are attended by community residents and by tourists, two audiences with differing expectations and impacts. Tourists tend to spend more money than local resident visitors. They are more likely to purchase gifts for others and for themselves. Tourists tend to be first-time visitors, whereas a large propor-tion of community visitors tend to be repeat visitors. Most tourists plan their destination sites; local residents may or may not have planned their visits far in advance. Tourists are likely to be seeking particular kinds of experiences and to have high expectations. Tourists also are attracted to so-called blockbuster exhibitions.

The tourism market is composed of several types of travelers: families, businesspeople, members of group tours, conventioneers, adult couples, and school groups. Museums are increasingly working with travel and tourist agencies and the hospitality industry to develop plans, promotions, and programs to attract tourism.

An early 1990s visitor survey in Great Britain estimated that tourists make up 44 percent of visitors at London's museums and art galleries and 26 percent of the visitors to British museums and galleries outside of London (Runyard, 1993, p. 9). The study of 1994 visitorship at the National Air and Space Museum reports that during the peak summer and fall seasons more than half of the visitors are from elsewhere in the United States and another 20 percent are visitors from other countries (Ziebarth, Smith, Doering, and Pekarik, 1995, pp. iv, 8). Another Smithsonian Institution visitor study reports that of the estimated ten million distinct visitors each year to Smithsonian museums, approximately 75 percent are tourists (Doering, 1995, pp. 3–4).

The National Trust for Historic Preservation (1994), a major nonprofit organization that manages and protects historic sites in the United States, forecasts that travel and tourism will become "the world's largest industry by the year 2000. It contributes almost $400 billion to the U.S. economy and is America's number one export." Among the factors boosting tourism are (1) rising incomes, particularly in Asian and Third World nations; (2) increasing leisure time among certain population segments, resulting from economic growth and an aging population; (3) improved transportation; (4) advances in information and communication systems; and (5) increasing social and political freedom, especially in Third World nations. At the same time, and on an episodic basis, certain forces, including political upheavals, natural disasters, economic recessions, inflation, currency differentials, clogged transportation systems, and slowdowns in investment in and expenditure on recreational sites, can depress tourism. Museums, to be sure, compete for tourists against other leisure activity providers, including shopping malls, national parks, and theme parks.

CHOOSING A MUSEUM VISIT:
STAGES IN THE DECISION-MAKING PROCESS

A museum visit is usually not accidental or unplanned; each visitor has made a choice among several competing forms of available leisure activity. Choosing to visit a museum is a selection of one particular set of expectations and values over others. That is why museum marketers have to focus on communicating the unique qualities and values that people find in museums that are not available in other recreational activities. Suppliers of leisure or recreational activities need to examine both the comparative demand and the changing demand patterns over time. For example, a British study (Woods, 1994) reported a declining use of public libraries between 1980 and 1992. This decline apparently resulted from the rise in home-based leisure activities such as viewing television and videos, using computers, and playing electronic games. Table 4.1 reports the frequency of participation in a variety of leisure-time activities on a particular weekend in 1992 in Washington, D.C.

Individuals and groups often follow an identifiable process to make choices among a variety of alternative goods, services, and activities, and marketing experts have developed several models of how consumers make decisions. To the extent that the decision process is deliberate, rather than impulsive, decision making involves five stages, as follows (Kotler and Andreasen, 1996, pp. 139–141):

Need arousal→ Information gathering→ Decision evaluation→
Decision execution→ Postdecision assessment and action

We will illustrate consumer decision making with the case of a family with children deciding how to spend a summer weekend. We assume that selecting a leisure activity is not fundamentally different from choosing a product or service in the marketplace. We also assume that the parents seek a recreational activity that will be active, sensorily rich, and educationally fulfilling.

Table 4.1. Participation Rates in Various Leisure-Time Activities in Washington, D.C., 1992.

Activity	Percentage of Respondents Participating
Visiting friends or relatives	86
Running errands	64
Exercising outdoors	59
Working in yard	47
Visiting shopping mall	37
Eating at a restaurant	34
Viewing a video	21
Going to a movie	15
Attending a musical concert	11
Taking a child to sporting event	10
Visiting a museum or art gallery	7
Fishing	5
Going to the theater	4

Source: "A Weekend in the Life of Washington," *The Washington Post* © 1992, Washington Post Writers Group. Reprinted with permission.

Need Arousal

The first task is to understand how consumers develop their initial interest in a type of recreational activity and what needs and wants underlie their decision making. Need arousal breaks down into three issues:

1. What factors initially trigger an interest in a particular recreational activity?
2. What deep-seated needs and values come into play when the consumer considers recreational activities?
3. What specific wants become activated by these needs?

Triggering Factors. The family's interest in a recreational activity can be stimulated by either *internal* or *external cues.* An internal cue is a person's feeling of a need for or readiness to do something. This cue might take the form of a physiological stimulus, such as hunger, or a psychological stimulus, such as anxiety or boredom. An external cue is an outside influence that stimulates a person's interest in a particular activity. The external cue can be *personal* (from a friend, coworker, or sales representative) or *nonpersonal* (from a magazine article or an advertisement). It can be either marketer controlled (advertisements and public relations personnel) or non–marketer controlled (friends).

An important marketing task is to survey consumers to learn the major types of triggers that stimulate their interest in a particular recreational activity. For example, consumers might be asked, "Recall what made you interested in this type of activity." Background factors, such social class, life cycle, and lifestyle, help shape a person's perceptions, attitudes, and motivations toward leisure activity.

In our case of the family engaging in recreational decision making, the following cues might stimulate family members' thinking about the type of activity they want to pursue:

During vacation periods, particularly in the summer months, children demand activity and parents seek to fill their children's time with both playful and learning activities.

The family hears from friends about their recreational choices and experiences.

Time is set aside for a recreational or outing experience and in the preceding days communication intensifies about the kinds of activities available.

Information is gathered about leisure activity offerings through the newspapers, magazines, guidebooks, and the like.

Deep-Seated Needs and Values. Triggering cues arouse a set of basic needs in an individual or a family. They do not create the needs; they activate existing needs. Psychologist Abraham Maslow (1954) held the view that people act to satisfy basic needs and that they typically act to satisfy lower-level needs before they satisfy their higher-level needs (see Figure 4.1).

People spend most of their time and energy satisfying their lower needs. A starving man first devotes his energy to finding food. He may then devote his energy to finding safety and security. Once these basic needs are satisfied, he may have more time and energy to devote to such higher needs as *belonging,* or *status,* or *self-actualization.* As each lower-level need is satisfied, it ceases to be a motivator and higher-level needs more and more define a person's motivation. In the context of leisure-time behavior and activity, Maslow's conceptual framework would predict that a person's free time would largely be devoted to the search for higher-level need satisfaction—that is, fulfilling needs for interpersonal relatedness and belonging, esteem needs such as recognition and status, and the self-actualization needs of achievement, intellectual growth, creativity, and generativity.

We can ask what basic needs are stimulated by the aroused interest in finding a suitable recreational activity. A major consideration is finding a safe and secure activity. The parents want the activity to take place in clean, comfort-

Figure 4.1. Maslow's Hierarchy of Needs.

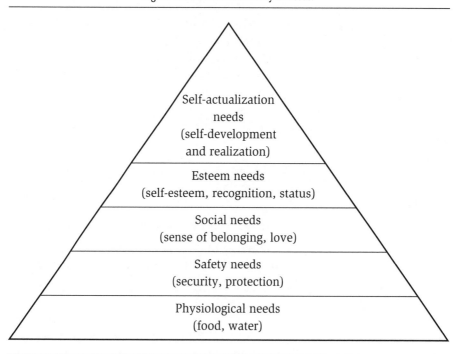

Self-actualization
needs
(self-development
and realization)

Esteem needs
(self-esteem, recognition, status)

Social needs
(sense of belonging, love)

Safety needs
(security, protection)

Physiological needs
(food, water)

Source: Maslow, 1954.

able settings. Parents seek relatedness with their children and activities that are both educational and entertaining. A particular outing experience might not fulfill all the needs families have, but certain needs might be given higher priority. A family's values come into play when choices involve conflicting activities. Values are the guiding principles that people employ to make choices among competing activities and ends.

Specific Wants. Whereas basic needs transcend particular products or services, wants are product or offering specific. Wants are identified when family members list specific recreational activities—going to a zoo, seeing a movie, visiting a museum, and so on—and confer or vote on which activity would most satisfy their needs. In stages, the family will move to a "purchase or buying decision," as it would be termed in commercial marketing.

Information Gathering

Consumers facing a leisure activity choice are likely to engage in varying degrees of information gathering, depending on the type of activity involved and their own level of need for information. As consumers gain experience and familiarity with particular types of exchanges, their decisions become simplified or routinized.

Consumer behavior specialists draw a distinction between *low-involvement* and *high-involvement* choices. High-involvement consumer choices occur when one or more of the following conditions exists:

- The behavior of the consumer reflects upon his or her self-image.
- The personal and financial costs of behaving "incorrectly" are perceived as high.
- The personal or social risks of a "wrong" decision are perceived as high.
- Group pressures to act in a particular way are strong, and the consumer's motivation to comply is strong.

Examples of high-involvement choices include choosing a college, choosing a career, changing nutritional and health habits, and contributing significant funds to a cause. Such choices are characterized by a high degree of information gathering, consulting with several and varied information sources, and evaluating and weighing alternatives. Low-involvement consumer decisions, by contrast, are treated as routine actions requiring little or no information gathering.

Consumer behavior specialists distinguish two dimensions of the information-gathering process: *information neediness* and *information sources*.

Information Neediness. Consumers vary greatly in their information neediness—ranging from those who jump right into a decision (as with impulse purchases) to those who spend days or weeks gathering information before deciding (as with major spending decisions). We can distinguish two broad levels of information neediness. The milder level is *heightened attention.* In the case of the family choosing a leisure activity to pursue, this might involve casual scanning of the newspapers to spot interesting activities. The more active level is *information searching* and involves making a focused effort to gather extensive information. A family member might do research at the library, phone recreational providers to ask questions, and so on.

Information Sources. Consumers can gather information from several sources: personal, non–marketer controlled (family, friends, reputable others); personal, marketer controlled (sales representatives, marketers); nonpersonal, non–marketer controlled (mass media); and nonpersonal, marketer controlled (catalogues, ads, in-house brochures). Normally, consumers will assign different influence weights to these sources. More weight is typically assigned to personal, nonmarketer opinions than nonpersonal, marketer sources.

Information sources vary also with the role the individual is playing in the group decision-making process, in this case a family's decision process. We distinguish five roles:

- *Initiator*—the person who first suggests the idea of engaging in a particular activity
- *Influencer*—any person whose views or advice carry influence on the final choice or decision
- *Decider*—the person who ultimately determines any part or the whole of the decision: whether to engage in an activity, which activity to choose, when to experience the activity, and where to experience it
- *Buyer*—the person who pays for the activity
- *User*—any person who engages in, consumes, or uses the activity

Consider the roles of the different family members in choosing a recreational activity. The mother might initiate the family's interest in a recreational activity by reporting that an aunt had recently visited an art museum and enjoyed it. The children might express a strong preference for going to the zoo. An older child advises a course of action that carries influence. The mother and father might make the final decision. The father might purchase the tickets. All the family members then engage in the recreational activity.

Marketers find it worthwhile to study the sources of consumer information. Identifying information sources and their respective perceived importance involves interviewing consumers to ask them how they learned about a particular activity: the sources of information they turned to, the type of information obtained from each source, the degree of credibility they placed on each source, and the extent of influence each source had on the final decision.

Decision Evaluation

As a result of gathering information, the family gains a clearer picture of the available choices. Certain alternatives might be eliminated at an early stage. We will examine how the family might narrow its choices of recreational activities. Table 4.2 shows a series of decision sets involved in the consumer decision process.

Our prototypical family has, theoretically, a wide range of choices in making a selection. The *total set* represents all the forms of leisure activity that exist. The awareness set consists of only those activities that the family members are currently aware of. Of those activities, the family may want to consider only a limited number; these constitute the *consideration set*. As additional information is gathered, certain choices will become more attractive, and these constitute the *choice set*. In the final stage the family will make a choice from the alternatives remaining in the choice set; in the example in Table 4.2, the family decided that visiting the science center would best satisfy their varying needs.

Examining consumer choices within this conceptual framework highlights the fact that any leisure activity competes with a large number of other activities. A museum's marketing task is to get its offering into the consumer's awareness set and hope it remains in the consumer's consideration and choice sets.

A central question is, How does the consumer—in this case, our prototypical family—make a choice among the final alternatives in the choice set? The simple answer is that consumers define certain attributes they are seeking and then determine which activity delivers the most of what they are seeking. Suppose that the family is trying to choose among a science center, zoo, aquarium,

Table 4.2. Decision Sets in Consumer Decision Making.

Total Set →	Awareness Set →	Consideration Set →	Choice Set →	Decision
Science center	Science center	Science center	Science center	Science center
Zoo	Zoo	Zoo	Zoo	
Aquarium	Aquarium	Aquarium	Aquarium	
Nature center	Nature center	Nature center	Nature center	
Theme park	Theme park	Theme park		
Pop music concert	Pop music concert			
Baseball game	Baseball game			
Swimming				
Art museum				

and a nature center. It places value on four activity attributes: location, cost, services, and interactivity. Figure 4.2 shows how the family might rate each recreational activity in satisfying each desired attribute. The numbers in the figure represent weighting alternatives in terms of how well they satisfy the attributes. The closer a number is to ten, the more a particular recreational activity satisfies that particular criterion. Thus the science center has the best location (it is closest to the family's home), a moderate cost and moderate services, and a high opportunity for interactivity.

Given the kind of information in Figure 4.2, how does the consumer actually choose? There is no standard evaluation process used by all consumers, or even by a single consumer, in all choices. One common model, however, is the Expectancy-Value Model. In this model, the consumer assigns importance weights to the attributes and then chooses the activity that maximizes the expectancy value. Suppose the family assigns the importance weights of .4, .3, .2, and .1 to the four attributes, respectively. That is, the family assigns 40 percent of the importance to the leisure activity's location quality, 30 percent to its costliness, 20 percent to its service quality, and 10 percent to its interactivity. To find the expectancy value for each leisure activity, these weights are multiplied by the ratings for each activity (illustrated in Figure 4.2). For the family, this process leads to the following expectancy values, and a prediction that the family will favor the science center, with the zoo as a close second choice.

$$\text{Science center} = .4(10) + .3(6) + .2(6) + .1(9) = 7.9$$
$$\text{Zoo} = .4(8) + .3(9) + .2(8) + .1(3) = 7.8$$
$$\text{Aquarium} = .4(6) + .3(8) + .2(7) + .1(5) = 6.7$$
$$\text{Nature center} = .4(4) + .3(3) + .2(10) + .1(8) = 5.3$$

Figure 4.2. A Family's Evaluations of Four Leisure Activities.

		Attributes			
		Location	Cost	Services	Interactivity
Leisure Activity	Science center	10	6	6	9
	Zoo	8	9	8	3
	Aquarium	6	8	7	5
	Nature center	4	3	10	8

Note: Ten represents the highest desirable score on each particular attribute. In the case of cost, a high score means a low cost, which makes an activity more desirable.

Alternative Model of Consumer Choice

Some marketing theorists prefer to emphasize the emotional and learning styles that undergird consumers' decision making. Three styles can be distinguished: (1) learn-feel-do, (2) do-feel-learn, and (3) learn-do-feel (see Ray, 1982).

In the *learn-feel-do* model the individual first learns about a leisure activity (or any product or service), then develops an attitude, or feeling-state, toward the activity, and then engages in it. This learning model is the most widely observed and researched model for explaining the behavior of consumers. The model achieves the best prediction results when two conditions are present: consumers are highly involved in the goal of engaging in an activity and they perceive clear differences between the various offerings available.

In the *do-feel-learn* model the individual tries an offering on a tentative basis; as a result he or she develops feelings about the offering. Then the individual starts learning more about the offering.

Finally, in the *learn-do-feel* model the individual chooses an offering on the basis of, say, exposure to repetitive messages through the media. She or he has not formed an attitude toward the offering and might not have a high degree of involvement with it. Once the individual has tried the offering, she or he will develop a set of feelings toward it.

Decision Execution

The evaluation stage leads the family to form a ranked set of preferences, normally choosing the most preferred alternative. However, at least three factors can intervene between an intention and its execution. The first is the attitude of others. Suppose the parents prefer a particular leisure activity choice, and the children, another choice. If the parents feel that it is important to satisfy their children, they may decide to sacrifice their own interests.

The second factor is the influence of anticipated or unanticipated situations. The former include such possibilities as changing expectations for family income and the expected cost of the activity. Unanticipated situations might intervene to prevent carrying out a choice decision. The family might discover that its automobile is not drivable or that the weather makes a visit difficult. Thus marketers observe that preferences and even intentions are not completely reliable predictors of actual behavior. They give direction to decision making but fail to take into account additional conditions that can exert a considerable influence on the final decision.

The third factor is perceived risk, which may cause the family to modify, postpone, or avoid a decision to visit a particular recreational site. Marketers have devoted a lot of attention to the risk aspects of consumer and buying behavior. Consumers cannot be certain about the consequences of their decisions, and this can produce anxiety. Perceived risk varies with the amount of money at stake, the degree of attribute uncertainty, and the amount of consumer self-confidence. Individuals develop certain routines for reducing risk, such as decision avoidance, information gathering from friends, and preference for brand names that tend to raise confidence levels. The marketer has to understand the factors that provoke a feeling of risk and find ways to provide information and support that will reduce people's felt risk.

Postpurchase Assessment and Action

As a result of visiting the science center, the family will experience some level of satisfaction or dissatisfaction. The family may encounter friendly or indifferent staff. The family may need orienting information, and the museum may or may not have orientation and information services. Museum signs and exhibit labels may be clear or confusing. Facilities such as a restaurant, rest rooms, telephone booths, and elevators may be ample or lacking. The museum's lighting may be bright or dull; its exhibitions easy or hard to view. G. Donald Adams, director of marketing at the Automotive Hall of Fame, in Dearborn, Michigan (interviewed on Feb. 6 and 20, 1996), argues that a family visit to a museum is an outing—a broad, interrelated experience. If certain aspects of the experience are perceived negatively, the other aspects, however pleasant or valuable, might also be diminished. Adams's recommendation is that museums assess in the broadest possible terms the characteristics of their visitors' experiences, along with travel to and from, and take steps to provide the highest-quality service at each stage and reduce, wherever possible, the psychic and physical costs involved.

What determines whether a consumer is highly satisfied, somewhat satisfied, indifferent, somewhat dissatisfied, or high dissatisfied with a given offering? There are two main theories about consumer satisfaction.

Expectations-performance theory holds that a consumer's satisfaction is a function of his or her expectations and the offering's perceived performance. If the offering or activity matches expectations, the person is satisfied; if it exceeds them, the person is highly satisfied; if it falls short, the person is dissatisfied. Visitors to museums form these expectations on the basis of messages and claims delivered by the museum and by other communication sources. If the museum makes exaggerated claims, visitors will experience *disconfirmed expectations,* and this can lead to dissatisfaction. A visitor's satisfaction or dissatisfaction will be greater the larger the gap between expectations and performance.

Cognitive dissonance theory holds that almost every purchase or adoption of an offering is likely to lead to some postpurchase discomfort. The issues are how much discomfort and what an individual will do about it. As Festinger and Branch (1962) write: "When a person chooses between two or more alternatives, discomfort or dissonance will almost inevitably arise because of the person's knowledge that while the decision he has made has certain advantages, it also has some disadvantages. Dissonance arises after almost every decision, and further, the individual will invariably take steps to reduce this dissonance."

According to this theory, we can expect members of our prototypical family to feel some postpurchase dissonance about their choice of recreational activity. They will then seek ways to reduce the dissonance because of the natural propensity "to establish internal harmony, consistency, or congruity among [our] opinions, knowledge, and values" (Festinger, 1957, p. 260). Consumers experiencing dissonance can resort to one of two courses of action. They may try to reduce the dissonance either by abandoning the activity or by seeking information that will confirm its high value (and avoid information that would disconfirm its value).

The family's satisfaction or dissatisfaction with its choice will influence its subsequent leisure activity behaviors. If the family is satisfied, the probability is high that it will undertake a similar activity on the next occasion. It will tend to say good things about the experience to others, and this in turn is likely to arouse other people to undertake a similar activity. Postpurchase assessments are important insofar as they can either encourage or discourage repeat visits. Museums would be wise to survey a sample of departing visitors to learn what they like and dislike about the museum experience.

FACTORS INFLUENCING MUSEUM-GOING BEHAVIOR

People vary in their awareness of museums, their interest in what museums offer, their attitudes toward museums, and their disposition to visit museums. Influencing the level of their interest, awareness, and disposition are an array of cultural, social class, socialization, and personality factors. An important challenge for museum marketers is to develop an understanding of how people's backgrounds and prior attitudes and perceptions influence their museum-going behavior.

Cultural and Ethnic Factors

Cultural and ethnic factors exert an influence on attitudes and behaviors toward museums. For example, it is frequently asserted that Europeans are more involved in the arts and in museums than people in the United States. They have a longer cultural history, and their monarchies and governments have long supported the arts. Cultural and ethnic identifications provide frameworks for socialization, value patterns, beliefs, and meanings. They influence tastes and preferences, attitudes and lifestyles, and disposition to participate in museums.

Urban centers in the United States and Europe have witnessed considerable population growth, immigration, and changing demographic patterns. Large numbers of newcomers are not familiar with museums and other cultural organizations. Many come from rural areas lacking museums. Members of certain ethnic groups have perceived museums as champions of European and Western cultural values and traditions and as having little relevance to their traditions. In response, large, urban museums, in particular, are striving to make their collections, exhibitions, and programs more broadly representative, and they have organized exhibitions focusing on non-European cultures.

Social Class Factors

Social class groupings show distinct consumer preferences in leisure activities. Individuals from the same social class tend to behave more alike than individuals from different classes. Upper-class consumers, for example, are more easily reached through magazines, whereas lower-class consumers are more easily reached through television and radio. Surveys indicate differences in perception of the value of the arts across different social classes. Visitor studies have consistently shown that audiences in history, art, and science museums are disproportionately upper-middle- and upper-class and well-educated (Falk, 1993, p. 20). In contrast, visitors to zoos tend to be more of a cross section of the community, wider ranging in education and social class.

Life Cycle Factors

People pass through several life cycle stages from childhood through adulthood. Their attitudes, motivations, and consumer choices are influenced by their age and their outlook at various stages in life. Thus, although upper-middle-class parents tend to take their younger children to museums, upper-middle-class teenagers are far less likely to participate in museums. Museum attendance is more likely among adults with grown children (the *empty-nesters*) than parents still raising children.

Lifestyle Factors

Individuals who share a similar subculture, social class, and occupational background nevertheless may be drawn to different lifestyles. One person might have a belonging and relationship-building lifestyle, preferring to spend a lot of time with family and friends. Another person might have a high-achiever lifestyle, investing a great deal in professional and material success, preferring to work long hours and play hard at sports, recreation, and travel. *Lifestyle* refers to an individual's pattern of living—interests, preferences, behavioral dispositions.

Individuals create their own lifestyles, and at the same time, lifestyles reflect personality characteristics. Some people, for example, exhibit a *learning lifestyle* with boundless intellectual curiosity; this leads them to be heavy consumers of continuing education courses, foreign travel experiences, arts performances, and museum visits. Marketing specialists have identified and studied a variety of *clusters* of people with similar lifestyles to predict their attitudes, behaviors, and consumption patterns (these are discussed further in Chapter Five). The names given to the clusters reveal the lifestyles involved: for example, Blue Blood Estates, Money and Brains, Gray Power, and Pools and Patios. Marketing professionals are able to provide individual consumers with pieces of the mosaic—events, happenings, activities, experiences—that fit into their lifestyles.

Reference Groups

An individual's reference groups (peer groups, adult influences) can have a significant effect on attitudes and behaviors. Reference groups include primary groups such as family or friends and secondary groups or associations such as neighbors, coworkers, members of a church, or colleagues in the same organization. Insofar as leisure activities have a strong interpersonal and social component, group affiliations and influences can influence whether an individual gets involved in museum activities as well as the extent of that involvement. Museum visitor studies demonstrate that word of mouth is one of the most significant channels for influencing people to visit museums, and therefore adult reference groups are a significant influence disposing people to visit museums. This suggests ways for museums to stimulate visits: promote participation among groups of similar people in the form of group admission sales—for example, to employees in a given corporation or members of a church or fraternal organization.

Socialization Factors

Social science research has found a statistical association between childhood experience and adult participation in cultural events. In a study commissioned by the Cleveland Foundation to develop profiles of population segments inclined to participate in the arts, respondents were asked about the factors affecting their attendance at cultural activities, including having visited an art or cultural institution as a child, having had art education instruction as a child, and as an adult having friends who participate in the arts. Each factor was examined for its effects, and the effects of the several factors were combined. The results are presented in Figure 4.3.

The survey shows that having art education and instruction as a child is a powerful factor in shaping attitudes toward participation in the arts as an adult. So is having adult friends who participate in the arts and cultural activities. Individuals involved in arts and cultural organizations are about twice as likely to have friends who participate in the arts as those who are not. The survey shows a strong interactive effect in having both early education in the arts and later having adult friends who participate in the arts. However, early exposure to the arts, in the form of visiting a museum or cultural institution as a child, appears to have a lesser effect on subsequent participation patterns. One can

Figure 4.3. Socialization Factors Affecting Attendance at Cultural Activities.

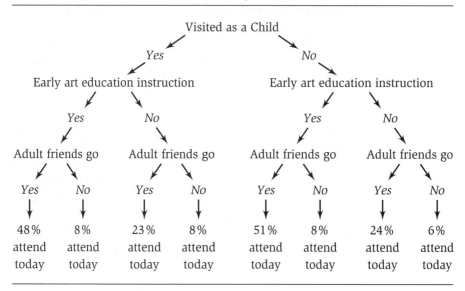

Source: *Marketing the Arts in Cleveland*, 1985.

speculate that infrequent or episodic childhood visits to a museum or to an art event are likely to have less influence than being involved in the activity on an ongoing basis, over an extended period of time.

Social Trend Factors

Social, political, economic, and technological trends can influence attitudes, values, and behaviors. Trend analyst Faith Popcorn believes that the following trends greatly characterize today's consumers (Popcorn, 1992, p. 22; see also Popcorn, 1996).

Cocooning. This is a tendency for people to look for a haven at home. It has manifested itself in skyrocketing sales of VCRs, take-out food, mail order goods, cellular phones and minivans (drive-time cocooning), and the fact that as of 1991, some 18.3 million people were working in home offices. Says Popcorn, "Don't expect consumers to come to you anymore. You'll have to reach them in the cocoon itself." This trend would seem to limit museum attendance, unless the museum itself is seen as a safe cocoon. Elaine Heumann Gurian, a former museum manager and now a museum consultant (interviewed Feb. 5, 1996), observes that museums attract certain visitor segments precisely because they are viewed as safe, secure places to visit. An alternative implication is that the museum should put more of its offerings on-line. Yet the fact that more people are working at home also suggests that they will want to get out once in a while to be part of the rest of the world.

Fantasy adventure. This is the desire of many people to have exciting exploits, heartfelt experiences, exotic adventures, and broad sensory and emotional experiences. This trend favors those museums that stir the imagination and transport the visitor to new experiences in a risk-free way. It points to the need for more interactive exhibits, including virtual reality.

Small indulgences. This trend is a response to the greed of the eighties, when people overextended themselves to buy showy luxuries. Today, people purchase accessories to update last year's outfit, a massage instead of a spa trip, a long weekend trip instead of a two-week jaunt to Europe—more incidental rewards and fewer big ones. For museum marketers, this trend suggests that people will focus on activities closer to home, as long as these promise to provide an engaging experience.

Egonomics. This trend reflects the consumer's need for customization and ego satisfaction. It suggests that people respond better to organizations that meet their personal and individualized needs. Museums can respond, for example, by soliciting a museum member's advice on exhibit ideas and by preparing alternative tours through the museum to cater to different member preferences.

The vigilante consumer. People want organizations to become more humane, value oriented, and responsive. Museums can take advantage of this trend by training their personnel to be visitor centered and service oriented.

Ninety-nine lives. This is the trend to try to do all and be all things simultaneously (work, be a parent, volunteer, travel, stay fit, achieve self-fulfilment, socialize, stay up to date, and so on). It suggests that museums should try to broaden their offerings to meet varied visitor needs and at the same time make themselves convenient so that people do not feel they are wasting precious time.

One of the best ways—in many cases, an indispensable way—for museums to identify, understand, and respond to their audiences is to incorporate into their organizations a systematic and comprehensive research process. This research process should focus on visitors and on people in the community who never or hardly ever visit. Information gathering and research are discussed further in Chapter Six. The Model Museum Practice on the Minnesota Historical Society, which concludes this chapter, illuminates the range of research applications and objectives in museums and the positive outcomes that research can bring.

SUMMARY

People who visit museums do so in their leisure time. They usually have a number of alternatives to a museum visit: cultural activities such as attending the theater or a concert; stay-at-home activities such as watching television, gardening, or entertaining friends; away-from-home activities such as going to a mall, hiking a nature trail, or attending a sports event; or substitutes for a museum visit such as browsing the museum's Web site or viewing an illustrated exhibition catalogue. To understand museum audiences, it is important for managers to learn why many people never visit, why other people visit occasionally, and why still others visit regularly. Managers must therefore investigate the process whereby museum audiences (and potential audiences) make decisions on how to spend their free time. Museums offer unique and distinctive activities and experiences, and managers have to increase the visibility and appeal of their offerings to compete with alternative leisure activities and attract larger and broader audiences.

○

MODEL MUSEUM PRACTICE

Using Audience Research to Create Engaging Museum Experiences: The Minnesota Historical Society

People are less interested in learning about facts and events in history than they are in experiencing how it felt living at a particular time.
—Marx Swanholm, senior exhibit curator,
Minnesota Historical Society, interviewed May 6, 1996

How people learn in museums is different from the way people learn in school. Museums offer visual experience rather than book learning. Visitors are self-directed. Influences are less cognitive and more emotional and intuitive.
—Barbara Franco, director,
The Historical Society of Washington, D.C., interviewed July 3, 1996

The Minnesota Historical Society (MHS) and its History Center, in St. Paul, undertake extensive audience research in planning exhibits and designing galleries. Staff continually ask the questions: What do visitors want to learn about history? How do they like to learn it? What makes exhibits lively experiences? What do families want out of their museum experience? How do schoolchildren connect their museum experience with their classroom experience?

MHS is a large museum complex with a central city museum and seventeen historic sites throughout the state of Minnesota. Its collections are extensive: 175,000 objects; 800,000 archeological artifacts; 5,500 artworks; 250,000 photographs; 37,000 maps; 38,000 cubic feet of manuscripts; and 500,000 books. MHS moved into an impressive new building of 45,000 square feet of exhibition area near the state capitol in October 1992. Once the move was completed, staff surveyed museum visitors, exploring their past museum experiences and their expectations for the new museum. Staff convened discussions internally and with outside consultants. The museum devotes two and a half staff positions to audience research. Formative and front-end studies help the museum shape new exhibits. Summative research, assessing exhibit outcomes, also is used, as is primary research exploring visitor's backgrounds, preferences, and views of museum services.

Research at MHS generated the finding that visitors have a strong interest in learning about the history of ordinary citizens and everyday life. Visitors expressed a strong interest in learning how past history shaped the choices people make in their present-day lives. These findings led staff to design exhibitions that encouraged visitors to see themselves as participants in and creators of history. Emphasis was given to making exhibit experiences personal and emotionally satisfying. The research found that visitors like to have choices of materials and perspectives, and the opportunity to interpret history for themselves. According to Maureen Otwell, assistant director for museums at MHS (interviewed Nov. 13, 1996): "The old model at history museums assumed that, with enough objects, materials, and interpretative texts, visitors would become uniformly well-informed. Exhibits tended to move along linear, chronological lines. However, visitors do not simply move along a single pathway; people think in different ways. Visitors want context (which is not the same as chronology). They want stories and ways to connect with history and to grasp personal associations and meanings."

A major direction was designing exhibits with a variety of presentational and interpretative elements to accommodate different visitor interests. Because the majority of visitors do not spend a lot of time viewing exhibit elements, MHS exhibits offer audiences reinforcing "messages" in multiple ways. In one part of the *Communities* exhibit, visitors can scan signs and text as if they were reading newspaper headlines. Other visitors can use large graphic books containing additional text and images. Staff also created a new method of presenting materials: plastic, three-sided cubes, known as *polygons,* that visitors can manipulate to find layers of texts and graphics. Visitors also can spend extended time in seating areas consulting printed and computer-generated information sources. Typical exhibits include video elements and hands-on interactive tools. In designing its new History Center facility, MHS gave major emphasis to the family-centered nature of the museum. A decision was made early on not to separate children's galleries from adult ones. Barbara Franco, former assistant director at MHS and currently director of the Historical Society of Washington, D.C. (interviewed July 3, 1996), observes: "Families in museums remind me of small hunting and gathering groups. Children take the lead, go off and forage for new things, unusual sights, and surprises, and then come back with reports for their parents."

MHS pioneered with exhibits that make history personal, immediate, relevant, and immersive. One means for doing this is *object theaters.* Currently, the History Center has two object theaters—small, intimate spaces with seating for twenty to fifty visitors each. In *Home Place Minnesota,* a rotating stage is filled with objects depicting different aspects of what it means to have a sense of place in Minnesota. A screen shows different localities and regions, voice-overs include narratives and quotations from diaries and literature, and sounds of places are heard (dogs barking, a train whistle, the sound of a stream). A narrator asks viewers, "But where is home in Minnesota? For many, it's wherever there is a bit of solitude, a bit of escape, our own personal versions of 'wilderness.'" Some words of Wallace Stegner's are read: "A place is not a place until people have been born in it, have grown up and lived in it, died in it." The second object theater, *Everything Must Change,* was developed for the *Families* exhibit, and deals with family life, relationships, and life passages (birth of a child, separations, the death of a family member). The theater offers visitors cathartic experiences in reliving common life and family experiences.

MHS's audience research closely informs its exhibit development and also generates modifications in existing exhibits. Feedback from visitors, for example, led to changes in *Communities*. Primary messages were clarified and better focused. Introductory panels were modified to improve conceptual orientation. The gallery's physical structure was improved for better visitor flow. Section headings were made visible from different vantage points in the galleries. Graphics were modified and interactive tools, improved.

Current MHS research examines the relationship of people's free-time choices and the types of museums they visit. Ahead are research programs to learn more about people as visual and experiential learners and a longitudinal study of children's attitudes toward learning history. Andrea Cutting, an audience research specialist (interviewed Jan. 24, 1997), argues for a focus on formative and front-end studies, given limited resources: "These usually do not result in big productions of findings but are the most effective in improving exhibits and museum services. If quick visitor studies exploration can prompt a slight adjustment at the beginning, we can save ourselves from major revisions later. Visitors studies should be a lubricant in the process of exhibit development rather than a crash test once the work is done."

The Minnesota Historical Society is reaping benefits from its investment in audience research. In the mid-1990s, staff expected typical visitors to spend 1.5 hours in the museum; visitors, however, are spending an average of 2.5 hours in the museum's galleries. Regular visitors are returning to the museum four times a year, whereas in the past these visitors had been returning two or three times a year. With audiences voting with their feet, visiting more often and spending more time, staff at the Minnesota Historical Society can take satisfaction in their investment in audience research.

CHAPTER FIVE

Applying Market Segmentation, Targeting, and Positioning

[O]rganizations will be required to demonstrate not only (a) that they can account for the resources entrusted to them, and (b) that they used those resources efficiently, but above all, (c) that they also used those resources effectively—that they used them to produce a positive outcome in the community they are intended to serve. . . . The museum . . . must be prepared to show in what positive ways its target community has benefited from its programs.
—Stephen E. Weil

Every organization soon recognizes that it cannot reach and appeal to all consumers in its marketplace. Potential consumers may be too numerous, widely scattered, or varied in their needs, wants, and preferences. Competitors are likely to focus on their own strengths and appeal to particular segments of consumers. Each organization, instead of attempting to reach everyone, will attempt to identify its most natural audiences and undertake specific efforts to reach and serve them.

In this chapter we will consider how a museum goes about identifying different groups with actual or potential interest in the museum's offerings and how it can build effective marketing plans to reach and serve them. We address these questions: What are the different approaches that a museum can make to its market? What are the main bases for identifying museum market segments? What criteria can museums use in targeting specific segments? How can museums position themselves to maximize their appeal to their target markets?

APPROACHES TO MARKETS

Treating all consumers in the same way may achieve economies of scale, but it ignores the diversity in most markets. Conversely, treating each person individually, in a customized way, is likely to be prohibitively expensive and impractical for most situations. The practical solution lies somewhere between the two extremes.

123

Historically, sellers of products and services had varied notions of how to approach a market. Their thinking evolved in three stages: *mass-marketing*, epitomized by Henry Ford and the Model T automobile, in which the producer sells a single product to all buyers, on the theory that this will lead to the lowest costs and prices and therefore result in the largest possible potential market; *product-variety marketing*, illustrated by General Motors's offerings of many different brands of automobiles, in which the producer offers a range of products with different features, styles, qualities, and sizes, on the theory that consumers have differing tastes and seek variety over time; and *segmentation (or target) marketing*, illustrated by Volvo and Mercedes Benz automobiles, in which the producer targets specific market segments and produces offerings for each segment.

Museums, similarly, can approach their market at the following four levels:

Mass marketing. Because mass marketing assumes that everyone is a prospect for the museum's offerings and services, the mass marketing museum pays little attention to differences in consumer behavior or preferences. The risk is that the museum's promotions and communications will be indiscriminate and scattershot, and resources are wasted. The other risk is that the museum will fail to develop strategies to attract specific groups that are likely to have a strong interest and bring advantages to the museum. The fact that the majority of people in any given community are non-museum-goers suggests that museums are better off to segment and target their audiences.

Segmentation marketing. Because segmentation marketing assumes that the market consists of distinguishable groups with varying behaviors and preferences, museums define groups that they want to attract and then run different programs for the targeted segments, such as families with young children, schoolchildren, senior citizens, ethnic groups, and so on. Segmentation marketing can cover several market segments.

Niche marketing. Niche marketing focuses on serving only one or a few groups rather than trying to attract a large number of segments. A museum with this approach will carefully focus its collections, exhibitions, and other programs to interest mostly the members of the niche. Examples of niche-oriented museums are golf museums, rare book museums, and U.S. Civil War museums.

Segment-of-one marketing. Segment-of-one marketing is practiced by museums that seek to know a lot about each member so as to serve that member better. A prime tool of this approach is to compile rich databases that include members' and donors' names, addresses, demographics, lifestyles, visitation history, donations, and other characteristics of interest. Segment-of-one marketing can lead to *customized marketing*, in which the museum customizes different experiences for different members and donors.

There are clear advantages to segmentation, niche, and segment-of-one marketing. Marketers can make finer adjustments of their offerings to match the desires of target consumers. Marketers can also fine-tune their prices, distribution channels, and promotional mix to each target segment. Instead of attempting to draw in all potential visitors with a shotgun approach, a museum can create several separate marketing programs aimed at specific markets and visitors.

BASES FOR SEGMENTING MARKETS

There is no one "right" way to segment a market. A market can be segmented in a number of ways by introducing different variables and seeing which ones shed the most light on the museum's market opportunities. Here we review the major geographical, demographic, psychographic, and behavioral variables used in segmenting consumer markets (see Table 5.1).

Geographical Segmentation

Geographical segmentation divides the market into local visitors, short-distance visitors, long-distance U.S. visitors, and overseas visitors. The assumption is that visitors from different localities will seek different offerings and have different needs. The museum can then develop different programs to attract visitors from different locations. (A variation on geographical segmentation, known as *geoclustering,* is discussed in a subsequent section.)

Demographic Segmentation

Demographic segmentation divides the market into different groups on the basis of variables such as age, sex, family size, family income, education, occupation, religion, race, and ethnicity. Demographic variables have long been the most popular bases for segmenting consumer groups. One reason is that consumer wants, preferences, and usage rates often are highly associated with these variables. Another is that demographic variables are easier to measure than most other variables. Even when the target market is described in nondemographic terms (for example, personality types), a link back to demographic characteristics is necessary in order to know the size of the target market and how to reach it efficiently. Here are some very basic examples of demographic segmentation.

Age and life cycle stage. A children's museum clearly aims its promotion at children and their parents, and a local history museum will typically focus on adults in the community. (One can only speculate on the age-linked audiences that visit the American Funeral Service Museum, in Houston.)

Sex. The Barbie Doll Hall of Fame, in Palo Alto, California, has greater appeal to girls than boys, but firearms museums and sports halls of fame tend to attract more males.

Income. A free zoo such as the Lincoln Park Zoo in Chicago is likely to attract more low-income, large families than is a zoo with an admission fee, such as the Brookfield Zoo, in a Chicago suburb.

Table 5.1. Different Bases for Market Segmentation.

Geographic

Region	Pacific, Mountain, West North Central, West South Central, East North Central, East South Central, South Atlantic, Middle Atlantic, New England
City or metro size	Under 4,999, 5,000–19,999, 20,000–49,999, 50,000–99,999, 100,000–249,999, 250,000–499,999, 500,000–999,999, 1,000,000–3,999,999, 4,000,000 or over
Density	Urban, suburban, rural
Climate	Northern, southern

Demographic

Age	Under 6, 6–11, 12–19, 20–34, 35–49, 50–64, 65+
Family life cycle	Young, single; young, married, no children; young, married, youngest child under 6; young, married, youngest child 6 or over; older, married, with children; older, married, no children under 18; older, single; other
Gender	Male, female
Income	Under $9,999, $10,000–$14,999, $15,000–$19,999, $20,000–$29,999, $30,000–$49,999, $50,000–$99,999, $100,000 and over
Occupation	Professional and technical; managers, officials, and proprietors; clerical, sales; craftspeople; professors; laborers; farmers; students; homemakers; unemployed
Education	Grade school or less, some high school, high school graduate, some college, college graduate
Religion	Catholic, Protestant, Jewish, Muslim, Hindu, other
Race	White, Asian, African American, Latino
Generation	Baby boomers, Generation X
Nationality	American, Brazilian, British, French, German, Italian, Japanese, and so on
Social class	Lower lowers, upper lowers, working class, middle class, upper middles, lower uppers, upper uppers

Psychographic

Lifestyle	Straights, swingers, longhairs, and so on
Personality	Compulsive, gregarious, authoritarian, ambitious, and so on

Behavioral

Occasions	Regular occasion, special occasion
Benefits	Quality, service, economy, speed
User status	Nonuser, ex-user, potential user, first-time user, regular user
Usage rate	Light user, medium user, heavy user
Loyalty status	None, medium, strong, absolute
Buyer-readiness stage	Unaware, aware, informed, interested, desirous, intending to buy
Attitude toward product	Enthusiastic, positive, indifferent, negative, hostile

Source: Kotler, 1997, p. 257.

Ethnicity and culture. The Metropolitan Museum of Art has pioneered in organizing exhibitions appealing to a variety of ethnic communities in the city and in motivating these communities to participate. In 1996, the museum's *Splendors of Imperial China* exhibition proved to be the best-attended museum show in the world that year, and of equal significance, the visitation of Asian Americans surpassed previous records (one in every five visitors). For its 1997 show *The Glory of Byzantium,* the museum devised a major ethnic marketing campaign to draw many of the 424,000 Armenians, Greeks, Russians, and Ukrainians in the greater New York area to the show and advertised heavily in ethnic media.

Psychographic Segmentation

People within the same demographic group can exhibit very different *psychographic profiles.* Thus museums can classify potential visitors on the basis of social class, lifestyle, or personality characteristics.

Social class. Social classes are relatively homogeneous and enduring divisions in any society that is hierarchically ordered, and class members share similar values, interests, and behaviors. Social scientists have identified six social classes, on the basis of income, occupation, education, and type of residence: (1) upper uppers (less than 1 percent); (2) lower uppers (about 2 percent); (3) upper middles (12 percent); (4) lower middles (30 percent); (5) upper lowers (35 percent); and (6) lower lowers (20 percent). Museums overall tend to attract visitors and members disproportionately from upper- and upper-middle-income and highly educated segments of the population. A study of museum-goers attending the King Tut exhibit held in New Orleans showed that, despite the effort at mass marketing, attendance came heavily from the upper and upper-middle classes (Robbins and Robbins, 1979, pp. 479–484).

Lifestyle. Even within a social class, different consumer lifestyles are found. Researchers can identify lifestyles by interviewing people about their activities, interests, and opinions and then clustering similar groups. Lifestyles can differ in terms of activity level, preference for outdoor versus indoor activities, attraction to the arts, and so on. Museums typically have an easier time attracting people with cultural, historical, and intellectual interests than with sports interests, for example. Increasing numbers of museums are targeting segments by lifestyle. Art museums, as an example, are expanding programs such as social events for young professionals, and thereby are segmenting by lifestyle, age, and life cycle.

Personality. Consumers exhibit different personality characteristics, such as dominance, dependence, gregariousness, introversion, and so on. Marketers have used personality variables to segment markets, and have then endowed their products with *brand personalities* (or *brand images*) designed to appeal to corresponding *consumer personalities* (or *self-image*). A firearms museum, for example, might segment its promotion not only to males but to males with a macho cast to their personalities. Advertising would then highlight features and offerings that appeal to this personality type.

Behavioral Segmentation

Behavioral segmentation divides consumers into groups on the basis of their knowledge, attitude, or use of a given set of products or services. Many marketers believe that behavioral variables are the best starting point for constructing meaningful market segments. Here are some behavioral variables that can be used.

Occasion. Consumers can be distinguished according to occasions when they engage in a specific activity. Some people visit a museum on the occasion of a family outing. Others visit because of a particular advertised exhibit or program. Still others visit because they are seeking something to do and prefer to be around other people. Some people come to museums because they are seeking a private quiet time for meditation or inspiration. Out-of-town guests are taken to museums to show them interesting institutions in the community. Single professional people might pay a visit to a museum after working hours to attend a singles social event. Occasions, happenings, and special events become the attractions in this kind of behavioral marketing.

Benefits sought. Consumers can be segmented according to the particular benefits or outcomes they are seeking in a product or an offering. A family might visit a museum as part of a broader outing experience—getting away from the house, traveling a distance, finding a new experience in an unusual setting. Another family might visit to bring their children in contact with a learning experience. Art lovers visit art museums to be inspired by masterpieces of visual art. People seeking an adventurous or thrilling experience are likely to visit an amusement or theme park.

User status. Consumers can be behaviorally divided by user status: nonusers, ex-users, potential users, and first-time users of a product, service, or museum offering. Similarly, markets can be segmented by light, medium, and heavy users. Heavy users may constitute only a small percentage of the consumer population but a major percentage of the use volume. Marketers attempt to identify the demographic and psychographic characteristics and the media habits of these different user groups (see Exhibit 5.1).

Loyalty status. Loyalty status describes the strength, from zero to absolute, of a consumer's preference for a particular organization or entity. Consumers can be deeply loyal to a brand (for example, Cadillac automobiles), an organization (Metropolitan Museum of Art), a place (New York City), a celebrity (Jasper Johns), and so on. A museum should research the degree of loyalty of its visitors and members. Four groups can be distinguished: (1) *hard-core loyals,* who are highly devoted to the organization; (2) *soft-core loyals,* who are devoted to two or three organizations; (3) *shifting loyals,* who are gradually

○○○○○

Exhibit 5.1. Museum Usage Rates: Nonusers, Light Users, Medium Users, and Heavy Users.

Museums have a strong interest in learning about the characteristics of nonvisitors (nonusers), light users, medium users, and heavy users. This information will help museums understand better who their audiences are and facilitate the conversion of nonusers into light users and light users into heavy users.

Nonvisitors. Museum visitation rates are not precisely measured, especially because many museums do not charge admission fees or use tickets, turnstiles, or other reliable means of counting. However, there have been enough studies at enough museums to roughly estimate proportions of nonusers and light and heavy users. A review of studies finds that infrequent visitation (at least once a year) accounts for less than 40 percent of the population. Frequent visitation (four or more visits per year to a single museum or group of museums) is estimated at 20 percent of the population. Nonvisitors, then, according to these estimates, account for approximately half of the population (Falk, 1993).

Adult museum nonusers tend to be in lower socioeconomic groups. Their lower educational level suggests they may identify museums with schooling, something that does not give them pleasure. Their work life might drain a lot of their energy, causing them to prefer to spend their leisure time more passively. Museum nonvisitors, in a study of leisure choices, tend to value highly leisure activities that are social and interactive, involve active participation, and let them feel comfortable about their surroundings. They tend to view museums, overall, as formal and inaccessible places that put restrictions on individual behavior and group interaction. There is evidence than nonvisitors lacked opportunities as children to visit museums or become socialized to using them (Hood, 1983, p. 54).

Light Users. Light users (some studies call them *occasional* or *infrequent visitors*) can be defined as people who visit a museum once a year. Light users tend to be middle class, with average educations and incomes. They respect education and learning but do not make it a central part of their lives. In attitudes toward leisure, they tend to be closer to nonusers than to heavy users. For example, light users tend to have been socialized as children into valuing group activity, entertainment, and active forms of participation. They prefer family-centered and group activities, and they place a high premium on relaxation rather than stimulation. Studies show that zoos attract members of the nonuser and light-user groups to a higher degree.

Heavy Users. Heavy users (*frequent* or *active visitors,* in some studies) are people who attend museums several times a year. Heavy users tend to come from higher socioeconomic groups. They tend to be highly educated, upper income, and professional. According to one significant study, heavy users scored high on six leisure values, chief among them learning, having challenging experiences, and doing something worthwhile. These people have had museum visits on their leisure agenda for a long time; they identify with museum values and methods, and they feel comfortable in the surroundings. Heavy users form the core of a museum's supporters. They can be counted upon to become members, sometimes join as volunteers, and to contribute to fundraising campaigns. Every museum should have a list of these members in its database and maintain a steady stream of communication with them.

○○○○○

moving from favoring one organization to favoring another organization; and (4) *switchers,* who show no loyalty to any organization. If a museum has a substantial membership base and most of those members are hard-core or even soft-core loyals, the museum is basically healthy. It might study its loyals to determine the basic satisfactions they derive from museum affiliation, and then attempt to attract others who are seeking similar satisfactions.

Stage of adopter readiness. At any point of time, people are in various stages of *readiness* toward adopting a product or offering. Some are unaware of the product or activity, some are aware only, some are informed, some are interested, some are desirous, and some intend to adopt it. The distribution of people over the different stages of adopter readiness has a major bearing on the design of a museum's marketing program. For example, if most of the potential market is unaware, the museum needs to mount a strong awareness-building, image-oriented communication and promotion program.

Attitude. Museums can divide a population according to people's attitudes toward a particular offering or toward the museum as a whole. People will fall along a continuum from *enthusiasts* to *positives* to *indifferents* to *negatives* to *hostiles.* Each group might have associated demographics and psychographics. A museum will want to focus on the enthusiasts and positives and possibly expend some effort to convert indifferents into positives.

Geodemographic Segmentation

Many of the previous variables can be combined to yield rich descriptions of specific groups and the geographical areas where they are found. Claritas Inc., a marketing consulting firm, has developed a geoclustering approach called PRIZM, which classifies U.S. residential neighborhoods and other localities into sixty-two lifestyle groupings (*PRIZM clusters*). The clustering is based on thirty-nine variables that fall into five broad categories: (1) education and affluence, (2) family life cycle, (3) urbanization, (4) race and ethnicity, and (5) mobility. The assumption is that people with similar backgrounds and interests tend to reside near to one another. Therefore clusters are identified by ZIP code, block, or census tract data. Individuals in each cluster tend to have similar backgrounds, lead similar lives, and enjoy similar interests. The clusters' titles convey their characteristics: for example, Blue Blood Estates, Young Influentials, Urban Gold Coast, Gray Power, Mid-City Mix, Pools and Patios, Shotguns and Pickups, and Towns and Gowns. A museum can use PRIZM to answer a variety of questions: Which clusters and neighborhoods contain our best prospects for audiences? How deeply have we penetrated our best prospect clusters? What is the best way to communicate with each cluster? Geoclustering has significant benefits for communication and promotion programs (see Exhibit 5.2).

When the National Symphony Orchestra (NSO), in Washington, D.C., profiled its ten thousand subscribers in 1985, for example, it discovered that four times more residents in Money and Brains neighborhoods attended concerts than did residents in Winner's Circle neighborhoods. The major difference is that the former cluster is composed of cosmopolitan singles and couples and the latter consists of affluent suburban families with young children. As a result the NSO's 1986 telemarketing campaign focused on cultivating certain previously ignored neighborhoods, like the Capitol Hill neighborhood, where the childless Bohemian Mix resides. In some of the targeted areas, subscription sales jumped 25 percent (Weiss, 1988, pp. 2, 15).

The Young Literati cluster, for example, is an attractive target for museums (see Exhibit 5.2). An understanding of Young Literati characteristics can help museum managers learn where best to reach these individuals with publicity and promotions, which exhibitions and benefits to promote, and even which corporations might be willing to sponsor a museum program targeted to the Young Literati.

Geoclustering is finding growing use as a segmentation tool due to three major developments. First, the Census Bureau reports are now releasing more detailed data at smaller and narrower geographical levels. Second, the U.S. population is growing in diversity, with faster population growth among certain ethnic groups, more women in the workforce, changing household structures, and changing size of age groups. Third, marketing to microsegments has become possible even for small organizations as database costs decline, personal computers proliferate, and software becomes easier to use.

Organizational Segmentation

Museums find it useful to segment organizations as well as visitors and members (also see Chapter Eleven). For example, an art museum development office might be seeking a small grant from an organization to support an exhibition of local student art. It will first distinguish between different organizations: foundations, government agencies, and corporations. If it decides to seek a foundation grant, it needs to distinguish between different sizes and types of foundations. For example, large foundations will not be interested in making small grants. Museums seeking corporate support will have to research the most appropriate industries and companies to cultivate, distinguishing them initially by size, location, product lines, and resources. Segmenting companies to identify potential museum sponsors is a major objective for museum development offices.

Museums are increasingly developing programs to attract new audiences through people's organizational affiliations. Museums can reach religious communities through churches and synagogues, senior citizens through community centers, and workers and professionals through employers. Promotion or membership programs can offer members of the targeted organizations such benefits as admission and gift shop discounts. The benefits to museums of organizational targeting are noteworthy: the ability to reach sizable numbers of

○○○○○

Exhibit 5.2. The Young Literati Cluster.

The Young Literati cluster consists primarily of upscale urban singles and couples without children, most of whom are college graduates; have professional, managerial, or other white-collar occupations; have a median household income of $52,100; and own (48.6 percent) or rent (51.4 percent) multiunit housing in urban uptown areas. The median home value is $245,200; 24.5 percent have moved within the past year; 14.3 percent last moved twenty or more years ago. Their predominant age ranges are 25 to 34 and 35 to 54, with a median age of 43.4. Among the Young Literati, 23.5 percent are married, 14.7 percent are married couples with children, 5.1 percent are single parents, and 56.8 percent are single. Here are some additional characteristics.

Ethnicity:

Ethnic Group	U.S. Population (percent)	Cluster (percent)
White	83.2	84.1
Black	12.4	7.4
Asian	5.4	14.9
Hispanic	9.9	9.4
All other	4.4	8.5

Lifestyle: More Likely to

- Rent foreign videos
- Travel to Japan, Asia
- Go jogging
- Spend $60/month + for dry cleaning
- Go scuba diving/snorkeling
- Attend live theater
- Use home pregnancy tests
- Play racquetball
- Buy hardcover books
- Go to the movies

Products and Services: More Likely to

- Have travel insurance
- Own state/local government bonds
- Own tax-exempt funds
- Have a gold/premium credit card
- Use an ATM card
- Own stock valued $10,000 +
- Own an Audi
- Buy a Mont Blanc/Waterman pen
- Own a Volkswagen
- Buy gourmet coffee beans
- Buy a $100 + sweater
- Drink imported beer often
- Own pagers/beepers
- Buy designer jeans
- Use olive oil
- Drink gin, low/no alcohol beer
- Eat Wheaties
- Buy Quaker Puffed Rice
- Own a CD player
- Buy Adidas shoes

Radio and TV: More Likely to

- Listen to progressive rock radio
- Watch the Travel Channel
- Listen to soft contemporary radio
- Watch BET
- Listen to contemporary radio
- Watch *The NewsHour with Jim Lehrer*
- Watch *Masterpiece Theatre*
- Watch Cinemax
- Watch *The Simpsons*
- Watch *Entertainment Tonight*

Print: More Likely to

- Read newspaper business section
- Read *Self*
- Read *Metropolitan Home*
- Read newspaper style/fashion section
- Read *Rolling Stone*
- Read *GQ*
- Read *Penthouse*
- Read *Elle*
- Read *Time*
- Read *Road & Track*

Note: A Claritas map shows that Young Literati clusters are most dense in northern and southern California, Minnesota, and Texas and in the greater metropolitan areas surrounding such cities as Boston, New York, Philadelphia, and Chicago.

Source: Prizm, Claritas Inc., 1994. Reprinted with permission.

○○○○○

potential visitors who are already segmented in terms of their interests and behaviors, and the ability to reach potential visitors who are opinion leaders in their respective organizations and communities.

Requirements for Effective Segmentation

There are many ways to segment a market. Segments turn out to be most useful when they exhibit three major characteristics:

- *Measurability.* The museum should be able to estimate the size of a proposed segment. For example, a natural history museum can estimate the number of teenagers living within a five-mile radius who might be attracted to a new exhibition on dinosaurs.

- *Substantiality.* The museum should find the segment large enough to be worth attracting. Given its limited resources the museum must focus primarily on attracting segments of sufficient size to make a difference.

- *Accessibility.* The museum should be able to communicate efficiently with the individuals in a chosen segment. For example, lists of high school teachers already exist, so a museum could promote its new dinosaur exhibition by sending announcements to local high school teachers.

TARGETING SPECIFIC MARKET SEGMENTS

Most museums welcome all visitors. The purpose of targeting is to attract and develop additional groups that might not come at all or might be less involved than desired in the museum's many activities. Deciding which groups to target, and how many, is a matter of *target market selection.* These are some target market issues:

- Should the museum try to attract the disabled? On the positive side this will attract a new audience that might also bring along friends who have not been to a museum. However, the museum will have to build special ramps, create large print material, and offer other services.

- Should the museum actively attract members of the gay and lesbian community? *Advertising Age* magazine in January 1993 reported that gays and lesbians are estimated to represent 10 percent of the U.S. population and to have a combined annual income of $514 billion. Furthermore, compared to the average American, gay men and lesbians are several times more likely to have traveled to Europe in the past three years, 6.5 times more likely to buy at least ten to fifteen hardcover books per year, and 10 times more likely to buy thirteen or more compact discs per year. This suggests that this market would have much more interest in museum attendance than the average American.

- Should the museum actively attract other groups who might be under-served, such as ethnic and cultural minorities, teenagers, and tourists from overseas? The issue is not whether a museum should welcome multiple and diversified groups but rather how to attract them so that the presence of one group will not interfere with the presence of others.

The actual choice of target markets depends on specific factors affecting the museum—its collections, subject matter, location, goals, and so forth. The more limited the museum's resources, the more likely it is that it can concentrate on only a few segments. The more homogeneous its market, the less the museum needs to diversify its offerings. If other cultural organizations have already captured the loyalty of certain segments, the museum needs to identify yet other segments to attract. Museums should focus on market segments that they have a good chance of attracting and a differential advantage in serving. The Model Museum Practice at the end of this chapter illustrates targeted outreach programs at the Johnson County Museums, in Shawnee, Kansas.

POSITIONING THE MUSEUM AND ITS OFFERINGS

Once a museum identifies relevant segments and decides which segments to target, it then has to deal with the matter of positioning. We define *positioning* as *the act of designing an organizational image, values, and offerings, so that consumers understand, appreciate, and are drawn to what the organization stands for in relation to its competitors.* Positioning a museum follows principles similar to positioning commercial products. The specific positioning that a museum adopts will depend on its analysis of its market segments; its strengths, weaknesses, and distinctive offerings; and its competition. As we have emphasized, the leisure, recreational, entertainment, and education sectors are highly competitive.

Each museum should strive to develop an identity in the public's mind so that its salient characteristics are clear and it is not confused with other museums and other leisure activity organizations. Consider a new science museum. It may have to decide about positioning itself as a museum with serious scientific exhibitions, as a museum designed primarily to engage young people, as a museum aimed primarily at adults who seek science literacy, or as a museum that achieves several such goals. When deciding on positioning, museums must consider the broadest range of offerings and benefits its visitors are likely to seek or expect. Because the public image of an organization is affected not only by image building and marketing but also by factors beyond its control, a disparity can develop between intended image and actual image. Museums must periodically monitor the quality of their actual images.

Measuring a Museum's Image

The starting point for any positioning strategy is to understand how the museum is perceived in relation to other museums and competing leisure activity organizations. This requires measuring the organization's image. *Image* can be defined as *the sum of beliefs, ideas, and impressions that people have of an entity.* (Note, however, that an individual's image of an entity does not necessarily reveal his or her *attitude* toward it. Two people may hold the same image of a museum and yet have different attitudes toward it, reflecting different interests, preconceptions, and priorities.)

Many methods are available for measuring images. We describe a two-step approach: first, measuring how familiar and favorable a museum's image is and, second, measuring that image along several relevant dimensions.

Familiarity and Favorability Measurement. The first step is to gauge how familiar the museum is to the members of a given group or segment and how favorably they feel toward it. To establish familiarity, respondents are asked to rate their own knowledge of the museum (often on a five-point scale such as "never heard of it," "heard of it," "know a little bit about it," "know a fair amount about it," "know it very well"). If most respondents place the museum in the first two or three categories, the museum has an awareness problem. Respondents who are familiar with the museum are then asked to rate how they feel toward it on another five-point scale ("very unfavorable," "somewhat unfavorable," "indifferent," "somewhat favorable," "very favorable"). If most respondents check the first two or three categories, the museum has a serious image problem.

Semantic Differential. In the next step, the museum researches the contents of its image. For this step, museums can construct a tool called a *semantic differential*, as follows:

1. *Develop a set of relevant attributes.* The research starts by having respondents identify the attributes they would normally use when thinking about the museum: "What attributes do you think of when you consider a museum?" If a respondent suggests "staff helpfulness," for example, this is converted into a bipolar adjective scale with "unhelpful staff" at one end and "helpful staff" at the other. It could be rendered as a five- or seven-point scale. (See Figure 5.1, which also shows a number of common useful attributes.)

2. *Reduce the set of attributes.* Here the number of attributes is kept small to avoid respondent fatigue. Image measurement researchers argue there are essentially three types of relevant scales: *evaluation scales* (good-bad qualities); *potency scales* (strong-weak qualities); and *activity scales* (active-passive qualities). By

using these new scales as a guide or by performing a factor analysis, the researcher can remove redundant scales (Osgood, Suci, and Tannenbaum, 1957).

3.   *Administer the instrument to a sample of respondents.* Here respondents are asked to rate one or several museums. The bipolar adjectives should be arranged so as not to place all of the negative choices at the same end of the scale.

4.   *Average the results.* Figure 5.1 shows the results of averaging respondents' images of Museums A, B, and C. Each museum's image is represented by a vertical *line of means,* which summarizes how the average respondent sees each museum. Thus Museum A is viewed very positively, Museum C is viewed negatively, and Museum B is viewed somewhere in between.

5.   *Check image variance.* Because each image profile is a line of means, it does not reveal how variable the image is among different respondents. Did respondents cluster around the mean, or was there considerable variation? In the first case the museum's image is well defined and in the second case it is not. The museum will want to analyze whether a variable image is the result of different subgroups of respondents rating the museum, with each subgroup having a different but consistent image.

Museums can acquire an image based on a distinctive collection. The Art Institute of Chicago, for example, has been singularly regarded over many years as having one of the world's greatest collections of Impressionist art. Less attention, in certain segments, is paid to the fact that it is an encyclopedic museum, with extraordinary collections spanning history, cultures, and geography. The Smithsonian Institution, despite its massive collections encompassing art, history, culture, science, and technology, is known by many people for particular treasures or icons, such as the Hope Diamond, Dorothy's red slippers from the movie *The Wizard of Oz,* and such historic machines as the Wright Brothers' flying machines and Charles Lindbergh's *Spirit of St. Louis.*

Figure 5.1. Images of Three Museums (Semantic Differential).

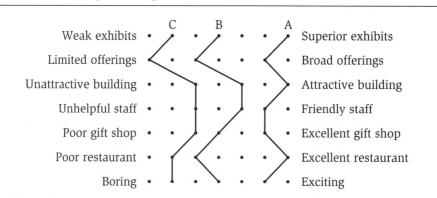

Source: Marketing Management (9th ed.) by Kotler, Philip, © 1997. Adapted by permission of Prentice-Hall, Inc., Upper Saddle River, NJ.

The Museum of Science, Boston. The museum's use of its new logo on store merchandise helps to build brand awareness and image.

Photo courtesy of the Museum of Science, Boston.

Museum images can be communicated by the merchandise sold in the museum shops. The illustration above shows goods in the Museum of Science shop, with the museum's brand image and its logo design (see the Model Museum Practice at the end of Chapter Nine).

Science and technology centers and natural history museums often position themselves according to the benefits they provide. The Denver Museum of Natural History invites visitors to "Entertain Your Brain," appealing to the fun and adventure of learning, as opposed to the fantasy and escapism that typify amusement and theme parks. Chicago's Museum of Science & Industry has used in the past the tag line "We've Got Fun Down to a Science!" The Carnegie Science Center has used the line "Fun at Your Fingertips" to highlight its interactive, participatory, and virtual reality experiences. Children's museums typically position themselves in terms of both users and benefits. The Children's Museum of Manhattan offers an "ideal setting to encourage toddlers to step out and explore, in a safe and stimulating environment." History and heritage museums are increasingly positioning themselves as places where visitors can participate in history, not just view the past. Historic sites offer immersion through *living history* experiences. At Harpers Ferry, West Virginia, the site of a major event triggering the American Civil War, visitors can immerse themselves in the historical period just prior to the war. Visitors stroll along streets with storefronts filled with workers engaged in mid-nineteenth-century trades. Guides are dressed in period costumes; they tell tales of what life was like and answer questions. Buildings are decorated as they appeared in that historical period. Sovereign Hill, in Ballarat, Australia, a reconstructed 1850s gold rush town, invites schoolchildren to spend two or three days as residents, dressing in period clothes, eating the food served in the 1850s, and simulating the experiences of those historic times.

Art museums have positioned themselves in several distinctive ways. Some seek to make their audiences feel comfortable with works of art, art history, and artists' lives and work. The St. Louis Art Museum, for example, invites visitors to probe and learn about particularly difficult art forms such as nonrepresentational art. New York City's New Museum of Contemporary Art seeks to demystify the esotericism, glamour, and precious values of established art and at the same time raise the visibility of avant-garde art forms. It also engages visitors in contemporary social issues, such as homelessness and drugs, raising consciousness through art. The Morris Museum of Art, in Augusta, Georgia, announces to its visitors, "As the home for a broad-based survey collection of Southern art, the Morris Museum is preserving and enhancing a cultural legacy." The museum highlights its purpose to "explore the art and soul of the South" both with collections that illuminate the history of America's South as well as with collections that offer artists' visions of contemporary Southern life and culture.

Positioning Strategies for Museums

Three main types of positioning strategies are available to museums:

- *Attribute positioning.* A museum describes itself in terms of some feature or attribute: for example, "the state's oldest art museum"; "the nation's most visited museum"; "the county's newest science museum."

- *Benefit positioning.* A museum describes itself in terms of some benefit it offers to visitors: for example, "the active hands-on science museum"; "a quiet museum for contemplation"; "a museum combining fun and learning"; "a museum for active, lifelong learners."

- *User positioning.* A museum defines itself in terms of the main intended users, visitors, or members: for example, "a leading African American museum"; "a children's museum"; "a community museum."

Choosing Positioning Variables and the Differences to Promote

If a museum takes the approach of positioning itself primarily as a provider of benefits, it has to determine further the range of benefits and the type of benefits it seeks to promote. For example, Museum A might decide it can promote itself as a museum with high-end services such as an elegant restaurant and a state-of-the art gift shop with the highest-quality goods; Museum B might decide it can position itself as a low-cost museum (with no admission fee or a low family fee and also free parking); and Museum C might decide it can position itself as a user-friendly museum with ample information, orientation, and support from guides and docents. Museums also can differentiate themselves in terms of the experiences they offer visitors for which they are best known. These are the experiences visitors can have from viewing particular exhibits or participating in particular programs or enjoying the museum's setting and surroundings. Some museums have taken great pains to distinguish their offerings from the offerings of theme parks and other mass entertainment organizations, generating the dichotomy of entertainment and education. This distinction, however, is simplifying insofar as a range of activities exists, some of which combine elements of entertainment and education. Museums, in thinking about their positioning, can benefit from assessing the range of recreational experiences they offer visitors and the position they occupy along this range. The categories, as shown in Figure 5.2, form a continuum, spanning visceral, emotional, and intellectual characteristics. These categories are illustrative and there is interaction and overlap between them. One museum, for example, can decide that the core experience it offers, that which distinguishes it from competitors, is in providing a contemplative environment, while a secondary experience it can offer is a learning experience. Another museum can decide that its core experience is an experience of amusement and combine this with learning experiences.

Museums, like other organizations, can differentiate themselves in terms of a variety of facets and features, such as offering exceptional quality, service, price, value, or uniqueness of experience. Increasingly, museums are assigning greater attention to *service* differentiation and positioning (high-quality information, dining and shopping facilities, providing child strollers, and so on); *personnel* differentiation (friendliness, caring, responsiveness, and competence of staff);

Figure 5.2. Range of Recreational Experiences.

Excitement	Amusement	Contemplation	Learning
Thrill	Fun	Musing	Curiosity and discovery
Adventure	Gaming	Meditation	Observation
Fantasy	→ Pleasure	↔ Reverie	↔ Pattern discernment
Immersive	Laughter	Pondering	Instruction
experience	Sociability	Aesthetic experience	Skill-building practice
	Diversion		Experimentation
	Visceral ↔	Emotional ↔	Intellectual

and *technological* differentiation (interactive tools, virtual-reality presentations, computer-generated information, Web sites, electronic maps to collections and galleries that enable visitors to design their own tours). The Chicago Historical Society uses a micropositioning approach for each of its four target segments: history lovers, heritage identifiers, the culturally aware, and entertainment- and experience-oriented visitors. It has identified the primary benefit each segment seeks, the demographics and size of each segment, and the kinds of services each segment looks for in a museum visit. For each visitor segment, it asks

- What is the customer's desire that will bring him or her to the museum?
- Will the museum's offering be highly valued by the customer?
- Will the museum's offering seem different and better than the competitors' offerings?
- Can the museum communicate its offering effectively to the customer?

Positioning, finally, requires museum staff to determine how many differences and which differences to promote in its positioning strategy. Many marketers advocate projecting a number of benefits to each target segment but emphasizing one as the core benefit; that one becomes the museum's *unique selling proposition.*

An excellent example of the work involved in positioning is evident in the planning at Chicago's new Museum Campus (see illustration in the Conclusion). The first objective of the planning and positioning efforts is a highly visible opening of the Campus, scheduled for June 1998. The second objective is to build and sustain an image and a brand identity for the Campus for subsequent years and to position the Campus's distinctive offerings and benefits to the target audience segments over the long term. The Museum Campus, covering nine acres of new parkland, was created after the city government rerouted a major highway that had divided three museums—the Field Museum, the John G. Shedd Aquarium, and the Adler Planetarium and Astronomy Museum—that have now been integrated and connected as a single destination site. The Museum Campus—the parkland around the museums—is being designed as a fourth destination, independent of the museums and yet reinforcing their value and attractiveness. The planning and positioning of the Museum Campus initially involves designing a distinctive image for the Campus itself. One remarkable facet of this planning is the close collaboration among the three museums involved.

The Museum Campus's preliminary marketing plan involves two phases: a phase of creating awareness and a phase of promoting activities and events. A team of professionals drawn from the three museums are designing an image-building program and establishing partnerships with the city government, the travel and hospitality sectors, schools and libraries, corporations, destination sites such as convention centers, and other appropriate groups. The team is also identifying the Campus's competition, which is a central element in a positioning strategy. In its preliminary plan, the Museum Campus team has identified among its competitors Navy Pier, largely a theme park similar to Baltimore's Inner Harbor, filled with shops and eateries, that also houses the city's premier children's museum; downtown Chicago, a few miles away, an area filled with leisure activity options; and Lincoln Park and Grant Park, two of the public parks where Chicagoans go to stroll and bike and relax. The planning also involves identifying audience segments and targeting the most promising ones (for example, employees and professionals who work downtown, who would be able to take lunch breaks at the Campus), developing pricing strategies (covering parking, public transportation, food services, admission to museums), and selecting communication vehicles and methods of promotion.

The Museum Campus will be a new attraction in a city already filled with activities and experiences for citizens and tourists to enjoy. That is why the planners are already working on differentiating the Campus from the competition. One concept under consideration is that the Museum Campus will offer visitors "intelligent entertainment"—a depth of content and a richness of design and aesthetic pleasures that few competitors can rival, a combination of intellectual and entertaining experiences, and a brand identity as the "smart choice" for Chicagoans' leisure time. By examining what competitors are offering, the Museum Campus team is raising the right questions, focusing on important issues, and marshaling resources to the task of designing an effective positioning strategy (interview with Christy MacLear, campus coordinator, Aug. 26, 1997).

SUMMARY

If consumer (client, visitor, user) orientation and service lie at the heart of marketing, one of the principal elements in marketing planning is the application of the principles of market segmentation, targeting, and positioning to a museum's strategic planning process. To build its audience, a museum has to identify the range of individuals and groups that would have an interest in its offerings and the other segments that might potentially have an interest if they were effectively approached. At a second stage, the museum has to determine which segments to focus efforts on both to attract new audiences and sustain existing ones. Museums, like other organizations, cannot be all things to all people, and they would be wasting resources if they tried to promote themselves to every group. However, museums should be broad in their offerings and focus on priority individuals and groups as target audiences. Once audience segments have been determined, the museum can design an image and a set of offering that will be appealing to its target audience and give the museum an advantage over its competitors.

O

MODEL MUSEUM PRACTICE

Building Community Involvement in the Johnson County Museums

Changes and trends at the Johnson County Museums (JCM), in Shawnee, Kansas, part of the metropolitan area surrounding Kansas City, illustrate the challenges affecting small and medium-sized museums in an increasingly competitive environment.

"JCM, in the first few decades, was narrowly focused," says Janet Bruce Campbell, the museum director (interviewed Apr. 22, 1996). "The museums' visibility in the community was low. In the early 1990s, the museum board launched a strategic planning process with the goal of building a strong relationship with the surrounding communities—strong enough to give citizens a sense of participation in the museums' activities."

Established in 1967 and housing a collection of twenty-five thousand objects, the Johnson County Museums are an agency of the county government, which provided in the mid-1990s approximately 70 percent of the museums' funding and the budget of $500,000. The museums also have a nonprofit unit that assists in raising private-sector support. A key part of the new strategic plan calls for a shift in the resource base from one of predominant government funding to a better balance between private- and public-sector support.

JCM, like other historical museums, has changed the way history is presented and interpreted. In the past, objects were the focus of attention and the ideas, events, and stories they represented had secondary status. Today, the museum focuses both on objects and on ideas and narratives. A JCM brochure, "Opportunity 98: A Community Legacy," announced plans for a new permanent exhibition on community life, describing the function of history as discovering "the individual and collective choices that have shaped our community over the last 150 years."

JCM has a major objective in building community support. One key program to accomplish this is a new permanent exhibition, *Seeking the Good Life.* Opening in 1998, the exhibition will explore "how ordinary Americans have envisioned and defined the 'good' life from 1820 to the present." Community residents have been invited to donate items of everyday life to the exhibit, objects that illuminate how their forebears lived. The spring 1996 issue of *Album,* the JCM newsletter, called on readers to "be a part of history," "put your family in the museum, and join the 'Community Collection Initiative.'" It also listed items sought for the restoration of a model home the museum has acquired: "upholstered 'barrel' style chairs," "27-inch Sylvania television with remote," "brass floor lamp with shade," "traditional-style sofa." "Our history is the story of ordinary and extraordinary families who have lived, worked, and played in Johnson County," the newsletter told its readers. "This story—your story—is the focus of the Johnson County Museums. We invite you to put your family in the museum and help us preserve the community's memory."

The exhibit planning process involved an estimated 250 people in the community, including community leaders, museum supporters, and educators and others who had not been active museum participants. According to Campbell, citizens "not only want the museum to be useful to the community, but they also want the museum to show how past history informs the choices and decisions that people have to make today in their own lives."

It was the community collection initiative, begun in 1994 with a grant from the National Endowment for the Humanities, that resulted in the museum's acquisition of the 1950s all-electric model house, a historic property that was part of a pioneering subdivision built near Kansas City. The house was donated by its owners after they learned about JCM's exhibition plans and interest in collecting recent community history. "The interpretation won't be that this house was typical," Janet Campbell remarked. "This house was the dream—that's what people aspired to." Built by the local electric company as a demonstration of the benefits of future electronic technology, the house contains many devices largely unheard-of at the time: a heat pump for central heating and cooling, a garbage disposal and indoor electric grill, built-in germicidal and fluorescent sunlamps in one of the bathrooms, a ceiling spotlight in the dining room that simulates candlelight, "moonglow lighting" along the floor, an electric garage door opener, and an instrument panel installed in the kitchen that allowed residents to monitor the lamps and appliances that were being used.

Several years ago, JCM restored a single-room schoolhouse, built in 1869, and furnished it with objects recreating the classroom experience as it existed in 1904. Docents at the Lanesfield School site dress in period clothing and offer both tours of the building and nature tours of the adjoining land, part of the historic Santa Fe Trail. The docents teach school lessons as they were taught at the turn of the century.

The Johnson County Museums are forging community relations in other ways. They are investing significant resources in designing exhibitions that highlight the contributions of various ethnic and cultural groups to the life of the community. For each exhibition, staff consult with community groups and call on members of the groups to contribute items and objects for the exhibitions. The 1996 exhibit *Shalom: Building a Jewish Community*, for example, highlighted the contributions of the Jewish community of Kansas City and Johnson County.

A regular feature in *Album* is "History Mystery," which invites readers to identify people and places shown in historical photographs. To help preserve people's sense of place, the museum is midway through a ten-year project to photo-document each structure built in the county prior to 1950. From this pool of photos, museum staff work with local planning offices and community volunteers to determine the key structures that provide community identity and develop strategies for their preservation.

Museum programs have increasingly focused on children and families with children. JCM offers workshops for parents and children in arts and crafts, research on family histories, nature study along the Santa Fe Trail, and workshops on local architectural styles and neighborhood history. Museum special events include Christmas activities, a May Day celebration, and a Prairie Sampler, which re-creates turn-of-the-century community life.

The Johnson County Museums have involved the community in planning and development to build a sense of ownership and investment in the museums' activities. Each program reinforces the theme of building a sense of community and projects an image of the JCM as an integral part of the community. In the long term, the museums' leadership hopes that the community will generate expanded private support. Like many other museums receiving public-sector support, JCM is anticipating a time when the museums no longer can depend on government funds as their principal means of support.

JCM's success with its community initiatives is evident in the doubling of its permanent collection between 1987 and 1994. In 1996, JCM welcomed thirty thousand visitors—about six times as many as visited in 1987. The number of tourists and of visitors from outside the metropolitan area is also increasing. Begun in 1988, the museums' membership program now numbers 415 members, and more than 100 people are serving as volunteers. Private support also has increased. In 1987, 100 percent of the museums' budget of $350,000 came from the county government. The county is still contributing at the same level, yet the budget has grown to $500,000 as a result of expanded private support and earned income.

PART THREE

STRATEGIES AND TOOLS
FOR MUSEUM DEVELOPMENT

CHAPTER SIX

Using Marketing Research and Information-Gathering Tools

An educator will tell you that "time on task" is a major factor in learning. How much time is spent on a subject or activity? How attentive is the student? The same factors are important in evaluating the effectiveness of museum exhibitions.
—Beverly Serrell

Museums attract different kinds of visitors having different kinds of interests. Some visitors to the Smithsonian Institution, for example, come primarily to view the treasures, like the Hope Diamond at the Natural History Museum, or memorabilia, like Dorothy's red slippers from the film *The Wizard of Oz* at the American History Museum. Other visitors are connoisseurs, scholars, and intellectuals. A study at the Smithsonian museums in the early 1990s estimated that 90 percent of visitors come with at least one other person and of these groups of two or more, about one-third include children (Doering and Bickford, 1994, p. vi). Museum evaluation experts like Beverly Serrell observe the behavior of visitors to museums—the length of time they spend in an exhibit hall, the number of elements in the exhibit they attend to.

Such observations and findings are of enormous utility to museum managers and help them answer important questions: Does the museum have worthwhile activities for visitors? Does it have objects that can be regarded as treasures but are not currently being promoted that way? How much time are visitors spending in the museum? Would the museum benefit if they spent more time? If so, what incentives are available to encourage visitors to extend their visits? Does the museum have enough social space and an attractive enough restaurant to welcome visiting couples or small groups? If the goal is to create as inviting and satisfying a museum-going experience as resources allow, museums would then employ systematic research to gauge visitor expectations, interests, needs, and satisfactions. The value of research lies precisely in collecting solid information to inform the choices that museum managers have to make. That is the substance of marketing research as it applies to museums.

Historically, museum managers have devoted their attention to managing their collections, facilities, funds, and staff and have paid less attention to another critical resource: information. In recent years, however, the emergence of sophisticated research methods and information technologies has revolutionized information gathering and analysis, making it accessible to the smallest museums.

Museums' need for market information is stronger than at any time in the past. Competition for the public's attention and participation is greater than ever. As market segmentation strategies become more sophisticated, museums need to learn more about the needs and preferences of more variegated markets. As consumers face a growing number of choices, museums find it more challenging to predict consumers' responses to different offerings, benefits, and appeals— unless they turn to marketing research. Marketing research can play a critical role in understanding consumer attitudes and behavior and in planning marketing strategy. What distinguishes marketing research from simple observation is that it is systematic and comprehensive. We define *marketing research* as *the systematic design, collection, analysis, and reporting of data and findings relevant to understanding market forces better and improving consumer satisfaction and organizational performance.*

In this chapter we examine five questions related to the efficient and effective use of marketing research: Why is there resistance to carrying on museum marketing research? What are the main museum applications of such research? What are the main data sources and tools? What is the budgeting procedure? What are the major steps in the research process?

RESISTANCE TO MARKETING RESEARCH

Although marketing research can benefit museums, its use is not widespread. There are several reasons.

Costs

Museums often see marketing research as an expensive undertaking. Yet it need not be. There are low-cost forms of effective research, such as systematic observation by volunteers or staff and the use of focus groups (Andreasen, 1983). Much can be learned from just observing visitors move through a museum or listening to visitor comments. Focus group discussions can yield a rich picture of visitor attitudes—often just for the cost of a complimentary admission or free purchase in the gift shop for the eight to ten participants. Another low-cost method is the analysis of currently available information, such as museum attendance figures by time of year, day of week, time of day, or audience segment. When a museum wants to conduct more thorough studies, it can get low-cost assistance from marketing students and professors at nearby universities; it can also invite a marketing research professional to sit on its board of directors.

Once managers realize the benefits gained by regularly administered, well-planned, and well-executed marketing research, they will value the process and budget for it. When the museum must make an important decision, spending money on preliminary research can be well justified.

Technical Knowledge

Unfamiliarity with the technical aspects of research can deter a museum from conducting research. Museum personnel who plan to hire marketing research specialists should acquaint themselves with the research process and the rudimentary principles of sampling, questionnaire design, and interpretation of results. They should be familiar enough with the methods and processes to communicate effectively with trained researchers and to know whether the museum's research needs are being adequately fulfilled. However they need not be focus group leaders, survey designers, statisticians, or computer experts themselves.

Professional Resistance

Some museum professionals fear that applying marketing research will compromise their museum's mission and integrity. A curator of medieval art who learns that the public shows little interest in this area might assume that this finding will lead to a budget reduction and that the museum's mission concerning medieval art might be compromised. But this curator is missing an opportunity to use research information to advantage (DiMaggio and Useem, n.d.). The research could reveal what different groups feel about medieval art and why they feel the way they do. It could provide clues about adding interest and excitement. It could result in a more focused approach to stimulating public interest in this area of art.

MUSEUM APPLICATIONS OF MARKETING RESEARCH

Marketing research aims to help managers make better decisions. Will a new costly exhibit attract the public? What will the impact be of a proposed 20 percent increase in the admission fee? Do families with young children perceive the museum as having adequate services and being responsive to their needs? Is a proposed program to attract more young professionals to the museum likely to succeed? Did the intended educational outcomes of a particular exhibit in fact occur? Answers to all such questions can only help the museum in its work.

Uses of Marketing Research

By using the various tools available to market researchers, museums can carry on a range of useful studies, which may have one or more of the following purposes: description, explanation, or prediction.

Description. Marketing research can tell museum management what the marketing environment is like: how many people from which demographic and psychographic profiles attend the museum, what factors led them to attend the museum, what exhibits they enjoyed most, and so on. Such descriptive data usually serve management in three ways: (1) they indicate whether strategy changes are needed, (2) they describe consumer segments, and (3) they report on the popularity of current exhibits.

Explanation. Usually a manager wants to know the forces that lie behind the descriptive findings. The simplest level of explanation is to discover what seems to be *associated* with what. For example, a museum manager may want to understand the common characteristics of museum members who allow their memberships to lapse. The findings will help management focus stronger appeals on the lapsing audience.

The next level of explanation is *causation*. Thus management may think that lapsed members were dissatisfied with the museum's programs. But it may turn out that these members were primarily unhappy with the attitude of museum personnel.

The ultimate level of explanation is to know not only that A caused B but *why* A caused B. Suppose many of these lapsed members had telephoned the museum for information but received poor or indifferent responses. Management can then put museum personnel who supply the public with information through a training program. Afterwards the museum can publicize stories of how helpful its staff is to visitors and to lapsed members.

Prediction. Descriptions and explanations can prove even more useful when they lead to prediction. Suppose management is planning to raise the annual membership dues from $40 to $50. It is useful to predict with some accuracy how many additional nonrenewals will occur as a consequence of the price increase and how this will affect revenue and costs.

Are Marketing Research and Museum Research the Same Thing?

Museums, particularly large, urban museums, have adopted research methods to assess the quality and effects of exhibitions and examine who the visitors are and how they feel about their museum experiences. To the extent that museum research and visitor studies seek to determine the quality of a museum's organization, programs, and personnel as perceived by audiences and stakeholders, a good deal of today's museum research can be considered marketing research.

However, traditional forms of museum research still survive, and they are different from marketing research in several respects: (1) marketing research tends to be systematic, strategic, and broad ranging, while traditional museum research often consists of ad hoc, piecemeal, and narrow-gauged studies; (2) marketing research tends to be regular and continuous over a period of time, while traditional museum research tends to be limited to single cases; (3) marketing research seeks to anticipate issues, events, changes, and emerging factors (and therefore often involves forecasting and trend analysis), while traditional museum research tends to involve "results data," facts of what already exists or has existed; and (4) marketing research in museums is likely to be more comprehensive in the range of factors it looks at.

Museums are typically involved in a broad range of relationships, more heterogeneous and demanding than the typical relationships in the business world. As a result, a museum can find it useful to undertake marketing research that scans the environment in which it operates and examines the full range of the publics the museum serves (the characteristics of all people who support it and what each group seeks in its exchanges and relationships).

The Importance of Organized Data

A museum's ability to learn about its publics and its markets depends on the availability of *organized* data. Many museums still keep written membership records, but these often are limited data sets, including demographic characteristics but excluding attitudinal and behavioral ones. A museum that seeks to examine visitorship changes needs a data series that measures visitorship over time. A museum that seeks to examine facility or exhibit utilization needs to count visitors reliably, and this will in turn require data from the issuance of tickets or the collection of admission fees. Museums that do not have admission fees and that depend on counting by security guards at the entrance are subject to relatively unreliable data collection.

Tickets can be coded—with the purchaser's ZIP code or telephone exchange, for example—to reveal various demographic or geographical characteristics. Museums can install computer screens at gift shop entrances and invite visitors to fill out questionnaires. A computer can also be used to allow visitors to provide feedback on satisfactions levels. A further justification for collecting organized data is that potential sponsors, such as businesses and corporations, usually want reliable visitor and usage data as a condition for their support.

Major Types of Museum Research

The following section offers a brief overview of the main types of museum research, along with some examples.

Exhibition Evaluation Research. A primary type of museum research is *exhibition evaluation research,* of which there are several forms. *Front-end evaluation* is used by exhibit developers to conceptualize and plan an exhibition; it involves a sample of museum-goers, who are asked for their reactions to exhibition concepts, goals, and plans. *Formative evaluation* involves surveying public responses to exhibition prototypes, as a way of assessing the effectiveness of exhibit elements; often this research focuses on discrete exhibit elements rather than the entire exhibit. A common form of exhibit research is *summative evaluation.* This research involves responses to exhibition design, elements, and other aspects in the context of the entire exhibition. This research is used to determine whether the objectives of the exhibition were in fact achieved. Occasionally, these research findings are the basis for modifying exhibition elements and features.

Beverly Serrell, the visitor studies specialist, examines the extent to which visitors use exhibitions—the time they spend viewing exhibitions, the number of elements (explanatory panels, paintings and other objects, display cases, dioramas, video monitors, and so on) they view, the elements they pay most attention to, and whether the visitors' reactions to an exhibition mesh with the designers' and organizers' intentions. Visitors normally spend a relatively brief time looking at an exhibit—about fifteen to twenty minutes in a typical exhibition hall. They spend less than a minute viewing a particular exhibit element and look at about one-third of an exhibit's elements. Studies also find that when exhibitions are smaller in scale, visitors tend to spend more time with each element than they would in larger exhibitions (Serrell, 1993).

There are various reasons why visitors spend limited time at exhibitions. Some come as part of a family or group and expect to spend time interpersonally and sociably as well as to view the museum's offerings. As part of a group, a visitor can be pressured to move through quickly. Visitors often like diversion between exhibits and may spend time in gift shops and restaurants as well as among the exhibits, even though they have only a limited time for their museum visit. Serrell (interviewed Apr. 29, 1997) points to another explanation: exhibits that are confusing or dull or of poor quality are not likely to attract much visitor attention. She observes: "Periodically I visit exhibits and can't tell what they are about, what's the beginning and what's the end, and what the organizers intended to accomplish. Visitors are likely to feel confused or uneasy if the idea of an exhibit is unclear and its design is ineffectual." Serrell has studied visitor utilization of the offerings at more than one hundred exhibitions and has analyzed factors and patterns that explain high and low use. She consults widely with museum professionals to help them create strong exhibitions or re-vise existing ones to make them stronger.

An excellent example of exhibition research is the Smithsonian research study of visitors to the *Ocean Planet* exhibition at the National Museum of Natural History (Bickford, Pekarik, Doering, and Yalowitz, 1996). Conducted in the fall and winter of 1995, this study involved a total of 978 visitors. Representative samples were surveyed as they entered or exited the exhibition or as they viewed exhibit elements. The study examined the goals of the exhibition's designers—their intended communications and learning effects—and compared these with the reactions of respondents. The study identified several learning outcomes, particularly the ways in which the exhibit expanded visitor awareness. The report stated: "The exhibition contents clearly modified the views of a number of visitors. Visitors left the exhibition more cognizant of the products that oceans provide, more aware of how human activities affect the health of the oceans, more willing to change their consumption patterns to help the oceans, and more pessimistic about the future of the oceans" (p. 6).

Visitor Studies. Museums have developed a large subfield of research known as *visitor studies,* or *audience research.* Visitor studies encompass a range of tools and objectives: demographic and psychographic surveys of visitors and nonvisitors; focus groups of active or infrequent visitors that examine feelings, attitudes, and preferences; tracking and timing studies that examine visitors' use of exhibition elements and the time spent in exhibits; extended primary research dealing with topics such as museum learning, visitor behavior, attitudes toward museum facilities, personnel, and services; and surveys of leisure-time behavior and choices and of attitudes toward museums in relation to competitor organizations.

Insights: Museums, Visitors, Attitudes, Expectations: A Focus Group Experiment was a pioneering visitor study—and an excellent example of primary research—sponsored by the Getty Center for Education and the J. Paul Getty Museum in the late 1980s (Walsh, 1991; see especially chap. 3). Cosponsored by several large U.S. art museums, the study involved 132 hours of focus group discussions with more than 220 visitors, 115 museum professionals, and a number of nonvisitors over a two-year period. It examined visitor expectations, the reasons people do not visit museums, visitor assessment of the museum experience, visitor attitudes toward museum services and staff (orientation, information, personnel, physical layout and design), and attitudes toward museum communications, advertising, and public relations. A major finding was the consistent and strong criticism expressed by the participants that museums, overall, provided inadequate information, orientation, and context for making visitors aware of and more appreciative and understanding of artworks and art experienced in the museum.

A growing number of visitor studies examine the learning or educational outcomes of exhibitions and programs. A series of studies at the Smithsonian Institution, conducted by Zahava Doering and her staff at the Office of Institutional Studies, have examined the cognitive dimension of museum education. One study concluded: "Schools are more effective than museums in providing cognitive learning. . . . Perhaps most fundamentally, the elaborate feedback system in the schools, in the form of tests, dialogue with teachers, work reviews, etc., makes students self-consciously aware of what they think and know, requires them to learn more, and encourages them to adopt alternative viewpoints. . . . [Another] reason that most people don't learn much new information in museums is that museum visiting is often a social activity with numerous distractions and a rather fast pace—more like watching satellite television with a remote control than like reading a book" (Doering and Pekarik, n.d., pp. 5–6).

A series of visitor studies has examined the behavior of families in museums: the interactions among family members and the effects of the museum experience individually and collectively. Minda Borun, director of research at the Franklin Institute, in Philadelphia, has developed an index to measure family learning outcomes in museums. The index uses seven indicators of family learning, reflecting the extent to which family members ask and answer questions, comment on exhibits, explain or demonstrate the use of interactive exhibit elements, and read labels and text silently and aloud (Borun, Chambers, and Cleghorn, 1995; see also Agustin, 1997, and Borun, Chambers, and Cleghorn, 1996).

Most visitor studies are systematic and quantitative; however, some qualitative studies have value. An example is a study by Russell J. Ohta (1996) of visitor reactions to *Old Glory: The American Flag in Contemporary Art,* after critics charged that some artworks in this 1996 Phoenix Art Museum exhibit demeaned and defamed the U.S. flag. The study's novelty lay in its method: using selected visitors' words, in the form of free association, to gauge visitor feelings, attitudes, and insights as these visitors moved through and experienced the exhibition. Ohta refers to this method as *continuous experiential reporting.* The study, however, deals in depth with only a handful of visitors.

One other type of visitor research warrants attention: broad-gauged studies that examine the behavior of people who visit museums and that of people who rarely or never visit museums and then compare the kinds of choices they make about their leisure activity. An excellent example is John Falk's study *Leisure Decisions Influencing African American Use of Museums* (1993). Falk analyzes the factors and conditions affecting the choices black Americans make in their leisure activities, the number who visit museums and who never visit museums, and the attitudes influencing those behaviors. He reports: "The first generalization this research clearly suggests is that African Americans, like Americans of all races, infrequently go to museums. . . . In terms of their overall leisure behavior and interests, African Americans fall so close to the norm of white America that they are virtually indistinguishable from them" (p. 73).

A classic series of studies comparing museum visitors and nonvisitors was produced by Marilyn Hood (1983). See Chapter Four for an additional discussion of visitor behavior.

Development Research. Larger museums that have a variety of membership and donor programs usually commission research that examines changing patterns of membership and donorship, levels of satisfaction, and preferences for modifying or expanding museum offerings. These museums often have a range of groups (members, donors, sponsors, and patrons, both individual and corporate) whose varying and changing opinions, needs, and attitudes warrant periodic examination.

An example of this *development-oriented* research (also called, *membership, donor,* or *sponsorship* research) is a project undertaken by the faculty in the Goizueta Business School at Emory University, in Atlanta, for the High Museum of Art. The museum board in 1994 recognized the absence of marketing research at a time when it was launching a new strategic plan. The museum, having had other relationships with Emory University, engaged three Goizueta school professors to undertake membership research among the eighteen thousand members, specifically to determine the reasons for nonrenewals, which were on the rise and at the time amounted to about one in three members.

Following a series of meetings with museum staff and review of museum records and data, the research team set out to define the research problem and objectives, design an appropriate research plan, determine the methodology, select survey forms and samples, and generate the types of desired data and analysis. The researchers decided on the following: (1) a quick telephone survey of lapsed museum members to get a sampling of their concerns; (2) a focus group study to test questionnaire items that would be used in the regular survey; (3) a pilot study with a sample of one thousand members to test the research vehicle; and (4) a broader survey of three thousand members, following analysis of the results of the pilot study. Early research revealed a number of potentially important factors and conditions that would be further examined in the larger survey. Thus the pilot study examined visitation frequency, benefit awareness, benefit use, ranking of benefits, satisfaction of expectations, and attitudes about membership, along with demographic data. Among the pilot study findings were relatively infrequent member visitation and participation, high benefit awareness yet low benefit use, and low satisfaction with interpersonal and social opportunities accompanying membership. With these findings in hand, the research group suggested that the museum organize more social-contact events and build a stronger sense of investment and participation in the museum. Subsequently, at the initiative of a new membership manager, the museum organized Artful

Friday Evenings, a series of social events for members that proved highly successful (Kroenert, 1995).

Organizational Research. Museums engage in varying forms of self-assessment and outside assessment of their management and governance, operations, collections, exhibitions and public programs, visitorship and usage, membership and community support, facilities, and services. One form of assessment occurs during museum registration in Great Britain and accreditation in the United States, when museums have to demonstrate compliance with a set of professional standards.

In 1981, the American Association of Museums (AAM) established the Museum Assessment Program (MAP), which is independent of AAM's accreditation program, to assist museums in reviewing their organizations, examining missions and goals, responding to environmental changes, and developing skills in assessment, goal setting, strategic planning, and implementing organizational change. The MAP program currently offers three levels of museum assessment: self-assessment, collections management assessment, and public service assessment. Assessment tools—institutional planning guidebooks and on-site visits by outside museum professionals (who compare their observations with the self-assessment data)—are provided to museums selected for the program, and the findings and recommendations are reported.

In the mid-1990s, the AAM set up the New Visions program. This program conceptualizes institutional self-assessment as a broad process of dialogue and communication that occurs among museum board members, officers, and staff and that embraces vision building, action and implementation plans, and change management. The program description says, in part: "Evaluation is built into every aspect of the New Visions approach. It provides information that enables you to gauge your progress and remain motivated to achieve results. Along with this basic structure [come] tools, examples, incentives, and assistance that will help your institution reach its potential for change. . . . The process invites a fundamental shift in the way museums operate as organizations, with an expanded audience focus, improved internal communication across departments, better external communication with the community, and greater commitment to diversity and inclusion" ("New Visions Basics," 1996).

In these ways and more, AAM museum assessment and professional development programs have been working successfully to diffuse knowledge and skills among museums.

DATA SOURCES AND RESEARCH TOOLS

Museums engaged in marketing research have many sources of data available to them and an array of methods of collecting that data. These data fall into two broad categories, *secondary data* and *primary data.*

Secondary Data

Secondary data consist of information that already exists somewhere, having been collected for another purpose. Marketing researchers usually start their investigation by examining secondary data to see whether their information needs can be partly or wholly satisfied without collecting more costly primary data. The rich variety of secondary data sources available can be divided into *external sources* (such as government publications, trade magazines, specialized journals and books, and foundation reports) and *internal sources* (museum financial statements, visitor data, membership data, and so on).

On occasion a foundation, a government agency, or a trade organization will undertake basic research on behalf of museums. Examples of strong secondary research data are the surveys and analyses sponsored by the Museums & Galleries Commission (MGC), the British government's advisory body that promotes museum and heritage organizations. MGC's study *By Popular Demand* (Davies, 1994) examines the market forces affecting museums (leisure time and activities, museum competition, demographic trends, demands on museum services) and the museum market (visitors, nonvisitors, patrons, stakeholders). Study author Stuart Davies advises museums to pool their resources and generate regional and national studies, standardize the content and format of survey research, and regularize research studies so as to produce periodic studies and benchmarks that could help many museums evaluate trends and changes over time. He also suggests making greater use of professional research consultants. MGC has also published *Museums and Tourism: Mutual Benefit* (Runyard, 1993), a study that describes the key players in the tourist industry, the composition of tourists as a group, tourist attitudes and preferences, and a series of successful museum programs to expand tourist visits.

Secondary data provide a starting point for research and offer the advantages of lower cost and quicker findings. However, the data needed might not exist, or existing data might be dated, inaccurate, incomplete, or unreliable. In this case, a museum will have to collect primary data—incurring greater costs and expending more time but probably gaining more relevant and accurate information.

Primary Data

Primary data consist of original information gathered for the specific purpose at hand. Most marketing research projects involve some primary data collection. When a museum manager thinks of carrying out primary research, the first technique that usually comes to mind is a field survey using questionnaires and conducted by mail, telephone, or in person. However, other techniques are available that may be more effective and efficient.

When planning a research project, the museum manager needs to know the array of available methodologies. Primary data can be collected in three broad ways: through *exploratory research, descriptive research,* and *experimental research.*

Exploratory Research. Exploratory research includes observation, individual in-depth interviews, and focus groups.

Observational research. Useful descriptive data can be gathered simply by observing the relevant actors and settings. Researchers might listen in on calls to the museum to learn what people inquire about or to hear how patrons talk about different exhibits and programs. Museums can also employ *mystery shoppers,* individuals who pose as visitors and rate staff performance and museum services. Researchers can visit a variety of museums to gain comparative perspectives, observing the different offerings and gauging visitor reactions by means of surveys or panel studies. Some museums use nonobtrusive methods to infer popularity of exhibits or parts of exhibits: for example, the degree of carpet wear or the quantity of noseprints on a sheet of glass (Webb, 1981). These are simple and inexpensive techniques for learning more about audiences and their reactions to offerings.

Individual in-depth interviews and focus group research. Individual in-depth interviews involve lengthy questioning of respondents one at a time. Focus groups involve bringing together groups of six to ten visitors, usually (but not always) relatively homogeneous, to discuss a specific set of issues under the guidance of a leader trained to stimulate and focus the discussion. Table 6.1 presents a range of conditions under which each technique might be selected.

The objective of both techniques is to get beneath the surface of an issue and beyond the preconceptions of museum staff. The findings can be used in designing a subsequent survey questionnaire. Exhibit 6.1 describes several techniques used by skilled interviewers and group moderators.

Descriptive Research. Descriptive research includes surveys, conjoint research, and panel studies.

Surveys. The survey is the most popular and widely used approach to examine, describe, and measure people's demographics, knowledge, beliefs, preferences, satisfaction levels, competitive choices, and decision-making processes. A museum can survey the views of its visitors, members, donors, and others about its programs and services. Questionnaires can be placed in the entry hall or mailed to random samples of current, past, or potential visitors and supporters. Surveys can also be administered on the telephone, providing a more personal and potentially more comprehensive response from respondents who agree to participate.

Conjoint research techniques. Conjoint analysis is a means of analyzing consumer choices. Traditional surveys inquire into consumer attitudes one item at a time and ignore the trade-offs among desired benefits. Conjoint research techniques capture the trade-off process, permitting analysts to estimate the importance to an individual or group of each attribute or factor and to project the likely success of varied offerings, each with a different set of attributes. Suppose a

Table 6.1. Which to Use: Focus Groups or Individual In-Depth Interviews?

Issue to Consider	Use Focus Groups When . . .	Use Individual In-Depth Interviews When . . .
Group interaction	Interaction of respondents may stimulate a richer response or new and valuable thoughts.	Group interaction is likely to be limited or nonproductive.
Group/peer pressure	Group/peer pressure will be valuable in challenging the thinking of respondents and illuminating conflicting opinions.	Group/peer pressure would inhibit responses and cloud the meaning of results.
Sensitivity of subject matter	Subject matter is not so sensitive that respondents will temper responses or withhold information.	Subject matter is so sensitive that respondents would be unwilling to talk openly in a group.
Depth of individual responses	The topic is such that most respondents can say all that is relevant or all that they know in less than ten minutes.	The topic is such that a greater depth of response per individual is desirable, as with complex subject matter and very knowledgeable respondents.
Interviewer fatigue	It is desirable to have one interviewer conduct the research; several groups will not create interviewer fatigue or boredom.	It is desirable to have numerous interviewers on the project. One interviewer will become fatigued or bored conducting the interviews.
Stimulus materials	The volume of stimulus material is not extensive.	A large amount of stimulus material must be evaluated.
Continuity of information	A single subject area is being examined in depth and strings of behaviors are less relevant.	It is necessary to understand how attitudes and behaviors link together in individual patterns.
Experimentation with interview guide	Enough is known to establish a meaningful topic guide.	It may be necessary to develop the interview guide by altering it after each of the initial interviews.

Table 6.1. Which to Use: Focus Groups or Individual In-Depth Interviews? Cont'd.

Issue to Consider	Use Focus Groups When . . .	Use Individual In-Depth Interviews When . . .
Observation	It is possible and desirable for key decision makers to observe consumer information firsthand.	Observing consumer information firsthand is not critical or observation is not logistically possible.
Logistics	An acceptable number of target respondents can be assembled in one location.	Respondents are geographically dispersed or not easily assembled for other reasons.
Cost and timing	Quick turnaround is critical, and funds are limited.	Quick turnaround is not critical, and budget will permit higher cost.

Source: Debus, n.d., p. 10.

museum is sponsoring a lecture series and needs to decide among the following attributes and levels:

Attribute	*Possible Levels*
Number of series events	4, 6, 8
Seating priority	Yes, no
Single ticket price	$5, $8, $12
Membership discount	30 percent, 15 percent, none
Evening of the week	Tuesday, Thursday

The researcher lists various full-profile alternatives: for example, one profile might be "four events, seating priority, $8, 15 percent membership discount, and Tuesday evening." In this instance, there are 108 possible combinations ($3 \times 2 \times 3 \times 3 \times 2$). Not all will need to be tested, however. Respondents might be asked to rank, say, eighteen full-profile alternatives in order of their preference. Conjoint analysis then determines which of the eighteen alternatives would be most popular and also the varying contribution of each attribute level to the ranked popularity. These results allow the museum to more carefully design its lecture series for maximum appeal to the target audience.

Panel studies. Museum researchers may wish to monitor the attendance, interests, and satisfaction of people signing up for the annual lecture series. They can recruit a sample of members who regularly attend the lectures and provide an incentive for these members to serve on a panel for a given period and answer

○○○○○

Exhibit 6.1. Suggestions for Soliciting Responses in Focus Groups and Interviews.

1. **Top-of-mind associations**   What's the first thing that comes to mind when I say "museum"? What else comes to mind? What comes to mind when I say "art museum"? "Contemporary art museum"?

2. **Constructing images**   Who are the people who like to go to museums? Why do they like museums? How do you feel when you visit a museum? Describe what you like and dislike.

3. **Asking the meaning of the obvious**   What does "avant-garde" mean to you? "Abstract art"? "Figurative art"?

4. **"Man from the moon" routine**   I'm from the moon; I've never heard of an art museum. Describe it to me. Tell me about the experience from the perspective of a visitor. Why would I want to visit one? Convince me.

5. **Conditions that give permission and create barriers**   Tell me about two or three situations in which you would decide to go to a museum and two or three situations in which you would decide to do something else.

6. **Chain of questions**   Why did you become a member of the museum? What do you like about being a member? Will you be renewing your membership? Why?

7. **Best of all possible world scenarios**   Forget about reality for a minute. If you could design your own membership plan for a museum, what would it be like? What other benefits would you enjoy? Use your imagination. There are no limits. Don't worry about whether it is possible or not.

8. **Sentence completions**   The ideal museum blockbuster exhibit is one that ... The best thing about this museum is that ... Attending this museum makes me feel ...

9. **Pointing out contradictions**   Wait a minute, you just told me you would like the museum to have more blockbuster exhibits, and now you're telling me that they can't be enjoyed because of waiting queues and crowds—how do you explain this?

Source: Adapted from Debus, n.d., pp. 132–133.

○○○○○

questions from time to time. Panelists might be asked about their interest in current or proposed exhibitions, their attitude toward alternative prices, their response to different ads, and other matters.

Experimental Research. The most scientifically valid research is experimental research. It calls for selecting matched groups of subjects, subjecting them to different treatments, controlling extraneous variables, and checking whether observed response differences are statistically significant. The purpose of experimental research is to capture cause-and-effect relationships by eliminating spurious or competing explanations of the observed findings. For example, a museum can send out two different brochures announcing a lecture series to two randomly selected groups of subscribers. The brochures are identical in all aspects except the price of the series. The museum can then analyze the impact of the price differential on the subscription rate. At the end of the research project, subscribers who paid the higher price are refunded the difference. If the test results are favorable, prices can be raised the following season for all subscribers. To the extent that the experiment eliminates alternative hypotheses, the research and marketing managers can have confidence in the conclusions.

MARKETING RESEARCH BUDGETING

Although marketing research should be an ongoing function, rarely are specific funds set aside for it. Too often it is treated as a discretionary activity rather than an essential tool for effective management. But sound budgeting is as much a part of marketing research as a solid understanding of the methods and tools we have been discussing.

A cost-benefit approach is the most effective method for determining an appropriate marketing research budget. Management specifies research needs for the forthcoming period and then costs out the research. These costs are then compared to the expected benefits. The specific steps are as follows:

1. Ascertain upcoming information and research needs and list all possible projects that might be undertaken in the planning period.
2. Estimate the costs for meeting the various information needs.
3. Estimate the value or benefit of each study in terms of the likely improvement in organizational performance.
4. Compare costs to expected benefits, and consider budgeting for all research projects where the latter exceed the former.
5. Reevaluate all ongoing research projects each year, and assess how to improve the effectiveness and efficiency of each project.
6. Use the total costs of both newly selected and ongoing research projects to constitute the year's research budget.

STEPS IN THE MARKETING RESEARCH PROCESS

This section describes the specific steps in applying the survey questionnaire, the most common instrument for collecting primary data.

Effective marketing research involves six steps: (1) defining the problem and the research objectives, (2) developing the research plan, (3) designing the questionnaire, (4) collecting and analyzing the data, (5) preparing and presenting the research report, and (6) evaluating and implementing the findings.

Defining the Problem and the Research Objectives

The first step involves defining the problem carefully and agreeing on the research objectives. Hundreds of things can be researched in any given problem. Unless the problem is well defined, the cost of gathering information may well exceed the value of the findings. Management should make clear to the researcher what the decision alternatives are and what research information is required to make those decisions. Management should also share with the researcher any financial, political, and other constraints that may affect the way the research is approached and evaluated.

Say that some board members at Atlas Museum (a hypothetical case) have suggested raising ticket prices 20 percent for the museum's annual lecture series on modern art. The lecture series director is concerned that her audience will find this price increase excessive, so she is considering cutting series costs instead, by presenting lesser-known and less costly lecturers. However, she also knows that less expensive lecturers will attract a smaller crowd. Thus either of the proposed changes is likely to reduce the number of subscribers.

Atlas Museum's first task is to make sure that either change will be compatible with the museum's mission. Its mission statement says, in part: "Atlas Museum is dedicated to presenting quality lecture programs on contemporary art that are accessible to diverse audiences in the greater metropolitan area." This mission allows Atlas Museum to present any lecture series as long as the program is of good quality. Nothing in the mission statement prevents the board from raising prices as long as the price does not substantially hurt accessibility.

Atlas Museum staff need to know several things before making a decision. They should

- Analyze ticket sales over the past two years to identify areas of strength and weakness

- Examine audience preferences and satisfaction levels for programs and prices

- Measure subscribers' preferences for different types of presenters and presentations

- Determine the current market's demographic and psychographic characteristics

- Study competitive offerings and prices

The marketing researcher and the museum manager need to determine which type of research will furnish the specific information needed to make a decision. For example, they may determine they need research to analyze the following: How many people will attend if they raise their prices 10 percent? 20 percent? 30 percent? Which lecturers are the most suitable to support the higher prices? The least suitable? Can prices vary with seat location? Can any amenities be added to soften the impact of higher ticket prices?

Developing the Research Plan

The second stage of marketing research calls for developing the most efficient plan for gathering the needed information. The manager cannot simply say to the marketing researcher, "Find some current subscribers and ask if they would come if we charged 10 percent, 20 percent, or 30 percent more." Research questions have to be defined carefully.

Designing a research plan calls for decisions on the *sampling plan, research biases, contact methods,* and *questionnaire design.*

Sampling Plan. A sampling plan determines *who* will be contacted (the sampling unit), *how many* people will be contacted (the sample size), and *how* the museum can obtain a representative sample of the target groups (the sampling procedure).

Sampling unit. The marketing researcher must define the target population that will be sampled. The answer is not always obvious. Atlas Museum decided to sample both frequent and infrequent current lecture series attenders. They also want to sample people who have not attended the series but who probably would enjoy it. *Snowball sampling* can be used to find nonattenders. In this method, current attenders are asked to suggest the names of others "like them" who could be contacted. This adds a group that does not have the familiarity biases of the first group but is likely to cooperate in the study (especially if the initial respondents allow their names to be used as references) and will closely match the first sample in socioeconomic characteristics.

Sample size. Large samples give more reliable results than small samples. However, it is not necessary to sample the entire target population or even a substantial portion to achieve reliable results. Samples of less than 1 percent of a population can often provide good reliability, given a credible sampling procedure.

Sampling procedure. To obtain a representative sample, a *probability sample* of the population should be drawn. Probability sampling allows the calculation of confidence limits for sampling error so that one could conclude that there is a 95 percent chance of being correct that attenders would prefer six lectures per year. There are three types of probability sampling:

- *Simple random sample.* Every member of the population has a known and equal chance of selection.
- *Stratified random sample.* The population is divided into mutually exclusive groups such as age groups, and random samples are drawn from each group.
- *Cluster (area) sample.* The population is divided into mutually exclusive groups such as city blocks, and the researcher draws a sample of groups to interview.

When the cost or time involved in probability sampling is too high, marketing researchers will take *nonprobability samples.* Some marketing researchers feel that nonprobability samples are useful in many circumstances, even though the sampling error cannot be measured. For example, if a museum's management is chiefly interested in frequency counts (say, of words used by museum-goers to describe the museum's offerings or of complaints voiced about staff), sampling restrictions need not be especially tight. Here are three types of non-probability samples:

- *Convenience sample.* The researcher selects the most accessible population members from which to obtain information.
- *Judgment sample.* The researcher uses his or her judgment to select population members who are good prospects for accurate information.
- *Quota sample.* The researcher finds and interviews a prescribed number of people in each of several categories.

In our hypothetical case, Atlas Museum's marketing director used a combination of nonprobability sampling techniques to provide the researcher with five hundred names and addresses of current subscribers and three hundred names of potential subscribers.

Research Biases. Research can be effective only if it avoids two major sources of error: *sampling error* and *systematic bias* (this description of research biases is largely adapted from Alreck and Settle, 1985, pp. 67–68).

Sampling error. No sample is likely to produce results that are precisely those of the entire population. It is always possible to pick, strictly by chance, a group whose members happen to be different in some important attribute from the population as a whole. When differences between the sample data and the population data result purely by chance, they are known as sampling error. Statistical findings from smaller samples are more likely than findings from larger samples to differ from population data, so smaller samples have more sampling error. The larger the sampling error, the lower the reliability; so the smaller the sample, the lower the reliability of the data.

Systematic bias. Systematic bias is more difficult to handle. It refers to extraneous sampling factors that affect survey results and reduce data validity. Systematic bias in a survey usually arises from one of the following sources:

- *Frame bias.* A probability sample is drawn from a wrongly chosen population. For example, estimating the proportion of people who like contemporary art by sampling solely spectators at a football game is likely to systematically underestimate the true number, because many people who like contemporary art may not be avid sports enthusiasts.

- *Selection bias.* The procedure for drawing actual sample members always excludes or underrepresents certain types of population members. This occurs, for example, when telephone interviewers only telephone during the day, thereby underrepresenting people who work. It also occurs in field surveys where the interviewers pick whom to interview. If all the field workers tended to interview only people who looked friendly, the findings would be biased.

- *Nonresponse.* The contacted people decline to participate out of lack of interest, antagonism, or busyness.

- *Interviewer bias.* An untrained interviewer deliberately or inadvertently leads the respondent to a particular response. This can occur, for example, when interviewers read or "clarify" a question in a way that suggests a particular answer is preferred.

- *Questionnaire bias.* Poor or confusing wording, leading questions, identification of the research sponsor when this information is to be withheld, and omission of important possible responses result in bias.

- *Respondent bias.* The respondent lies or unwittingly distorts an answer. Often this source of bias manifests itself when respondents exaggerate their income, educational level, or frequency of attendance.

- *Processing bias.* The interviewer or respondent writes down the wrong answers, the office enters the answers into the computer incorrectly, or the computer analysis is programmed incorrectly.

Catching all these glitches is not easy. It takes careful attention to the design process, to interviewer training, to checking on data processing, and to reviewing reports for errors. Research funds are often better spent on catching systematic errors than on increasing the sample size.

Contact Methods. Museums can contact respondents by mail, program inserts, telephone, or personal interviews.

The *mail questionnaire* is the most cost-effective way of reaching a large number of people. It is also the best way to reach individuals who will not give personal interviews or whose responses might be biased or distorted by the interviewers. However, the mail response rate is usually low or slow, or both. Alternatively, a museum can give questionnaires to people directly. For example, Atlas Museum could insert its questionnaires in the lecture program guide and collect them after the talk. This has all the advantages of mailed questionnaires but reduces the problem of low or slow response rates.

Telephone interviewing is an effective method for gaining information quickly; the interviewer is also able to clarify questions if they are not understood. The response rate is generally higher than in the case of mailed questionnaires. However, the sample size will necessarily be much lower because calling is time intensive. Furthermore, telephone interviews have to be short and impersonal.

Personal interviewing is the most versatile of these methods. The interviewer can ask more questions and can record additional observations about the respondent, such as body language or dress. However, personal interviewing is the most expensive method and requires more administrative planning and supervision. It is also subject to interviewer bias or distortion.

Personal interviewing takes two forms, *arranged interviews* and *intercept interviews.* In arranged interviews, respondents are randomly selected and are either telephoned or approached at their homes or offices and asked to grant an interview. Intercept interviews involve stopping people in public—say, at a shopping mall or in the museum—and requesting an interview. Intercept interviews have the drawback of using nonprobability samples, and the interviews have to be brief. Often a small payment or incentive such as a museum admission or gift shop discount coupon is presented to respondents in appreciation of their time.

Designing the Questionnaire

Questionnaires need to be carefully developed, tested, and debugged before they are administered on a large scale. See Exhibit 6.2 for several types of errors that may be found in an unprofessionally prepared questionnaire.

In preparing a questionnaire, the marketing researcher must develop the question content and also pay close attention to question form, wording, and sequence.

Questions Asked. A common error is including questions that cannot, would not, or need not be answered and omitting questions that should be answered. Each question should be checked to be certain that it contributes to the research objectives, does not require too much time, and does not strain respondents' time and patience.

Museum managers should be given the opportunity to review the questions in advance so they can spot problems. For example, some questions can set up

○○○○○

Exhibit 6.2. A Questionable Questionnaire.

Suppose a museum asked respondents the following questions. Think how various respondents might react to each question before you read the comment in italics.

1. What is your income?

   People do not generally want to reveal their exact income. Broad categories should be provided so people can indicate their income range. Furthermore, a questionnaire should never open with such a personal question.

2. Are you an occasional or a frequent museum-goer?

   How are you defining occasional versus frequent attendance? What seems frequent to one person may be considered occasional by another.

3. Do you like this museum? (Check yes or no.)

   "Like" is a relative term. Besides, will people answer this honestly? And is a yes-no answer a useful response to the question?

4. How many advertisements have you read or heard on the radio for this museum this season?

   Who can remember the number?

5. What are the most salient and determinant attributes in your evaluation of new exhibits?

   What are "salient" and "determinant" attributes? Don't use big words (or museum in-house jargon). Ask clear questions if you want clear answers.

6. Don't you think it is outrageous for the government to cut NEA funding for the arts?

   Loaded question. Don't ask questions with built-in biases.

○○○○○

unrealistic audience expectations, resulting in disappointment. Thus one museum director requested that researchers exclude a question asking museum members if they would like three evening openings a week, a benefit that he was not prepared to offer. Management participation in the design decision has other advantages. It serves to win managers' support of marketing research and deepens their understanding of research details. Participation also sensitizes all concerned to the study's limitations. The researcher has to recognize what types of research information have highest priority for decision makers and leave out other lines of inquiry.

Form of Questions. The form of a question influences the response. Marketing researchers distinguish between *closed-end* and *open-end* questions. Closed-end questions are accompanied by several possible answers, and respondents choose among them. Closed-end questions are easy to interpret and tabulate. Open-end questions allow broader answers and are especially useful in the exploratory stage of research, when the researcher is looking for insight into how people think rather than measuring how many people think in a certain way. Exhibit 6.3 provides examples of some commonly employed forms of closed-end and open-end questions.

Sequencing of Questions. Care should be exercised in the sequencing of questions. The lead question should create interest. The questions should follow a logical order. Difficult or personal questions should be asked toward the end. Questions designed to classify the respondent are asked last precisely because they are personal.

Wording of Questions. Care should be taken to use simple, direct, unbiased wording, and questions should be pretested for effectiveness before the final questionnaire is drawn up. Exhibit 6.4 shows some questions that might be used to ascertain interest in a proposed new lecture series.

Collecting and Analyzing the Data

The data collection phase is generally the most expensive and the most liable to error. First, data from an adequate sample must be obtained, as described earlier; then pertinent findings must be extracted. The researcher tabulates the data and develops frequency distributions, averages, and measures of dispersion. The researcher then analyzes these results in terms of the managerial decisions to be made and forms a series of recommendations.

Here, for example, is what happened at Atlas Museum. The eight hundred recipients of the mailed survey were given an incentive of $5 off from any purchase at the museum's gift shop as a thank-you for filling out the survey. There

○○○○○

Exhibit 6.3. Examples of Types of Survey Questions.

Closed-End Questions	*Examples*
Dichotomous. A question offering two answer choices.	Is this the first time you have attended this museum? Yes___ No___
Multiple choice. A question offering three or more answer choices.	With whom are you attending this museum? No one___ Spouse___ Other relatives/friends___ Business associates___ An organized group___
Likert scale. A statement with which the respondent shows a specific amount of agreement/disagreement.	Good critical reviews are an important factor for me in choosing to attend a new exhibit at the museum. 1 = strongly disagree, 2 = disagree, 3 = undecided, 4 = agree, 5 = strongly agree. 1___ 2___ 3___ 4___ 5___
Semantic differential. A scale is inscribed between two bipolar words, and the respondent selects the point that represents his or her opinion.	High ticket prices . . . Low ticket prices Top speakers . . . . Good speakers
Importance scale. A scale that rates the importance of some attribute.	Ticket exchange privilege to me is . . . 1 = extremely important, 2 = very important, 3 = somewhat important, 4 = not very important, 5 = not at all important. 1___ 2___ 3___ 4___ 5___
Rating scale. A scale that rates some attribute from "poor" to "excellent."	The quality of our exhibit is . . . 1 = excellent, 2 = very good, 3 = good, 4 = fair, 5 = poor. 1___ 2___ 3___ 4___ 5___

Exhibit 6.3. Examples of Types of Survey Questions, Cont'd.

Intention-to-buy scale. A scale that describes the respondent's intention to buy.	If subscriptions were offered for packages of 6 lectures, I would . . . 1 = definitely buy, 2 = probably buy, 3 = not sure, 4 = probably not buy, 5 = definitely not buy. 1___ 2___ 3___ 4___ 5___
Open-End Questions **Completely unstructured.** A question that respondents can answer in an almost unlimited number of ways.	***Examples*** What is your opinion of Atlas Museum?
Word association. Words are presented, one at a time, and respondents mention the first word that comes to mind.	What is the first word that comes to your mind when you hear the following? Museum _____ Atlas Museum _____ Contemporary art _____
Sentence completion. Incomplete sentences are presented, one at a time, and respondents complete the sentence.	When I choose a lecture series to attend, the most important consideration in my decision is _____ _____

○○○○○

was a healthy response of nearly 25 percent, or two hundred completed responses returned by the cutoff date, about six weeks after the mailing.

Based on the pricing questions in the museum survey, the researchers determined that 80 percent of the patrons were willing to pay 20 percent more for the lecture series, as long as quality presenters were continued. There would probably be a nonrenewal rate of 25 percent, but this gap could be filled by promoting the lecture program to new audiences. Detailed analyses were also made on the pricing sensitivity of different demographic groups.

Preparing and Presenting the Research Report

The researcher also prepares a report that summarizes the research results and conclusions. It begins with an *executive summary* in a few succinct pages. This is followed by the detailed findings. The research report should be clear and ac-

○○○○○

Exhibit 6.4. Assessing the Interest in a Proposed New Lecture Series: The Buyer Intention Survey.

One way to form an estimate of future demand is to ask a sample of target buyers, either individually or in focus groups, to state their buying intentions for the forth-coming period. Respondents can be asked:

> If you hear about an interesting lecture series on contemporary art at the Atlas Museum will you . . .
>
> ___Definitely attend
> ___Probably attend
> ___Probably not attend
> ___Definitely not attend

Researchers feel that the *definitely attends* would be fairly dependable as a mini-mum estimate, and some fraction of the *probably attends* could be added to arrive at a forecast.

This can be followed by additional questions:

> What two or three factors would *encourage* you most to subscribe to the lecture series on contemporary art at the Atlas Museum? (Check up to three items that you consider to be most important.)
>
> ___Discount ticket prices
> ___Membership newsletters
> ___Restaurant or parking discounts
> ___Guaranteed priority seating
> ___Special ticket exchange privileges
> ___Desire to support the institution
> ___Guaranteed ticket availability
> ___Ability to attend with friends more easily
> ___Interest in particular speakers
> ___Ease of ordering tickets

> What two or three factors would *discourage* you most from subscribing? (Check up to two items that you consider to be most important.)
>
> ___Too much money to commit at once
> ___Too much advance planning required
> ___Unfamiliarity with speakers
> ___Limited interest in attending so many performances of certain speakers
> ___Limited interest in the particular selection of speakers
> ___Too inconvenient (live too far away, difficulty leaving the house at night, and so forth)

○○○○○

curate, well presented, and attractively designed because in the final analysis, no matter how well all previous steps have been done, the project will not be successful unless the report is an effective communication vehicle.

Evaluating and Implementing the Findings

Now that the findings have been presented, management must digest the conclusions and decide on any appropriate actions. Some museum personnel, especially those who dislike the conclusions, may dispute the validity of the findings, criticizing sample size, the questionnaire, or other aspects of research design. The researcher must acknowledge the possibility of error.

It is always desirable to evaluate any research process just undertaken. The researcher and the museum manager should ask whether there were any ways in which the research could have been carried out better. Only through evaluating and improving its research process will a museum get the most benefit out of its research investments.

SUMMARY

Marketing research is the systematic design, collection, analysis, and reporting of data and findings relevant to understanding an organization's consumers, the environmental factors influencing the organization, and ways to improve consumer satisfaction and organizational performance. Museums are increasingly using types of market research in the form of visitor studies and exhibition evaluations. Marketing research differs from simple, casual observation insofar as it is systematic, comprehensive, and thoroughly evaluated in its methods. It can take the form of focus groups, surveys done with visitors at museums, mail and telephone surveys, and panel studies. The research process involves careful examination of sampling size, survey instruments, and areas of possible bias. Because marketing research is expensive, the first step is for a museum's management, along with marketing researchers, to define the issues the research is intended to address and the objectives the managers have in mind. Having staff trained to some degree in the methods and processes of marketing research can lead to greater confidence in the research and in tailoring the research to the museum's needs.

CHAPTER SEVEN

Developing Attractive Offerings

Exhibitions, Programs, Experiences, Services

Visitors do not expect intellectual thrills from attending a museum.
They are, rather, hoping for surprise and excitement as they escape temporarily
the predictable confines of existence. . . . [W]hat the audience expects from
an art museum is, above all, a magical transformation of experience.
—Mihalyi Csikszentmihalyi

All museums face the challenge of deciding what to offer to their visitors. After all, there are a variety of ways to design an exhibition hall or to present objects. Museums have choices of the programs they offer and the services they provide. A museum's offerings consist of a mix of at least five basic elements. First, there is the museum *setting* itself, the exterior and interior architecture and designed space (discussed in Chapter Eight). Second, there are the *objects, collections, exhibitions.* Third, there are interpretive materials such as labels, texts, and catalogues. Fourth, there are museum *programs* (sometimes called *ancillary services*), such as lectures, performances, and social events. Fifth, there are the museum *services,* such as reception and orientation, food service, shopping, and seating.

Some observers suggest that there is a sixth element in the mix of museum offerings: the extent to which the museum organizes or fails to organize the visitor's time, activity, and experience. Certain museums even today offer visitors the most minimal responses. In such a "nonresponsive" museum, for want of a better term, a visitor can enter the building, walk around unguided and unaware of the museum's offerings and what a museum is, never see or talk with a museum employee, and leave the premises in a state of bewilderment.

According to Alan Andreasen, professor of marketing at Georgetown University (interviewed Oct. 31, 1994), museums can productively learn about customer service from the Disney organization. Disney manages the visitor's time, keeps the visitor from being bored, offers a friendly and comfortable setting, maintains a clean environment, watches over the visitor, and undertakes extensive research to keep informed about a visitor's expectations, needs, and preferences. Organizing a visitor's time and activity does not mean controlling that activity. A museum visit is a voluntary endeavor. What organizing a museum visit involves is furnishing a visitor with, at a minimum, a welcome, orientation, and services that will facilitate the museum-going experience.

G. Donald Adams, director of marketing and visitor programs at the Automotive Hall of Fame, in Dearborn, Michigan, and a longtime museum professional (interviewed on Feb. 6 and 20, 1996), offers the view that the experience of a visit to a museum is not limited to viewing exhibits on the premises. The museum-going experience is a broader one that includes leaving home, driving to the museum, parking, being greeted at the entrance, the visit itself, and the return home. A museum cannot control every facet of this outing, but it can view its responsibility broadly, encompassing the services and surrounding experiences as well as exhibition content.

Yet another way to view a museum's offerings is to take a historical view. Originally, museums were noted for their collections and rare objects and the distinctive obligation they had to care for and conserve these collections and pass them along to future generations. Beginning in the twentieth century, museums began to elevate their information and education role, and this has continued to be a high priority in most museums ever since. In recent years, museum leaders and staff have awakened to the museum's role in providing experiences, on the assumption that visitors expect this of a museum visit. Museums have also awakened to their community role. Each of these attributes, as they have unfolded historically, constitutes a type of museum offering.

It is important to a museum's success that management and staff examine the full range of the museum's offerings. Museums often focus on their core collections. But if they neglect ancillary services or fail to provide an attractive setting, they may disappoint their visitors. Given the budgetary constraints facing all museums and the competing interests of different staff members, issues of what to offer audiences are likely to be a matter of constant tension. Therefore it is all the more important for the museum's leadership to develop a vision, a strategic view, of the optimal mix of offerings and carefully allocate resources accordingly. The further challenge is to create a good mix of offerings to satisfy disparate visitors who have a variety of expectations and needs.

As Mihalyi Csikszentmihalyi observed in the quotation introducing this chapter, museum leaders are well served by assessing their museum offerings from the point of view of visitors and consumers and not merely from the vantage point of program staff. In this chapter we will examine three types of museum offerings: first, a museum's existing exhibitions, collections, and programs; second, a museum's development of new exhibitions, programs, and other offerings; and third, museum services.

ONGOING COLLECTIONS AND EXHIBITIONS

A museum's collections and exhibitions are its core offerings, the distinctive elements that few other organizations can provide; therefore, maintaining and managing the quality of ongoing exhibitions is a first priority in a museum. Each museum should identify what makes it distinctive. For example, large art museums are likely to have distinctively encyclopedic collections, while other art museums may be distinctive for specialized collections. Contemporary art museums can focus on twentieth-century art or post–World War II art.

History museums like the National Museum of American History include every aspect of a nation's material culture: portraiture and artworks, handicrafts and consumer goods, inventions, machines, and technologies, objects of everyday life, treasures and icons, books and manuscripts, stamps and coins, films and recordings, and objects of notoriety associated with famous individuals and families. Other historical museums are distinctive in representing particular aspects of a society (for example, the American West, baseball and football, rock and roll music) or the products of particular industries (automotive, banking and finance, transportation) or famous figures in popular culture (Elvis Presley's Graceland, in Memphis, Tennessee).

Some museums, science and technology centers, history centers, and children's museums are not built primarily around collections of rare or authentic objects. These museums can focus on science experiments as learning experiences, designed settings and hands-on activities as means for young children to develop motor skills, and historical exhibitions as narratives that help visitors experience different historical eras. Today, the trend is toward structuring exhibitions with themes, contexts, and points of view.

Regardless of the kinds of exhibitions a museum offers, staff can continuously improve the way exhibitions are designed, presented, and interpreted. Robert Sullivan, associate director of public programs at the National Museum of Natural History, in Washington, D.C., helped develop a list of guidelines for exhibitions at his museum that has applicability in other museums (interviewed on Oct. 1, 1997). The following guidelines are the outcome of visitor research.

1. *Remember the audience.* Exhibitions should be audience focused. Identify the primary and secondary audiences early, to be certain that your goals are appropriate. The thinner you can slice the target audience segment, the more likely you are to achieve your objectives.

2. *Exhibitions don't tell, they show.* As visual media, exhibitions work best when they are object and image centered. Long, unbroken blocks of copy do not get read. Most visitors sample at random. Read each label and ask yourself, Is this the voice of someone I would like to sit

next to at a dinner party? You don't have to dumb down, but you do have to liven up.

3. *Exhibitions are provocative, not comprehensive.* You do not have to tell everything you know about a topic; rather, you have to provoke the visitor to want to find out more. The exhibit experience should be seen as a threshold to learning, not an end point.

4. *A good question is better than a declaration.* Learning should be thought of as a looping process, not a linear one. Asking a provocative question in a banner line will open up that interactive loop, and that will motivate a visitor to look harder and read deeper. Asking unexpected and provocative questions is a good way to pique interest in a topic visitors may not be predisposed to.

5. *Interaction, unexpected connections, surprises, and even humor are all pluses.* Interaction does not mean blindly pushing buttons; it means the effective combination of hands-on action with minds-on learning. Asking visitors to do things and make connections can be very effective. Visitors will spend more time learning if they feel they have initiated or participated in the information process.

6. *Match media with message.* The statement of purpose is where you identify the function, objectives, and audience for the exhibition. It is also where you determine if the correct medium for delivering the message is indeed an exhibition, rather than a video or a book. In short, exhibitions are object-centered, multisensory and multimedia, nonsequential, provocative learning avenues.

A British study of visitors' reactions to old and new exhibitions to determine what visitors thought of as "ideal" qualities of exhibitions led to a list of thirteen qualities, including "It makes the subject come to life," "It gets the message across quickly," "You can't help noticing it," "It involves you," "The information is clearly presented," and "It's clear what you're supposed to do and how to begin" (Serrell, 1996, p. 46). A study of visitors at the Brookfield Zoo, in the Chicago area, yielded the following list of attributes of strong exhibitions: "It is memorable," "It's an experience that involves your senses," "You are gently guided to make discoveries," "It is a personal experience," and "You get lots of opportunities to investigate and make observations" (pp. 46–47).

Museums have improved their ongoing offerings in various ways in recent years. History museums have made great efforts to connect visitors with historical experiences. Exhibitions increasingly deal with family and community history. The Minnesota History Center (MHC), in St. Paul, has pioneered in presentations that engage visitors emotionally as well as intellectually. Exhibitions on family, community, and regional history serve as bridges to exhibitions on national and world history and the history of great leaders and events. (MHC exhibitions are discussed further in the Model Museum Practice at the end of Chapter Four.)

As museums eschew their traditional position as temples, with interpretative resources handed down from above, they are becoming forums for the presentation of multiple perspectives. As museums move away from the tradition of placing objects in exhibition cases with a minimum of label text and interpretation, they are more and more using objects and exhibitions to tell stories that capture the context and meaning behind the objects as well as the richness of the objects themselves. An example is the United States Holocaust Memorial Museum (USHMM), in Washington, D.C. The museum's high degree of conceptual and presentational skill is worth examining by other museums. Some analysts argue that USHMM is as much a theatrical stage as it is a collections-based museum; that is, the objects are largely tools for illuminating the experiences of a historical era rather than ends in themselves. USHMM makes use of a variety of presentational forms and media. Visitors encounter information in a various ways, in both the exhibitions and the archival resources available on a computer database. Visitors hear the voices of Holocaust survivors, view photographs of Holocaust victims, and read their letters and poems. Motion picture, video, and audio recordings re-create the experience of the Holocaust. Ethical and philosophical perspectives, in the form of an exhibit on heroes who rescued Jews, and texts that stimulate inquiry and reflection draw visitors to think about enduring human values.

Museums in recent years have experimented with different presentational and design forms, and this has resulted in considerable innovation. A successful example is found at the National Zoological Park, in Washington, D.C., a leading zoo and research center. Management and staff created exhibitions and activities that would better inform visitors about the zoo's research enterprise. So they created two floors of science galleries that allow visitors to view through a glass partition a series of laboratories where scientists work. In the Biodiversity Lab, a scientist can be seen using a scanning electron microscope to probe the structure and function of an organism. In the Molecular Genetics Lab, visitors can view the technology and equipment for examining genetic materials. Down the hall is the Nutrition Laboratory, where researchers analyze food and animal diets. And farther along, the Behavior Lab, where researchers study animal sounds and communication by means of tape recordings, video monitors, and computers. Visitors can find information on computer screens in front of each of the labs and read *equipment guidebooks* that explain the machines and technologies. Researchers will periodically mingle with visitors to discuss the work they are doing. The National Zoo has also transformed animal habitats into learning and behavioral study areas. Visitors can view orangutans walking up towers and moving across cables as well as sitting at computers and solving problems. Visitors can view cheetahs racing across a terrain engaging in behavioral experiments.

Kevin Moore (1997) points to another engaging element in museum offerings: offering visitors "real people" and "real places" as well as "real things." Interaction with curators and docents is one manifestation of this technique, as is listing the names of the curators and designers who are responsible for an exhibition. Historical reenactments and immersion experiences are another form. Reenactments of American Civil War battles, for example, take place at historic sites where the battles occurred or in a museum-designed environment that simulates those war scenes. Staff at some historic sites (Colonial Williamsburg is one prominent example) dress in period clothing, offer dramatic readings, tell stories of the times, demonstrate cooking and occupational activities of the period, and re-create musical performances as they occurred in bygone days.

Museums that explore different cultures and offer cross-cultural experiences have found that audiences value the opportunities to learn about other cultures through indigenous voices as well as curatorial ones. The Smithsonian's Festival of American Folklife, held each summer on the National Mall, in Washington, D.C., was one of the first cultural exhibitions to move outside museum walls. It pioneered in the presentation of cultural experiences from the point of view of members of cultural groups. In 1995, the festival featured four programs— *The Cape Verdean Connection, The Czech Republic, Voices of First Nation's Women,* and *Russian Roots, American Branches*—in which indigenous people told their stories, showed their ways of life, performed their music, demonstrated their arts and crafts, and offered their culinary specialties. The 1996 *Stories of the People* exhibition, organized by the National Museum of the American Indian as a special exhibition in the Smithsonian's Arts and Industries Building, is another example of innovative presentation of cultural experiences. The exhibition communicates entirely through the voices of Native Americans, some of whom are museum curators and some tribal leaders and members. Several different American Indian nations speak to visitors through objects, interpretative materials, and graphics. In each section, an individual is shown in a photograph and identified as the spokesperson of the Indian nation represented. The text recounts, in personal terms, the spokesperson's experience and knowledge of the Indian nation's history and culture. All 190 objects in the exhibition were selected by the spokespersons, who are perceived as tribal authorities. The effect on visitors is engaging, personal, and emotional.

Art museums are augmenting their exhibitions with family and children's programs that introduce visitors to studio arts through hands-on creative interaction. The Walker Art Center, in Minneapolis, invites visitors one Saturday each month to work with materials, play roles in theater pieces, and listen to musical performance.

Museums have augmented exhibitions and other offerings by means of electronic information technologies—interactive computer screens, audiotapes, and hand-held audio-video guides running on CD-ROMs—that supply pictures, sounds, and information databases to enlarge visitors' experiences. An example, from the National Museum of Natural History, is the interactive computer screen "How to Become a Fossil." The interactive screen is located just inside the paleontology halls and fossil exhibits, and it is especially helpful for young people. The computer asks the user, "What is a fossil?" and invites the visitor to imagine what becoming a fossil is like. Participants are told that the chances of becoming a fossil are scant, and the computer illustrates the various obstacles, such as being eaten or being dismembered, crushed, worn away by weathering, or decomposed by burial. The user is then invited to take a chance at becoming a fossil and may choose to be a plant, an invertebrate, or a vertebrate. Finally, a "wheel of chance" determines whether the user has achieved fossil status. This interactive screen is a very popular destination that prepares visitors for viewing and appreciating real fossils in the adjoining halls.

Young children often feel that museums are uninviting places, built largely around visual experience and offering few of the tactile experiences children enjoy. Science centers are known for providing interactive tools as well as multimedia demonstrations. The Carnegie Science Center in Pittsburgh employs high-school students as docents to share with visitors, particularly young people, a variety of objects to touch and view close up, including live snakes and other small animals. More and more history museums are featuring special galleries in which youngsters can handle artifacts, tools, and machines. Art museums are organizing weekend programs that allow children and their parents to work with art materials. Children's museums such as the Children's Museum of Indianapolis and the Please Touch Museum in Philadelphia offer young people tactile and kinesthetic activities, hands-on objects and tools, games and puzzles, performances, storytelling, and demonstrations.

Museums' exhibitions should not remain unchanged through time. They lose their appeal both to active visitors who sample them repeatedly and to new visitors who might find them stale, old-fashioned, or uncommunicative. The main way to fight the cycle of decline in exhibits is to refresh the content periodically. Consider the recent developments in dinosaur exhibits at natural history museums. The Field Museum, in Chicago, was one of the first U.S. museums to exhibit the bones of dinosaurs. Owing to the popularity of the movie *Jurassic Park* and its sequel, children have become even more interested in dinosaurs, and the Field Museum responded with a new exhibit that includes mechanically operated dinosaurs in primordial settings replete with explosive movements and sounds. These new exhibits have drawn enormous crowds. The Field Museum in 1997 purchased the most complete *Tyrannosaurus rex* dinosaur ever found, and this addition is likely to reinforce the fascination that visitors have.

Updating exhibitions costs money, however. The National Museum of Natural History (NMNH) in the early 1990s struggled to find resources with which to replace aging exhibitions, some of which dated back forty or so years. Robert Sullivan, the museum's public programs officer, was recruited with the mandate to organize a major overhaul of the galleries and exhibits. Sullivan has estimated that a substantial renovation of the museum, with two hundred thousand square feet of exhibit space, would cost as much as $450 per square foot, or $150 million. Lesser degrees of overhaul would cost less. NMNH has adopted a plan to renovate exhibitions and galleries in stages, and new galleries and exhibitions, including the Janet Annenberg Hooker Hall of Geology, Gems, and Minerals, are winning considerable praise.

Art museums typically rotate their exhibitions by means of traveling exhibitions, loans from other museums, and modifying exhibitions of permanent collections. Science museums refresh exhibits regularly, to keep up with scientific advances as well as to stimulate visitor interest.

Many museums are establishing exhibition teams to plan new exhibits and upgrade existing ones. Typical teams consists of a curator, a designer, an educator, a writer, and an audience, communications, or marketing specialist. Some responsibilities are individual; others are shared. Curators have major responsibility for creating exhibit concepts and content, selecting objects, and overseeing interpretation. Other team members are expected to represent the point of view of audiences. The design and presentation side often involves a sharing of expertise among curators, educators, and audience-oriented specialists. Promotion and positioning of an exhibition are largely the responsibility of the communications and marketing specialists. Teams of this kind have been productive in revitalizing old exhibitions and bringing forth new ones with innovative features.

ONGOING PROGRAMS

Many museum offer ongoing supplemental programs such as lectures, classes, and tours. Musical, theatrical, and film programs can also augment the visitor's experience in encountering art, history, and science. An expanding museum activity consists of continuing education classes and workshops, which appeal to museum members and to older, retired citizens and are often means to convert museum visitors into members. These educational programs can be closely related to specific collections and exhibitions or to a museum's subject matter, as in the case of studio arts classes at art museums. Some museums have teamed up with outside educational organizations; for example, the Minneapolis Institute of Arts and the Minneapolis College of Art and Design together offer a range of art and studio courses.

Museums are increasingly in the business of organizing social, recreational, and celebratory events and happenings that are not necessarily directly connected with their collections and exhibitions. History museums and historic sites organize holiday and seasonal events as ways to reach larger audiences, build community support, and raise revenue. Art museums have typically launched new exhibitions with opening-night events for selected audiences. A growing number of art museums have created another category of event, social gatherings for target groups, such as young professionals, who can enjoy the special ambience of an art museum, meet like-minded others, and socialize over food and drinks and musical and theatrical performances. The Art Institute of Chicago, for example, one Thursday evening a month hosts a social event for young professionals known as "After Hours." The Corcoran Gallery of Art, in Washington, D.C., has created a variety of social programs combined with educational features that are targeted to several groups: senior citizens, African Americans, young professionals, and active arts and culture consumers. Natural history and science museums, in particular, have upgraded educational programs, incorporating decidedly recreational features. They offer overnights and summer camps for children.

DEVELOPING NEW OFFERINGS

Many museums are actively engaged in upgrading their existing exhibitions and programs (offerings that might be in place for an extended period of time)—for example, renovating galleries, expanding signage, improving exhibition design, and augmenting exhibitions with educational and multimedia programs. In addition to managing existing offerings, museums also have to develop new offerings—new forms of exhibitions, new ancillary programs, or both. The line separating existing offerings from new ones is not always clear, yet it is useful for museum managers to think about both. Moreover, whatever its offerings, a museum's managers are well advised to think about them from the point of view of visitors and consumers (see Witteborg, 1981).

Developing new offerings helps a museum reach and appeal to a larger and broader audience. New offerings can be developed specifically to attract underserved segments, such as families with young children or members of ethnic and cultural groups who do not currently participate in the museum. For example, an urban art museum in a U.S. city that has a large Western European collection is likely to want to expand its collection to include works by Hispanic and African American artists and art that reflects the life of these communities. These new offerings have the potential to broaden the museum's audience and its programming. New offerings can also appeal to regular visitors and museum members, who are likely to welcome new things on subsequent visits. Museums that are oriented strongly toward members are expected to generate new types of ancillary programming. In large art museums, blockbuster exhibitions have provided novelty and drama, as well as aesthetic experience.

The following are a sampling of new offerings at U.S. museums that illustrate the benefits and objectives. The Johnson County Museums, in Shawnee, Kansas, formerly attracted an upper-middle-class Protestant segment of the community. In the 1990s, the museums began to broaden their collections to include artifacts and records reflecting other ethnic and cultural groups in the community, immigrants as well as the native born, and members of different social classes. The museums then extended the scope and subject of their exhibitions to embrace all segments of the community.

The Missouri Historical Society, in St. Louis, in addition to its collections and exhibitions depicting local and regional history and culture, has in recent years added a new dimension: coverage of urban issues that encompass neighborhoods, the central city, the metropolitan area, and the surrounding region. The society's mission has expanded considerably to represent and interpret the present and the evolving future as well as the past and to deal with human concerns, problem solving, and public policy that extend far beyond the primarily collections-oriented activities of past years.

In the mid-1990s, Chicago's Museum of Science and Industry opened an exhibition on HIV/AIDS titled *AIDS: The War Within* that featured a number of innovations. Design and presentational elements presented multiple perspectives, personal narratives, clinical experiences, and multimedia presentations, the combination of which has had a forceful effect on museum visitors and has attracted new audiences. Visitors can learn directly from individuals (speaking on videos and CD-ROMs) about their experiences of coping with AIDS; play the role of clinical researchers and learn about the biochemistry and physiology of the disease using microscopes, digital scanning devices, and photographs; view breakthrough experiments that have resulted in new treatments for AIDS; and view time lines and maps that show the history and spread of the disease worldwide.

Two examples of new offerings at art museums illustrate other possibilities for revitalizing museum offerings. James Robinson, a curator of Asian art at the Indianapolis Museum of Art, has experimented with inviting comments and reactions from visitors to the Asian art galleries and also from scholars and connoisseurs regarding the artworks, labels and texts, design elements, and the gallery setting and has posted these in or near the galleries. Visitors to the Krannert Art Museum, on the campus of the University of Illinois in Champaign, can arrange for tours with museum curators, educators, and docents (in the case of schoolchildren, with specially trained teachers) to extend the experience of viewing art as an interpersonal and interactive process. Using an approach known as *visual thinking strategies,* small groups of people take the tours, focus on a single object or a few objects, and share perspectives, thoughts, and feelings among the group and with the guide. Some museums have occasionally invited visitors at a designated time to meet with other visitors and museum staff to talk about and share their overall museum-going experiences.

Museums have developed a variety of ancillary programs as ways to refresh and augment the museum-going experience: behind-the-scenes tours for members to view the collections in storage, in the conservation labs, and as subjects of research; ethnic and cultural festivals that include arts and crafts demonstrations, storytelling, musical and theatrical performances, and food services; sleep-overs at the museum; holiday events; and special family-oriented programs.

The challenge for museums is to provide a range of museum-going experiences that appeal to the spectrum of visitors. Most museums lack the scale and resources to be all things to all people (and such a strategy can be self-defeating even for the largest); yet museum managers and staff should reflect periodically on the types and quality of experiences their museums offer. Regular self-assessments can be productive, leading to answers to the following questions: Does the museum offer sufficient learning experiences, and to what groups are these targeted? Are there an adequate number of celebratory experiences? Can visitors enjoy interpersonal and social experiences at the museum, and are the facilities and services conducive? Does the museum have exhibitions that are enchanting?

SERVICES

Today's museums offer their publics a variety of services, including orientation and wayfinding information, places to sit and relax, food services, shopping in gift shops, rest rooms, facilities to change infant's and children's clothes, water fountains, and lost-and-found and other security functions.

Museum visits can be tiring. In addition to requiring much walking around and standing, museums can be crowded and hard to negotiate. The visual stimuli can be overabundant. Objects and exhibitions may be unfamiliar and strange. Families with children must divide their attention in order to help the children have good and safe experiences. Even veteran museum-goers often can be heard complaining that they have energy only for a single exhibition or a specific set of galleries, and after some time need relaxation and diversion. Visitor studies indicate that many visitors find museums disorienting or uncomfortable. It is in this context that museums have to try to provide ample services.

Characteristics of Services

Museum managers should pay particular attention to the four main characteristics of services: intangibility, inseparability, variability, and perishability.

Intangibility. Most services are intangible and cannot be seen, tasted, felt, or heard before they are consumed. Suppose a museum visitor decides to attend a lecture titled "Picasso's Blue Period"; the title is promising, but the visitor cannot be sure of the lecture's quality in advance. The lecturer may turn out to be articulate or inarticulate, fascinating or dull, learned or superficial. Visitors may have a set of expectations, information they may have heard from others, images and notions, however incomplete or inaccurate, of what to expect.

Because services are basically intangible, museums find it useful to make their intangible offers tangible. They can do this by showing photos of a lecturer, of their restaurant, or their exhibition halls. They can influence visitor expectations by the design of the building, by the guards' uniforms, by the advertisements they create. Museums can design their brochures in ways that convey excitement, adventure, and important learning experiences. A museum's logo can serve as a tangible manifestation of the services and experiences a museum provides.

Inseparability. Most services are inseparable from a provider. Medical service is rendered by a physician, and haircutting by a barber or beautician. A person who wants to enjoy the full services of a museum must visit the museum site; electronic media offer only a limited experience. The full experience is inseparable from the gallery.

Museum services are rendered directly by museum employees: a docent leading a tour, a guard answering a question, a telephone operator listing the museum's hours of operation. Therefore a critical part of ensuring satisfying museum visits consists of effectively training and motivating these employees (providers) to be friendly and responsive to visitors. Good marketing cannot be provided by the marketing department alone. If the rest of a museum is not responsive to the visitors, then the museum will fail in its marketing mission. A museum must carry out internal as well as external marketing. Internal marketing involves selecting friendly and helpful employees, giving them customer training, encouraging employee feedback and ideas, and running recognition award programs for good service.

Variability. Service quality is more variable than product quality, insofar as the providers vary more than the products. Service quality in a museum depends on who provides it and on when, where, and how it is provided. An art museum docent can be cheerful on Monday, matter-of-fact on Tuesday, and grumpy on Wednesday. Furthermore, service quality fluctuates with the levels of museum attendance. Staff resources are often stretched to the limit at peak periods, and service quality is likely to fall. In science museums during busy periods, there are likely to be long waiting lines and equipment breakdowns. Given that museums are open to the public virtually every day of the year, operating from 9 A.M. to 5 P.M. and sometimes in the evening, proper museum maintenance taxes the ability and the mood of management and staff.

Service-oriented organizations take a number of steps toward achieving quality control in their services. Not only do they invest in employee training and provide incentives by recognizing and rewarding excellent staff behavior but they also make employees available to answer questions and respond to customer concerns. They establish regular procedures for receiving customer's suggestions for service improvements. They create complaint systems and customer surveys to ensure responsiveness to customer needs.

Perishability. Services are perishable—they cannot be stored for later sales or use. Visitors to Washington, D.C., during the week of December 18 to 25, 1995, could not see the famous Vermeer exhibition at the National Gallery of Art, even if they had advance tickets, because of the government budget crisis and shutdown. Similarly, those who missed the blockbuster Monet show at the Art Institute of Chicago will never see it; it cannot be stored, certainly not experientially, even though it can be reproduced on videos and computer screens.

Service perishability is more of a problem when demand is unsteady. The scale of service is usually geared to normal attendance, and services are strained and service quality deteriorates in periods of overdemand. Conversely, a museum might be overstaffed during periods of lower than normal attendance.

Service organizations employ several strategies for producing a better match between demand and supply. On the demand side, museums have the option of charging different admission fees at different times to help regulate demand between peak and off-peak periods. When overdemand might result from a major exhibition, museums can require advance ticket purchase and regulate admission at different designated times. On the supply side, museums can hire additional part-time employees to serve at periods of peak demand. During peak periods, employees can be given only essential tasks to perform. Outside contractors can be hired to manage specialized services, thus freeing the time of the regular staff. In slow periods, employees can catch up on work that they put aside during the rush period.

Specific Museum Services

Let us consider the management of specific services offered by museums.

Visitor Orientation and Information Service. Countless audience surveys have pinpointed visitor orientation and wayfinding information as a critical need in museums. Visitors have a particularly hard time navigating large museums; all visitors need information, ranging from where to find objects and exhibits to where to find services such as cafeterias and rest rooms. Many of today's museums provide visitors printed guides and maps, and a growing number provide computer screens with the museum information. The National Gallery of Art, in Washington, D.C., opened in 1996 an impressive electronic information gallery called the Micro Gallery. Visitors can use it to locate artworks and shows and create self-directed tours and print out tour maps.

Visitors often seek information from museum staff. Museums in the United Kingdom—such as the Colchester Museums, the Doncaster Museum and Art Gallery, and Glasgow City Museums—have taken the lead in training staff at all levels to be information and orientation providers. Security guards can serve both security and information needs. Guards and other front-line staff are being trained broadly to serve as welcomers, informants, spokespersons, and motivators. The Canadian Museum of Civilization's pioneering work in guest services focuses on training staff in visitor services, providing visitors with all the information and orientation they require, and having tools to monitor and evaluate the quality of the services provided.

Seating and Relaxation Spaces. Traditional museums rarely provided seating for visitors. Today's museums recognize the need for seating and for spaces where visitors can relax and enjoy some diversion. The Baltimore Museum of Art lets visitors borrow folding chairs to use in the galleries. Infirm visitors can use walkers of various kinds. The Oregon Museum of Science and Industry, in Portland, added a space where visitors can sit at tables and relax with card games, checkers, and dominoes. Marilynne Eichinger, the museum president at the time (interviewed May 7, 1996), observed that many visitors come as extended families, with children, parents, and grandparents. Grandparents could occupy themselves while parents dined and children visited the galleries. The National Gallery of Art, in Washington, D.C., provides its members and patrons with a special lounge for relaxation. The Field Museum in Chicago offers visitors study rooms, filled with books, periodicals, and videos, next to certain galleries, allowing visitors to learn more about the museum's collections in a relaxing setting.

Courses, Clinics, and Research Services. Art museums today are offering collectors special courses and clinics to improve their skills in collecting. An example is the Expertise Clinic offered at the Minneapolis Institute of Arts. Curators and other experts meet with the public at designated times to examine objects and artworks brought in. Different sessions are held for paintings, Asian art, African art, Native American art, decorative arts, and photographs. Specialists discuss the history and age of objects, historical or artistic significance, and the condition of objects, but the clinics do not deal with appraisals.

Some museums are able to market research services. History museums, for example, can perform historical research for individuals and organizations, reproduce documents, and distribute photographs. Large research museums such as the Field Museum provide special services to visiting scholars and researchers, often free of charge or subsidized by fellowships and grants. More museums are charging for these services and keeping a close eye on the prices they charge.

Food Service. Museums are giving greater prominence in their planning to food service and restaurants. Food is always a critical need where groups of people assemble. Larger museums in the past provided modest and utilitarian cafeterias for visitors who were, for the most part, informally dressed and not part of family groups. The thinking was that pricey restaurants or cafés were impractical and unnecessary. Today's museums, however, have discovered the benefits of providing different types and levels of food service. Museum food service ranges from cafeterias, to food courts, to cafés and upscale restaurants. The Guggenheim Museum's upscale café is managed by one of the leading culinary firms in New York City. Baltimore's Walters Art Gallery provides an upscale restaurant with a separate street-level entrance in addition to the museum entrance. Some museum restaurants offer live music. Museums should segment their audiences and provide a range of food services and dining facilities that match the needs of different segments.

PURCHASABLE PRODUCTS

Many visitors like to leave a museum with a souvenir of their visit. It could be a book illustrating the museum's collection, an art poster, a T-shirt with the museum's name on it, or some other memento. Museum pamphlets and guides often make good souvenirs. Not surprisingly, museums established gift shops early on. They were typically small, out-of-the way places managed by volunteers and offering limited merchandise reflecting the museum's collections. Eventually, the shops added more items—a wider selection of books, jewelry, children's games, and so on—and what had begun as a small service to museum-goers became a major activity and a significant source of income. Art museum shops specialize in art catalogues and books and personal items bearing images from famous artworks. Natural history and science museum shops tend to specialize in rocks and minerals, specimens, microscopes, telescopes, and science learning games. The shops at the National Air and Space Museum have extensive inventories of model airplanes and kites. The gift shops at large museums have become large-scale operations, often employing professional managers and buyers.

The shop at the entrance to Chicago's Art Institute, for example, offers a broad range of merchandise connected to the collections and exhibitions or else bearing little connection. The shop offers ample spaces for browsing and buying and well-lit and well-designed areas for shopping. Divided into a series of boutique-like areas, it contains a bookstore, a gift shop, a jewelry shop, a section selling personal items such as ties, scarfs, and clothing, a section with art reproductions and prints, and other areas. Today, major museums have opened shops in off-site locations, such as airports, train stations, and shopping malls. They also have mail-order catalogues to reach a geographically broader audience. During the Smithsonian's 150th anniversary year, in 1996, the U.S. cable television channel QVC, which calls itself the "electronic retailer," featured not only tours of several Smithsonian museums but also Smithsonian museum shop merchandise that viewers could purchase by telephone.

Some museum programs are also in a sense purchasable objects and services. Large museums offer members an array of study tours and travel packages. The Smithsonian Institution, for example, markets its study seminars and tours, in the United States and overseas, as high-end educational tours, differentiating them from regular commercial tours. Accompanying these tours are curators, scientists, and experts in the areas visited and subjects covered, and the schedule often includes formal classes, lectures, and workshops.

People like to purchase things, and museums are increasingly meeting this need. It is a mistake not to bring modern retailing principles to bear on gift shop operations and other museum sales. Gift shop managers need good service policies and skills in merchandise development and selection, shop design and flow, merchandise presentation, and customer-oriented staff training. This becomes increasingly important as new competition, such as the Museum Company, emerges in the private sector.

SUMMARY

A museum's offerings usually involve a mix of five elements: the physical facilities, the collections and exhibitions, the interpretative materials (labels, texts, brochures, catalogues), supplemental programs (lectures, performances, social events), and services (information and orientation, food service, gift shop). Some analysts argue that museums should also facilitate visits by providing orientation, seating, rest areas, comfortable spaces, good management of visitors' time, minimum congestion, and enough of interest to prevent visitors from being bored. Museum offerings can also be viewed from another perspective. Museums offer collections, usually of rare objects, that are maintained not only for use in the present day but also for the enjoyment of future generations; they offer information and education; they also offer distinctive destination-style experiences that go beyond gathering information; and they can play an important role in the community and offer community services. Museums should continuously monitor their offerings, improving them, expending them to capture the interest of new audiences, and updating or replacing long-standing exhibitions and programs to keep them from becoming stale and unappealing, especially to regular visitors and to members.

O

MODEL MUSEUM PRACTICE

Pioneering in Education and Community Outreach: The Newark Museum

Nine decades ago, The Newark Museum was founded by John Cotton Dana in downtown Newark, New Jersey, specifically as an educational and community institution. As Dana ([1917] 1988) noted, with an eye on other, more traditional museums: "The new museum . . . examines its community's life first, and then straightway bends its energies to supplying some of the material which that community needs" (p. 11). It has remained true to Dana's vision. Even when racial riots racked the central city in 1967, the museum board never wavered in its loyalty to Newark. The then director, Samuel Miller, insisted: "We're not just the beacon or oasis here. In this old, old city, even with a middle class on the run, we're part of a fabric, not the temple in the park" (Cohen, 1991, p. 94).

The Newark Museum has evolved into one of the premier U.S. museums, combining in a unique way a world-class collection with vigorous community, multicultural, and educational outreach. Its collections include 87,000 art objects (exceptional examples of American paintings, sculpture, and works on paper; African, Tibetan, Chinese, Korean, and Japanese art; decorative arts; classical antiquities), 70,000 natural science specimens, a planetarium, a small-scale zoo, and 15,000 objects of the original "Lending Collection," first assembled by Dana for the loaning to schools. Decorative and industrial arts, taxidermied birds, architectural models, clothing from bygone eras, and a two-thousand-year-old crocodile mummy are among objects delivered by a van to schools both in Newark and statewide—an average of two thousand loans a year. Dana's collection for school use was intended, in his words, "to give pleasure, to make manners seem more important, to promote skill, to exalt hand-work and to increase the zest for life" (Dana, [1917] 1988, p. 8). At the museum's founding in 1909, the city had a large immigrant population from European countries; today, the great majority are from African American, Hispanic, Korean, and Portuguese ethnic backgrounds.

John Dana proudly contrasted The Newark Museum as a "living museum" with museums in nearby New York City, with their grand marble buildings, precious high-priced collections, and high-status patrons and visitors. Museums of the future, Dana wrote, would become "living organisms, with an abundance of teachers, with ample workshops, classrooms and spaces for handling the outgoing and incoming of objects which they lend" (pp. 11–12).

According to the museum's present director, Mary Sue Sweeney Price (interviewed Mar. 11, 1996, and Feb. 27, 1997), the twenty-first-century Newark Museum will continue the traditions set down by Dana, particularly the goals of accessibility, outreach, and education. "Some people mistakenly think, in hearing about The Newark Museum's active outreach, that the museum is primarily an art or science center, lacking in outstanding collections. In fact, the two are joined together. The museum's democratic ideal of making its resources widely accessible was linked to an ideal of excellence—anchoring the museum programs in research and scholarship, world-class exhibitions and collections, and proven instructional principles and methods. The founding belief was that the museum had to make its resources accessible if it sought to inspire excellence."

Education in The Newark Museum reflects the twin emphases on active learning (experiments, hands-on activities, demonstrations) and visual learning (utilizing objects, collections, and material culture generally). Young people are encouraged to use the museum's resources for inquiry, experimentation, and discovery and meld everyday experiences with museum resources to acquire problem-solving skills. The museum shapes its educational program around both instruction and enjoyment. And children and their families continue to be a focus of museum programs. In a recent study, The Newark Museum ranked twelfth of 170 U.S. art museums in the size of its educational budget, placing it in the company of such large museums as New York's Museum of Modern Art and the Art Institute of Chicago in actual dollars spent annually on education (Association of Art Museum Directors, 1997).

The Junior Museum was an innovation when it first opened in 1926: a free-standing educational center to serve as an adjunct to school-based learning. It has evolved into a multifaceted education department with five separate programs, including teen art shows, along with workshops, hands-on activities, and classes. Membership still costs only 10 cents a year in dues. The group fosters a sense of ownership and participation in the museum. Young people participate in meetings and trips and help with various museum departments, including the Junior Gallery. Exhibits in the Junior Gallery involve visitors in experiential learning. An example was the exhibit *Stepping into Ancient Egypt: The House of the Artist Pashed,* which consisted of a full-scale installation of a three-thousand-year-old Egyptian artisan's house. Visitors were invited to lie in a bed, try on robes, and grind the grain.

During the summer of 1996, the museum offered eleven- and twelve-year-olds a workshop titled "Paints, Pots and Prints: Art Around the World." Young people learned about the art of different cultures and received training in creating a Japanese folding screen, dyeing a fabric with Ghanaian symbols, and crafting Pueblo-style coiled pottery. Eight workshops for children of different age segments, ranging from three to sixteen years, were held that summer. The education department also offers all-day junior camp during summer months and in collaboration with community organizations provides children's programs after school and during school vacations.

The Newark Museum's outreach programs, while available regionally and statewide, are mainly centered on the Newark community. Education staff take natural science and planetarium programs to local schools. The Community Gallery provides space for local artists to show their works. An annual parade and fair are centered on an unusual part of the museum's collections, fire trucks and equipment. The museum hosts recognition events and graduation ceremonies for Junior Museum members, as well as jazz concerts and children's theater. It offers Newark's only continuing education program for adults in crafts and fine arts. Several activities highlight the community's multicultural characteristics. The annual Black Film Festival has generated a significant following. The Korean American community helped support *Explore Korea: A Visit to Grandfather's House,* a 1995 special exhibition for young people that highlighted Korean culture. A 1996 photographic exhibition highlighted Portuguese culture and traditions, offering comparative perspectives on traditional and contemporary culture in Portugal and in Newark and helped shape discussion on issues of immigration and assimilation.

Artworks, exhibits, and related public programs at the museum generate community discussion of contemporary social and cultural issues. An exhibit on Nubian art featured a forum that vetted intensely held beliefs about cultural origins. The artwork *Badge of Honor,* by Pepon Osorio, illustrating communication between a son and an estranged father in jail, led to a forum on raising families. A large challenge is fostering cross-cultural experiences in which different cultural groups participate not only in activities reflecting their own culture but also in activities involving the other cultures.

The Newark Museum's successes are accompanied by ongoing challenges. The museum derives the majority of its funds from government grants and appropriations; yet as public-sector budgets are reduced, the museum is working hard to raise new private funds. Although Newark's downtown area is being redeveloped (a new performing arts center is being built near the museum), residents of local suburbs are still reluctant visitors because of their perceptions of central city crime. Tour operators need to be persuaded that their tourists will enjoy the museum visit. Yet The Newark Museum attracts an estimated 250,000 visitors annually, reaches more than 80,000 metropolitan students and an additional 150,000 in off-site programs, and has built a solid reputation in the community as a place particularly for young people to learn and develop and to spend time after school, during school breaks, and on the long summer holiday. The museum has challenges ahead. Yet its focus on education and community life has generated remarkable community support, which serves to anchor and cushion it during rough times.

CHAPTER EIGHT

Distributing the Museum's Offerings and Services

*To build and sustain a relevance to a truly representative population
of museum users, the Institution must seize the opportunities offered by
new technologies to bring museums to those who cannot come to them.*
—Commission on the Future of the Smithsonian Institution

Travelers disembarking at Gate 4, Concourse E, of the Miami International Airport in early 1997 passed a full-size museum exhibition as they moved toward the baggage claim area. The exhibition, titled *Coral Reefs: Caribbean Connections,* was produced by the Smithsonian Tropical Research Institute, in the Republic of Panama, and was the first major exhibition focusing on coral reefs. After Miami, it traveled to a variety of locations in the Caribbean and Central and South America.

On the other side of the United States, in the town of Bellevue, Washington, the Bellevue Art Museum has for nearly two decades leased and occupied fifteen thousand square feet on the upper story of the Bellevue Square Shopping Mall, an upscale mall near Seattle. Although the museum lacks permanent collections, it organizes an average of eight exhibitions a year and attracts an estimated fifty thousand visitors annually.

People usually think of a museum as a physical entity located in a specific place, whose benefits are primarily available to those who make the effort to visit its premises. But this is too limited a view of a museum's distribution possibilities. A museum's main facility must be designed to offer maximum accessibility and convenience to visitors. At the same time, museums have the opportunity to deliver their offerings and services far beyond the bounds of that physical structure. A museum's ability to distribute its resources depends on the type of museum it is and the nature of its collections. Science centers, for example, often have an easier time transporting a selection of their resources than art museums, whose old, rare, or high-priced art requires climate-controlled environments, specialized packing, and high rates of insurance. Nothing, of course, prevents art museums from distributing reproductions of great artworks, on the theory that reproductions in classrooms are much preferable to having no artworks at all.

Museums can make their exhibitions, programs, and other offerings available in a variety of ways (see Exhibit 8.1). Distributing museum offerings as far and as wide as possible is highly desirable and goes to the heart of a museum's educational mission. Large numbers of people are not able to visit museums. Museum resources in many countries are concentrated in urban centers, at a distance from the suburban, exurban, and rural communities where the majority of people live. A lot of people even today do not feel comfortable visiting museums. To change these patterns and make museums more accessible, museum leaders have taken actions to eliminate barriers, including programs to bring resources to where people live and work.

Peter van Mensch, a Dutch museologist, has observed that museum buildings are objects and they shape the ways visitors see things. The museum experience, van Mensch observes, is foremost a visual learning experience made available through design, training, and professional skills. The museum experience can conceivably take place in any time or setting. Van Mensch uses the example of Dutch windmills. When a growing number of windmills deteriorated from lack of care and use, a group of conservation-minded citizens organized a campaign to rescue at least the most historic and best-preserved examples. Some windmills have been restored to working condition and, indeed, are operating windmills. Many of their materials, however, are new. Other windmills have been restored with original materials but not to operating standards. Van Mensch (1989) argues that both types can be regarded as museum objects: the operating windmills with reproduction elements as *process museums;* the authentically restored, nonoperating windmills as *fabric museums.* Both offer visitors, who are given adequate interpretative background and context, significant museum-going and visual experiences.

There are good reasons to justify the cost and trouble in moving around and dispersing museum collections and exhibits. Yet there are critics of off-site distribution. Their argument against moving highly fragile objects has credibility. Every time a fragile object is moved, some deterioration takes place. Certain art objects, such as works on paper, would be better off in proper storage, with occasional displays under controlled conditions. And museums must balance the value of distributing collections to a large number of people in the present day against the value of conserving these collections in the best state for future generations. Critics of off-site museum activities point to still another drawback. Viewing objects in a museum setting is a distinctive experience. Certain objects, separated from the larger collections and shown piecemeal or electronically, can lose meaning out of context. However, digital scanning and computer modeling

○○○○○

Exhibit 8.1. Eight Ways to Distribute a Museum's Offerings.

1. Art museums offer their members the benefit of reciprocal memberships at other leading art museums. This gives a museum member options as a tourist and builds the museum's visibility. An example is Atlanta's High Museum's Contributing Membership, which includes reciprocal memberships at thirty-five leading U.S. art museums.

2. Corporations, serving as sponsors of museum programs or as marketing partners, offer their employees gift memberships or free passes to a museum. The Eli Lilly Company, in Indianapolis, Indiana, offers discounted memberships and free passes to the Indianapolis Museum of Art.

3. Curators at the Art Institute of Chicago offer lectures and slide shows at downtown headquarters of participating corporations and associations in a program called "Art-Express." Employees get together with a curator over a brown-bag lunch to discuss a collection, exhibit, or other museum attraction. Employees are offered free passes, discounts in the museum shops, or discounted memberships.

4. Forty thousand schoolchildren visit the Denver Art Museum every year on field trips. To bring home to parents, each student is given a "family pass" that is good for free admission for two adults and up to four children. The pass is written in English on one side and Spanish on the other.

5. Museums can have branches to reach larger and more variegated audiences. The museum's collection can circulate among the branches. The Guggenheim Museum, on Fifth Avenue in New York City, has a branch in lower Manhattan called the Guggenheim SoHo. It also has branches in Venice, Italy; Bilbao, Spain; and Berlin, Germany.

6. Cities, counties, and regional governments, as well as tourist associations, publish guides to museums and cultural institutions in their localities. The city of Atlanta, along with the convention and tourist bureau, the mass transit agency, and other entities, makes available eight different brochures promoting Atlanta's cultural life, including the "Culture Card" (a pamphlet describing and listing museums, performing arts organizations, and recreational offerings) and the mass transit system's map, which identifies the location of museums and their proximity to transit stations and bus lines.

7. Museums organize marketing partnerships with hotels, airlines, restaurants, and other organizations to build a critical mass of culture and recreation to attract tourists. A special museum exhibition can serve as a hook for a partnership program. Tourists can obtain a package of benefits, including discounted rates on hotel rooms, discounts at restaurants, discounted tickets to concert or theatrical performances, and free admission to museums. The Philadelphia Museum of Art offers packages in cooperation with an airline and a railroad, eleven hotels, a car rental firm, and fourteen performing arts organizations in the city.

8. A museum can distribute its offerings on the World Wide Web and reach a large number of people anywhere in the world. A museum home page on the Web can include general museum information, educational materials, images from the collections, maps of galleries for future visits, and even merchandise for sale in the museum shop that can be ordered directly on-line. An example is the home page of New York City's American Museum of Natural History (http://www.amnh.org).

○○○○○

techniques now permit a person to view an entire exhibition and its gallery site and even to manipulate the image of an object from any angle on a computer screen without leaving home.

Museums are under pressure to expand the reach of their offerings. Museums that receive considerable public-sector support are increasingly asked to justify that support in terms of the numbers and the diversity of the people they reach. Even museums that are privately supported are under pressure to expand their reach. Corporate sponsors are heavily influenced by marketing factors; number of visitors, composition of visitors, proportion of families with children, the image a museum has among the people in the surrounding community. An exhibition that opens in one museum and travels to museums in several cities is more likely to obtain corporate support, all things being equal, than an exhibition shown in only a single place for a limited period. Exhibitions that travel to schools and community centers are more likely to find support among local legislators than exhibitions that stay put in a museum building.

A museum that seeks to distribute its resources beyond the museum walls, and to do so in the most efficient and effective way possible, needs to address several key questions:

- What are the goals of outreach and distribution?
- What are the target audiences for outreach and distribution?
- What types of distribution (or *channels*) are most appropriate to the goals and the target audiences?
- How well are the distributed offerings working? Whom are they reaching? How is effectiveness measured?
- What are the relative costs and benefits of several distributional methods?

In this chapter we examine the many opportunities museums face in distributing their offerings to as broad an audience as possible. We examine the decisions that museums can make with regard to six major distribution channels: the main facility, branch museums, traveling exhibitions and loans, off-site programs, publications, and electronic distribution (see Exhibit 8.1).

THE MAIN FACILITY

The place where most of a museum's offerings are distributed is the main museum building. Museum buildings vary in terms of accessibility, attractiveness, and atmosphere. When we encounter a specific museum in a specific location, we may wonder how it came into being. Most museums get started in one of three ways. In the first case, someone in a community owns a valuable collection of objects (paintings, antiques, butterflies, old medical instruments) that the person or community believes should be preserved in a museum, existing or new. The Phillips Collection, in Washington, D.C., one of the earliest modern art museums, was established by the Phillips family in their home. Two of Chicago's largest museums—the Field Museum and the Museum of Science & Industry—were built by wealthy businesspeople who sought to create great educational institutions that would feature the collections amassed at Chicago's 1893 World Fair, known as the World's Columbian Exposition.

In the second case, an individual, group, or community decides that the community needs a museum to add stature, visibility, or pride to the community. In the late twentieth century, major urban U.S. museums have come to symbolize a high quality of life and an incentive attracting newcomers and new businesses to the area. Cleveland's $92 million Rock and Roll Hall of Fame and Museum, designed on a lakefront site by renowned architect I. M. Pei, catapulted the city into the first rank of cultural and tourist destinations when it opened in 1995. The new museum has brought prestige, glamour, and economic development value to Cleveland and will serve as a magnet for further attractions. A community may also contain an idle facility—an old mansion, an abandoned railroad station, an empty department store—that would serve admirably as a museum. Several U.S. cities with historic train stations in varying degrees of decay have transformed them into museums. An example is the new science museum being created in the restored historic Beaux-Arts train station in Kansas City, Missouri.

A third motivation for starting a museum has been more evident in Europe and Asia than in the United States: amassing a collection of art, history, science, and technology that celebrates and extols the achievements of a people and a culture, brings glory to a nation, and advances the aims of government. The Louvre in Paris, the British Museum in London, and the Prado in Madrid are examples of institutions sponsored by rulers and governments originally for ideological and nationalistic ends.

Once a museum gets established, it must make the best use of the physical facility. This facility is not always well designed from the point of view of either museum's staff or visitors. If the building was taken over from another use, it may need a great deal of work to set up galleries, administrative offices, a restaurant, a coatroom, a gift shop, and rest rooms.

Even if the facility was originally designed as a museum, problems will inevitably arise. The roof may leak; the carpeting will likely need frequent replacement because of heavy traffic; and heating, cooling, and other environmental control systems will have to be replaced and updated. As the museum's visitors and collections grow, the museum will soon run out of exhibition and storage space. Management will begin to think about adding a wing, if there is sufficient land. The museum will have to undertake a special fundraising campaign, hoping to find a donor for whom the wing can be named.

Many museums have undergone several additions, modernizations, and expansions, making the original building almost unrecognizable. Then the day may come when the current building can no longer serve the museum's purposes, and the museum lays plans to build an entirely new building. One dramatic example of a new museum building is the J. Paul Getty Museum (part of the Getty Center), built on a ridge of the Santa Monica Mountains in the Brentwood section of Los Angeles. The original Getty Museum, a re-creation of a Roman villa and estate, is being renovated and will reopen as a classical antiquities museum. The new Getty Center complex opened in December of 1997. Designed by the world-famous architect Richard Meier, it has won major acclaim as a "tour de force" and an "incredible creation." Resembling a citadel on a hill and offering breathtaking views of Los Angeles, the ocean, and the mountains, the complex is estimated to have cost nearly $1 billion (Hales, 1997).

Many factors affect the building that any museum comes to inhabit. There are external factors (architectural features, surroundings) and internal factors (entranceways, corridors, stairwells, galleries and other display spaces, storage). In considering space and design, museum managers have to grapple with significant challenges that few other institutions face. Museums maintain and preserve the record of human, natural, and cultural history. They protect original objects that in most cases are irreplaceable and are expected to maintain these objects so that future generations can enjoy them.

Managing a museum facility properly is essential to carrying out the museum's ongoing balancing act between using its objects to satisfy present and future needs. It is a structural imperative that museum architecture facilitate the care and conservation of objects. Environmental and climatic controls are critical, especially in art museums. Cases have been reported in which large crowds of visitors on rainy days have boosted humidity levels in galleries to unacceptable levels. Museums on occasion have had to close down galleries to protect the paintings. A second structural need is to design galleries large enough to accommodate sizable crowds, so that visitors do not physically interfere with objects and exhibitions.

Museum managers have to take into account the importance of making their facilities presentable and comfortable. They must therefore consider how the main facility looks from the outside and the inside.

How Does the Museum Look on the Outside?

Museum buildings come in all styles—some were built to look like Greek temples, some were originally mansions (in various states of repair), some were once department stores, and some were built as landmark examples of modern architecture. Museums built in the nineteenth and early twentieth centuries were designed to communicate respect, authority, solidity, and grandeur. Because the museum as an institution has classical antecedents, it is not surprising that a large number of major museum buildings have been built in the classical style. Daniel Burnham, who supervised the design and building of Chicago's Columbian Exposition and later designed the Field Museum was inspired by the Erectheum, a temple that forms part of the Acropolis in Athens.

Yet museum managers have to consider the impact of the museum's external appearance in inviting people to enter or discouraging them from approaching. As long as museums disproportionately attracted the affluent, high-born, and educated classes, their physical appearance of solidity and grandeur was appropriate. However, when museums sought to attract a diverse cross section of the community, including newcomers who never had set foot in museums and people from low-income communities, the grand appearance of museums became a barrier. The Greco-Roman marble-columned style of museums such as the Metropolitan Museum of Art, the Art Institute of Chicago, and the Philadelphia Museum of Art was designed to inspire awe and respect and deliberately set museum-going apart from routine, day-to-day activities. Yet many museums today wish to balance an image of seriousness and grandeur with an image of pleasure and enjoyment. Even museums designed in the imposing classical style can be made more inviting. This can be accomplished by humanizing activities. Every year, the Cleveland Museum of Art holds for young people a chalk-drawing contest on its terrace. The Field Museum organizes on the grounds ethnic celebrations featuring music and cuisine.

Some museums in the classical style constrain visitors with physical handicaps. The main entrance to the Philadelphia Museum of Art, on the museum's eastern side, features an imposing set of marble stairs that visitors with even the slightest of handicaps can find daunting. Making matters worse from the standpoint of physical accessibility is the fact that the museum is surrounded on this side by a curve of fast-moving highway that visitors have to negotiate. The east entrance to the Philadelphia Art Museum is thus among the most beautiful museum facades in the world but also one of the hardest to reach. The western side of the museum has a street-level entrance that is easier to approach but more remote for visitors on foot. Museum managers have recognized the accessibility issues and have placed abundant signage at key points directing visitors with physical handicaps to this second entrance.

The design of a new museum building will inevitably make a statement about the museum. The new J. Paul Getty Museum in Los Angeles is likely to become one of the world's most celebrated destinations, by virtue of its peerless architecture, landscape, vista, collections, and the allure of its remote hilltop location. Consider the challenge of designing the building for a museum of contemporary art. One school of thought holds that the exterior should be contemporary, with flair, a taste of modernity, a provocative statement of design and fashion. New York City's Guggenheim Museum is such an example and has become a major icon of twentieth-century architecture. The San Francisco Museum of Modern Art, which opened in January 1995, combines the classic and contemporary: a massive, fortress-like structure with an airy, bright, exuberant interior featuring a giant cylindrical light shaft. Situated close to downtown San Francisco, it is easily accessible from the street, despite its somewhat daunting appearance.

How Do Functions and Flow Work on the Inside?

The way a museum is organized on the inside and the way it appears to visitors is partly a function of its architecture and design. It is also a reflection of a museum's mission and the particular concept the museum's leaders seek to project. There are two basic views of what a museum's interior design and organization should be like. The traditional view emphasizes the special character of a museum as a lofty institution of learning that offers visitors a rare aesthetic, intellectual, contemplative, or spiritual experience. According to Otto Mayr, former director of the Deutsches Museum in Munich, Germany (interviewed June 6, 1995), a museum in a large building can be thought of as a "secular church," and its interior design should be "a solemn space." It should not under any circumstances resemble an amusement center or treat its visitors in a condescending way. Visitors to museums, at least in the past, expected a museum to offer a grand setting and an out-of-the-ordinary experience that provided relief from the humdrum, routine circumstances of daily life. A good museum, according to Mayr, while offering visitors clean, comfortable facilities, should not be a congested and noisy place; nothing should interfere with the visitor's focus on the collections and exhibits. The museum should instill in visitors a sense of physical and psychological well-being.

The other view of museum design, which predominates today, gives priority to an inviting, informal appearance and a functional, user-friendly design. A good museum, in this view, is well lighted and well ventilated; has well-maintained furnishings, carpets, and decorations; provides an accessible, inviting, and ample entryway and foyer and ample seating and nongallery spaces for visitors to relax in; and furnishes abundant signage, orientation, and wayfinding services, particularly directions to rest rooms, restaurants, and shops. Even Mayr concedes that even though museums are old-fashioned institutions, they should have modern facilities. The grandest museum buildings today are being renovated with an eye toward better lighting, ventilation, wayfinding, and functionality, including access for handicapped individuals.

Some interior design problems may be inherent in an inherited building and can be altered only at great expense. Some may be easily fixed. There is, however, no easy solution to the common challenge that major museums face: staying open to the public virtually every day of the year, operating from morning to evening and on some days during the evening too, and facing major crowds repeatedly at particular times and seasons. The National Air and Space Museum, for example, the most heavily visited museum in the world, with an estimated nine million visitors a year, spends a significant portion of its budget just to maintain the interior facility.

The central point about distribution of a museum's offerings is this: managers must view the museum's interior through the eyes and experiences of visitors as they move through the museum. As numerous studies have shown, museum visitors are as concerned about physical facilities and ambience as they are about offerings.

A museum has many options for its interior. It can cram many paintings on each wall to show more of its collections or hang fewer paintings so that the room is airier and each painting commands greater attention. It can place cushioned benches in every gallery or leave visitors standing through most of their museum experience. A science museum can create silent exhibits or noisy exhibits; it can fill its interior with neon lights and stimulating graphics and create multiple theaterlike spaces for demonstrating science. The subject of *atmospherics* deals with the question of how a place should feel to its visitors, and how this feeling is best delivered through the choice and arrangement of three kinds of cues: sensory, auditory, and visual (Kotler, 1973–1974).

One of the toughest issues facing larger museums is providing good-quality visitor orientation and wayfinding. A major criticism of museums, commonly expressed in visitor surveys, is that visitors are often unable to find their way around. They say things like "I was kind of nervous because I really didn't know where to go"; "I asked about tours. No one could give me a definite answer when they were or if they were"; "More direction [is needed] at the beginning when you first walk in the door" (Walsh, 1991, pp. 18, 20).

Sometimes architectural elements stand in the way of getting around. The Science Museum of Minnesota, in St. Paul, for example, consists of two skyway-connected buildings, each with an entrance. The entrance to the newer building offers high-quality visitor information and orientation; the entrance to the older building lacks space, lighting, and orientation. In response to visitor surveys, the museum is modifying the older entrance to make its interior design more consistent with the main entrance.

Another factor interfering with wayfinding is the tendency at some museums to keep signage at a minimum. Art museums in particular minimize signage, wall text, and labels so that graphics and text do not interfere with visitors' experiencing the works of art. Through the early 1990s, visitors at the Hirshhorn Museum & Sculpture Garden, in Washington, D.C., could enjoy the exterior architecture—a circular building surrounded by lovely terraces filled with sculptures—but found little information or orientation on the inside. The museum's orientation space was located on a lower level, near the gift shop and rest rooms. Museum managers, however, recognized the inadequacies from the visitor's point of view. The Hirshhorn entrance today has an information desk offering maps and orientation materials, as well as a glass-enclosed gift shop, where additional staff are available to answer inquiries.

Museums nowadays are doing a better job of welcoming visitors with information and orientation. Boston's Museum of Science, for example, has established color-coded directional signs at the entrance and at key points in the museum to guide visitors to each of three main sections of the museum. Museums provide other orientation tools: computer screens with maps indicating the locations of key collections and exhibitions, volunteers at kiosks who greet visitors and answer questions, orientation galleries that run short videos describing the museum and its collections, and even sophisticated electronic aids that print out customized maps and provide electronic tours.

BRANCH MUSEUMS

Boston's Museum of Fine Arts was one of the first U.S. art museums to create a branch operation in a nontraditional setting, at the Faneuil Hall Marketplace in downtown Boston. Developers of that restored former warehousing area invited the museum to convert a second-story space into an exhibition hall. The developers sought a distinctive feature to bring novelty and visibility to the new mall. Museum managers wanted to reach out to newcomers and nonvisitors. The two-year experiment, from 1979 to 1981, was a great success. The exhibition hall attracted an estimated 300,000 visitors the first year and 200,000 the second. The popularity of the mall led the developers to increase the rents, and the museum's short-term lease came to an end.

The Guggenheim Museum opened in 1992 a branch museum in a restored nineteenth-century building on Broadway in lower Manhattan's SoHo district, one of the city's liveliest and most colorful neighborhoods, filled with artist's studios, theaters and performing arts sites, shops, restaurants, and cafés. The SoHo museum's distinctive café, Time for T, does a brisk business, offering a tea emporium, a wine and sherry bar, and gourmet cuisine. The branch museum's exhibitions are intentionally avant-garde. The Guggenheim is, as mentioned earlier, establishing satellite museums around the world—in Venice, Bilbao, and Berlin to date. The Guggenheim museums, remarkable for their architecture, style, and prestige, represent a bold effort at establishing a distinctive and universal museum brand identity.

Branches are more common for history museums and historic sites. The Museum of Television and Radio, based in New York City, has opened a branch in Hollywood, California, and thus now operates in the two hubs of U.S. broadcasting. The Minnesota Historical Society operates seventeen historic sites and homes throughout Minnesota, including the Oliver H. Kelley Farm, an 1860s-era working farm and living history site; Historic Fort Snelling, a re-created military fort that is a setting for re-creations of significant U.S. battles; the Forest History Center, a living history site depicting frontier life; and the Split Rock Lighthouse on Lake Superior. Ohio's Center of Science and Industry (COSI), a highly successful museum in Columbus, is opening a satellite museum in Toledo.

Some of the world's largest museums, including the Louvre and the Smithsonian Institution, are museum complexes, consisting of multiple freestanding museums and research facilities. The Smithsonian Institution distributes its collection of 140 million artifacts, specimens, and objects among sixteen museums and the National Zoological Park in the nation's capital and in New York City. Some of the museums in the complex have their own branch operations. The Renwick Gallery (across the street from the White House), which collects and exhibits decorative arts and crafts, is a branch of the National Museum of American Art. The Carnegie complex in Pittsburgh, Pennsylvania, is also a multimuseum institution, consisting of the Carnegie Science Center, the Carnegie Museum of Natural History, the Carnegie Museum of Art, and the Andy Warhol Museum.

TRAVELING EXHIBITIONS AND LOANS

In the museum world, one of the most important ways to distribute and disperse exhibitions and collections, so that the public in different towns and cities can enjoy them, is by means of the traveling exhibition or by loaning particular objects that flow from one museum to another. Such practices are increasing, partly as a result of the growing visibility of museums and the appeal of their collections and exhibitions and partly as a result of the growth of museum collections, the great majority of which are placed in storage for lack of exhibition space. Associated with this, museums with large collections are eager to share these with other museums in order to alleviate crowding and reduce storage costs. Traveling exhibitions and loans are also increasing as public agencies and private sponsors press museums to make their offerings available to more people and in more places.

An effort is under way in the United States to help smaller art museum acquire loans from large museums and at the same time help defray the costs of loan transactions. Many large museums have not analyzed the extent and nature of their collections completely; they may be unaware that they have items that they can easily share with other museums. And smaller museums that have particular needs for works to fill gaps in their exhibitions often lack information regarding which museums have the items they need and how to arrange for the loan of these items.

Two leading foundations, the John S. and James L. Knight Foundation, in Florida, and The Pew Charitable Trust, in Philadelphia, have teamed up with administrative support at the Massachusetts Institute of Technology to create the Museum Loan Network. Financing is expected to be on the order of $3 million a year. The program will provide incentives to large museums to cover the cost of loans and incentives to small museums for shipping, conservation, and exhibit costs and also the costs of technical assistance. The network is building an electronic database of art collections in museums across the United States and the status of loans, condition of art objects, and other relevant information.

Another new program to lend objects and collections is the Smithsonian Institution's Affiliations Program, initiated in September 1996. The Smithsonian will work with other museums and communities that are interested in acquiring Smithsonian collections on an extended-loan basis. Recipient museums have to cover the costs of the loan transactions and ensure the care of objects. One of the first affiliation agreements was reached in 1997 among the Smithsonian, the city of Bethlehem, Pennsylvania, and the Bethlehem Steel Corporation. It involves creating in Bethlehem the new and wholly independent National Museum of Industrial History, to open in 2000. The corporation will convert three of its former manufacturing plants into a museum and family entertainment district. The Smithsonian will offer long-term loans of objects that reflect the industrial history of the site. Among the objects are an 1876 Jupiter steam locomotive, a Frick Eclipse portable steam engine, a Cameron steam pump, and a Nasmyth steam hammer. The partnership will also include the sharing of curatorial expertise; Smithsonian professionals will work with the new museum's staff to design the galleries, install the exhibitions, and create interpretive materials.

One of the largest traveling exhibitions ever organized in the United States was put together by the Smithsonian to celebrate its 150th anniversary and to share Smithsonian treasures with the American people in communities across the country. Titled *America's Smithsonian,* the 1996 exhibition toured several U.S. cities, set up in convention centers rather than museums due to its size. The exhibition included General George Washington's sword and President Abraham Lincoln's top hat; paintings by Georgia O'Keeffe, Edward Hopper, and Thomas Eakins; Dizzy Gillespie's trumpet, Arthur Ashe's tennis racket, and the microphone used by President Franklin Roosevelt in his legendary "fireside chats"; the *Vin Fin,* the first airplane to fly across the United States; fossilized dinosaur bones, meteorites, and butterflies and beetles; a 1948 Tucker sedan, one of the most famous automobiles ever built in the United States; and jewels, including a 182-carat blue star sapphire known as the Star of Bombay, given to the museum by the estate of actress Mary Pickford. Exhibition objects were periodically changed, reflecting concerns for their fragility and tolerance of light and climatic conditions; and objects with special significance for, say, Texas found their way into the Houston exhibition, just as objects with significance for Minnesota found their way to the St. Paul venue.

The public response to the traveling Smithsonian exhibition was overwhelming. More than two million people visited it during 1996. Press attention was considerable. In certain cities, mayors, local councils, and businesses organized high-level public relations and promotion events. Financing for the traveling exhibitions was initially provided by four U.S. corporations—Intel, Discover Card,

MCI Communications, and Trans World Airlines. When the original corporate support for *America's Smithsonian* ran out, the Smithsonian asked the cities subsequently hosting the exhibitions to cover the cost, an estimated $4.2 million.

An innovation in distributing museum offerings throughout a given city is the idea of the *museum without walls.* An example is The Contemporary, based in Baltimore. The Contemporary consists of a group of museum professionals who organize exhibitions across the city, at places ranging from schools, libraries, and community centers to corporate headquarters and municipal buildings. The Contemporary has an administrative structure but has no building of its own and no permanent collection. The shows it organizes contain objects and collections that are assembled from museums, collectors, and corporate owners. The Contemporary has an advantage in not having to deal with the overhead costs of acquiring, maintaining, and storing collections or operating a facility. Another advantage is bringing exhibitions to places where people live and work.

Another unusual way of taking art to the public is Artrain, a five-car train and a locomotive that is leased or donated by local or national rail operators (Bond, 1996). It is managed by Artrain, a nonprofit organization in Ann Arbor established initially by the Michigan Council for the Arts to serve Michigan communities. Later, Artrain became national in scope. In April 1996, for example, Artrain arrived in Edenton, North Carolina, a town of 5,300 people in the northeastern part of the state not far from Kitty Hawk. The onboard exhibition featured prints by artists such as Georgia O'Keeffe, Alexander Calder, and glass artist Dale Chihuly. The towns that Artrain reaches are expected to make modest contributions to finance the operations; corporations generally provide the bulk of these funds.

Major art, history, natural history, and science museums in the United States, Canada, and Europe have set up large departments devoted exclusively to the design, development, and financing of traveling exhibitions. The Smithsonian Institution Traveling Exhibition Service (SITES) is one of the largest. Since 1952, SITES has distributed several hundred exhibitions to museums, libraries, science centers, historical societies, schools, and community centers in towns and cities around the country. Exhibitions in 1995–96 included *Jazz Age in Paris, New Jamaican Art, How Things Fly,* and *After the Revolution: Everyday Life in America, 1780–1800* (a small-scale replica of the large permanent exhibit of the same name in the Smithsonian's American History Museum). Exhibitions are generated both at the Smithsonian and at other museums.

Museums and organizations receiving SITES shows pay a participation fee, although the exhibitions are also partly financed by federal appropriations. Other U.S. museums' traveling exhibitions are typically financed by corporate or foundation sponsors, by fees contributed by receiving institutions, and occasionally local or state governments. There are also commercial firms that build and organize traveling exhibitions.

In the mid-1990s, two U.S. art museums developed what may become a new form of distribution, combining branch operations, traveling exhibitions, and marketing partnerships. The Whitney Museum of American Art, in New York City, with one of the leading American art collections in the world, established a long-term partnership with the San Jose Museum of Art, in Northern California. The Whitney will provide San Jose with four eighteen-month-long exhibitions of portions of its permanent collections, and in return, San Jose will pay the Whitney several million dollars. The Whitney's management recognized that although the museum had roughly eleven thousand pieces in its collection, only 2 percent were on view at the museum. Further, art objects in storage are less likely to receive conservator and restorative care than objects on display. Whitney leaders also recognized that many of its objects are world famous, of great value, and capable of drawing large audiences. On the San Jose side, the museum and the city establishment have for years aspired to rival San Francisco and Los Angeles as an arts and cultural center. The city had a major museum facility but lacked great works of art. It was determined that a series of important museum shows and events could elevate the city's and the museum's prestige and appeal. The city redevelopment agency contributed $3 million to the transaction. The loans to San Jose will represent 4 percent of the Whitney's collection, and the exhibitions are being jointly mounted by Whitney and San Jose curators. Since the first show, attendance at the San Jose Museum of Art has increased by one-third, generous grants have been received from foundations and corporations, and major gifts to the museum's collection have increased sharply. Along with the significant revenue gain on both sides, the collaboration has had a positive effect in helping Whitney staff rethink the role and value of the museum's permanent collections and the range of audiences the museum seeks to attract. The Whitney is organizing a series of collection-based shows in New York in the light of the popularity of its collections in San Jose (Kino, 1995).

Another example of a collaboration to distribute museum offerings is the 1991 agreement between Boston's Museum of Fine Arts (BMFA) and the Foundation for the Arts in Nagoya, Japan. BMFA holds one of the world's greatest collections of Japanese and Chinese art; it has a long-standing tradition of consulting with and advising Asian museums; and it has a reputation for authority and scholarship. The Nagoya foundation is building a new museum, to open in 1999. Known as the Nagoya/Boston Museum of Fine Arts, the new facility will function as a sister museum to BMFA with exclusive rights to show BMFA collections. The partnership will continue for twenty years and will consist of small shows every two years and a series of major five-year exhibitions. The inaugural exhibition will be *Art of the Ancient Mediterranean World,* featuring BMFA's collections of Egyptian, Greek, and Roman art (Boston Museum of Fine Arts, 1995). BMFA has not officially reported the fee it will receive from Nagoya; it is said to be in the neighborhood of $40 million.

OFF-SITE PROGRAMS

Museums are information and education centers, and there is little preventing them from distributing materials to other locations. Off-site museum activities often involve education. The Virginia Museum of Fine Arts (VMFA), in Richmond, was established by the Virginia legislature to provide art experiences and education to communities across the commonwealth. The VMFA has two major outreach programs. One is the museum's partnership with twenty-six museums, art centers, and regional and local art associations to arrange loans and exhibitions, lectures by visiting curators, workshops for educators, and technical and consulting services to member museums. The VMFA also actively distributes video, slide, and other curricular and instructional materials to schools throughout Virginia. (The VMFA's outreach programs are discussed further in the Model Museum Practice at the end of this chapter.)

The Pacific Science Center, in Seattle, Washington, has organized a statewide service, known as Science on Wheels, that distributes science exhibits, demonstration kits, and educational resources to schools and communities. Twenty-five teachers work in the program each year, traveling on one of several vans that operate throughout the state. The Museum of London, the historical museum of the city of London, England, has an active resource outreach program, known as Museum on the Move, in which vans distribute museum collections, exhibits, and educational materials to outlying museums and community facilities. The Field Museum, in Chicago, offers its members a variety of educational and recreational programs, including nature walks and camping experiences at various sites in the metropolitan area. The Art Institute of Chicago conducts education outreach activities in senior citizen centers throughout the city.

Museums are establishing partnerships with school systems, combining object-based education with classroom teaching. Museums have developed extensive educational materials that are used in classrooms and are also obtainable by electronic means. A new development is the establishment of magnet or charter schools devoted to the arts and to object-based visual learning. In 1995, a consortium of four New York City museums (the Brooklyn Museum, the Jewish Museum, the American Museum of Natural History, and the Children's Museum of Manhattan) joined with the city's school system to establish a "museum school" for middle-school students. These young people study all the subjects in a regular curriculum and also make use of museum resources. Three days a week, students visit one or more of the affiliated museums; the other two days they spend at their home school (O'Donnell, 1995). Other museum schools can be found in Fairfax, Virginia, and in St. Paul and Minneapolis. The Natural History Museum in Battle Creek, Michigan, decided to organize exhibitions at a popular shopping mall precisely because students frequently hang out there. The museum set up a hologram show at the mall site and several months later also put its insect collection on view there. The response from young people and parents was very positive.

Off-site programming can also focus on promotion, public relations, and marketing, along with education. The Henry Ford Museum & Greenfield Village has had small-scale exhibits of antique cars at the Detroit Metropolitan Airport. Travelers can obtain museum information and sign up for museum memberships. Conner Prairie, in Indiana, offers visitors on group tours orientation videos that they can view prior to arrival. A growing number of hotels offer guests videos illustrating local cultural and recreational opportunities, including museums. The Art Institute of Chicago has experimented with ways to broaden its audience and in the early 1990s designed the program known as ArtExpress to reach young professionals working in downtown Chicago and encourage them to become active members. Curators take slide shows and museum materials to business offices during lunch periods and discuss a variety of art- and museum-related topics. Participants in these brown-bag lunches are given incentives to become museum members.

Yet another type of off-site museum activity is commercial: the growing practice of operating museum gift shops in retail centers, shopping malls, and other public places such as convention centers and airports. New York's Metropolitan Museum of Art has operated stores in shopping malls that carry merchandise similar to that sold at the museum shop on Fifth Avenue. The Smithsonian Institution in 1997 opened a store in the new terminal building at the Washington, D.C., National Airport. As off-site museum stores succeed, museums have experimented with adding exhibition-like features and collections to the stores, on the theory that such distinctive museum features enhance the shopping experience and heighten the consumer's sense of value. Off-site museum stores can also prove useful in promoting visits to museums and making the museum experience more familiar to non-museum-goers.

PUBLICATIONS

Museums have traditionally distributed their offerings through publications. Museums can produce as many as seven different kinds of printed publications:

- "Coffee table" books describing a museum's history and illustrating its collections and departments (for example, the book commissioned by the Smithsonian Institution for its 150th anniversary celebration; Conaway, 1995)

- Books, pamphlets, and catalogues on special exhibits (for example, the catalogue for the 1996–1999 traveling exhibition *Masterpieces from Central Africa,* organized by the Royal Museum for Central Africa/Tervuren Museum, in Belgium)

- Card and board games based on the museum's collection
- Members' newsletter (for example, *Magazine of Cooper-Hewitt, National Design Museum, Smithsonian Institution*)
- A magazine or journal (for example, *Curator,* published by the American Museum of Natural History; and *American Art,* published by the National Museum of American Art)
- Children's guides to museums (for example, *A Kid's Guide to the Smithsonian;* Bay, 1996)
- Annual reports, distributed to corporate sponsors and other donors

Catalogues of museum exhibitions have been the mainstay publications of art museums. They are less used by historical museums; an excellent example of a historical museum catalogue, however, is the National Portrait Gallery's *1846: Portrait of the Nation*, produced for the 1996 exhibition by that name. An exhibition may last three to six months, but the catalogue is available for a lifetime. Catalogues have been significant educational resources insofar as exhibits are likely to have limited labels and texts, descriptive and contextual information. Catalogues typically include biographical essays on artists, time lines, scholarly essays, memoirs, diary entries, artists' letters, and photographs, and of course large, highly professional reproductions of works of art. In the early and mid-1990s, however, the publishing market for catalogues declined. They are costly to produce and fewer visitors appear interested in purchasing them. The catalogues that have maintained their market are ones produced in connection with blockbuster exhibitions.

Smaller-sized, illustrated but less costly books describing a museum or a special collection have maintained a good market, especially among visitors who want a souvenir of a visit. A good example is the museum guide *Musée Canadien des Civilisations/Canadian Museum of Civilization,* featuring side-by-side French and English texts and stunning photographs of the exhibit halls, collections, and facilities and of events such as musical and dance performances.

Museums are publishing more materials for membership groups and promotional pieces for targeted audiences. The Corcoran Gallery of Art, along with the Corcoran School of Art, provides members with the bimonthly newsletter *Night and Day,* promoting a rich menu of continuing education, concerts, music and art forums, and weekend and evening events.

As large museums broaden their scope and offerings, they have to communicate information to the audiences they are seeking to attract. Museum visitor research confirms that word of mouth is a primary means of recruiting new visitors, and visitor information and membership publications serve as tools to attract newcomers. A museum membership group is typically provided with an appealing newsletter. An example is *Zoogoer,* a bimonthly publication of the National Zoological Park's support group, Friends of the National Zoo. An attractive, sophisticated, and informative thirty-page publication, the magazine is mainly devoted to articles about conservation, zoo collections, new types of research, and educational programs. Calendars of events are left to occasional mailings. The magazine has attracted advertisements from major corporate sponsors.

Publication programs can be viewed as investments in attracting visitors, members, and patrons and sustaining their interest and involvement. They may run at a loss, but this is not always the case. A museum has to examine at least these basic questions concerning publications:

- What types of publications should the museum launch?

- How can a museum do a better job of circulating and promoting its publications beyond the museum's walls?

- Should the museum run a publication program at a loss, to cover costs, or to earn revenues? How can publications become a revenue center for the museum?

ELECTRONIC DISTRIBUTION

The Metropolitan Museum of Art, in New York City, in December 1996 launched a new membership category called "Met Net," one of twelve membership groups. Met Net is geared to cyberspace visitors, and its special membership benefits are available only via the Internet, upon entry of a member's access code. Members pay an annual fee of $50. In addition to free admission to the museum building, use of member facilities, and distribution of the museum's mail-order catalogues, Met Net members get exclusive benefits: the ability to download the museum's computer screen saver (featuring a colorful image of the museum entrance), offers of special merchandise that can be purchased only by members at the Web site, and digital visits to exhibitions and views of objects in the collections, along with audio-assisted guides provided to members reaching the Web site with an access code but not to other Internet visitors. The museum is also considering for Met Net members having real-time discussions with curators and setting up a "chat room" to communicate with other members on-line. The Met Net membership category is an excellent response to devoted museum followers who live at a distance from New York, even across the globe, who want to maintain contact with the museum and continue to support it. This membership service does, however, take the museum experience far away from the traditional museum-going encounter in viewing rare objects in person in a museum setting.

The Metropolitan is not alone in extending its offerings and services to a much broader audience, in fact, a world audience. Any person who has access to the Internet and the World Wide Web can visit many of the world's great art museums on the computer. Museums of all types are building Web sites ("home pages") that enable people anywhere in the world to visit museums digitally, tour the facilities, view collections, and even make purchases on-line (see "Perfect Site," 1997). (Exhibit 8.2 presents a list of selected Web sites.) In one sense, people are able to do the same thing by purchasing a museum catalogue or visiting the public library. A museum catalogue can provide a more comprehensive and in-depth view of a museum than a Web site can. But the Internet makes the museum's information available twenty-four hours a day, seven days a week, anywhere in the world. Home pages can supply images of superb quality and even videos, sound, and other multimedia applications. Furthermore, the browser can visit many more museums than are likely to be found on the shelves of a public library.

The cost effectiveness and efficiencies of Web sites are extremely high. In 1996, it was estimated that maintaining and upgrading a modest Web site cost between $5,000 and $6,000 annually—far less than a one-time single-page ad in the *New York Times*. And Web sites provide feedback: museum managers can learn how many users have visited the site (in Internet parlance, how many "hits" the site has had), which parts of the site command the most attention, how long visitors stay at the site, and whether they dialed up over commercial, educational, or international lines. As the Internet develops, advertising will become a more pervasive feature, supporting the costs of maintaining Web sites and the operation of the system. Museums will be able to finance their Web sites by finding sponsors. In August 1996, at the time of the Smithsonian Institution's 150th anniversary celebration on the National Mall, the Smithsonian's Web site had four million hits.

There is much for museums to consider regarding the cyberspace environment. Until computers and access are more widespread in society, cyberspace visitors will be a self-selected group and not representative of the general public. Yet the self-selectivity of cyberspace visitors may not be so different from the self-selectivity of museum visitors. Museums expect some significant portion of cyberspace visitors to become converts to real-time and real-space museum visitors. The reasoning is that electronic information will familiarize people with museums, make their collections and activities more familiar, and in doing so will help make museum-going more desirable. It is still too early to determine with certainty, however, the effects of the Internet environment on users. Some early evidence shows that Web sites can become revenue generators for certain types of museums and cultural institutions, but they are not a majority of cases. New browsing software ("Web crawlers") is helping to resolve one issue by making it easier for Internet users to find their way to desired sites.

Besides the digital environment of cyberspace, museums have abundant opportunities to engage in electronic publishing and distribution: films, videos, cable and broadcast television, satellite-based communication, and CD-ROMs.

○○○○○

Exhibit 8.2. Selected Museum Web Sites.

Many museums throughout the world are accessible by computer through their addresses on the Internet and World Wide Web. Museum Web sites vary in how much information they provide and how many images of their collections, exhibits, and galleries they present. Here are some major examples.

Metropolitan Museum of Art. The Web site of the Metropolitan Museum of Art, in New York City [http://www.metmuseum.org], provides users a full array of information as well as images from the collections, of special exhibitions, and of museum facilities and galleries. Its menu includes information about new exhibits and programs (along with a calendar of events) and orientation to the galleries and visitor services (along with a floor plan); information about ticketing, membership, and educational programs; frequently asked questions; a library catalogue listing; a page identifying museum sponsors and patrons; on-line shopping; and a chat room in which users communicate with curators and museum staff. At the beginning the Web site identifies new programs and services: on a recent screen, for example, were mentioned a new membership program for young professionals, new exhibits, and new benefits of membership programs.

Michael C. Carlos Museum. The Web site of the Michael C. Carlos Museum in Atlanta, Georgia, a museum of classical art, anthropology, and ethnography [http://www.cc.emory.edu/CARLOS/carlos/html], offers extensive information on museum staff, their work, and museum operations, in a section titled "Behind the Scenes." The information on the museum's Public Services Department, as an example, offers photographs of the three staff members; identifies functional areas; describes management goals and priorities in each area; provides phone, address, and e-mail contacts with department heads; and lists the range of visitor and public services at the museum.

The Exploratorium. The Web site of the Exploratorium, in San Francisco [http://www.exploratorium.edu/], in addition to regular museum information, offers an extensive inventory of exhibition information, including cross references to past and current exhibitions and interactive programs at the museum.

Museum of Paleontology. The Web site of the Museum of Paleontology, at the University of California, Berkeley [http://ucmp1.berkeley.edu/], offers considerable visual information from its collections and research programs and, additionally, provides hyperlinks to other natural history museums and research centers, which can be reached by a simple click of the mouse.

Carnegie Museum of Natural History. The Web site of the Carnegie Museum of Natural History, in Pittsburgh [http://www.clpgh.org/cmnh/], along with a full menu of information, provides the name of its Webmaster and contact information so that users can ask questions about problems they are having using the site.

Exhibit 8.2. Selected Museum Web Sites, Cont'd.

Canadian Museum of Civilization. The Web site of the Canadian Museum of Civilization, in Hull, Quebec [http://www.cmcc.muse.digital.ca/], is a large cyberspace site divided into the following areas: Virtual Museum (a collection of information and images chosen from across the museum and changing frequently); What's New?; About the Museum; Calendar of Events; Gallery Tours; Children's Museum; Public Programmes, Facilities and Services; CINEPLUS (Omnimax theater information); Museum Collections; Behind the Scenes; and Get Involved? (membership, sponsorship, and volunteer information). The Web site in addition features an extensive shopping service (Cyber Boutique). Users can call up images and information on over 250 items in the museum stores (as of mid-1997), select products for purchase, complete an on-line order form (that calculates taxes and shipping charges as well as prices, both retail and for members, who have a discount), indicate preferred method of payment, and confirm their purchases on-line twenty-four hours a day. Actual payment is by credit card, and for security reasons, that information is transmitted only by telephone, fax, or mail. Orders can be filled in all major nations of the world.

Croydon Clocktower. The Croydon Clocktower is a British museum in the London borough of Croydon that has a small collection and that organizes exhibits with borrowed objects around themes it selects. Its Web site [http://www.croyden.gov.uk/cr-fcloc.htm] provides users with exhibit images and descriptions, and in the Pictorial Guide to the museum, browsers can view nearly the entire interior space, using interactive cues to access photographs that incorporate views from a variety of angles. Users can browse the entrance foyer, library, escalator leading to upper-story galleries, several galleries, and other facilities.

Webmuseum. An unusual art museum Web site is the Webmuseum, headquartered in Paris [http://sunsite.unc.edu/wm/]. Nicolas Pioch, the site's founder and Webmaster, welcomes users to the site, informing them that he created the site as a partnership among many art museums in the world in order to make art accessible to as many people as possible. Established in March 1994, the Webmuseum links museums in many countries. In mid-1997, it offered users a section called Famous Paintings, which showed full-screen and detailed images of famous paintings, a special virtual museum exhibition on Cézanne, and an exhibition on medieval manuscripts, among other exhibitions and collections. Each Web site section includes extensive information on artists, artworks, historical and geographical context, critical opinion, and other art history information.

○○○○○

A growing list of CD-ROMs includes major museum collections in the United States and abroad (recent productions have included *Uffizi,* the collections of the great museum in Florence, Italy; *Taking Art Apart: An Interactive Guide to the World of Art,* from the Portland Art Museum; *European Portrait Miniatures in the Metropolitan Museum of Art*; and the Barnes Foundation's CD-ROM, titled *A Passion for Art,* produced in partnership with Corbis, Inc.). CD-ROM technology offers great potential for projecting the museum-going experience into the home or office. A company in North Carolina has created a CD-ROM product that can scan a museum's interior spaces and galleries and then allow the viewer to shift perspective as if walking around, take a closer view of an object, and even manipulate the image from any angle—something a visitor to the actual museum cannot do. However, it is still unclear whether a viable CD-ROM market exists, given the high costs of production.

Films and videos are a mainstay of art education and a principal means for museums to distribute educational materials to schools. Cable television in the United States—with its specialized stations such as the History Channel; Ovation, an arts channel; and the Discovery Channel, with a focus on science and nature—offers increasing opportunities for museums and other cultural organizations to communicate with larger audiences. Museums, in addition, are using teleconferencing and satellite transmissions to reach educators, classrooms, and other targeted audiences. Multisite transmissions, linking students and teachers in several cities with a museum facility and its staff, have become a significant outreach activity at the National Museum of American History's Lemelson Center for the Study of Invention and Innovation.

Museums will increasingly be dealing with the question of how to disseminate resources to a larger audience, most of whom may never have an opportunity to visit the museum facility. Given the range of electronic information products and distributional channels, however, museums have to consider which products and vehicles are appropriate to their audiences and which are most cost-effective in achieving the goals of education and public service. Museums are addressing the following questions in connection with electronic distribution:

- Should a museum set up a Web site, and if so, what should the site feature?
- What can a museum do to get more people to view its Web site?
- Will viewing the museum's Web site increase or decrease interest in visiting the museum?
- What degree of control will the museum have over the quality of the images and the interpretation in labels and text as they are transmitted in cyberspace?

SUMMARY

More and more museums are eager to expose their offerings (exhibitions, collections, lectures and events, merchandise in the gift shop, interior design, exterior architecture) to a broader range of people and to larger audiences, including individuals who are not able or not inclined to visit the museum building. People can experience a museum's offerings not only by visiting the museum but also by viewing a traveling exhibition at a convention center, examining museum objects in a classroom, viewing a museum video, or accessing the museum's Web site via the Internet. Museum offerings can be distributed at branch or satellite museums, museum gift shops in retail centers and airports, traveling exhibitions, and educational outreach activities in schools. Whatever the vehicle of distribution, offerings should be distributed and made available in a way that is pleasing and convenient and also reflects the museum visitors', members', and patrons' points of view, interests, and needs.

○

MODEL MUSEUM PRACTICE

Distributing Offerings to a Wider Audience: The Virginia Museum of Fine Arts

The Virginia Museum of Fine Arts, in Richmond, with eighteen thousand artworks in its collections, offers visitors a visual feast that rivals in range and quality collections found in large urban museums. The museum is nearly encyclopedic, containing ancient, medieval, and modern art; collections of African, Asian, European, and American art; and examples of the fine arts and the decorative arts. A notable feature of the museum's exhibitions and galleries is the juxtaposing of artworks in different media and the proximity of artworks of different societies and civilizations. Galleries are arranged by culture, period, and occasionally by theme (portraits and landscapes). Many contain paintings and drawings, sculpture, furniture, and works of decorative art. The museum's building, with four wings added to the original structure, houses galleries of varying and notable architectural and historical styles.

The Virginia Museum of Fine Arts (VMFA) was founded in 1934 as an agency of the Commonwealth of Virginia to promote the arts and art education throughout the state as well as in Richmond, the state capital. It was the first state government-supported art museum in the United States. Its full-time staff of 170 are state government employees; the board of trustees is appointed by the governor. The museum has also created a nonprofit foundation (Virginia Museum of Fine Arts Foundation) that oversees development activities (annual giving campaigns, restricted funds, and portions of the endowment), membership groups, and specialized collections-based support groups.

The museum had 423,000 visitors in 1995 and reached an additional 360,000 citizens across the state through its extensive outreach programs. The museum budget, in fiscal year 1994–95, was just over $12 million. Appropriations from the Virginia legislature accounted for $6.9 million, or 54.7 percent of total revenues. However, the museum encountered a 21 percent cut in state appropriations in the years 1989 to 1995. This resulted, among other things, in scaling back statewide programs. By 1996, the museum had convinced the legislature that further reductions would derail the programs bringing museum resources to Virginia's communities; the legislature, as a result, restored some earlier cuts and boosted museum spending.

VMFA's statewide outreach programs have long been recognized as a standard among American museums. The legislature mandated the museum to devote a portion of its resources (staff, collections, publications, funds) to bringing the art experience to schools and communities across the state. Three programs have accomplished this: an affiliate program, in which the museum has formed partnerships with twenty-six museums, art centers, and regional art associations across the state, providing loans, educational resources and teacher training, and technical museum and exhibit support; a traveling exhibition and media services program, providing exhibits and educational materials; and an artmobile program, employing three specially equipped tractor trailers to transport objects and small-scale exhibits to outlying communities. The media services, with one of the nation's largest art film and video collections, reached 1,200 client organizations and an estimated 400,000 people in the mid-1990s. These audiovisual resources, along with the slide sets, teachers' kits, discovery kits, and educational posters also loaned through this program, are extensively used in the schools. In addition, approximately fifty crated exhibits a year are sent to small, outlying communities. The artmobile program was discontinued in 1994 because the equipment, maintenance, and fuel costs proved too expensive. In its place, VMFA is accelerating the distribution of educational materials and is also sharing museum resources digitally over the Internet.

The museum's statewide programs have proved popular and effective. However, the museum also faced a challenge closer to home. The population of metropolitan Richmond is approximately 30 percent African American and yet the museum by the late 1980s had a relatively small number of African Americans as visitors, members, and patrons. Museum staff had identified neighborhoods in the city and suburbs that were underserved. Their years of experience reaching out to communities across the state became a platform for building relations with diverse communities within the museum's own neighborhood.

During much of the museum's history, African Americans living in Richmond faced considerable barriers to participation. The museum, at its opening in the 1930s, was a segregated institution, like other state-supported institutions. In the post–World War II period the African American community perceived the museum as a place reserved for Richmond's elite groups. Indeed, many had perceived the museum as primarily a preserve for wealthy, high-status Richmond citizens. To change these perceptions the museum created in 1984 a multicultural advisory committee. A breakthrough in museum-community relations occurred when the museum applied for and obtained a $1.44 million grant from the Lila Wallace–Reader's Digest Fund for the express purpose of significantly increasing African American visitation and participation, including recruitment of additional African Americans to the staff and board and as members and volunteers. A component of the grant was used for audience research and program evaluation and for enhanced marketing communication efforts, including advertising, promotion, and community relations.

A vehicle for outreach to the African American community was the development of a major new exhibition, supported by the grant and drawn from the permanent collection of African art. Titled *Spirit of the Motherland: African Art at the Virginia Museum of Fine Arts,* the new exhibit opened in 1994 with a wide range of collateral programming such as lectures, school tours, workshops, catalogues, videos, and educational materials. A smaller version of the exhibit, along with marketing, evaluation, education, and community relations components, traveled to two of the museum's affiliates in the state.

A major factor in successfully reaching the African American community was the hiring of a talented, respected, and energetic professional to coordinate the community relations activities. Grant funds supported this position, which, together with an assistant's position, formed the museum's first community relations department. African American members of the museum's board worked to ensure the support of the museum's management and staff. The community relations director, working with trustees and museum staff, won the participation of African American community leaders and generated partnerships with schools, churches, community organizations, and the business community. One of the direct results of the community relations initiative was the formation of a new support group, the Friends of African and African-American Art. Through its membership, programs, and fundraising activities, the group is extending the reach of the museum into the African American community.

The Lila Wallace–Reader's Digest Fund grant came to an end in October 1996, but its effects have been far-reaching. Katharine Lee, director of the Virginia Museum of Fine Arts, describes the many positive outcomes. African American attendance increased from base attendance of 7 percent to a peak of 21 percent during the *Spirit of the Motherland* exhibit. Membership increased from a baseline of 1.1 percent (152 members) to 2.8 percent (500 members). More African Americans participated in the museum's volunteer group. Four African Americans joined the museum staff as a result of positions funded under the grant and made permanent through other funds. The Friends of African and African-American Art became a strong force for community involvement, numbering 275 members at the end of 1996. Most important, the grant enabled the museum to make a commitment to reaching the African American community, and this contributed to building a new feeling of trust between the museum and the community.

The Lila Wallace grant also had a positive impact on the museum. Innovations in *Spirit of the Motherland* were partially supported by the grant—a video theater within the exhibit; the museum's first use of interactive videos, contextual photographs, and audio recordings; the museum's first series of popular handbooks on its collections, beginning with the African collection; the use of gallery diagrams and maps; and production of a Family Gallery Guide, with information and learning games derived from the exhibit. These innovations contributed to the development of subsequent exhibits of high quality.

Staff were trained in community relations, communications, marketing, and evaluation, and they developed motivation and skills that made a difference in later museum programs. A seasoned professional was recruited to head up a new department of communications and marketing. In communicating effectively with Richmond's African American community, museum staff reinforced the museum's long-standing commitment to distributing offerings as widely as possible. The grant also led the museum to make visitor research and evaluation a solid part of programming.

The results of the Lila Wallace grant were sobering, too. Kathleen Schrader, associated director for collections management and resources (interviewed Feb. 25, 1997), observes:

> The three-year planning and implementation, under the Lila Wallace grant, gave us a much-needed jump start; but it represented only a beginning. We learned that changing the way our visitors think about us is a slow process. It takes time to change perceptions, and it takes time to convert nonparticipants into participants. Perhaps the best thing the grant accomplished was to help train our staff and build our confidence level that, indeed, we have the ability to broaden our audience and make our resources widely accessible. We could reaffirm our mission of providing education in the arts to everyone in the commonwealth of Virginia.

CHAPTER NINE

Communicating and Promoting

Image and Brand Building, Advertising, Public Relations, Direct Marketing, and Sales

*It is also possible for an organization to mature at a level way below
its maximum potential. Its books balance very nicely with income. . . .
This will satisfy the accountant but it should not satisfy you because
your aim must be to sell everything you have to sell.*
—Keith Diggle

In this chapter we discuss communications and promotion and how museums can more effectively use four major tools for communicating with their publics: advertising, public relations, direct marketing, and sales promotion.

IMAGE BUILDING AND BRAND IDENTITY

Before a museum or any other organization can determine which communication and promotion tools to use, it has to have an image or message for a product, service, experience, or organization to promote. This image must be something that consumers will respond to, find appealing, or want to purchase or participate in. An image of a product, service, or organization (sometimes called a *brand image*) is also a shortcut to attracting attention and building familiarity and trust. People generally do not want to spend a lot of time learning about products and organizations or doing comparison shopping. The image of IBM or Intel, for example, is one of quality and reliability; it conveys a promise, a sense of trust, and an expectation of benefit. An effective image works like a funnel, directing the flow of attention and regularly bringing consumers to an organization's or product's corner whenever the consumer has a need for that type of product or service.

Museums in recent years have complained that although blockbuster exhibitions draw large audiences, once an exhibition is over, the audience drops off until the next big show. Some museums, like Boston's Museum of Science, have devoted considerable resources to creating a brand image and identity that attracts people to the museum not just for blockbusters but anytime, as a place to spend free time, have fun, or have a great experience (Finke, 1996). In some cases, a museum might not be familiar to some people in a community; in other cases, a museum might have a dull image that stands in the way of building an audience. An effective image or brand identity can entice people to visit a museum; many may ultimately become regular visitors.

An image or brand identity is created after considerable consumer research. It takes the form, as a communication and promotion tool, of a visual symbol or logo and a message, conveyed in a slogan or tag line, that work together to attract attention. The image should be simple, direct, appealing, vital, and memorable. Once a brand image becomes familiar, it becomes associated in the consumer's mind with a set of positive expectations and benefits (quality, reliability, trust, anticipation of future benefits, and so on).

A brand name or brand identity is a particular dimension of image building. The logo of Boston's Museum of Science, a two-color symbol of a plant in orbit, along with the museum's name and the slogan "It's Alive," is communicated widely in the media and appears on shopping bags, items in the gift shop, brochures, membership cards, stationery, and other museum materials. A brand image is a promise. An organization with a brand identity is expected to live up to the expectations and benefits it has promised; part of this is managing the brand and matching the consumer's experience of the brand with the brand image. (The success Boston's Museum of Science has had with its brand identity is discussed further in the Model Museum Practice at the end of this chapter. For further information on image building and measuring image effectiveness, see Chapter Five.)

Communication and promotion objectives are highly variable, and therefore a museum has to use a mixture of communication tools, tailoring them to audience and message objectives. Table 9.1 illustrates the variety of available tools.

ADVERTISING

Advertising can be defined as *any paid form of nonpersonal presentation and promotion of products, services, ideas, persons, or organizations by an identified sponsor.* Advertising can add value to a museum's efforts in several ways: as a long-term buildup of the museum's image *(institutional advertising)*, a buildup of a specific collection or exhibit *(product advertising)*, the dissemination of information about a particular event *(classified advertising)*, or an announcement of a new membership drive *(promotional advertising)*.

Museums generate advertising in newspapers and magazines and on billboards, radio, and occasionally television. Museums also print brochures, mail

Table 9.1. Some Common Communication and Promotion Tools.

Advertising	Public Relations	Direct Marketing	Sales Promotion
Print and broadcast ads	Press kits	Direct mail	Gifts and premiums
Packaging	Speeches	Telemarketing	Exchange privileges
Mailings	Seminars	Integrated direct marketing	Discounts
Catalogues	Annual reports	Database marketing	Tickets
Newsletters	Sponsorships		Gift shop redemption coupons
Brochures and booklets	Publications		
Posters and leaflets	Community relations		
Directories	Lobbying		
Reprints of ads	Media relations		
Billboards			
Display signs			
Point of purchase displays			
Audiovisual materials			
Symbols and logos			

letters, and make phone calls to solicit memberships and donations and advertise in other ways.

Advertising as a medium of communication offers the advertiser a set of advantages. It permits a high level of control over the message content and over the choice of the medium, plus substantial control over the scheduling of the message. The fact that advertising is public suggests that the advertised product is standard and legitimate. Because many people see ads for the product, consumers know that purchasing the product will be publicly understood and accepted. Advertising allows an organization to repeat a message many times. It lets the receiver compare the messages of various competitors. Large-scale advertising says something positive about the advertising organization's size, popularity, and success. Advertising is expressive, allowing an organization to dramatize its products through the artful use of print, sound, and color. Advertising is used to build up a durable image for a product or service. Advertising can reach masses of geographically spread out people at a relatively low cost per exposure.

Advertising also has shortcomings. It reaches many people quickly, but it is impersonal. It cannot be as persuasive as a personal communication from an organization's representative. It is scattershot and blunt, reaching far beyond an organization's targeted audiences (compared to direct mail, for example, which can be selective and fine-tuned to fit different segments). Advertising carries on only a one-way communication with an audience, and the audience does not feel that it has to pay attention or respond. Advertising also can be costly. Some forms, such as newspaper and radio advertising, can be done on a small budget, but others, such as television advertising, require very large budgets. Another problem is that it is difficult to assess the actual impact of paid media advertising because the feedback is usually delayed and because other factors also affect consumer response.

In museums, advertising is normally handled by communications or marketing personnel who work in concert with an advertising agency. Museum personnel propose the budget, approve advertising agency ads and campaigns, and handle direct-mail advertising, displays, and other forms of advertising. The advertising agency's task is to create effective ads and advertising campaigns and to select and purchase media.

Developing an effective advertising program involves the following steps: (1) setting the advertising objectives, (2) deciding on the advertising budget, (3) designing the message, (4) deciding on the media, (5) deciding on media timing, and (6) evaluating advertising effectiveness. Exhibit 9.1 illustrates many of these steps within the context of the advertising strategy of the Art Gallery of Ontario for a major exhibit.

Setting the Advertising Objectives

The first step in developing an advertising program is to set the advertising objectives. These objectives must flow from the museum's prior strategic planning decisions on the target market, market positioning, and the marketing mix. A complete statement of objectives includes four components:

- *The target:* Who must we reach?
- *The position:* What are the offering's merits and its point of difference from competitive offerings?
- *Response desired:* What audience response is being sought?
- *Time horizon:* By what period should the objectives be achieved?

The more carefully the specific objectives are defined, the more effective is the advertising communication likely to be. Objectives are tied to the types of responses an organization seeks to elicit from the subjects of advertising.

Awareness. A museum first may find it necessary to build awareness in the community. Some groups, especially newcomer and ethnic groups, may not be fully integrated in the community's communication web. Awareness can be built initially with recognition of the museum's name or logo. Recognition has to be

○○○○○

Exhibit 9.1. Advertising Strategy of the Art Gallery of Ontario: Building Awareness of the Barnes Exhibit.

The Barnes Exhibit, one of the finest collections of Impressionist and Postimpressionist paintings ever to come to Toronto, was shown at the Art Gallery of Ontario (AGO), in Toronto, from September to the end of December 1994. The AGO knew that it was a critical exhibition and that a balanced, integrated communications campaign would be essential for success. The target attendance objective was to presell fifty thousand tickets and achieve total sales of half a million tickets. Success was measured in terms of audience, by ticket sales, but attention also was paid to hotel occupancy and other indicators of spin-off economic activity.

Prior to the development of advertising strategy and execution, a feasibility study was commissioned to determine the best price range of tickets and the best operating hours, to forecast attendance, and to determine what would be the best way to motivate ticket sales. It was decided that the Barnes Exhibit would charge $15 per ticket and that the gallery would be open for eleven hours per day.

Advertising the exhibit presented several challenges. First, there was low consumer awareness and interest, both about art and galleries, as well as the show and the artists. Moreover, research indicated that consumers were intimidated by the whole affair. People did not think they could have a good time at a gallery, regardless of the content.

The communication strategy was to turn the Barnes Exhibit into a "must see" event. To do this, the advertising campaign needed to increase awareness and build excitement in the exhibit and the artists, then sustain that interest and excitement over a nine-month period, from the preshow publicity through to the event's conclusion.

The advertising budget for the Barnes was set at approximately $1 million. Of that, 70 percent had to be spent outside the Metropolitan Toronto area as part of an agreement with the Ontario government to make this a provincewide event and attract out-of-town visitors. The original name of the show was "From Cézanne to Matisse: Great French Paintings from the Barnes Foundation." The feasibility research and focus group testing indicated this title would be unwieldy, even counterproductive in the broad consumer market it was intended to reach. As a result, part of the strategic decision was to shorten the title to "The Barnes Exhibit." This was done to help make the show's name memorable.

Black-and-white newspaper ads became the primary medium in order to stretch the media dollars. Ads were displayed in various sections of the newspapers, including general news and entertainment sections. Approximately three ads per week ran, with varied headlines to give the campaign a broad range of appeal and coverage. Focus groups indicated consumers were polarized when it came to art. "Still life" people are less inclined to like "nudes," and vice versa. Therefore, another strategic decision was made not to show the actual art in the newspaper ads to avoid alienating segments of consumers. This added a creative challenge to the print portion of the campaign: marketing a major art exhibit without showing the art.

Transit and television advertising started in August as part of the prelaunch and launch stages, and, overall, the look of the advertising campaign never varied. Every execution, regardless of medium, was designed to generate further consumer interest. The media attention that was generated helped build the momentum, and word-of-mouth and recognition helped make the event the "must see" that was intended.

The Barnes Exhibit became the hottest event in town. *Five times* the target fifty thousand tickets were presold, and nearly six hundred thousand were sold overall—nearly 20 percent above target. The Barnes Exhibit generated spin-off tourism and economic activity in Toronto; 60 percent of Barnes Exhibit visitors were from out of town, and hotel use exceeded the forty-two thousand rooms forecast. Retail sales at the AGO were excellent and also above the forecast. (A reproduction of a Barnes Exhibit advertisement appears later in the chapter.)

Source: Adapted from Canadian Congress of Advertising, 1995, pp. 222–232.

○○○○○

reinforced through a series of simple messages over time repeating the name and the logo or a thematic message.

Knowledge. The knowledge objective builds on the awareness objective and offers more complete information. For example, a museum that offers a social evening for young professionals will design communications that emphasize the interests of the target audience, such as contemporary art, jazz and other musical programs, performances, food and drink, socializing opportunities, and shopping and parking services.

Liking. Another communication objective is to build a positive feeling for the museum. For example, the museum can invite the culture editor of a newspaper to review a strong exhibition and obtain endorsements from well-known figures to convey people's excitement and satisfaction with the exhibition.

Preference. A museum's target audience may like the museum but prefer other activities, such as staying at home, going to movies, or attending sports events. Here, advertising seeks to build a stronger image of the benefits that flow from visiting the museum, benefits that outweigh those derived from alternative pursuits.

Intention and purchase. An important advertising objective is to stimulate the target audience's intention to visit the museum soon or even immediately, not at some distant, deferred time. The advertising should emphasize, for example, the importance of visiting the museum before a special exhibit closes down.

The setting of clear advertising objectives played a role at Boston's Museum of Science (MOS). MOS is a highly respected U.S. science museum, with 1.6 million visitors annually, nearly two-thirds of whom are families with children. Research showed that a large number of households felt intimidated by science and therefore by MOS. Furthermore, the museum was not reaching growing ethnic communities. Museum communications subsequently combined messages and images of learning and skill building with messages of entertainment and excitement, the point being to persuade people that science is fun rather than frightening. Another objective was to portray the museum as dynamic and lively rather than static, in tune with contemporary issues and concerns. Yet another objective was to communicate the museum's competence and authority in interpreting and communicating science.

Deciding on the Advertising Budget

The most effective way to set an advertising budget is the objective-and-task approach. Staff are called on to define their specific market-related objectives, determine the tasks that have to be performed to achieve those objectives, and estimate the cost of performing the tasks. The sum of these costs is the proposed promotion budget. A frequent concern in any museum is the weight that should be given to promotion in the total marketing or planning mix, as distinguished from adding better services and programming, doing more research, or organizing stronger exhibitions. The answer depends on the particular circumstances of a museum, how well positioned it is, and the kinds of visitors it seeks to attract.

Museums have to allocate advertising spending carefully to different market segments, geographical areas, and time periods. These questions frequently arise: What is the best time period for advertising (preceding major new exhibitions, coinciding with anniversary periods, during the weaker seasons)? What will be the target groups, and how many will there be? How much should be allocated to reaching current patrons and how much to new markets? What should a museum's advertising budget be in relation to competitors' advertising budgets?

Museum staff will propose a number of projects requiring advertising. A case should be made for the importance of each project, its cost, and its likely results (including means to assess results). These projects can then be ranked according to a set of criteria and the highest-ranking one selected, up to the limit of the budget. (Also, a museum should not pass up an opportunity to collaborate with other museums and cultural organizations in joint advertising. In this way the dollars of each museum will go further.)

Designing the Message

After determining the objectives, the target audience segments, the desired audience response, and the budget, the museum has to develop an effective message. An effective message will capture attention, hold interest, arouse desire, and elicit action. Effective ads contain several elements. Bud Schulberg suggests five rules: (1) begin strongly, (2) have a single theme, (3) use simple language, (4) leave a picture in the viewer's or listener's mind, and (5) end dramatically (Zarco, 1993, pp. 10–12). Creativity is an important feature. An ad needs an attention-getting device; it also should have built-in associations familiar to the target audience, so that individuals can process the message more easily. The Barnes Exhibit advertisement on the next page exemplifies the factors of success.

Formulating the Appeal. The communicator has to develop an appeal, theme, idea, or *unique selling proposition.* An ad should capture a person's attention, offer reasons why that person should respond, and motivate the person to respond in desired ways. Formulating the message will require a number of decisions: what to say *(message content)*, how to say it *(message structure)*, how to say it symbolically and imaginatively *(message format)*, and who should say it *(message source)*. Another consideration is what type of appeal to use in an advertising message and image. It might be largely rational (directed at a person's self-interest), emotional (emphasizing such feelings as desire, nostalgia, or pride), or moral (reinforcing a person's sense of what is right and proper).

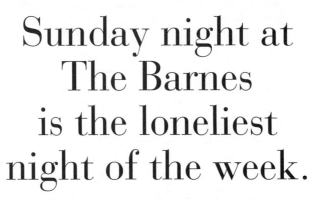

Sunday night at The Barnes is the loneliest night of the week.

The loneliest nights are actually the best nights
to see the Picassos, Monets, Renoirs and Cézannes.
No crowds. No hassles. Just great art.

For same day tickets, come to the Art Gallery of Ontario.
Box office opens at 9:30 am.

Tickets for Sunday nights are available at the Gallery
or call TicketKing: 1-800-461-3333

Great French Paintings from Cézanne to Matisse

The Barnes Exhibit
Art Gallery of Ontario

Never before. Never again.
Until December 31, 1994

Gluskin Sheff

The Sponsor of The Barnes

Special funding provided by the Ontario Ministry of Culture, Tourism and Recreation.
Additional support from the Government of Canada, the Municipality of Metropolitan Toronto and the City of Toronto.

Art Gallery of Ontario, Toronto, advertisement for the Barnes Exhibit. This simple yet effective ad, which appeared in newspapers and on mass transit posters, combines an attention-getting message with an inviting selling proposition.

Copyright 1994: Art Gallery of Ontario.

Choosing the Execution Style. Any message can be presented in different *execution* styles:

- *Slice of life.* The message shows people experiencing a museum offering. The cover of a brochure may show a family viewing an exhibition.
- *Lifestyle.* The message emphasizes how the offering fits in with a lifestyle. An ad to attract singles as museum members may show young adults conversing in small groups and sipping wine during a members-only reception.
- *Fantasy.* The message creates a fantasy around an offering or the occasion of its use. In promoting a new dinosaur exhibit, one natural history museum called on visitors to "experience yourself at the dawn of history."
- *Mood or image.* The message builds an evocative mood or image around the offering. An ad for the Japanese Garden in the Chicago Botanical Gardens evokes serenity and perhaps love, showing strolling couples in the garden, lost in their thoughts.
- *Evidence of expertise.* The message conveys the expertise of the museum and its researchers and curators.
- *Testimonial.* The message features a highly credible, likable, or expert source endorsing the museum's offering.

Designing Print Ads. Research on print advertisements indicates that the *picture, headline,* and *copy* are important, in that order. The picture must be strong enough to draw attention to the ad. The headline must be effective in propelling the person to read the copy. The copy itself must be well composed. Even then, a really outstanding print ad will be noted by less than 50 percent of the exposed audience; about 30 percent of that exposed audience might recall the headline's main point, about 25 percent might remember the advertiser's name, and less than 10 percent will have read most of the body copy.

Format elements such as ad size, color, and illustration make a difference in impact. Designers can make minor rearrangement of mechanical elements within the ad to improve its attention-getting power. Larger ads gain more attention, though not necessarily in proportion to their higher cost. Color illustrations are more effective than black and white.

Creative people must find a *style, tone, words,* and *format* for executing the message. All of these elements must deliver a coherent image and message. Because few people read the copy, the picture and headline must summarize the selling proposition.

Sometimes an ad can be most effective when it is suggestive. Rather than stating specific benefits or attributes, a suggestive ad allows the consumers to imagine the benefits or attributes meaningful to them. The decision of the Art

Gallery of Ontario (Exhibit 9.1) to avoid advertising that categorized the art in the Barnes Exhibit is one example of this technique. Another example comes from the Buffalo Bill Historical Center in Cody, Wyoming—a complex of four museums (Buffalo Bill Museum, Whitney Gallery of Western Art, Plains Indian Museum, and Cody Firearms Museum) and a library (Harold McCracken Research Library)—which uses "Discover Your Place in the West" as its theme for print ads, billboards, and brochures. Its advertising aims to build a sense of identification with and participation in one of America's most powerful and romantic ideas. The American West is a historical, intellectual, and emotional reality; the concepts it embodies have come to have mythic force in the culture. Today it is also a commercial reality and a leading industry. Therefore museum advertising calls on participants to become members to "help preserve and celebrate the West of imagination and reality . . . [and] join those who are striving to keep the mythic and factual West alive."

Designing Radio Ads. Well-written radio ads can lead listeners to imagine themselves at a place or event and enjoying its ambiance. Experts recommend a direct approach in radio advertising. The announcement must be entirely geared to developing response. If the objective of a commercial is to elicit requests for a brochure, the commercial should talk about the brochure. If a sixty-second commercial is selling a membership, this should be clear throughout the entire sixty seconds. A radio ad should be written as if addressing one person alone. Here are some additional tips:

- Mention your organization's name several times.
- Include a deadline, the time by which the listener must respond. ("Only two days left to purchase the few remaining tickets to the biggest event of the season!")
- Recognize that the most important part of a radio ad is the ending. Everything should build up to it.
- Repeat the telephone number three times. End the ad with the third repetition, because the last sounds of an ad will linger in the listener's mind for a few seconds.

Chicago's Museum of Science & Industry (MSI) in the mid-1990s invested heavily in advertising, particularly radio ads, that proved successful in achieving the museum's objectives. In recent years, four new local and regional science centers opened that compete with MSI. Since the 1980s, MSI has used three slogans in its advertising: "The Museum That Smiles," "We've Got Fun Down to a Science," and most recently, "An Ever Changing Adventure." MSI's radio ads seek to accomplish multiple objectives: reach underserved ethnic groups and children and young people, communicate the excitement of new exhibits and films in the museum's Omnimax theater, and highlight interactive and participatory experiences. Let us look at two examples.

The following sixty-second ad ran in 1995 and had the sound of a 1950s-style detective movie:

> DETECTIVE: "It was a sweltering summer day in Chicago. My partner and I were driving north on Clark when the call came in.
>
> DISPATCHER: Big cases unfolding at the Museum of Science & Industry.
>
> DETECTIVE: We headed south on Lake Shore Drive. . . . A crowd was already milling around. . . . Some were sifting for clues hidden deep in the Mystery Maze. Others were cracking the case of 'Whodunit?' . . . No one needed our help. So we slipped away to watch . . . the mysteries of the Titanic on the big Omnimax five-story screen. . . .
>
> VOICE-OVER: Come be a detective for a day at Mystery Summer.

This next fifteen-second radio ad also ran in 1995 and focused on MSI's Omnimax Theater: "Dive head first into a breathtaking underwater adventure. Immerse yourself in a five-story screen. While Meryl Streep tells you all about *The Living Sea*. With music by Sting. *The Living Sea.* Now playing at the Omnimax Theater at the Museum of Science & Industry."

Deciding on the Media

Because message design is affected by the medium to be used, thought has to be given to the most effective media for delivering the message to the target audience. Media selection involves three steps: choosing media categories, choosing specific vehicles, and scheduling.

Choosing Media Categories. The first step calls for allocating the advertising budget to the major media categories. In decreasing order of advertising volume, the media are newspapers, television, direct mail, radio, magazines, and outdoor advertising. Social Marketing for Change (SOMARC) has summarized the advantages and disadvantages of the major media, as shown in Table 9.2. Marketers selecting media should consider the following variables.

- *Target audience media habits.* A museum may seek to attract a particular underserved ethnic community or age group and thus will place its ads in media channels that reach the target groups, such as community radio stations and newspapers.

- *Product or service.* Media categories have different potentials for demonstration, visualization, explanation, and believability. A color ad in a magazine may be the most effective medium to show off a newly renovated auditorium; however, a short television ad may be an effective way to promote interest in an interactive new exhibit.

- *Message.* A message announcing an upcoming lecture by a celebrated scientist requires newspapers or radio to reach an appropriate audience. A message containing a list of next season's lectures might require direct mailings or special newspaper inserts.

- *Cost.* Television is very expensive; newspaper advertising is relatively inexpensive. What is most important, of course, is which medium will yield the highest return per dollar spent.

Media categories should be examined for their capacity to deliver reach, frequency, and impact. *Reach* is the number of different persons or households exposed to a particular message at least once during a specified time period. *Frequency* is the number of times within the specified time period that an average person or household is exposed to the message. *Impact* is the qualitative value of an exposure and the fit with a target audience (thus an art museum's ad in the *New Yorker* or *Esquire* will likely have a greater impact than it would in *Good Housekeeping* or *Police Gazette*).

Media selection involves finding the most cost-effective media package to deliver the desired number of exposures to the target audience. The media planner must consider trade-offs. With a given budget, What is the most cost-effective combination of reach, frequency, and impact? *Reach* is especially important when announcing a new exhibit or going after new target markets. Museums can maximize reach by advertising on several radio stations at the same time or by advertising on one station at several different times of day.

Frequency is more important where there are strong leisure-time competitors, a complex story to tell, or high consumer resistance. It is most effective when museum visits are not planned by the target audience, when there is low interest and loyalty, or when the museum's offering is new. Advertising repetition offsets the tendency toward forgetting; it gets the message back into memory. Many advertisers believe that certain audiences need a large number of exposures for the advertising to work. Too few repetitions can be a waste, because they will hardly be noticed. Herbert Krugman (1975, p. 98) favors three exposures to an advertisement:

> The first exposure is by definition unique. As with the initial exposure to anything, a "What is it?" type of cognitive response dominates the reaction. The second exposure to a stimulus . . . produces several effects. One may be the cognitive reaction that characterized the first exposure, if the audience missed much of the message the first time around. . . . More often, an evaluative "What of it?" response replaces the "What is it?" response. . . . The third exposure constitutes a reminder, if a decision to buy based on the evaluations has not been acted on. The third exposure is also the beginning of disengagement and withdrawal of attention.

Here Krugman is describing three *advertising exposures;* that is, the person actually sees the ad three times. These are not the same as *vehicle exposures,* the number of times the person has been exposed to the vehicle carrying the

Table 9.2. Strengths and Weaknesses of Alternative Media.

Strengths	Weaknesses
Television	
• High impact	• High production costs
• Audience selectivity	• Uneven delivery by market
• Schedule when needed	• Up-front commitments required
• Fast awareness	
• Sponsorship availability	
• Merchandising possible	
Radio	
• Low cost per contact	• Nonintrusive medium
• Audience selectivity	• Audience per spot small
• Schedule when needed	• No visual impact
• Length can vary	• High total cost for good reach
• Personalities available	• Clutter within spot markets
• Tailor weight to market	
Magazines	
• Audience selectivity	• Long lead time needed
• Editorial association	• Readership accumulates slowly
• Long life	• Uneven delivery by market
• Large audience per insert	• Cost premiums for original or
• Excellent color	demographic editions
• Minimal waste	
• Merchandising possible	
Newspapers	
• Large audience	• Difficult to target narrowly
• Immediate reach	
• Short lead time	
• Market flexibility	
• Good upscale coverage	
Posters, Billboards	
• High reach	
• High frequency of exposure	
• Minimal waste	
• Can localize	
• Immediate registration	
• Flexible scheduling	

Source: SOMARC Practical Guide Series: Practical Advertising—Media Planning (Washington, D.C.: The Futures Group Intl, 1995).

ad. If only half the readers look at the ads, or if readers look at the ads only every other issue, then the advertising exposures are only one-half of the vehicle exposures. The museum has to buy more vehicle exposures than three in order to achieve Krugman's three hits.

Assume a Chicago museum places ads in three local newspapers. The *Chicago Tribune* has circulation of 710,000; the *Chicago Sun Times*, 625,000; and the *Chicago Reader*, 137,000, for a gross audience of 1,472,000. Reach and average frequency can be calculated as follows. Assume that there is overlap of readership between the *Tribune* and the *Reader* of 80,000, and between the *Sun Times* and the *Reader* of 40,000, and virtually no overlap between the *Tribune* and the *Sun Times.* By subtracting this duplication (120,000) from the gross audience of 1,472,000, one derives a *reach* of 1,352,000 people or households. Average frequency can now be computed. Assume the ad is placed once a week for three consecutive weeks. The gross audience over that time equals the gross audience for one ad multiplied by the number of times the ad runs (1,472,000 × 3 weeks × 4,416,000). However, the average *frequency*, then, is the gross audience over three weeks divided by the reach (4,416,000 ÷ 1,352,000 = 3.27). Thus the three-vehicle schedule provides 4,416,000 exposures, reaches 1,352,000 different people or households, and (with some of those households taking more than one paper) reaches those people or households an average of 3.27 times.

To determine the impact value of each vehicle, the Chicago museum conducts an audience survey. It discovers that more visitors read the *Tribune* than the *Sun Times* and that frequent arts attenders are more likely to seek out the *Reader*—a free weekly distributed in bulk to various locations. Therefore the *Tribune* and the *Reader* have a higher impact value (higher advertising exposure per vehicle exposure) than the *Sun Times* for this museum.

Advertisers have long debated the trade-offs in budgeting for reach versus frequency versus impact. Until recent years, it was common to favor a reach approach. Today, with the increased targeting of messages to different groups, the preference is for narrow casting over broadcasting. Museums tend to choose media with the best impact on the target group without going for either broad reach or high frequency. In addition, multimedia advertising is considered usually more effective than single-media advertising. For example, radio ads can run just before and after brochures are mailed to sell memberships. A radio ad can direct listeners to see a print ad for details. Referring to a print ad is especially useful when the radio spot is short and the print information is extensive.

Selecting Specific Media Vehicles. The next step is to choose the specific media vehicles within each media category that will produce the desired response in the most cost-effective way. The wide array of radio stations, television channels, daily and weekly newspapers, other publications, and Internet sites spells a condition of extreme *media fragmentation,* which may allow advertisers to reach special interest groups more effectively but raises the cost of reaching general audiences. In making media choices, the media planner relies on media measurement services that estimate audience size and composition and media cost. Creativity is clearly needed in choosing media. Hard data will not be available to answer all questions, and museums finally must make judgments about a vehicle's effectiveness. It is useful to construct a scenario of how consumers go about choosing cultural activities and the role of media in their choices. The scenario can suggest when, how often, and where the museum's messages should appear.

Deciding on Media Timing

In determining the timing of media messages, the advertiser faces a macroscheduling problem and a microscheduling problem. The macro problem is *cyclical* or *seasonal* timing. Audience size and interest vary at different times of the year. Most marketers do not advertise when there is little interest but spend the bulk of their advertising budgets just as interest in the offering begins to increase and when it peaks. If a museum has no new exhibit, a diet of steady advertising serves to remind people of the museum's existence. If a museum has put together a special exhibit, the advertising issues are more complex. The museum may want to build up heavy early attendance that could grab headlines, generating free advertising and good word of mouth. If the crowds continue to come at a capacity level and face long queues and congestion, the museum's marketers will be wise to reduce the advertising intensity.

The microscheduling problem is to allocate expenditures within a short period so as to obtain the maximum impact. How should advertising be spaced during a one-week period, for example? Consider three possible patterns. *Burst advertising* concentrates all the exposures in a very short time, say, in a single day. Presumably, this will attract maximum attention and interest, and if recall is good, the effect will last for a while. *Continuous advertising* schedules exposures evenly throughout the period. Continuity may provide the highest level of exposures and reminder value but also carries the greatest costs. *Intermittent advertising* schedules small bursts of advertising interspersed with brief periods of no advertising *(flighting)* or continuous advertising at low weight levels reinforced periodically by waves of heavier activity *(pulsing)*. These intermittent strategies draw on the reminder value of continuous advertising but at lower cost, and many advertisers feel they provide a stronger message than a continuous approach.

Evaluating Advertising Effectiveness

The final step in the effective use of advertising is *advertising evaluation*. The most important components are copy testing, media testing, and expenditure- and sales-level testing.

Copy Testing and Media Testing. Testing can be done both before an ad is put into actual media (copy pretesting) and after it has been printed or broadcast (message and media posttesting).

Copy pretesting. In order to improve the advertising copy to the fullest extent possible prior to its release, an ad should be pretested on a sample audience to see how well it meets the following criteria:

- *Attention:* How well does the ad catch a person's attention?
- *Comprehension strength:* How well does the audience understand the words and sentences?
- *Follow-through strength:* How well does the ad lead the reader to read/listen further?
- *Cognitive strength:* How clear is the central message or benefit?
- *Affective strength:* How effective is the particular appeal or emotional tone?
- *Behavioral strength:* How well does the ad suggest follow-through action?

An effective ad must score high on all these properties if it is ultimately to stimulate buying action. Too often ads are evaluated only for their attention-getting or comprehension-creating abilities. To gather pretest information, a panel of target consumers or advertising experts may be shown or mailed a set of alternative ads and asked, "Which of these ads do you think would influence you most to buy the offering?" Another approach is to pretest with focus groups. The latter technique has these advantages: its synergism can generate more reactions than a one-on-one session, it is more efficient in that it gathers data from several people at once, and it yields data relatively quickly. Because pretesting is judgmental and less reliable than the harder evidence of an ad's actual impact on target consumers, it is more helpful for screening out poor ads than for identifying great ads.

Message and Media Posttesting. Message and media posttesting assesses whether the desired impact was achieved. There are two approaches. One is to measure whether the communication objectives have been achieved; the other is to measure the sales impact.

To test communication effectiveness, regular consumers of the media vehicle may be asked to recall ads contained in the publication or broadcast (ad recall) or to point out what they recognize as having seen or read before (ad recognition). But these methods test only *cognitive* outcomes of advertising. To posttest the sales effectiveness of various messages and media, their actual impact on *behavior*, the advertiser will have to do one or more of the following:

- Place mailback coupons in the advertisement. Each coupon should carry a code or department number that varies by message and medium.
- Ask target audience members to mention or bring in an advertisement in order to receive special treatment (such as a price discount or free parking).

- Ask individuals to call for further information (on which occasion they can be asked where they saw the ad and what they remember).

- Stagger the placement of ads so that this week's attendance or sales can be attributed to ad A and next week's can be attributed to ad B.

Expenditure- and Sales-Level Testing. Measuring the purchase, sales, or visitorship impact of advertising is harder than measuring the communication effect. The purchase or consumption of something is influenced by many factors besides advertising. Commercial firms have used a variety of methods (model building, historical data, experimental data) to measure sales impact. The point for museums is to determine the effectiveness of advertising in relation to actual reach and visitorship per dollars spent. The purpose is to learn whether they are overspending or underspending on advertising. One experimental test is to vary advertising volume in two test markets or geographical areas; if the high-spending area yields significantly higher visitorship, the museum might conclude that it is underspending in that particular area.

PUBLIC RELATIONS

In a recent survey of five hundred arts presenters, unpaid promotion (public relations) was ranked as the third most effective marketing tool, closely following first- and second-ranked direct mail and paid advertising (Association of Performing Arts Presenters, 1991–1992, p. 45). As advertising costs continue to rise and the advertising audience reached continues to decline, as increasing advertising clutter reduces the impact of each ad, and as marketers continue to place more emphasis on *marketing public relations* techniques, it is anticipated that before long, PR will exceed advertising in effectiveness.

Historically, public relations arose primarily as a *reactive* function. Public relations personnel got out press releases as needed, fought the brush fires of unfavorable publicity as they emerged, and coped with individual and group complaints on an ad hoc basis. This *reactive* stance has many negative consequences. The environment rather than the organization sets the public relations agenda, the organization's image is defined by its response to special situations rather than by the creation of a carefully crafted image over a long period of time, and the organization's responses to crises are not guided by a long-term strategy.

An *active,* market-oriented public relations stance avoids these problems and ensures that the organization has control over how others see it. Tom Harris (1991, p. 12) defines marketing public relations as "the process of planning, executing and evaluating programs that encourage purchase and consumer satisfaction through credible communication of information and impressions that identify organizations and their products with the needs, wants, concerns, and interests of their publics."

Whereas the main function of marketing is to influence *behavior,* the task of public relations is to form, maintain, or change public *attitudes* toward the organization or its products, attitudes that in turn will influence behavior. Thus public relations also can be defined as a management function of a continuing and planned character, by means of which organizations seek to win and retain the understanding, sympathy, and support of those with whom they are or may be concerned.

Public relations and marketing are complementary functions. It can be argued that PR, through the attention, visibility, and news that it generates, provides the conditions, the atmosphere and environment, that make effective marketing possible. It is also clear that PR and marketing have separate, though linked, domains of responsibility. PR is responsible for generating favorable publicity, images, and attitudes, particularly in relation to patrons, sponsors, stakeholders, and visitors, in the case of museums, while marketing is responsible for attracting and satisfying the same patrons, sponsors, stakeholders, and visitors.

Benefits of Publicity and Public Relations

Public relations has several qualities that make it an important part of the marketing function. First, it may have higher credibility than advertising because it appears as news and not as sponsored (paid-for) information. Some experts say that consumers are five times more likely to be influenced by news and editorial copy than by advertising. PR can catch the attention of people who avoid paid messages. PR also extends the reach of advertising, breaks through commercial clutter, and makes news before advertising. PR can complement advertising by reinforcing messages and legitimizing claims and by telling the story in greater depth. It has high potential for *dramatization* in that it can reveal a noteworthy event and thus arouse attention.

PR comes at a fraction of the cost of advertising. The museum pays only for the staff who develop and circulate the stories and manage the publicity for events. The museum does not pay for the media space or time. If the museum develops an interesting story, it may be picked up by all the news media, and this could be worth a great deal of money in equivalent advertising. PR is also less expensive than direct mail. The smaller the museum's promotion budget, the stronger the case for using PR for a larger portion of the promotion activity.

A Museum's PR Constituencies

Museums direct their PR to several audiences. These include their members and donors on which they are heavily dependent for earned income and gifts. Museums also depend on their local communities and agencies of government for support; therefore a portion of their PR has to be directed to political and governmental leaders. Furthermore, journalists, critics, and editorialists increasingly are generating information and opinions that can affect the public response to an exhibition and, indeed, a museum's goodwill, support, and patronage.

Marketing PR Tasks

Marketing public relations falls into the following three distinct categories.

Image PR. PR's central concept is that of image building and image management. Image PR tries to shape the impressions that people have of an organization. It will go after two kinds of impressions:

Revitalizing a museum's image. The Victoria and Albert Museum, for example, one of the world's great museums, is engaged in a PR campaign to modernize its image and appeal and correct erroneous perceptions. Most Londoners have heard of the museum, but few are able to recall any of its superb collections, and many have never visited it, thinking of it as an "old dowager" museum with many objects locked inside glass cases.

Building an image of consumer confidence and trust. PR can disseminate rave reviews about blockbuster shows, develop stories around the activities of a museum's director or curators, and position the museum as a leader and expert in its subject matter. It can also generate news stories with community leaders who articulate the important role the museum plays in the community.

Routine PR. PR also requires routine, day-to-day efforts to promote the museum and its collections, exhibitions, events, and programs. Routine PR has a variety of aims.

Introducing new products. Advance media articles about upcoming exhibitions are critical for building interest and excitement and for selling tickets before a show opens, reviews are printed, and word of mouth has a chance to spread.

Communicating benefits. An article might describe the various benefits that museum members enjoy that go beyond the normal experience of one-time visitors.

Raising the visibility of special or specific collections. The museum might invite outside photographers to take pictures of the collections and grant permission to use them in news stories.

Cultivating new markets. The PR department, in conjunction with marketing, can develop lectures, events, and tours designed to attract a specific market segment.

Crisis PR. Crisis PR attempts to protect the museum and its management, staff, and board members from adverse publicity that could undermine the museum's image, reputation, and support. It helps museums anticipate and deal strategically with the media and stakeholders when serious problems arise. One observer advises, if the museum is not currently in a crisis, it should consider itself in a "pre-crisis situation" and prepare for the crisis that looms on the horizon. Crises can result from a range of internal and external factors and events, including mismanagement; inappropriate policies, strategies, and practices; scarcity of financial resources; sudden economic, legal, or political changes; credit squeezes; new market competition; sharp drops in attendance and in sales levels; labor strikes; and loss of credibility with consumers. Museums have faced crises over organizing exhibits that interpret history, displaying art criticized as obscene, and several other core museum activities. Because crises tend to be highly publicized, crisis management has grown as a specialty area within the public relations function (Reinhardt, 1987).

G. Donald Adams (1983) was one of the first museum managers to write a book devoted exclusively to museum PR. He observes that since museums depend on their publics and constituencies at so many levels, there is the potential for PR problems on a daily basis. He recommends that museums give priority to setting up procedures for dealing with crises and monitoring their crisis responses. Procedures include diagnosing the nature and magnitude of a problem, determining whom to communicate the problem to, taking account of all views involved, and having an appropriate mechanism for resolving crises. Museum management can anticipate crises by distributing guidelines for dealing with them to all employees, assigning staff responsibilities in the event of a crisis, and constructing a list of possible crisis scenarios and of the actions that could be taken to respond to or resolve each crisis. Finally, Adams counsels museum leaders and staff in most instances to establish a policy of openness toward the media and museum constituencies, communicating quickly as problems arise and describing the steps that will be taken.

Tools of PR. Public relations managers can use several tools in their image- and visibility-building efforts. The primary tools are events, community relations, media relations, press releases, public service announcements, interviews, photographs, speeches, and brochures.

Events. Events are planned happenings that aim to communicate or deliver something to target audiences. Public relations departments arrange press conferences, grand openings, public tours, and other events. In addition, museums can sponsor events as programs, including exhibition openings, art fairs, and art competitions. Planned and managed events have several advantages:

- They draw news coverage. When a museum makes an event of the opening of a new museum wing, for example, the success of the event is measured by how widely it is reported.

- They celebrate a museum's history or commemorate an anniversary that generates widespread interest in a community.

- They dramatize a particular program or personality. A science museum may sponsor a book signing by a famous Nobel Prize–winning scientist.

- They bring people together on social or other occasions and bond them to the museum.

PR managers can both *create* and *enlarge* events. Thus the opening of the traveling exhibition *America's Smithsonian* was marked in each tour city by formal dinners that included Smithsonian leaders and local political, corporate, and cultural leaders. The formal dinner in Houston, for example, was attended by former President George Bush and his wife, the state governor, and a large number of the city's economic and political elite. The media in each of the cities covered these dinners and the other events surrounding the exhibition as major news items, and the publicity contributed to the large turnout for the shows.

Community relations. Community support for museums is crucial, and museums are building closer relations with their communities for several reasons. As federal and state funding diminishes in the United States, gaining community financial support becomes ever more important. This involves enlisting more members and patrons and soliciting various types of direct municipal support. Museums that in the past appealed to small constituencies are endeavoring to reach out to new underserved communities. Some museums are launching community advisory boards to help them plan future collections acquisitions, exhibitions, and other programming. The Virginia Museum of Fine Arts initiated a significant community relations program in the mid-1990s to involve members of the city's African American community in the life of the museum (see the Model Museum Practice at the end of Chapter Eight).

Community relations campaigns at museums aim to

- Identify local opinion leaders and build relationships with them and their organizations

- Make museum facilities available for community events

- Arrange museum open houses and tours for local residents and community leaders

- Host special community events such as holiday observances and parades

- Create community advisory boards as consultants on programs and as mediators when museum-community conflicts arise

- Organize a speakers' bureau so that museum leaders can participate in outside lecture programs sponsored by community organizations

- Develop educational programs at schools

Community relations programs can be more costly than other public relations activities because they can require more staff support and use of facilities. A museum will have to estimate the amount of publicity and favorable community attitudes that each project is likely to generate in order to find the best mix and the most cost-effective PR programs.

Media relations. Getting news items to run in the local press or on television or radio is a marketing PR task. The publicist must start with the immediate audience—the media. She or he must understand what the media are looking for in a news or local interest story. People used to believe that there were a limited number of events in the world. Says historian Daniel Boorstin (1992): "There was a time when the reader of an unexciting newspaper would remark, 'How dull is the world today!' Nowadays, the reader says, 'What a dull newspaper!'" (p. 7). The enterprising reporter is expected to find a story and relies in part on public relations personnel to provide material. The public relations director can assist the reporter by setting up interviews, identifying human interest stories in commonplace events, and helping a reporter discover the "news behind the news." The better the PR director is able to meet the media's needs, the more likely she or he will be to meet the museum's PR goals. Museum PR staff should be in regular contact with key columnists, critics, and editors in the community to build relationships and keep them informed about the museum's activities and accomplishments. Long-term cultivation of media gatekeepers helps ensure that news items are reported and coverage is positive and consistent. Preexisting favorable attitudes among gatekeepers can be particularly valuable when a crisis occurs.

Many critics and reviewers are sensitive to cultural organizations' pressures and issues. They are generally receptive to receiving information that keeps them current on these organizations, their programs, and their people. However, they also appreciate a PR person who understands and works to meet media needs. Among the prime characteristics journalists seek in a story are the audience's potential interest in the subject, the possibility for dramatization through pictures and first-person live interviews, the clarity and comprehensiveness of the information provided, a limited need for further "digging," and the possibility of exclusive coverage—for either the entire story or a specific angle. Exhibit 9.2 lists several tips for working with the media.

Although the public relations function has grown in impact in recent years, the media resources available to arts publicists have dramatically shrunk. Looking at the situation from the media end, *New York Times* editor James Oestrich says, "I really feel sorry for these [PR] people. . . . There are just not that many publications around, and I can't be all things to all people. I feel every day of my life in this job that I am letting down publicists, artists, writers—I'm letting down everybody, because I don't have the space to do more" (Boorstin, 1992, p. 7). Looking at the situation from the PR person's end, publicist Alix Williamson graphically describes the frustrations of her job: "I get an idea. Then I write a letter about that to a given editor. I don't get an answer, so I start to call him. I call him not once but twelve or fourteen times. He never returns the call. Finally one day I'm lucky and get him on the phone, and he asks what I'm calling about. I tell him, "It's about the letter I wrote to you on such-and-such a day." "Well, what was it about?" he asks, and I repeat the gist of it. "Well," he says, "that sounds like a good idea—would you mind writing me another letter about it?" So I write another letter, and I go through another sixteen calls" (Boorstin, 1992, p. 7).

○○○○○

Exhibit 9.2. Tips for Working with the Media.

- Do advance planning. Prioritize the events and issues that best meet the organization's goals.
- Know the media—read, watch, listen—and become familiar with style, orientation, strengths, and limitations. Know the reporters, columnists, and editorialists. Know which columns and broadcasts are appropriate for the museum's events. Know the audiences each media professional specializes in. Do not call all media with each new idea; the story must be compatible with the medium.
- Be selective. Not all events call for a full-scale campaign. If the museum overemphasizes a minor story today, it may have trouble getting coverage for a genuinely newsworthy story tomorrow.
- Know each medium's deadlines and preferred formats for information submitted for calendar listings and articles. Coordinate your deadlines to take advantage of media deadlines.
- Do not send uninvited publicity faxes to the press; many journalists do not accept them because they can tie up their fax machines and keep them from getting important news.
- When phoning a journalist to make an initial contact or to follow up on a mailed release, find out first if the journalist is free to talk and then be brief and to the point. Figure out before the call what you can say in ninety seconds that will spark the person's interest, possibly adding a new twist in a follow-up call.
- When making an exploratory call to a journalist, try to have three or four different story ideas, so you have a better chance of providing something of interest. Journalists know the interests of their publics and may have personal preferences that affect their responsiveness to various ideas.
- Once you have been turned down, even for an important story, do not argue. If you discover a new angle to the story, test it out on some colleagues to make sure it is really different and meets the organization's needs—then call the journalist again and make your new pitch.
- Never tell a media person what to write. However, develop a sense for the kinds of stories each one likes to cover. Send a written suggestion pointing out interesting aspects of a production, event, or human interest story. Develop opportunities for the journalist to contribute his or her own *spin* to the story. Know which journalists like to dig further to cover a story well and which do not.
- Have one, and only one, person from your organization as your media contact, so that the media are not deluged with different requests, releases, and even arrangements for buying space or time from the same organization. Such confusion reflects badly on the organization. However, make key people in the organization available to the journalist when requested. Sales and financial information in the public domain should be readily given to journalists upon request.
- Schedule events to take advantage of slow news days such as holidays. Opening-night invitations should go out to the media three to four weeks in advance.
- Send a yearly press kit or letter to reporters and editors listing your name, address, and daytime and evening phone numbers. Include a short description of the organization, its offerings, and upcoming annual programs.

Sources: Adapted from Chreiber, 1987b, pp. 39–41; Bissell, 1985, pp. 51–55. Used with permission by the League of Chicago Theatres.

○○○○○

To save time, canny critics and editors typically press down on the envelope of a press release to see its headline and toss it if it is of no interest. Others automatically throw away any envelopes addressed mechanically. So the more sophisticated PR people individually typewrite or handwrite envelopes to the most important members of the press.

Creative public relations managers have found other solutions to shrinking arts coverage. One approach is to place stories in alternative newspaper sections such as the sports, business, food, or home sections. A natural history museum exhibit dealing with the workings of the digestive system, for example, might be the basis for a story in the food section. Another solution is to promote several museums jointly; this might get more media attention. PR managers can also publicize museums in souvenir programs for sporting events, on bus benches, on taxi panels, on community bulletin boards, in church and synagogue bulletins, in chamber of commerce publications, and in service club newsletters. Companies and individuals that support a museum can publicize it through their internal business documents and even in headers on their fax memos. Major corporations might insert museum leaflets in billing envelopes.

Press releases. Press releases are the basic tool for communicating with the media. The press release has a style and form all its own; it should never resemble an ad or feature story. A press release's job is not to sell or entertain but to inform; it should be concise, to the point, and free of filler. It should avoid hyperbole but take advantage of favorable reviews or notices from leading critics. An endorsement from a reputable third party always lends credibility to your claims. Each press release competes with dozens of others each day. Unless the message is clear, it will be passed over in favor of one more readily understood. A cluttered, ill-organized release also looks unprofessional. PR staff should learn whether a given press release had an impact. For example, they can send stamped, preaddressed postcards with each press release, eliciting whether the media professional plans to use the release, needs additional information, and so forth. Exhibit 9.3 describes the main components of a well-prepared press release.

Public service announcements. Although airtime on radio and TV is expensive, broadcast media are usually willing to give free airtime for public service announcements (PSAs). There was a time when radio and TV stations were required by the Federal Communications Commission to give airtime to nonprofits. Although this is no longer the case, the broadcast media like to be seen as good community citizens and to have community material that interests and informs viewers.

Airtime is highly coveted, and the number of organizations competing for it is tremendous; therefore only properly prepared material will be considered for use. Many local and national advertising agencies and production houses are willing to donate their services for developing PSAs. Whether PSAs are prepared in-house or by an outside agency, use the following guidelines:

○○○○○

Exhibit 9.3. Main Components of a Well-Prepared Press Release.

- *Name of organization.* Whenever possible, send press releases on letterhead; otherwise, type the name of the organization in the upper left-hand corner of the page.

- *Contact name and phone number.* Underneath the organization's name, type your own name or the name of the person who will be available to answer follow-up calls. If you list another person, be sure that she or he has read the release before it goes out. Type the correct phone number clearly underneath the contact name; do not expect the recipient to search the letterhead for the number.

- *Date.* Type the date on which the release is sent out in the upper right-hand corner.

- *Exclusivity notice.* Situations that call for exclusivity are rare. If you do have a story that lends itself to an exclusive approach, send the prospective journalist a standard press release, then contact him or her in person or over the phone to offer the additional exclusive information. An alternative is to type "<u>EXCLUSIVE TO</u>" (all caps and underlined) followed by the name of the person and the name of his or her organization immediately below the contact name on the unique press release. This should be included only if you are offering the information to a single source. Never mark anything exclusive if you intend to send the same information—even in an altered form—to anyone else. If you do, you will damage your own credibility and that of your organization.

- *Release date.* If you want publication of your release to coincide with a specific event, or if there is a tie-in with a particular date, say so clearly. Type in either "For release on or after [date]" or "For immediate release." If your event is a special announcement, say, the naming of a new museum director, do not provide the journalist with any information that you would not want publicized in advance. The journalists' job is to report anything newsworthy as soon as they hear it, and their preference is to be the first to do so.

- *Headline.* The headline should include as much vital information as possible (without assuming paragraph proportions) and should clearly express the tenor of the story to follow. It should be written in the present tense, even if the report is of a past or future event and should use the active rather than the passive voice.

- *Body copy.* In organizing your release, follow the journalists' rule of thumb, the inverted pyramid. Include all the critical information (the who, what, when, where, and why) in the lead or opening paragraph, then move through the rest in descending levels of importance, concluding with the least essential points in the shortest paragraphs at the end. This structure is helpful to copyeditors, who, when pressed for space, can simply cut copy from the bottom, assured that the crucial information will remain intact. Always double-space and leave wide margins. Use only one side of the paper. Be sure to cover the following points: name and address of organization; name of new exhibit; opening and closing dates; brief description of exhibit; ticket prices and special rates (where applicable); and box office hours, address, and phone number.

If you use more than one sheet of paper, type "—more—" on the bottom of the page, number all the pages, and at the conclusion, type a series of # # #, the journalistic symbol for "the end."

○○○○○

- Offer several PSAs of differing lengths. The more variations you submit, the better your chances of getting on the air. Indicate the reading time at the top of the page: "10 seconds (25 words)," "20 seconds (50 words)," and so on. Never send anything without reading it aloud and timing it carefully. Names that might be mispronounced should be followed by a phonetic respelling in parentheses.

- Check deadlines. Most stations require a long lead time, often as much as six weeks.

- Check with each station's public affairs director for its PSA policies. Some stations air PSAs randomly throughout the day; others have community calendars or bulletin boards that air announcements collectively. Cable stations in particular use this latter format, and many have forms that must be filled out and submitted with the PSA.

- Remember that it is against the law to mention raffles, door prizes, and lotteries as promotional incentives.

Museums can offer incentives to radio and television stations to run their PSAs. For example, the museum can offer to trade a certain number of memberships for a certain number of announcements. The station can use these memberships as prizes in contests it is sponsoring or as gifts to employees or advertisers. The station benefits, and the museum gets not only the PSAs but a chance to increase its membership (Newman, 1983).

Interviews. An often effective vehicle for publicity is the media interview. It was recently reported that there are 4,250 local news and talk shows on 988 television stations in the United States. On these shows, 10,200 guests appear annually (Manners, 1985, p. 1). Television public access channels are particularly eager to find and use such guests: celebrities or newsworthy individuals, experts on a subject, artists, scientists, or people with a story to tell. Anything offbeat generally has a much better chance of getting time or space than a subject already well worn in the media. To successfully pitch a story to a talk show producer or guest coordinator, follow these guidelines:

- Keep pitch letters to a single page.

- Use background information and statistics to show how and why your idea is important to the audience. Provide brochures, news clippings, and similar brief items that show the idea is timely and provocative.

- Suggest a few thought-provoking questions that could be asked during the interview.

- Follow up with a phone call to the producer or coordinator and be prepared to sell your idea.

Museums can also send stations a list of possible discussion topics and names of experts to deal with each one. Some stations keep expert lists on file so they know whom to call locally for information and quotable views on topics in the news.

Once your interview has been approved for airing:

- Bring along visual aids or props to help enliven a television segment.
- Make sure your guest or representative sees or hears the show before the day of the interview.
- Routinely remind the talk show contact that you exist and that your people are available.

Photographs. Photos are more than visual supplements to features and reviews; quite often a photo and its caption tell a complete story. When pitching a story to the press, be sure to alert the photo desk to the photographic opportunities. In some cases, coverage results exclusively from the interest of the photo editor. Try to come up with a visual angle for every museum event or program. Whether the media send photographers or not, have your own photographer on hand to record such events as opening night parties, a visiting celebrity, special announcements by the museum director, or an enthusiastic standing-room-only audience. Keep a photo archive for future promotions and publications.

Speeches. Public relations managers can generate many firsthand contacts by providing museum leaders as public speakers. A large museum may have its own speakers' bureau and provide this service on an ongoing basis. To develop speaking engagements, consider the following:

- Identify the potential audiences in your area, such as service clubs, cultural associations, social clubs, churches, business associations, schools, and libraries. Your chamber of commerce may have local listings of such organizations.
- Develop a list of speakers in your museum and their possible topics.
- Send information about your speakers' bureau to program coordinators for your potential audiences. Include them on your mailing list when publicizing your programs and fundraisers and sending direct-mail pieces.
- Develop a comprehensive worksheet for each speaking assignment; it should specify the date, location, start time, program length, audience size, whether to expect a question-and-answer session, and the name and phone number of the contact person.
- Capture for the museum's mailing list the names and addresses of people who attend these speaking engagements.

Museum brochures and newsletters. Museums often make heavy use of internally generated publications such as brochures, pamphlets, and newsletters. The can serve multiple purposes, including public relations, advertising, community relations, and direct marketing.

For example, the richly colored brochure "After Hours at Pacific Science Center" features information and endorsements regarding the center's facility rental program for corporate events, employee parties, holiday parties, and convention receptions. The brochure of the Children's Museum of Indianapolis, which bills itself as "The World's Largest Children's Museum," captures in cartoons and eye-catching graphics the kinds of experiences visitors can have.

The New York Hall of Science, in Flushing Meadows, offers several brochures aimed at different constituencies. "Services for Schools & Teachers" deals with the science center's variety of instructional programming, such as workshops for students and teachers, and its services, such as classroom science kits, CD-ROM kits, and computers that schools can rent to demonstrate interactive lessons, curriculum materials, and student activities. The "Youth Programs" brochure lists activities that include science demonstrations, hands-on activities, special weekend events, intern and apprenticeship programs, Science Club membership, center sleepovers, high school prom programs, and day camp programs.

The Public Relations Manager

Most museums handle all of their public relations in-house; some hire an outside PR agency. One of the biggest mistakes a museum can make is to underestimate the amount of time and planning that goes into successful public relations. Therefore a museum that chooses to do publicity in house with an already overextended staff may work against its own best interests. Either adequate time must be allotted to an in-house person to handle the myriad PR details on a timely basis or a professional PR person or agency should be hired. In any case the ultimate responsibility for the planning and direction of all publicity efforts belongs to the museum.

When hiring an outside publicist, look for someone with a proven track record with cultural organizations—someone who clearly understands the special needs and opportunities. In order to avoid any gaps or overlaps in service, spell out in a written agreement all responsibilities and fees. Designate one member of the in-house staff to act as liaison to avoid the confusion that inevitably results when two or more people are involved. The liaison person should assemble a calendar indicating deadlines for press releases, photographs, PSAs, opening night invitations, and so on; help the publicist develop story ideas and identify audiences that are to be targeted for specific exhibits and events; and meet regularly with the publicist. The work must focus both on publicizing current exhibits and events and on planning strategies for upcoming exhibits and events (Bissell, 1985).

There are several precautions every publicist should take to ascertain information is correct and that there will be no awkward questions later. Gather the information for press releases, PSAs, and other publicity materials in writing. Follow up all conversations, both within the organization and with media, by writing confirming memos. When other people in the organization have to approve publicity material, ask them to initial it. When quoting a person in a news release, be sure to send the person a copy ahead of time (Yale, 1991).

Public relations is a critical part of a museum's communication mix. Its effectiveness depends upon close cooperation between the public relations manager and the museum's other key managers. Public relations is the museum's primary tool for shaping public opinion and, when integrated with advertising, direct marketing, promotion, and other marketing tools, it can boost the museum's audience, support, and community relations.

DIRECT MARKETING

Advertising and PR, in spite of their reach, have limitations in meeting a museum's strategic communication goals. Mass media advertising and promotion are broad in scope, reach a diverse audience, and can miss significant segments of the target market. Furthermore, advertising and PR generally lack addressability and customization to specific groups the museum wants to appeal to.

Direct marketing, accomplished through direct mail, telemarketing, and personal contact, is often a more effective way to nurture patrons, donors, members, and visitors. Selling via personal communication has been used successfully by people throughout the ages, and with telecommunication tools, personalized computer-generated letters, and the many applications of a customer database, the scope of direct-marketing techniques is nearly limitless. In this section we describe how museums can use the tools of direct mail, telemarketing, integrated marketing communications, and database marketing more effectively.

Advantages of Direct Marketing

Museums are major users of direct marketing. They mail out announcements of new exhibits and lecture series, invitations to become members, donor solicitations, and other items. They also run telemarketing campaigns to recruit members and solicit donations. Direct marketing offers several advantages over other modes of communication:

- *Prospect selectivity.* Museums can send one letter to nonvisitors, another to frequent visitors, another to new donors, and still another to major donors. The museum can buy mailing lists containing the names of almost any group it would like to attract: people who subscribe to art or science magazines, high-income members of selected ethnic communities, new empty-nesters, and so on.

- *Personalization.* Museums can customize messages to different persons and groups. A new dinosaur exhibit can be promoted to elementary grade school students in one way and to college science majors in another way.

- *Relationship building.* Museums can build a stronger relationship with each visitor and member. Through direct marketing, a museum can encourage a first-time visitor to consider becoming a member and get a regular member to become a high-end member or a volunteer. By appealing to individual needs and preferences, marketers can increase consumer interest, attendance, and contributions.

- *Timing.* Museums can time direct marketing more precisely than advertising to reach prospects at the best moment. If tickets for attending a major lecture at the end of the week are selling slowly, for example, telephone calls can be used to stimulate interest quickly.

- *Attention.* Museums' direct-marketing material receives higher readership than ads because it is directed to more-interested prospects. Consumers are also more likely to pay attention to messages specifically directed at them. The targeted approach reduces the waste inherent in mass media advertising campaigns and often results in lower marketing costs.

- *Research opportunities.* Museums can test alternative direct-marketing media and messages (headlines, salutations, benefits, prices) to find the most effective approach. Moreover, the museum knows whether a direct-marketing campaign has been profitable because the response can be measured.

Managing Direct Mail

Direct mail is commonly used to sell an offering, usually a membership or subscription; collect or qualify leads for further follow-up; communicate interesting news about an event, an award, or a rave review of an exhibition; or solicit donations for an annual or capital campaign. Well-conceived, well-executed, and well-targeted direct mail is the primary tool for membership retention and renewal. In a survey of five hundred performing arts presenters, direct mail was found to surpass all other marketing methods in effectiveness, followed by paid advertising, unpaid promotions, telemarketing, posters and handbills, and direct sales (Association of Performing Arts Presenters, 1991–1992, p. 45). Direct mail is a frequent component of telemarketing campaigns and even advertising campaigns.

Target Consumers. In preparing to use direct mail, a museum's direct marketer needs to determine the characteristics of the museum audiences and of the member and donor prospects who would be most able, willing, and ready to visit, participate, and support. Bob Stone (1979, 1988) recommends applying the R-F-M formula *(recency, frequency, monetary amount)* for rating and selecting consumers from a list. The best targets for museums are their members, individuals who visited most recently, those who visit frequently, and those who are active customers in the museum shop. Points are assigned for the various R-F-M levels, and each consumer is scored; the higher the score, the more attractive the consumer.

Names of prospects may also be selected from among the museum's own lists, from lists exchanged with other cultural organizations, or from lists purchased from mailing-list brokers. Organizations typically first obtain a subsample of names from a potential list and do a test mailing to see if the response rate is high enough. For targeting new prospects, the marketer can use various segmentation criteria. Good prospects can be identified on the basis of such demographic variables as age, gender, income, education, and where they live and work. Geodemographic list building allows a museum to target different consumer lifestyle segments, such as the culturally and socially active, for whom its offerings would be appealing.

Elements of Effective Direct Mail. The first task of the museum's direct-mail marketer is to interest the recipient in reading the mailed piece. Yet the most common consumer response to typical direct mail is to throw it away! A recipient spends about twenty seconds deciding whether to give a mailing serious attention. These twenty seconds have been carefully studied by direct-mail researchers, and much has been learned about effectively using the key elements and guidelines of a direct-mailing program: envelope and contents, cover letter, brochure, and response card.

Envelope and contents. Mail recipients first see the outer envelope. The first challenge is to stimulate enough interest with the envelope's exterior that people will be motivated to open it. The envelope should therefore convey a message that is clear, compelling, and brief. A marketer may put the headline or main selling proposition right on the envelope or arouse reader curiosity with teaser copy. Envelopes are more likely to be opened if the addressee's name is handwritten and if a postage stamp is affixed.

On average, recipients take about eight seconds to scan and open the envelope. For the next four seconds, enclosures are unfolded, and the reader builds up judgments about the contents even before a single word has been read. The final eight seconds consist of the first run-through: reading the pictures and headlines, finding short answers to such unspoken but already present reader questions as: "What are the benefits?" "Does this offer apply to me?" "Is it better than other offers?" "What will it cost me?" (Vsgele, 1992, pp. 86–88). The marketer should be sure to use pictures, headlines, captions, and other methods for expressing the offer's advantages as strongly and succinctly as possible. If the package has survived the first twenty seconds, the recipient is likely to undertake a more comprehensive process: reading blocks of text and gathering information in greater depth. This is when the body copy of the letter or the brochure's descriptions are put to the test. After reading the copy in some detail, the reader will do one of three things: throw it away, place an order, or file it away for later reconsideration. Putting it to the side is better than throwing it away, but what is out of sight is also out of mind. Responses usually require a new external stimulus. That is why a museum often does a second and a third mailing.

Cover letter. If the direct-mail piece is thought of as the modern-day equivalent of the personal sales call, then the letter represents the *contact stage.* Because of the importance of this stage, direct-mail packages, even those with elaborate brochures, almost always bring in a higher number of responses when they contain a separate letter. Bob Stone (1988, p. 344) offers this seven-step formula for writing a successful letter:

- *Promise a benefit in the headline or in the first paragraph.* Most people will not read an unsolicited letter unless they see a clear benefit.

- *Enlarge on the most important benefit.* If the lead is relevant, you can build interest without reader diversion.

- *Give details about basic product or service features.* If you expect readers to take action, they must know what they are getting.

- *Support your statements with proof.* You can dispel the normal reader's skepticism if you can support your claims with demonstrable facts.

- *Tell readers why they should act.* By introducing a sense of urgency, you can put the readers in a receptive frame of mind before you get to the close.

- *Rephrase prominent benefits in your close.* By summing up the main benefits, you reinforce preferences built previously.

- *End with a call for action.* Use a strong, urgent close. This is your moment of truth.

The headline. Some letters carry headlines, good attention-getters when they are succinct, catchy, and to the point. The headline makes sure that the offer's highlights and benefits are not buried in copy (Hatzenstein and Sachs, 1992).

The salutation. One of the first things the reader sees is the salutation. The museum should customize the salutation for each target group: for example, "Dear Friend of the Museum" or "Dear Newcomer to the City."

The body copy. On reading the letter, the recipient immediately has questions, forming a kind of inner dialogue: "What will I get out of this for myself?" "Is this right for me?" "Will I find it comfortable and enjoyable?" The marketer should always give an answer that either spells out the benefits or arouses curiosity. A museum's claim that "we are the best" is sensible only when the reader can also perceive a personal benefit. The letter should be long enough to do the selling job but not so long that the reader loses interest. It should have a personal tone, creating a bond of familiarity between sender and receiver.

The letter's opening paragraph gets the most reading. It should introduce the main theme and create a desire to continue to read. A membership solicitation letter might open with a benefit promise or an interesting statement: "10,000 people are enjoying the privileges of membership. We would love to have you enjoy them too." The letter's body copy can then enlarge upon the subject, present data to support the selling proposition, and urge the reader to take immediate action. The end of a cover letter should give clear and compelling instructions (the call for action):

"See for yourself by filling in the reply card and returning it today."

"Pick up the phone and call our members' hotline at . . ."

The recipient's job of responding should be as simple as possible. The forms should require little effort. Postage-paid reply envelopes should be provided whenever possible.

The postscript. Research indicates that readers start at the top of the letter and look at the salutation but then turn to the end of the letter to see who is writing to them. At this point, most eyes are drawn to the postscript (P.S.) because of its proximity to the signature—with more than 90 percent reading the P.S. before moving back to the top. With this in mind, some direct-mail professionals compose the P.S. first and then move on to write the letter's lead. The most effective P.S. is a succinct statement of the overall offer, the concept and theme. The focus should be on the reader's anticipated benefits.

The brochure. A museum brochure is an effective complement to a direct-mail letter. The brochure's success is largely dependent on outstanding copy and graphics. As for controlling costs, an arts organization does not need to print a fancy four-color brochure in order to get results. A well-conceived two-color brochure that says the right things and has broad distribution may be equally effective. Once a brochure is designed and printed, the costs for producing extra copies drop dramatically. One indication that it is time to stop using a specific brochure for direct-marketing purposes is a negligible response from a variety of mailing lists that received the brochure.

Response Rate and Response Card. It is difficult to provide a general answer to the question, What constitutes a good response rate to a mailing? There are so many variables. Does the museum have a loyal, long-standing membership base? Does it have a good reputation, or is it little known? How selective is the mailing list?

From the most selective lists, new subscriber response may be as high as 2 to 3 percent. When marketers lower their requirements for list quality in order to increase their reach, the response rate is much lower. With a 2 percent response rate, the marketer may conclude that 98 percent of the campaign effort was wasted. However, that is not necessarily the case. The direct-mail package presumably has some effect on awareness and possible interest. It may enhance the museum's image. It may educate and inform the recipients and prepare them for later action. The recipients may become more attentive to the museum's mass media advertising, to reviews and PR, to word-of-mouth recommendations, to telemarketing strategically timed to follow up direct-mail efforts, and to future direct-mail efforts.

Mailing a colorful, general-interest brochure filled with details may not be the most cost-effective mailing for the purpose of attracting new members or donors. If people have not visited the museum and are unfamiliar with it, information about all the programs, benefits, and membership levels can easily overwhelm them. A response card that provides an opportunity for prospects to request more information is a more effective way to reach these prospects at a lower cost. Once a person has responded in some way, he or she has taken a step, however small, toward some level of interest.

The response card can range from a flashy, four-color, three-fold piece to a one-color postcard. It highlights information. The easier the card is to fill out, the higher the response rate will be. The respondent should be asked to fill in his or her name, address, and daytime and evening telephone numbers (rather than using a peel-off label) so that the museum can capture the phone numbers. The museum's telephone and fax numbers should be in bold print. The return section should be perforated so that the respondent does not have to search for scissors, and it should have prepaid postage (Wade, 1992).

Managing Telemarketing

A direct-mail piece can deliver detailed information to segmented groups; it cannot deliver the exact information each individual might need. Telemarketers, however, can talk to prospects, distinguish between offerings, and help prospects make an appropriate selection. They may deliver less information overall, but they can deliver the exact information a specific prospect most wants. Telemarketers can also solicit current members to share their concerns and ask questions, and thereby increase their likelihood of renewing membership or making a donation. Telemarketing's success at selling memberships or renewing contributions is based upon the simple fact that it eases the decision-making and purchase process. The telemarketer describes the benefits in a concise and attractive manner and then answers the respondent's concerns.

The amount of emphasis to place on telemarketing depends on several factors. How routinized is the renewal process among current members? How strong is the current membership base? Given the higher contact cost for telemarketing, privacy issues, and the multitude of organizations using telemarketing, precise list selection and targeting is critical. This section considers some characteristics of the caller and the call and the legal issues telemarketing raises.

The Caller. Effective telemarketing depends on choosing the right telemarketers, training them well, and offering them effective incentives. Stephen Dunn, whose firm supervises telemarketing at many arts organizations, rarely if ever hires individuals who are trained in selling stocks, aluminum siding, and the like over the phone. Rather, his firm advertises in the local paper for articulate, motivated people who have a knowledge of the particular field and an interest in the arts organization. Applicants hired might include high school students, actors, musicians, professionals between jobs, and retired people. They are screened twice: once over the phone to determine if they have pleasant voices and sound enthusiastic, then in more depth in person.

Training the callers is an important and ongoing part of a successful telemarketing campaign. Providing incentives is also critical. Telemarketing is hard and often stressful work, creating frequent turnover. It is not unusual for a telemarketer in an eighteen-to-twenty-week campaign to quit work after only six to ten weeks. Therefore incentives that can keep callers sharp and motivated are worthwhile. For example, the telemarketing supervisor can build up enthusiasm by offering prizes to top performers or to the first one who gets an order. Larger museums often employ professional firms to hire, train, and monitor callers and to manage the telemarketing campaign day to day. Smaller museums tend to conduct their own in-house campaigns. One advantage smaller museums have is that given their more limited aims and their close-knit community, they can rely on patrons and members to assist in telemarketing efforts.

The Call. The opening lines in the telephone call are critical; they should be brief and lead with a good question that catches the listener's interest. The call should be made at the right time; the best time to reach households is usually between the evening hours of seven and nine. Individuals can be called at dinnertime, but to mitigate the intrusive timing, they should be asked, "Is this a good time to talk?" Most important, a customer service approach should be maintained. Whatever the response of the person called, the contact should always be courteous and informative. Responsible organizations should go to the trouble of deleting from telemarketing lists anyone who asks not to be contacted by phone.

The telemarketer also needs to know how to end the conversation if the prospect seems to be a poor one. However, Joseph White, president of a telephone fundraising firm, believes that considering no a final answer could be a major mistake. For three nonprofit organizations, White sent follow-up letters to current and lapsed members who had refused to pledge support during a phone call. The letters, mailed within three weeks of the call, generated a 9.9 percent, a 4.9 percent, and an 8.6 percent response. The telephone contact, though not successful at the time, nevertheless generated a delayed reaction. Although these efforts were mainly to gain contributions, the same principle can work for membership campaigns as well. Each letter should be mailed soon after the telephone contact. It should thank the prospect for accepting the phone call and should reinforce the offer's highlights and major benefits. The package should include a detached reply device and a preaddressed, postage-paid business reply envelope. Also, if the person was obviously angry at being called, the letter should include an apology—followed, of course, by an invitation to become involved (White, 1994).

Telemarketing and the Law. The Federal Trade Commission is now engaged in reviewing various aspects of telemarketing, namely hours of calling, the use of disclosure scripts that require the caller to say by whom he or she is employed, a ban on the use of automatic dialers (which use computer messages and random dialing), and the creation of a national *do not call* list against which all telemarketing lists will have to be purged. Nonprofit organizations will be exempt from these regulations for the near future, but in a few years this exemption will probably disappear. Yet any organization will retain the right to contact its members (those who have expressed interest in its product or service) in any manner it wishes, including the telephone. So no matter what restrictions come from the FTC, a museum will retain the right to call people in its in-house file who have provided their phone numbers. Museums should plan for this eventuality by developing a prospect campaign as a key element of their direct-marketing strategy (Dunn, 1992).

Integrated Direct Marketing

Too often, direct marketers rely on a single advertising vehicle and a one-shot effort to reach and sell a prospect. For example, a *single vehicle, single-stage* campaign might send a one-time mailing to enlist new members. And a *single-vehicle, multiple-stage* campaign might send successive mailings to the same prospect. (Each successive mailing must be considered effective enough to justify its cost for the mailings to continue.) However, a third approach is to run a *multiple-vehicle, multiple-stage* campaign, a technique called *integrated direct marketing.* Consider the following sequence:

Paid ad with response mechanism → Direct mail →
Telemarketing → Ongoing communication

The paid ad creates product awareness and stimulates inquiries. The museum then sends direct mail to those who inquire. Within forty-eight to seventy-two hours following mail receipt, a telemarketer phones, offering to give further information, and encourages a purchase. Even if the prospect is not ready to become a member, there is ongoing communication. This *response compression,* whereby multiple media are deployed in a tightly defined time frame, increases message awareness and impact. Multiple media are used because they reach different people who respond to different media (Roman, 1995).

Developing a Marketing Database System

A *customer database* is an information-intensive and long-term marketing tool. Many marketers confuse a customer mailing list with a customer database. A customer mailing list is simply a set of names, addresses, and telephone numbers. A customer database contains much more information, including customer lifestyle, demographics, and financial information; purchase transactions; and promotion and media response characteristics. The customer database can be the museum's cornerstone for planning its current and long-range marketing efforts.

Ways to Use a Database. When a marketing communication program is database driven, it is customer driven: the museum's marketer can target the correct offer to the correct consumer. Jackson and Wang (1994, chap. 4) have identified the following ways to use a database as the central tool of marketing communications.

Identify your best consumers. A database allows the marketer to look at consumer data using recency, frequency, and monetary (R-F-M) analysis to determine the most supportive visitors and members.

Develop new consumers. By analyzing information about the current consumers, the marketer can develop a consumer profile and use it to identify other people whose characteristics closely match those of current consumers.

Enhance available information. Database enhancement is an overlay of information that supplements consumer and prospect records. Consumer data can be enhanced with demographic data (compiled by such companies as Donnelley Marketing, Metromail, and R. L. Polk) and with psychographic information (such as provided by the PRIZM clusters described in Chapter Five). For example, assume a museum is planning to sponsor a singles evening once a month for young professionals working near the museum. By enhancing its currently available customer information (name, address) with U.S. Census Bureau data, it can identify the people who travel thirty minutes or more to work. Other data sources can be used to add information on occupations, age of family members, and so on. The marketer may even want to research the brand names of cars owned or athletic shoes worn by singles working near the museum, to help attract corporate sponsors.

Deliver a message consistent with product usage. The database allows the marketer to target communications based on usage patterns. New and infrequent patrons can be stimulated to more frequent attendance by mailed announcements. Moderate-usage patrons can be encouraged to play an active part in the organization.

Develop complementary-sell opportunities. By analyzing past purchase behavior, the museum may discover, for example, that people who like dinosaur exhibits are the most likely to attend a series of lectures on ecology. The museum can then use this information to develop new programs for specific target markets or advertise specific programs to the best prospects.

Identify ongoing research opportunity. A well-run database program allows the marketer to easily and regularly access in-depth information about individual consumers and research their responses to various marketing efforts. This, in turn, allows the marketer to improve subsequent marketing decisions.

Integrate functions. Too often, the databases of a marketing department and a development department are incompatible. They should be linked so that the museum can get a picture of the total involvement of each patron or member in the museum's various activities.

Development and Maintenance Costs. Specially designed database systems are expensive. According to Andy Brolin, director of marketing for Prologue Systems (a major provider of arts marketing and fundraising database systems), the start-up costs for licensing software and purchasing and installing hardware for a typical eight-user-station system is approximately $75,000. However, before managers of lower-budget organizations despair over such numbers, they should consider the following factors.

New revenue. A database is a highly effective tool in increasing attendance by current members and in building new audiences and membership. The increased revenue can often pay for the database system many times over.

Collaborative opportunities. The most expensive portions of the database system are software licensing and the server (which centrally stores the information). According to Brolin, if ten small organizations were to share these costs and have one or two workstations each, the cost to each would approximate $20,000.

Corporate partnerships. A museum might find a corporate partner willing to subsidize some or all of the costs of database marketing.

Adaptation of existing software. Many museums that cannot afford a specially designed system have ready access to such standard software as Lotus, Excel, or Quattro Pro. Technical assistance will be necessary to encode levels of information, and access and data integration are much more difficult to achieve, but even a relatively simple system based on this standard software is far better than no system at all. Two critical ingredients in making database marketing work are (1) getting top management to approve the investment and ongoing cost and (2) getting organizational acceptance and support for the new way of doing marketing. Once a database is set up, the museum must continually upgrade its data and its database management system, to keep pace with the dynamic market environment.

Developing Lists. In order to promote its offers to appropriate current and potential audiences, the museum needs to maintain a full range of lists and update them regularly. The main lists are house lists, external lists, and specially created lists. Museums that do not charge admission fees or require tickets and those that lack membership programs are in a compromised position as far as obtaining supporter and visitor information. Tickets for special events can be helpful in building lists of local residents, but tickets for blockbuster shows often are purchased by out-of-towners, who may be less inclined to support the museum at a distance. Gift shop and restaurant purchases, if made with credit cards or checks, are also an important source for visitor information. A growing number of museums invite people to participate in brief visitor information surveys on interactive screens placed at museum entrances and exits. (The surveys can use the same screens that display museum information and orientation.)

House lists. House lists are generated from the museum's current members, patrons, and active visitors. They should be broken down as follows:

1. Single-ticket purchasers at museum events and special exhibitions should have their names, addresses, and phone numbers added to the database, along with information on the events or activities attended.

2. First-year members are more likely to lapse at renewal time and should be given special attention.

3. Long-term members and patrons should be accorded special attention as the most likely source for gifts and volunteering.

4. Lapsed members should be tracked to learn why they dropped out and whether they contributed or participated actively in the past, and this information can help in efforts to recapture their attention.

5. Active gift shop customers sometimes constitute a separate list from those who visit the museum galleries or participate in special programs and events.

External lists. Museums can obtain additional lists from a variety of sources.

- *Exchange lists.* Museums and art organizations are increasingly reaping the benefits of exchanging lists with one another, realizing that the most satisfied patrons are those who frequent multiple organizations. When selecting organizations to contact for list sharing, the marketer should match up as many prospect characteristics as possible.

- *Rental lists.* A musical instrument museum might rent a list from Blockbuster Video of people who rented *Amadeus* or *Chopin.* Or it might rent lists of subscribers to classical music magazines.

- *Mail-order buyers.* A museum might be interested in renting lists of names of the young, upscale, active people who purchase from Lands' End and similar catalogues. For an art-loving market, the museum store of the Metropolitan Museum of Art has a prime list.

Creating Lists. Museums can create their own lists by generating leads in a variety of ways. These lists have a great advantage over external lists because they consist of people who have already expressed interest in the museum's offerings. *Lead cards* (or *name cards*) can be placed on tables in the lobby or near exhibition entrances with a sign reading, "Please leave your name and address so that we can notify you of our future programs." Lead cards can also be placed in brochures or program notes, distributed at corporate sponsors' offices, and distributed in other ways. Ads with coupons can generate names for the database. Radio broadcasts can make similar offers, providing telephone numbers for listeners to call and thereby generating additional data from respondents (Stephen Belth, personal communication).

Mailing List Selectivity. When conducting a major new membership or fundraising campaign, the museum should prioritize its lists according to the likely response rate but not necessarily eliminate the lists with the lowest rates. According to Stephen Belth, marketing director for the Los Angeles Philharmonic, a 0.5 percent response rate is considered good for direct mail; a 1 percent response rate is profitable in the first year. For telemarketing, which is more costly to implement, a 3 to 4 percent response rate is profitable. Remember that the profitability of a one-year subscribership is only a small fraction of the lifetime value of each subscriber who stays with the museum. Even if the museum spends, say, $50 or more to attract a $60 subscription, the annual renewals, contributions, gift shop purchases, and potential for bringing new people into the organization can far outweigh this cost.

As organizations collect lists from multiple sources, they should check for duplications. The more duplication there is between the lists, the more likely it is that those people will be good prospects. It is advisable to test a suspect list before doing a full-fledged mailing or telephone campaign. It is not unusual for 25 percent of addresses to change each year, so if a list has not been updated annually and if the names have not been merged and purged, its worth will be greatly reduced.

SALES PROMOTION

Sales promotion consists of using short-term incentives such as coupons, discounts, exchange privileges, and gifts and premiums to encourage adoption or purchase of a product or service. A variety of sales promotion techniques exist, but they all have three distinctive characteristics:

- *Communication.* Sale promotions capture public attention, or the attention of a particular segment, and usually provide information that can lead to a purchase.
- *Incentive.* Sale promotions incorporate some concession, inducement, or contribution that gives value to the consumer.

- *Invitation to purchase.* Sales promotions represent an invitation to engage in a transaction at a given time rather than putting it off indefinitely.

The incentive is the core benefit of sales promotion. It is something of monetary or symbolic value that is added to an offer to encourage a particular behavior on the part of the individual. The challenge is to design an incentive that attracts and satisfies the target audience and at the same time accomplishes the museum's revenue, attendance, and other goals.

Museums can make good use of sales promotions in four particular areas: to attract first-time visitors, to attract underserved segments, to distribute audiences more evenly across peak and off-peak periods and eliminate overcrowding, and to expand the membership, including encouraging existing members to renew and to become higher-end members.

Sales promotions should receive adequate planning. A first step is to determine the *objective(s)* for which an incentive is offered. A museum that has off-peak periods, when visitorship is low, can offer discounted group tickets to tour operators to attract tourists, or free or discounted tickets to local residents, tied together perhaps with special programming of particular interest to this group. When the Walker Art Center opens its doors for free once a month on Saturdays, it has the specific goal of attracting families with young children to special programming directed at young people. A sales promotion also might be directed at people who have never visited museums (combining free or discounted tickets with coupons redeemable in the gift shop) or at museum members who have failed to renew (offering them an additional membership benefit such as a tote bag or other gift). Museums that have social events for targeted groups sometimes offer free or discounted tickets that encourage people who sign up to bring a guest.

Several decisions are required in developing sales promotions. First, the recipient must be determined, whether individuals, family units, membership groups, or touring groups. Next the *form* of the incentive is identified: free or discounted tickets, a special event, or a gift. Then the *amount and duration* of the incentive is decided. Too small an incentive is likely to be ineffective, but an overly generous one will be too costly.

A growing number of museums are using sales promotions to raise their visibility, reach underserved or target groups, and *close sales* on museum visits. Museums that have free admission and free exhibits or that anticipate large crowds can require visitors to obtain tickets, even free tickets. Tickets are incentives to participate and to participate at a definite time as well as a means of crowd control. The *America's Smithsonian* traveling exhibition required tickets for entrance, free if picked up at the exhibition site and at a nominal fee if ordered by phone or mail. The tickets raised the exhibition's visibility and desirability and at the same time served to minimize crowds and congestion. As described in Chapter Ten, the Philadelphia Museum of Art during its 1996 blockbuster

Cézanne exhibition pioneered new types of sales promotion by offering ticket purchasers a package of additional benefits, bundling the exhibit catalogue and an audiotape tour with the ticket for a single discounted price. The Philadelphia Museum also organized an alliance with airlines, tour operators, hotels, restaurants, and businesses such as banks and credit card companies to maximize publicity and market the exhibition. These allies publicized the show and the offers in their own promotional materials, enabling the museum to reach a much larger audience than it could on its own. For example, downtown hotels offered special discounts on two-day, single-night visits. Visitors using a sponsoring bank's credit card were offered major hotel discounts on a second and third night's stay. A major airline offered special fares for exhibit visitors, as did Amtrak for rail passengers. Fifteen local restaurants offered dining discounts. The mass of publicity, the multiple marketing channels, and the variety of benefits offered in this marketing and sales promotion alliance helped generate the highest attendance and single-show receipts in the museum's history, as well as considerable income and revenue for the city.

Because shopping can represent a considerable part of a museum experience, museums increasingly are making use of gift shop coupons as incentives to boost museum visitation. Museums with an admission fee have the choice of discounting the fee or maintaining the set fee but providing a gift shop discount coupon with the ticket.

Museums also are collaborating with other museums to expand the benefits they offer members by granting exchange privileges that are available at all the museums in the network. The Museum of Discovery and Science, in Fort Lauderdale, Florida, offers upper-tier members a membership in New York City's American Museum of Natural History, along with a subscription to the latter's distinguished magazine. Considering that many New Yorkers spend their winter vacations in Florida, it makes sense to build a collaboration between two kindred museums in New York and Florida, thereby reinforcing the appeal of each one. Similarly, eight downtown Philadelphia museums have organized a marketing alliance and joint sales promotion that offers visitors the benefits of experiencing several different museums at discounted prices. This critical mass of varied museum offerings can also result in more tourist trade than the offerings of a single museum. These are all examples of short-term sales promotion incentives to encourage people to visit, participate in, and support museums.

SUMMARY

Many museums in the past found it unnecessary to promote themselves or to explain their value to the public. These museums were often supported by patrons, appealed to a specialized audience, and offered limited programs. Today, museums of all types seek wider audiences and offer a greater number of programs. They are more subject to competitive pressures in attracting visitors and raising support. They recognize the importance of image building, communication, and promotion. Thus museums are engaging in advertising, public relations, direct mail, and sales promotion to boost their visibility, communicate their distinctiveness, and build public support. Each communication tool or channel has advantages and shortcomings, and the choice will depend on the specific objectives, the target audiences, and cost effectiveness considerations. A mix of tools and messages is sometimes appropriate. Regardless of the communication programs, museums will find it prudent to pretest messages and tools and establish procedures for evaluating outcomes, effectiveness, and impact.

O

MODEL MUSEUM PRACTICE

Image Building, Communications, and Media Partnerships at Boston's Museum of Science

The Museum of Science (MOS), situated on the Charles River in Boston, attracts 1.7 million visitors annually. Two-thirds of these visitors are families with children. Eighty percent of the museum's budget derives from admissions fees and earned income.

Museum management in the early 1990s launched a strategic planning process, reviewing the museum's strengths and weaknesses, public awareness and perceptions, competitive advantages and disadvantages. "When I first came to the museum," David Ellis, a former college president who became the museum's director (interviewed May 6, 1997), recalls, "I asked people in the community what they thought of the museum. Several said to me, 'What's the next show?' I was struck that few had a sense of the museum as a whole and its value to the community. Their focus was on shows. I concluded that one thing the museum needed was a stronger public identity."

One focus of the planning process dealt with promotion and communication. In previous years, MOS management had communicated images and messages built around particular, changing offerings such as special exhibits and Omnimax films. Yet, according to Elinor Selame, a corporate identity consultant: "Institutions will build major, expensive edifices . . . choose a wonderful, visible location and bring in world-class exhibits. But when the exhibit is gone, there's nothing left but a tired building with a tired image. Just like a store, an institution should have a name and an identity that gives people a sense of what it stands for" (Finke, 1996, p. 138).

Science museums and science and technology centers enjoy some advantage over art and history museums insofar as the demand for science literacy and learning is high. Parents are more likely to focus on science training for their children than training in art or history. A parent may not understand what science is, yet recognize its prestige and value. Science museums can motivate young people and families as a result of their association with science education. Yet, according to Joyce Gardella, former MOS vice president of marketing and head of Gardella Associates, a nonprofit consultant (interviewed Jan. 21, 1996), "science museums in the past had image problems with young people. They often perceived science museums as gigantic science tests, more likely to be failed than to be passed, much less enjoyed. Our goal at the museum is to reach all kids and parents who are convinced they cannot do science."

Planning at MOS led to a shift in the communications program—from focusing on short-term offerings, which spoke primarily for themselves, to building a long-term image of the museum, of which the offerings and programs were expressions.

The museum's communications program had two main objectives: first, create an organizational image that is relevant and accessible—intellectually welcoming as well as physically and economically accessible; second, create an anchoring image that is consistent and ongoing, rather than generating a novel image for each new exhibit, film, or planetarium show. Specific offerings then became means for promoting the museum, rather than having the museum promote specific offerings. These offerings become the emblem of the museum's ongoing promise to provide the highest-quality experiences and education available.

MOS created an image that combines excitement, energy, learning, and a sense of change. The museum's logo says "Museum of Science: It's Alive." The logo shows a red planet revolving in a gray orbit, with the lettering "Museum of Science" in white on a black background. MOS has transformed the image into the equivalent of a brand name, and this brand name communicates excellence, accessibility, reliability, and a distinctiveness that competitors cannot match.

Building and maintaining a brand image involves using that image consistently in the media, in the museum brochures and literature, at the entrance and in areas throughout the museum, in the gift shop and restaurant, and on the tote bags, wrapping papers, T-shirts, and other signature products that the museum sells in its shops and catalogues. The museum logo, tag line, and image then become a cue, calling up previous satisfactions at the museum and enhancing future expectations. Maintaining the brand identity behind the image involves maintaining the quality of the museum and its offerings and making sure the experience of the museum matches the image. MOS's brand image resulted from market research that revealed the positive and negative elements in public perceptions of the museum.

Gardella is convinced museums have to compete with entertainment-centered popular culture and leisure activities and organizations. Museums have to go after broad audiences rather than narrow segments. And they have to be accessible and relevant in people's lives. Organizations like Disney, Blockbuster, Fox, and Sony have brand images and ample resources to promote themselves and their products. So, too, do museums have to create brand names to reach large, diverse audiences. Brand images are solutions in media-dense societies. They are a low-cost way to raise public visibility and presence in people's minds.

MOS, having developed a brand image, found other relatively low-cost ways to promote and communicate. It formed partnerships with television and radio stations in the Boston area, and one TV station agreed to broadcast a certain number of promotional spots during selected periods—a media campaign the museum could not have afforded on a commercial basis. The spots highlighted the museum's offerings, particularly the Omnimax Theater and the new exhibitions and learning technologies. In exchange, the museum featured the television station's logo and recognition of its support in its advertising, on museum signage, and in the brochures and publications. MOS obtained an additional benefit from the partnership: the station provided marketing information on the types of promotional spots that were most effective and the population segments that were reached. The museum also launched billboard advertising to communicate MOS's brand identity.

Today the Museum of Science is reaching a larger and broader audience, partly as a result of its image- and brand-building and promotion campaign. Repeat visits have also increased, along with membership development, corporate support, and museum store sales. The moral, as Elinor Selame, likes to say: "Build a brand, and they will come."

CHAPTER TEN

Setting Pricing and Revenue-Building Strategies

Prices are not just expenses, from the consumer point of view. They also serve as a reference point against which to measure perceived benefits or values, as a means of reallocating expenditures, or reducing the purchasing decision's complexity.

From an organization's point of view, pricing differentials represent a spectrum designed to fit different market segments. Prices should be designed to capture the different perceived values of the offering among the segments served.
—Dan Nimer

There was a time when pricing was not a relevant or important tool for museums. Most museums opened their doors to the public without a charge; they were sufficiently funded by donor groups and government agencies. In recent years, under the pressure of declining grants and subsidies, rising costs, and the need to expand private revenues, museum administrators have begun to examine with care the ways of raising revenue through earned-income sources, notably admissions, special exhibit and event fees, and gift shop sales. As a result, pricing has become a sophisticated practice in a growing number of museums. Pricing has also influenced museums to think more clearly about the benefits they offer the public and what the public perceives as the value of a visit or a membership.

Many people both inside and outside museums, however, have opposed the new emphasis on revenue raising. They argue that museums serve public and educational purposes and have a distinctive fiduciary role of protecting national and local treasures for future generations. Therefore museums are public assets to which the public has the right of free and unlimited access. In Great Britain, in particular, there were heated debates in the early 1990s about establishing admission fees. The British Museum has thus far held out, but the Victoria and Albert Museum and several other British museums have adopted admission fees. The Smithsonian museums remain free to the public, but a majority of U.S. museums now charge admission or else request a donation at the door.

Museums have discovered that charging an admission fee and setting prices for other services can be compatible with keeping their organizations accessible to people with limited means; free days, passes, and discounts can be used to maintain access for all people. Moreover, earned income for many museums no longer is a discretionary choice but rather a matter of necessity. U.S. museums in 1988 reported $1.1 billion in earned income (nearly one-third of their total aggregate operating income) (American Association of Museums, 1994, pp. 84–85, 89). Clearly, earned income has become an important source of financial stability. The question then is not whether to raise earned income but how to do it in ways that are congruent with a museum's mission and needs and the community's expectations.

Consider the hypothetical example of a large, urban museum that has recently adopted a policy of charging admission. There are at least three pricing issues the museum must consider. The first is to determine what among its offerings can command a price, or put in another way, what the public or specific segments of the public perceive to be of sufficient value and benefit to dispose them to pay a fee. In many cases, before the public ever perceives a value in museum offerings, the museum has to persuade (communicate to) the public that a value exists. Then museum staff have to determine how much weight that value has among various segments, relative to the perceived value of similar offerings elsewhere or offerings by competitor organizations. Second, the museum has to determine its pricing policy for various audience segments. Should everyone pay the same price, or should admission be priced lower for certain groups such as students and seniors? Should one or more free days or discounted events be set aside to serve those who have limited means? Third, the museum must determine what proportion of total revenue will be contributed by earned income. That is, how much total earned income will the museum need to raise in a given year?

The pressure for attracting more revenue has led museums to exercise pricing decisions in a number of areas: pricing admission, pricing loaned objects and traveling exhibitions, pricing special exhibitions and events, pricing memberships, pricing items in the gift shop, pricing rental of museum facilities, and pricing donor support.

PRICING ADMISSION

Museums, like public libraries and public schools, look upon themselves as performing valuable public-interest activities that deserve community support. The fact is, however, that both public treasuries and donor groups are under intense pressure to support many worthwhile causes. As museums and other nonprofit organizations respond by developing additional revenue-generating sources, one of their first steps is typically to establish an admission fee.

Alternative Admission Fee Systems

Museums face several alternatives in setting admission fees (these choices are of course not mutually exclusive):

- Charge the same price to every visitor
- Charge different prices to different classes of visitors (*multiple pricing*)
- Establish a membership program so that members are admitted free and only nonmembers are charged
- Request visitors to contribute whatever they wish (by dropping money into a box near the entrance)
- Post suggested admission prices or donation levels, but allow free entry or discretionary payment
- Charge a price, but establish one or a few free days or blocks of time and make available free passes or discounts to targeted groups
- Charge different rates for different seasons, days of week, or times of day

Many museums first introduced pricing by encouraging voluntary contributions. Some set up an out-of-the-way contribution box so as not to embarrass those who chose not to pay. Others placed the contribution boxes near to entrances or entry turnstiles. Some museums seeded the boxes with $10 or $20 bills, a practice that has been shown to encourage visitors to make donations and to boost the level of those donations.

Museums that now charge for admission often establish a pricing schedule, charging less to children, students, and sometimes seniors. For example, the Miami Art Museum, in Florida, charges $5.00 to adults and $2.50 to seniors and students; children under twelve are admitted free. One of the highest-charging museums, the Florida International Museum, in St. Petersburg, has charged $14.50 for adults, $13.25 for seniors, and $5 for youngsters five to sixteen, with no charge for children under five. Today, a large number of museums operate with differential charges but also have a free day and a membership program in which members pay no admission fee.

Museums are recognizing that price can also be used to regulate attendance levels. Museums that have an active season when attendance is pressing against capacity can, in principle, raise their admission charges during the peak season. This reduces wear-and-tear on facilities and at the same time increases per visitor revenue. By the same token, during slow seasons, charges can be lowered, and incentives such as discounts or free passes offered to attract visitors.

Nevertheless, in general, museums want to keep admission charges as low as possible so as not to discourage attendance. Low admission fees are viewed not only as the socially responsible thing to do but also as making good economic sense if the demand is highly elastic and fluctuates with price. That is, the museum's revenue may be greater if the museum charges a low price but receives many visitors than if it charges a high price but receives fewer visitors. The relationship between price and demand has not yet been sufficiently researched. There is some evidence, however, that the public reacts negatively to frequent price changes and to overly complex pricing systems. And there is evidence that when a major museum first introduces admission fees, a drop-off in visitation takes place that may last several months, after which visitation levels return to pre–admission fee levels.

No museum likes to increase its price. There is the risk that demand will fall by an amount that will leave the museum with the same revenue as before the price rise or even less. Much depends on the price sensitivity of the target market. To reduce visitor price sensitivity, a museum may decide to introduce several small price increases instead of one large one. Small price increases are hardly noticed and seem justified in the face of rising costs. Most organizations prefer to pass on small price increases on a regular basis than to make large price increases on an infrequent basis.

Some museums have set up a process for monitoring and revising their pricing. An example is Canada's National Museum of Science & Technology, in Ottawa. It examined attendance and gross revenue at several price levels and identified an optimal price that maximizes both visitation and revenue. It found that an $8 admission price was the *break point* beyond which its public showed resistance. One means of researching such price inhibition is to observe the rate of *customer turnaround:* namely, how many visitors enter the museum and upon seeing the admission charge, decide to leave. This tends to happen more in locations where there are alternative leisure-time activities at hand. The museum could set a lower price and then observe whether the number of turnarounds decreases significantly.

Surveys have been conducted on how people feel about the prices they have to pay for other cultural activities and whether these prices have inhibited attendance. The questions are whether price is a barrier to attendance, and if so, for whom is price important? Some interesting performing arts research has been done that might have bearing on people's decision to attend a museum as well. For example, in a study of 1,298 regular performing arts attenders in Great Britain, Walshe (1991) found that price was not a major factor behind nonattendance and that the decision to attend or not to attend bears less on price than on other considerations. Only 4 percent of the respondents mentioned cost as a barrier to attendance. Walshe concluded that the potential for price increases is substantial, although he warned that such price increases can be disastrous unless accompanied by efforts that maintain or improve the event's value to the market.

Other performing arts studies show that price is typically a second-tier issue. If the subject matter, performance, and performers are of high quality, then price is less of a barrier. At the same time, price increases can have a significant impact on certain audience segments (groups with moderate or low interest), who react to price increases by attending fewer performances. For the purpose of analyzing pricing among nonattenders, Walshe drew a distinction between *nonintenders,* nonattenders for whom pricing is not the central issue, and *intender-rejecters,* those who express interest in attending but become alienated as a result of pricing policy. To show how people considered performing arts attendance in relation to price, Walshe developed the decision-making model displayed in Figure 10.1.

Walshe's analysis indicates that for the vast majority of people, rejection sets in *before* price becomes a consideration, because these people have a probably irreversible barrier: lack of interest. There is, to be sure, an alternative hypothesis: lack of interest among the majority can mask a lack of information, and awareness, if aroused, would generate interest and motivation. As a cultural organization

Figure 10.1. Decision-Making Model for Performing Arts Attendance.

Source: Walshe, 1991.

reaches out to a broader audience, one can assume that price becomes a factor even if interest in participation exists. A conclusion can be drawn: there is little point in major price cuts to reach the mass market; price cutting will not generate significantly greater attendance. And a second conclusion can be drawn: pricing strategies should be based only on segments, not on the public at large, and perhaps specifically on the intenders—those who express an interest in attending a specific event.

Pricing policy also has to reflect the fact that there are costs or barriers to visitation besides admission fees. The consumer may face the cost and time of driving to the museum and paying for parking, of standing in a long line (especially for special exhibitions), of hiring a babysitter for younger children, and of paying admission fees for older children. Museum marketers face the challenge of raising the perceived benefits of attendance in the minds of potential visitors in order to lower the importance of such actual and perceived costs. Some costs, such as babysitters and traffic conditions, are beyond the marketer's control. However, the museum can help visitors lessen related costs. It can provide free parking, discount parking coupons, or a guide to nearby commercial parking facilities. Reducing the waiting time in lines, providing good dining and rest room facilities, furnishing strollers for children, and taking similar steps all work toward reducing perceived costs and heightening the visitors' satisfaction. In general, visitors who have formed an expectation of good value for their money will come and be satisfied.

As for perceived value, it varies by audience segment. For example, many mature audiences value what Abraham Maslow called self-actualizing experiences. A couple in their fifties or older may take coupons to the grocery store to save $3 or $4, then spend $200 that evening at a fine restaurant and a concert. They may drive a car that has clocked over 100,000 miles and that they hope to keep longer, yet spend $12,000 on a trip to Asia or Europe. Although they may spend tightly on goods and services necessary to *maintaining* a lifestyle, they are likely to spend loosely on products and services that *enhance* lifestyle (Wolfe, 1993, pp. 124–128). This segment places a high value on cultural experiences. For certain segments, factors other than price are so central to creating value that prices can be raised significantly without eroding their participation. This underscores the need for an organization to know as much about its consumers as possible.

Contrasting Objectives for Setting Admission Fees

A museum needs to clarify its objectives when setting its admission fee. The following section describes alternative objectives.

Charging to Maximize the Number of Visitors. Many museums favor the objective of audience maximization because it is likely to create two additional benefits.

The larger audience will generate more positive word of mouth—assuming that the museum experience meets or exceeds expectations. A larger audience also increases the number of people who might make purchases in the museum gift shop and restaurant, take out memberships, or make donations to the museum. Thus the Millicent Rogers Museum, in Taos, New Mexico, specializing in the art of northern New Mexico, offers special group and group tour prices in a region that is especially appealing to tourists. However, when the objective of audience maximization is secured by free admission or a low fee, the museum gives up the tangible revenue that would result from higher admission charges and also forgoes the incentive that encourages museum-goers to take out a museum membership. Most museums prefer the tangible revenue flow from a solid admission charge to the less tangible revenue effects of word of mouth. Moreover, audience maximization may not be a sound objective if crowds create a lot of property wear-and-tear and if they rob visitors of a satisfying experience due to long queues, less visible exhibits, noise, and other inconveniences. Art museums, particularly, guard the quality of the setting and the ability of audiences to take long, comfortable, leisurely views of exhibitions. These considerations favor higher admission charges to restrain visitor levels. However, too high an admission charge could lead to criticism that a museum is exclusive and elitist.

Charging to Maximize Cost Recovery or Surplus Building. When the museum is trying to maximize its cost recovery or even build up a surplus, price setting is a matter of viewing price for its impact on revenue and demand. The museum's admissions revenue is its price times the number of visitors; the issue, then, is visitor sensitivity to price. If the museum has great treasures, offers a lot of experiences, and attracts many out-of-town visitors, it is able to charge a higher price and not lose visitors than a museum in the opposite circumstances. In fact, the more the museum can build up its visibility and reputation for being distinctive, the higher the price it can charge. Moderating the temptation to set a high admission fee is the nonprofit, publicly funded museum's vulnerability to criticism that low-income people (especially with large families) cannot afford visits and therefore the museum is behaving inappropriately to the extent that it impedes access. Although there is understanding, among the public as well as government officials, that subsidies cannot cover all the revenue museums require, the environment and set of expectations in which museums operate serve to place limits on the amount that can be charged for admission, alongside the constraints the market itself places on admission fees.

It is important for museums to recognize that, whatever the level of admission fees, visitation rates will have an effect on other sources of revenue. Visitors typically enjoy having a meal or making purchases in a museum gift shop as well as visiting galleries and exhibits. For this reason, price setting has to take into account the effects of an admission price on both visitor levels and visitor propensity to make purchases. The Art Institute of Chicago found that during its 1995 blockbuster Monet exhibition, the resulting jump in attendance generated significant increases in shop and restaurant revenue, in memberships, in gifts, in facility rentals, and even at off-site shops, all attributable to the elevation in image and visibility that resulted from the exhibition.

Charging What Comparable Museums Charge. A museum might want to take its pricing cues from what comparable local museums are charging. If most local museums charge $6 for admission, another museum can feel justified charging $6—but not much more. The museum-going public will be accustomed to paying $6 for admission to comparable museums but may balk if one or another of the museums charge more.

Charging What Other Leisure Activities Charge. Another approach to admission price setting is to examine what other leisure-time activities and organizations charge. People are quite willing to spend $7 to see a ninety-minute movie. They will spend $20 to watch a baseball game, $30 for a seat at a symphony or a live theatrical performance, and $37 to spend a day at Disney World in Orlando, on top of lodging, dining, and travel costs. The question becomes, What is the museum experience comparable to? Whatever a given museum's answer, it is quite clear that charging $4 to $7 for museum admission is not out of line; most people seem to be willing to spend at least that and often much more for other leisure-time activities. In one sense, museums have been disadvantaged by their history of charging little or nothing for admission. They must therefore emphasize the value of their offerings to alter perceptions and expectations.

Some visitors relate the admission price to the length of their museum visit. Although it is difficult to generalize, research has shown that an average museum visit tends to be only a few hours long, and that includes dining, shopping, and rest room stops as well as viewing exhibits. Museums that have found ways to encourage visitors to spend more time than the average are therefore in a position to raise their fees accordingly.

An innovation at large, urban museums is the bundling of the admission fee (usually the fee that tourists pay) with other related offerings, such as a visit to the museum's Omnimax theater and the rental fee for audio tours. For its 1996 Cézanne exhibition, the Philadelphia Museum of Art bundled its admission fee with purchase of the exhibition catalogue and the renting of an audio tour. The assumption is that in offering extended benefits as a package, a museum can charge a higher, though discounted, price and thereby obtain greater revenue. Such packaging of benefits (which could also include discounts on air travel, lodging, and restaurant meals) also helps simplify the decisions tourists have to make about various options, thereby defraying some of the psychic and other costs associated with a museum visit.

Dan Nimer, a leading U.S. pricing expert (interviewed Mar. 12, 1997), suggests that museums consider three ideas in determining their pricing objectives and programs. First, museums could segment their pricing (for admissions or for special exhibitions and events), tailoring prices to the capability of various segments to pay and to the perceived value of benefits. Charging a single, uniform price overlooks the ability to pay and fluctuations in demand. Second is the idea of unbundling or uncoupling prices and benefits. Museums have a variety of offerings and services, each of which, if appropriately communicated, could be perceived as having a particular value and benefit. Charging one overall price is then equivalent to lumping these various benefits together. However, if benefits were differentiated, each might command a separate price. Ironically, museums, especially those with multiple membership levels, have recognized the variety of benefits they offer, relating tiers of membership benefits to pricing tiers. Yet the same museums fail to apply this idea to their admission, exhibition, and event areas. In a similar sense, in determining prices to charge for donor gifts, museums can segment donor benefits (name on a plaque with others, name on a plaque alone, name on a gallery for a period of time, name on a gallery indefinitely, sponsoring a free museum day open to schoolchildren, sponsoring an exhibition opening), in effect segmenting prices according to perceived values and benefits.

Nimer's third idea is to link prices to incentives as well as costs. An admission price of $10, for example, that confers no benefits other than admission could be perceived as more costly than a price of $12 that includes free parking nearby. The latter, in reducing the psychic cost and adding convenience value, offers a greater benefit and incentive and can therefore be perceived as a reasonable price for the value. Similarly, a museum that offers a package of benefits tied to admission is offering extra value that can be perceived as justifying a higher price. Such *product bundle pricing* is a means to boost incentives, although the price charged for each individual benefit in the bundle would be less than if priced separately. Bundles or packages are similar to the subscription tickets used by performing arts organizations and season tickets used in professional sports.

Nimer suggested, for example, that a museum could set an admission price (say $10) that included a certificate worth $4 either for purchases in the gift shop or restaurant at a certain level. Alternately, visitors could be charged $7 for entry without the certificate, establishing a $4 value for a $3 incremental fee. Those visitors who pay the $10 fee, and use the gift shop or restaurant, would probably spend more than the $4, the equivalent of the certificate, and would perceive a greater value in the higher fee, based on Nimer's experience. At the same time, the museum derives considerable benefit from generating incremental income from those visitors using the certificates to make purchases they might not otherwise have made. Nimer has other pricing suggestions. On its free day, a museum could organize a jazz concert to attract different visitor segments and capture additional revenue. He suggests that museum admission prices could be higher on weekends because people have a greater need then for cultural and recreational activities. Moreover, competitive offerings, such as movies, theater, and concerts also command higher prices.

Charging to Maximize Revenue. Keith Diggle, a leading arts marketing consultant in Great Britain, is a strong advocate of arts organizations and museums charging admission fees at a level comparable to other leisure activities. According to Diggle (1984, p. 92; see also Diggle, 1995, pp. 32–33):

> We should always charge as much as we can *get.* If we charge more than people will pay then we get nothing and that is very uncommercial. . . . Because we are supported by public subsidy we also have an obligation to the community at large . . . [and] to those who want what we have to sell but cannot afford to buy it at prices that are acceptable to the majority. The mistake which is sometimes made is to behave as though the *whole* community cannot afford to pay our prices and so to keep prices far below the level of general public acceptance.

Diggle observes that a common assumption is that free admission maximizes museum attendance. He suggests that museums overlook the differential ability of various segments to pay fees and asserts that charging for admission could help a museum achieve greater attendance as well as expand revenue. Diggle advances two arguments. First, he holds that people, especially in certain segments, tend to undervalue services provided free or nearly free; cost-free and low-cost museums are generally thought to be of less value than destinations or activities that command a price. Second, he argues that most people most of the time have few incentives to visit a museum (especially one that is free or lacks special exhibitions) because it can be visited at any time at the same cost and for the same experience. That explains why a museum visit tends to be treated differently from a performing arts event, which is scheduled for a particular time and for which tickets may be purchased in advance. A performing arts event, in addition, occurs in a place that has a limited number of seats. Once a ticket is purchased under conditions of scarcity, the ticket holder is likely to attend the event at the given time. Museums can match the characteristics of performing arts organizations by offering special exhibitions and events.

Diggle advises museums to accept the idea of charging for admission, treat programs as scarce events, tailor prices to various segments, and link incentives to the prices charged. Further, museums should adopt the habit of requiring tickets for admission and of scheduling events and selling tickets in advance. This gives potential visitors an incentive to schedule a visit soon rather than delay it and to take advantage of programs that have a limited life, thereby raising the perception of scarcity in relation to museum offerings. Museums can then transform permanent exhibitions into special, changing, short-term exhibitions for which tickets are required. Museums can also organize special tours of the collections led by curators, behind-the-scenes visits, or lectures by well-known authorities, each of which constitutes an event that can be perceived as having added value and for which a price can be charged. To attract low-income groups and others lacking the means to pay, museums can offer vouchers or discounts. Building demand for participating in events, using tickets, and charging fees requires, to be sure, prudent planning and image building, along with advertising and promotion (see Chapter Nine).

Charging the Socially Justified Price. Even when charging admission, museums carry a social and public purpose. Normally, they do not intend to make a profit or to recoup total museum costs but to meet a fraction of their many expenses. Museums would normally rather charge on the low side than the high side, given that they believe this will attract more people to enjoy their treasures. Like so many decisions in the museum world, pricing admission is partly a matter of striking the right balance between contrary and competing goals. The goal of raising revenue must be balanced with the goal of reaching out to new or underserved audiences. Raising revenue for present use must be balanced with the need to raise revenue for future use (the preservation of collections and their accessibility for future generations). Raising revenue to stave off underinvestment and eroding museum resources must be balanced with achieving wide museum usage in the short term. If a particular museum is compelled to become creative in finding ways to raise sufficient earned income to survive (assuming the museum has reasons and resources that justify survival), then the museum has an obligation to generate fiscal stability and at the same time keep its visitors and supporters.

Museums should be especially sensitive to the admission price they charge school tours and young people generally. The museum of course wants to encourage students to visit. Most museums establish lower admission prices for students in groups than for individual students, recognizing that the paying party is likely to be the public school system. Museums are sometimes able to find government agencies, corporations, or patrons who will underwrite school visits and school-museum programs.

PRICING OBJECTS LOANED TO OTHER MUSEUMS

When the Art Institute of Chicago mounted its famous Monet show, it had to solicit paintings from many other museums and private collections. Museums customarily loan objects to other reputable museums. They may also develop traveling exhibits that combine objects in their own collections with objects on loan. Natural history museums often loan specimens for research purposes. Loans typically fill in gaps in exhibits and research. Museums that hoard their collections, on the other hand, rarely making loans to others, cannot expect others to make loans to them when the need arises.

Loans involve expenditures and can involve revenues. A loan of an artwork, for example, involves staff time and other in-house costs (processing applications, facilities reports, use assessments, testing the ability of objects to withstand travel, sign-off procedures, and so on). There are costs of packing, shipping, and insurance, which normally are paid by the borrowing institution. Risks accompany loans of rare and precious objects. Loss and damage can occur, and these considerations are uppermost for museums, an overriding purpose of which is to build and preserve collections for all time. Lending museums have to be confident of the borrower's ability to care for and safeguard loaned objects. Art museums, particularly, are cautious about lending objects and do so when they judge the public service benefits to outweigh the risks. Art museums typically do not charge lending fees in loan transactions and absorb the in-house processing costs on the assumption that one museum's request for a loan will be offset by the loan request of one's own museum. In recent years, however, large art museums with rich collections have begun to charge lending fees to cover in-house costs and even to discourage the frequency of loan requests. A lively debate has arisen between small and medium-sized museums that frequently make loan requests to fill in gaps in their collections and exhibits, and large museums that perceive themselves as shouldering excessive processing costs. Museums are public-service institutions that can justify lending objects for the purposes of educating the public by means of quality exhibits and interpretive materials and providing scholars with a range of objects to study. Once a threshold of care and safety is satisfied, museums are expected to make their objects as accessible as possible.

Museum loans may sometimes be sources of revenue. The Whitney Museum of American Art, for example, has raised considerable revenue from large-scale, long-term loans to the San Jose Museum of Art. Big, circulating exhibitions that travel to several venues and include popular treasures can resemble commercial transactions, given the high costs, potential visitor demand and ability to charge special fees, and comarketing arrangements. The market for museum loans also involves companies in the leisure and entertainment sectors that package large-scale shows in nonmuseum settings. Local governments also may seek to use museum objects to build convention business and tourism; icons and "blockbuster" shows can raise visibility and demand. Lending museums, once satisfying thresholds of care and safety, may have to consider differential pricing for loans of the latter kind. In any case, the pricing and fee-structure for loans of museum objects is likely to become a bigger concern in the future.

PRICING SPECIAL EXHIBITIONS AND EVENTS

Museums that have mounted a special exhibition at considerable expense often establish a special admission fee beyond the general admission charge. Museum members can view the special exhibition at no cost (one of the privileges of membership), but nonmembers must pay a separate charge.

The special exhibition charge will vary with the quality and prestige of the show. The Philadelphia Museum of Art charged $12.50 to visit the Cézanne show. That price was in line with the pricing of previous comparable blockbuster shows at the museum and exhibitions at other museums in the region. Marketing staff had suggested a higher price, but the museum management insisted on keeping the price within a certain range. There is evidence that a price of $15 or more would have had no appreciable effect in discouraging visitors, especially since the viewing audience was predominantly upper-income and devoted to art. Thus from a narrow marketing perspective, the price of the Cézanne exhibition could have been raised. However, from a broader perspective, and considering the balance of constituencies and interests that a museum represents, the price for a blockbuster show has to be calculated at a level that will not unduly discourage citizens of limited means, or some proportion thereof, from visiting.

Museums also sponsor special events such as opening night receptions and dinners, social gatherings for young professionals, anniversary parties, celebrity receptions, and celebratory events marking major holidays and the change of the seasons. Such events present good opportunities for earning additional income. Museums can set prices for individual attendees and for tables, for example, $150 per individual and $1,000 for a table of ten. These prices cover the cost of keeping the museum open, hiring staff, purchasing and serving food, and so on—expenses that might amount to half of the price charged. When several hundred people attend, the museum can easily make a profit of $20,000 to $70,000 on a one-evening event. It would take a lot of visitor admission fees to equal the level of revenue arising from a special event. Special social events on weekend evenings, furthermore, do not interfere with customary museum operations and hours; and event participants typically represent a segment different from the regular museum-going visitor.

Conner Prairie, in Fishers, Indiana, offers dozens of special events (seasonal events, themed events, musical and theatrical events, holiday events) throughout the year. For some events, visitors pay an additional charge; other events are free, and yet others are offered at a discount to members. Some museums prefer not to sponsor too many events, lest their supporters and members feel imposed on, events show diminishing returns, and the museum's facilities experience excessive wear-and-tear. (The Model Museum Practice at the end of this chapter examines events, revenue growth, and business development at the Genesee Country Village & Museum, in Mumford, New York.)

PRICING MEMBERSHIP

Most museums have established membership programs. (Chapter Eleven provides an extended discussion of their characteristics.) They have two purposes: first, to involve people more actively in attending and supporting the museum and, second, to provide an independent revenue stream. Most museums establish a price difference between single memberships and family memberships and charge a lower membership fee to students. Membership fees tend to be in the neighborhood of $30 for single membership and $50 for family membership. The Minnesota Historical Society charges individuals $35, households $45, and seniors $30. It also offers an associate membership at $100 that has virtually the same benefits as regular memberships but provides the opportunity for a segment of members to contribute something extra to the society's support. The Museum of Contemporary Art in Chicago has seven membership categories, ranging from $30 to $175, and also single-year and double-year membership prices (the latter offering a discount).

In recent years, museums have created additional membership categories to reach different segments with different benefit packages. Virtually all membership programs offer members, at a minimum, two privileges: unlimited free admission to the museum and a discount (usually 10 percent) on museum gift shop purchases. At higher membership levels, members receive invitations to special programs, behind-the-scenes tours, meetings with directors and curators, and sometimes free exhibit catalogues and other gifts. Table 10.1 shows, for example, the membership levels and benefits at the Adler Planetarium, in Chicago.

Museums promote memberships at the door and through the mail. Visitors upon entering the museum might have the option of paying the admission fee or purchasing a membership on the spot. Museums run periodic membership drives, usually in the form of a direct-mail campaign. Depending on the quality of the mailing list and the benefit package, a museum might get a response of 0.5 to 2 percent.

One of the best times to sell memberships is during a blockbuster exhibition. Many more people are visiting the museum, and the general excitement makes it easier to convert visitors into members. A case in point is the Monet exhibition at the Art Institute of Chicago. Tickets became so scarce that the museum decided to make the remaining tickets available only to members. Many out-of-towners who were keen on seeing the show willingly bought memberships. The museum then faced the challenge of maintaining a high percentage of these out-of-town members when their memberships were up for renewal.

PRICING GIFT SHOP ITEMS

Museums have not always had museum shops. At some point, museums began to set aside a small space for the sale of gift items, recognizing that visitors were interested in purchasing souvenirs and mementos of their visit. Thus the Bergstrom-Mahler Museum, in Neenah, Wisconsin, which features one of the world's great paperweight collections, specializes in the sale of paperweights in the gift shop. Similarly, natural history museum shops feature books on nature, minerals and fossils, and ethnographic objects.

Table 10.1. Adler Planetarium Membership Levels and Corresponding Benefits.

									Adler Associates		
	$30 Individual 1 Year	$45 Family 1 year	$55 Individual 2 years	$85 Family 2 years	$100 Mercury Club	$250 Venus Club	$500 Mars Club	$1,000 Jupiter	$2,500 Saturn	$5,000 Halley's Comet	$10,000+ Solar System
Unlimited free admission to Sky Shows and the museum	*	*	*	*	*	*	*	*	*	*	*
15% discount on Adler store purchases	*	*	*	*	*	*	*	*	*	*	*
Discount on courses	*	*	*	*	*	*	*	*	*	*	*
Newsletter and Skywatcher's Guide subscription	*	*	*	*	*	*	*	*	*	*	*
Free coat and stroller checking	*	*	*	*	*	*	*	*	*	*	*
Invitations to Members' Only events and parties	*	*	*	*	*	*	*	*	*	*	*
Exclusive travel opportunities	*	*	*	*	*	*	*	*	*	*	*
Use of planetarium library	*	*	*	*	*	*	*	*	*	*	*
Invitation to annual meeting					*	*	*	*	*	*	*
Listing in annual report					*	*	*	*	*	*	*
50% discount on courses						*	*	*	*	*	*
Free admission to Sky Show for up to 5 guests						*	*	*	*	*	*
Invitation to black tie event							*	*	*	*	*
Recognition on the donor wall								*	*	*	*
Invitation to a behind-the-scenes tour									*	*	*
Discount on rental of the museum										*	*
Invitation to president's dinner											*
Non-tax deductible portion of membership is . . .	$30	$45	$55	$85	$100	$100	$100	$100	$100	$100	$150

Source: Reproduced from the Adler Planetarium & Astronomy Museum's membership brochure.

Many museum gift shops were drab areas devoid of retail flair and stocked with a limited number of items. They were tucked in out-of-the-way locations, as if the shops somehow defiled the educational and research aims of a museum. Museum shops were typically managed by volunteers who lacked entrepreneurial and merchandising skills. Those days are gone. Today, museum gift shops are being sited near museum entrances and in other prominent locations, and they are expanding in size.

Some large museums have contracted out the management of their gift shops. Others have created distinctive inventories that have gained a following among consumers. Still others have created shops that cater to out-of-town tourists rather than local visitors. In 1997, the Smithsonian Institution's National Museum of Natural History opened a major new shop near a main entrance. The old shop was small, crowded, dark, and out of the way; the new one is large, well lighted, and impressively designed, featuring collection pieces and artwork as design elements. The new shop carries a vastly expanded inventory, and visitors have responded enthusiastically. The shop has significantly boosted the museum's revenue.

Entrepreneurs have recognized that museum gift shops constitute special market for souvenirs, novelties, gifts, art, and educational games. This has led new firms such as The Museum Company to capitalize on this market, specializing in reproductions of museum objects. Lines of items are being developed that are identified in the consumer's mind with a particular museum and its collections or particular fields of art, history, and science. Investing objects with added historical or aesthetic value can boost their price. Colonial Williamsburg, for example, has partnered with several manufacturers to produce a line of branded goods (furniture, glassware, tableware, linen, lamps, and the like), which are sold in special department store boutiques known as Williamsburg Shops. Product licensing and development has become a growing part of large museum operations. The Smithsonian Institution, with its massive collections of gems and minerals, fossils, antique automobiles, furniture, clothing, ethnographic objects, images of stars and the universe, and scientific tools, is in a strong position to license a wide range of consumer, gift, and educational products. And each product line can include high-end, intermediate, and low-end goods. Museum shops in ethnic museums have discovered strong markets for ethnic art and artifacts and objects and materials relating to cultural traditions. An example of a successful gift shop of this type is the shop in the Mexican Fine Arts Center Museum, in Chicago.

One of the first museum directors to recognize the revenue potential of museum gift shops was Thomas Hoving, director of the Metropolitan Museum of Art from 1967 to 1977. Hoving increased the amount of space in the Met's gift shop, and soon the museum carried not only souvenirs and books but also replicas of artworks, large counters of jewelry, and even clothing. The Met hired merchandising consultants to design the shop and create a special shopping ambience.

Specialists were used to determine the inventory. As the number of items carried by the Met grew, the museum established a mail-order and catalogue operation. Museum shops run by the Met, the Art Institute of Chicago, and other large museums now operate in shopping malls and airports.

The Met's pricing of items in its gift shops and catalogues follows a few basic principles. Items that are exclusive to the Met are priced on the high side because they are available only from the Met. The higher price reflects the smaller volume of sales expected and the special character of the items. Items commonly carried by several museums are priced at the level of museum-goers' expectations formed from visits to other museums and other similar stores. Items also found in department stores are priced close to the department store price. If the latter items are priced too low, merchants would complain about unfair competition. If they are priced too high, museum-goers would think them overpriced.

Another pricing principle to which most museums adhere is offering a discount to museum members, and this can considerably increase the volume of gift shop purchases. Many museum members prefer to purchase items at the museum, both because of the price discount and because of the desire to support a worthy institution.

Along with gift shop pricing, museums also have to focus on the types of merchandise carried in the shop. Museum gift shops are expected to carry items that reflect the collections in the museum. Souvenirs, gifts, novelties, books, and educational games are also typical. They should also stock items that appeal to particular types of tourists and other visitors. Merchandise can be varied to reflect the season and typical audiences at different times of the year. Museum gift shop managers can contact tourist and convention bureaus to ascertain which groups are scheduled to visit at particular times. Gift shops at large, urban museums that normally attract tourists should then plan to carry the special items that appeal to particular groups of visitors—conventioneers, tour groups, participants in political rallies—and reflect their demographics, lifestyles, and interests. The goal is to tailor merchandising to target audiences.

Today, managing a large museum gift shop is big business; it requires experience in purchasing, merchandising, and interacting with customers. Many museum gift shops are using computers to facilitate transactions and to build a customer database to stimulate further sales and store loyalty. Large museums are increasingly building off-site distribution channels, selling through stores in shopping malls, mail-order catalogues, and Web sites on the Internet. To further their development, museum stores have banded together in the Museum Store Association, headquartered in Denver, Colorado.

There are, to be sure, constraints on business development at museums because museums are typically operated as nonprofit organizations. Commercial competitors have periodically put pressure on the Internal Revenue Service (IRS) to curb the tax-exempt and charitable-giving privileges that museums enjoy.

Competitors seek to restrain museum store expansion, inventory expansion, and off-site expansion. The IRS frequently audits museum gift shops to ensure that they sell only items that are related to the museum's collections or that have educational value. Some museums voluntarily make payments in lieu of taxes on items they recognize as only marginally related to the museum or its mission, under a provision known as the Unrelated Business Income Tax (UBIT).

Despite the many requirements of running a modern gift shop, museums that still have small, drab shops that carry uninspired items are missing an opportunity for revenue generation as well as for building member and visitor loyalty.

PRICING THE RENTAL OF FACILITIES

Museums have discovered that their facilities are attractive to a variety of groups and organizations. The Lincoln Park Zoo, in Chicago, did not realize this until an enterprising consultant suggested holding a corporate dinner for one hundred people in the zoo's lion house. There, seated at candlelit tables, sat one hundred guests enjoying filet mignon as huge feline beasts pranced in their cages. Many receptions and dinners are held in the main hall of the Field Museum, in Chicago, where the diners sit among the giant remains of dinosaurs. Chicago's Shedd Aquarium hosts events where the guests dine surrounded by tanks featuring some of the world's most exquisite tropical fish.

Long before that consultant discovered the special ambience and value of dining at the Lincoln Park Zoo lion house, the great museums built in cities throughout the world had already commanded attention as grand settings and places to be seen. Today, museums regularly rent out their facilities for events. Some museums are blessed with extraordinary architecture and design (the East Building of the National Gallery of Art, in Washington, D.C., designed by I. M. Pei, is a good example). Such settings are sought after by associations and corporations willing to pay a premium price to host a social or business event. The facilities of other museums may not have world-class features but may nevertheless be remarkable for their communities. Even museums that lack unique settings may have large galleries, auditoriums, and other spaces that can be rented to outside groups. Conner Prairie, with its several hundred acres of lovely rolling fields interspersed with historic homes and villages, has in recent years specialized in renting out its spaces for corporate, business, and association picnics for groups ranging from 75 to 7,500. The museum's kitchens provide the food service, so the combined revenue generated by a picnic event is far higher than the rental fee alone would be. A large part of Colonial Williamsburg's revenues, in the neighborhood of $150 million annually, derive from the hotels and restaurants it owns, many of which are organized under a for-profit subsidiary.

A museum's costs in renting out facilities vary with the occasion. The daytime use of a lecture hall that would otherwise be empty hardly adds any cost; in fact, renting it could benefit the museum by bringing in first-time visitors. However, the evening use of a large museum space for a large party entails much more cost. Extending the museum's hours requires guard and maintenance services, as well as heating and lighting; there might also be catering and cleanup costs. In renting its facilities a museum will normally want to cover the variable costs occasioned by the event. Beyond this, to earn something for its efforts, it could establish a standard markup over the actual cost. As an alternative, it could price each event in terms of the sponsor's resources and perceived value. That is, it would make a difference to the pricing whether it was IBM, the American Heart Association, or a small corporation that wanted to sponsor a museum dinner for one hundred guests.

While recognizing the potential rental value of their facilities, museums should be careful not to rent facilities out too frequently. The hotel and restaurant industry resents this competition, especially given that museums are publicly supported and enjoy tax advantages. Low pricing of rental facilities could be viewed by competitors as a museum subsidy. The price a museum can command for facility rental depends on its distinctiveness. Museums that rent out facilities during regular visitor hours have to minimize disruptions to their operations and their core mission.

PRICING OF DONOR SUPPORT

Most museums establish a development office whose task it is to raise money from individuals, foundations, corporations, and government agencies. Government grant proposals must be drafted with a price tag attached to them. The price tag represents the estimated cost of achieving the proposed objectives and normally includes coverage of the museum's operating and fixed expenses as well.

In pricing donor support from individuals and corporations, museums usually develop tiers of prices and tiers of benefits. Wealthy and even middle-class museum supporters are often receptive to making donations and gifts beyond regular membership fees. Museum development specialists need information on target donors and donors' giving preferences. Museum leaders have to determine their marketing objectives and the benefits they are willing to offer donors. Donor benefits could include names on individual or group plaques, names as sponsors of special events or as patrons of specific museum galleries, and names on galleries for a limited period or permanently. In raising corporate donations, museum staff should be aware of the alternative cultural and educational organizations companies might choose to support. Pricing donations and gifts from individuals and companies should be informed by the principles of segmentation, positioning, and tailoring incentives to donations. (Donor marketing is discussed further in Chapter Eleven.)

SUMMARY

Museums offer a range of benefits and value (learning, recreation, sociability, experiences), each of which can command a price in the marketplace. Often a museum will overlook some of the benefits it offers or lump together disparate benefits that should be treated separately. Museums in the past were often free to the public, and museums were reluctant to put a price on the goods and services they offered. Today, museums that are compelled to raise revenues in the marketplace to supplement or replace subsidies and public-sector support have to address questions of revenue-raising objectives, the variety of ways in which to raise revenues, the costs involved, and the prices to charge for various revenue streams (museum admission, special exhibitions and events, sales in gift shops, rental of facilities, and so on). Pricing strategies should reflect the ideas of segmenting and targeting, pricing in relation to competitors, and linking prices to specific benefits and incentives. Most museums operate as nonprofit organizations and are subject to tax, charity, and other regulatory rules. Though they may be in a position to generate considerable revenue and may need as much revenue as they can raise, museums also have to consider their objectives carefully and often have to balance revenue-raising and pricing objectives with their educational and public service missions.

O

MODEL MUSEUM PRACTICE

Business Development at the
Genesee Country Village & Museums

"Museums that don't receive public-sector funding and that charge admission fees learn quickly how to measure the success of their performance," says Douglass McDonald, chief executive officer at the Genesee Country Village & Museums (GCVM), in Mumford, New York (interviewed Jan. 24, 1997, and Mar. 11, 1997). "Museums that depend on private and earned income discover what their visitors and supporters value and what they regard as program quality. This keeps us competitive and accountable."

The Genesee Country Village & Museums is situated on four hundred acres of land in upstate New York and has fifty-seven historic structures built between 1795 and 1880—making it the third largest collection of historic buildings on a museum site in the United States. GCVM has a collection of 25,000 objects, historic buildings, an art gallery, a nature center, several miles of nature trails, restaurants and shops. Its season is limited to the period between mid-May and mid-October, owing to the harsh winters. It opens for a few weeks before Christmas, a week at Halloween, and for three weeks in April during the weekdays for school tours.

GCVM faces the same need to increase earned revenue as other museums, and it has the added challenge of having to raise that revenue during roughly six months to support year-round planning and development along with forty full-time year-round staff and two hundred seasonal staff. Business development practices at this museum illustrate the opportunities and obstacles other museums face in building earned income.

GCVM's earned income accounts for a significant portion of the museum's total revenues: 18 percent from retail sales; 16 percent from programming revenue (special events, continuing education classes, a lecture series, nature programs, day camp fees); 17 percent from admission fees; and 49 percent from memberships, donor support (individual, corporate, foundation), and endowment. The museum has 150,000 visitors a year, drawing 33 percent from the nearby city of Rochester, 30 percent from the city of Buffalo, and 36 percent from tourism.

GCVM's ability to raise private and earned-income revenue depends on two critical factors: creating new experiences and programs that visitors value, without sacrificing existing quality; and controlling costs. "Museums that lack adequate accounting practices," McDonald observes, "are not able to determine which of their programs are earning net revenue and which are too costly to operate. The key is for every museum department and program to report both the direct and indirect costs involved in generating its revenue and the ratio of cost to income."

GCVM's management examines carefully the revenue streams of each of the programs and whether these have sufficient margins. Each program is subject to a profit-and-loss analysis that includes the revenue margin per participant. If a program projects a surplus, it is likely to receive additional funds to invest in development. Programs that project losses, conversely, are likely to find their spending levels reduced. This accounting practice enables the museum to make comparisons across program areas. Without such strict accounting a museum will find that hidden costs are exerting financial pressures on the museum as a whole and draining strong programs while rewarding weak ones. Further, it is important for any organization, whether a business or a nonprofit, to relate program performance to staff performance and to use incentives to make improvements. GCVM's CEO points out that sound accounting practices in museums depend on the ability to measure visitation levels and program usage.

Between 1990 and 1996, GCVM's earned-income revenue doubled (from $74,000 to $150,000). Retail sales in the shops and restaurants showed modest increases, but income derived from program fees doubled. New programs include a day camp, continuing education (for example, classes in hearth cooking and in horticulture), nature education activities, and special holiday and seasonal events.

GCVM's special events account for a large part of its earned income. Six special event programs are held annually that attract twenty-three thousand participants. They include a Christmas yuletide festival, an agricultural fair and a fall festival, and an Independence Day celebration (which features a nineteenth-century parade, readings, and orations). One of the most popular events each summer is the Civil War Battle Reenactment, which draws eight thousand people over a weekend. The special event programs have multiple benefits for the museum. Special celebratory events build a sense of community and community support. A large portion of the audiences drawn to the special events are newcomers, so the events help build visitorship and membership. Events like the Civil War Battle Reenactment spur local media attention, build the museum image, and draw audiences.

One further benefit of the special events has not gone unnoticed by museum management: the greater the number of visitors entering the gate, the higher the level of shop and restaurant sales. Average admission fee revenue on a regular July weekend, without a special event, is approximately $6,000; the Civil War Battle Reenactment weekend generates on the average $34,000; the July Fourth weekend celebration, $18,000. The museum is exploring other special events to capture the multiplier effect that seasonal events represent.

GCVM is planning to expand the museum's rental fee income. It is negotiating with business firms to rent the museum facilities for corporate retreats and business and social events. The museum's vast and attractive acreage, along with its restaurants and catering capabilities, make it an attractive site for sponsored events. Two constraints on rental events are that they compete with regular visitors and programming and that the museum is only open roughly half the year.

Not all of GCVM's earned-income programs are working as successfully. Gift shop revenue has remained flat in recent years, which has led management to examine the age and quality of its inventory and redouble efforts to improve the shop's merchandise and services. Less expensive items, overall, sell best. GCVM's shops are also limited by a lack of computerized data on purchases and purchasers. One earned-income source the museum is not currently pursuing is product licensing and development. Although the historic buildings contain furniture and interior designs that can be used as product designs, management does not think the museum has yet achieved a high enough recognition level to support product development. At the same time, GCVM is tackling image and visibility with a program to generate media stories and advertisements regionally and nationally.

As the museum's earned-income sources are developed further, another area of business analysis likely to gain prominence is pricing. GCVM charges adults a $10 admission fee, and it prices a family membership at $75. The museum expanded its membership to 2,300 people in 1996. Members who use the museum regularly have found that purchasing a membership is less costly than paying admission fees for each visit. According to McDonald, local residents think the museum prices are high, but tourists think the prices are reasonable. Some museum staff want to experiment with pricing; for example, raising the admission price to $12 and giving $2 coupons to residents, which in effect would maintain the existing $10 fee. Staff reasoning is that having a coupon in hand will create an added incentive for local people to make visits to the museum. Coupons also can be structured around off-peak visitation periods. An alternative also under discussion is to make coupons available that link museum visits to discounts on purchases in the shops. GCVM offers, in any case, discounted prices for senior citizens and young people.

The Genesee Country Village & Museums is an example of a museum organization that works hard at building support in the short term as well as the long term and at balancing its public service mission with the needs of raising self-support. A large corporation in nearby Rochester asked its employees about the extent to which they participate in local museums. The survey revealed the largest number of employees participated in GCVM programs (although it is not the largest museum in the area), and employees reported high levels of satisfaction. These employees furthermore indicated that GCVM is a significant contributor to their quality of life. The survey findings influenced the corporation to boost its donations to the museum. GCVM has responded to corporate goodwill by organizing *corporate appreciation days*, during which employees of sponsoring corporations are invited to the museum free of charge.

CHAPTER ELEVEN

Attracting Resources

Building Member, Volunteer, and Donor Support

*. . . [T]here is the role of the private donor, that essential wellspring
of generosity without which most museums would stop growing
(and many would not survive). . . . Frankly, the people we do
reach are often the privileged. . . . To a striking degree, then,
we have always been and still are by and for the privileged.*
—Franklin W. Robinson

Franklin Robinson, director of the Herbert F. Johnson Museum of Art at Cornell University, candidly observes that art museums, historically, paid a lot of attention to their art patrons and supporters. In recent years, however, art museums have had to square their preoccupation with patrons with the demands made on them by the public and museum visitors, demands for orientation and information that require different services. Museums and other nonprofit organizations continually confront the challenge of attracting resources. This chapter will focus on the efforts of museums to attract and sustain supporters and the involvement of *members, volunteers,* and *donors.*

ATTRACTING AND DEVELOPING MEMBERS

Many museums have created membership programs as a way of building long-term relationships with visitors and members of the community and as a critical means for raising funds. Museums would like to convert visitors into members because members have a more permanent link to the museum and their support can be channeled and regularized. Museums would also like every existing member to become more active. In practice, only a small percentage of the membership of any organization shows a high level of enthusiasm and involvement.

Members typically fall into three groups: *high actives,* who contribute most of the time, money, and energy to the museum; *moderate actives,* who participate frequently but who do not get highly involved; and *inactives,* who participate infrequently but maintain their memberships. It is useful to track a museum's proportion of inactives, moderate actives, and high actives. A high or growing number of inactives is a sign that the museum is not creating high value for these members. The museum should survey the three groups to find out what facets of museum membership are satisfying and dissatisfying. By monitoring attitudes, the museum can take steps to improve members' satisfaction.

Membership organizations typically face such problems as too few members overall, a poor mix of members, too many inactive members, or too many non-renewing members. *Membership development* is the general name given to the task of creating a healthy membership program. Here we examine the four main tasks in membership development: defining membership, attracting members, motivating members, and retaining members.

Defining Membership

A museum's first task is to define the different levels of membership and their corresponding benefit packages. Table 11.1 shows the range of benefits that museums can offer their members in such categories as admissions, discounts, conveniences, events and programs, and gifts. A museum is likely to offer a varying mix of benefits, with upper-category members receiving a fuller range than lower-category members (see Table 10.1 for an example of membership categories).

Membership benefits and levels can be better understood in the context of membership programs at particular museums. Chicago's Museum of Science & Industry offered in the mid-1990s three basic membership categories: an individual membership at $45, a family membership at $60, and a lifetime single-payment membership at $1,500. Yet the museum provides a wide range of benefits covering each category. Special features of membership include free tickets to the museum's Omnimax theater (along with a ticket reservation service) as well as free general admission, free admission to more than one hundred other U.S. science museums, and use of a members' lounge for relaxing and meeting other members. The Maryland Science Center had six membership programs in the mid-1990s—family (two adults and children between the ages of four and seventeen) ($57); individual ($35) or senior individual ($30), couple ($50) or senior couple ($42), sustaining ($90), contributing ($150), and patron ($500). The museum also had a special category for honors students at local schools, who were active during the summer months. The museum invites the patrons to have lunch with the museum's executive director and offers a variety of special events. The membership program at the National Zoological Park, in Washington, D.C., is managed by an affiliated organization, the Friends of the National Zoo (Fonz). Fonz members typically pay a fee of $45 and receive discounted prices for children's and adult courses and children's summer camps; they are also invited to participate in social events, special evenings at

Table 11.1. Varieties of Membership Benefits, by Category.

Free admissions
- Admissions to museums, special exhibits, Omnimax theaters
- Reciprocal admissions to other museums

Discounts
- 10 to 20 percent discount in shops and restaurants
- Discounts at special events, continuing education classes, lectures, concerts, special exhibit tours, travel tours, seminars
- Discounts on photographic, photocopy, and other museum services
- Discounts on participation in other cultural activities, cultural organizations, and sometimes wider dining, recreational, and hospitality services in the area

Conveniences
- Free parking
- Free coat room services
- Access to members' lounge
- Free children's strollers
- Reservation booking for special exhibits and no waiting-line guarantee
- Access to museum library (visitors require appointments)

Social events
- Special exhibit preview and opening-night events
- Members' nights
- Members' camp-in for families with young children
- Holiday events
- Auctions
- Monthly singles' or young professionals' evening gatherings
- Dinner with museum director
- Membership council or board meetings

Education
- Continuing education classes, lectures, workshops
- Special exhibit tours
- Meetings with curators
- Programs for collectors
- Travel and study tours

Information
- Monthly or quarterly newsletters or magazines
- Special membership mailings
- Advance notices on exhibits and programs
- Wall calendars

Recognition
- Recognition in the museum's annual report, newsletter, and special recognition brochures
- Recognition on wall panels at museum main entrance
- Recognition ceremonies

Gifts
- Tote bags for new members
- Plastic membership cards
- Raffle prizes
- Guest passes

the zoo, members-only behind-the-scenes tours, and nature- and conservation-oriented tours in the United States and abroad.

Attracting Members

Most museums open their membership to anyone who wants to join. A museum can recruit new members in two basic ways. The first is *a mass marketing* approach, in which membership recruitment brochures are mailed or distributed widely. The second is a *segmenting and targeting* approach, in which the museum solicits memberships from specific groups.

In any given community, the majority of residents are not disposed to join a museum's membership. For this reason, the targeted approach is more appropriate. The museum has to identify a range of prospects, from those who show the most interest and can afford the annual membership fee to those less likely to be interested and able to pay. Museums can purchase lists of people who have joined other cultural organizations or who have attributes such as interest in cultural activities. It can then direct appropriate communications to the best prospects. The best source of members is current visitors and active participants in museum programs. Some museums have developed marketing databases that identify groups who use museum shops and restaurants; others use questionnaires and surveys to ascertain who the frequent visitors and strong prospects are.

A museum should interview a sample of prospects to ascertain their reasons for joining or not joining. Usually the nonjoiners fall into three groups: *resisters, indifferents,* and *un-informs.* Resisters are opposed to joining a museum. Among the reasons they give are these: "I disagree with the museum's policies"; "I don't find it a pleasant place"; "I don't think the staff are friendly." The museum can try to answer these objections, but if resisters' views have any basis in truth, the museum will gain little by pursuing this group. Indifferents do not see much benefit to joining or perceive the cost of joining to outweigh the benefit. They say, "The membership fee is too high," or, "I don't have time to spend at the museum." This group includes *free riders,* those who obtain the benefits of the museum without becoming members. The best approach to indifferents is to make the benefits of museum membership more vivid and attractive. Un-informs know little about the museum. They typically say, "I guess I don't know the museum," or, "I need more information." The best approach to the un-informs is to provide appealing information to stimulate their interest.

Potential members differ in what might interest them in the museum. Some may be interested in the educational programs; others in the interpersonal and social opportunities. Zoological parks, for example, can appeal to potential members with interests in conservation, the natural world, environmental protection, and saving endangered species. History museums can attract people to whom history and heritage are important elements of community life. Museums have to probe the values, benefits, and satisfactions potential members seek.

Museums in the 1980s and 1990s have endeavored to broaden their appeal, attract members of underserved groups, and at the same time deepen their community support. Some museums focus their recruitment effort among older adults, who represent a growing segment of the population. They offer programs such as studio arts and continuing education courses as well as group experiences that include travel and social events. Other museums focus on young adults with children, offering them expanded educational programs, workshops and camps, and interactive and performance events for children and their parents. Urban art museums have focused their recruitment efforts on the young adult and young professional segments of the population. These groups represent a large proportion of urban and central-city populations. They have relatively high levels of disposable income and tend to be single and to be active socially and recreationally. Museums have recognized that young adults place a premium on settings and situations that offer group experiences and allow them to meet others like themselves. Young professionals have for years been the marketing targets of bars, restaurants, and fitness centers; museums have discovered that they too have advantages to offer this group: elegant settings, ample space for parties, stimulating visual sights, status. Museum managers are also acknowledging that delight in viewing exhibitions is compatible with the social pleasures of parties and events. The Corcoran Gallery of Art, in Washington, D.C., for example, has been highly successful at building membership and visitorship with a focus on young adults. The Memorial Art Gallery, in Rochester, New York, has also been very successful in organizing events for young professionals and singles as a way to combat a decline in membership and to build new support among young prospects. A friends group of young adults, known as the Averell Council, has taken on the responsibility of providing support for museum programs, recruiting new members, and sponsoring social and educational activities. The council raises some $125,000 a year for important museum programs. In the first years of operation, the monthly First Friday social events have attracted hundreds of participants and have generated more than 10 percent of the museum's membership each year.

Museums in urban centers are also giving attention to building membership among ethnic and cultural groups that have not been involved in the past. The Los Angeles County Museum of Art, for example, found in 1990 that only approximately 4 percent of the museum's membership base of ninety thousand was Latino. Yet in the Los Angeles metropolitan area, an estimated 14.3 percent of households earning $60,000 or more were of Latino origin. Seeking to improve its standing with this segment of the community, the museum organized a major exhibition, *Mexico: Splendors of 30 Centuries.* It also organized a substantial marketing campaign that led to a successful outcome: during the exhibition an additional 5,800 people of Latino background became members, bringing the Latino proportion of total membership to nearly 6 percent.

Motivating Members

Douglass McDonald, CEO at the Genesee Country Village & Museum, in Mumford, New York, observes that the members of his museum are very conscious of the benefits they enjoy as members. A large number of the museum's active visitors have been motivated to enroll as members because they perceive it to be less costly than paying admission fees to events they frequently attend. (The Genesee Museum is discussed in depth in the Model Museum Practice at the end of Chapter Ten.)

Museums have a strong interest in motivating their members. The Art Institute of Chicago established a membership group of young professionals and young single people, known as the Evening Associates, that has become a major player in raising funds and hosting events. Leaders are responsible for recruiting members and raising funding support. The Minneapolis Institute of Arts (MIA) organized in the early 1990s two higher-end membership groups (Collectors and Connoisseurs) for supporters who sought more active engagement in museum acquisitions and collections. Out of these resulted a series of small-scale membership groups, known as *curatorial councils,* consisting of patrons who are major art collectors and who are inclined to support the museum in significant ways. The councils cover the collections areas of distinction at the museum. Curatorial council members participate in lectures, social events, and travel. They advise curators on acquisitions and provide support for acquisitions. The museum also sponsors monthly Expertise Clinics at which curators examine objects brought in by members and offer advice on age, condition, significance, and authenticity.

Retaining Members

The ultimate indicator of a failure to satisfy members is a high or growing non-renewal rate. Renewal rates are an annual market test, in which each member votes on whether the "product" is worth the cost or involvement. Museums invest a great deal of energy in encouraging renewals. Therefore museum staff need to determine the main reasons why members do not renew. A health club once discovered that four reasons accounted for 80 percent of its membership dropout: move to a new community, membership switch to another organization, dissatisfaction with the facilities and conditions, and light use or nonuse of facilities and services. An organization cannot prevent members from leaving a community, but clearly it can do something about the condition of its facilities and the quality of its programs.

Membership development and maintenance involve considerable cost. Staff have to monitor membership rolls continually to maintain the existing membership. Members require a lot of information and printed materials like newsletters. Free admission benefits represent revenue losses. Servicing a membership involves staff resources. For all these reasons, museums are well advised to monitor membership program costs and the revenues they generate (Labyak, 1995).

Yet membership programs can yield significant benefits and advantages. They build community support. A museum with a large number of influential members has an easier time winning support from local and regional governments. Members contribute fees, make extensive use of gift shops and restaurants, and are potential contributors to annual giving, capital campaign, and planned gift programs. There is always an opportunity to influence members in low-end categories to increase their membership support and join high-end groups. There is also the possibility of converting a member into a volunteer who contributes time, service, and expertise to a museum. The Art Institute of Chicago, with 150,000 members in the mid-1990s, one of the largest membership programs in the country, has had many long-time museum members assume active and full-time roles as volunteers. Many of these later contribute collections and gifts to the museum or designate the museum a beneficiary in their wills. In periods of economic downturn and fiscal stress, members are also a group to turn to for immediate and urgent support. The advantages are well worth the costs of running an active membership program.

ATTRACTING AND DEVELOPING VOLUNTEERS

The United States throughout its history has depended on volunteerism, especially at the community level. In 1991, some 94.2 million Americans, or 51.1 percent of adults eighteen years of age or older, reported volunteering an average of 4.7 hours per week. That volunteer time amounted to 20.5 billion hours. Volunteers at nonprofit organizations contributed the equivalent work of nine million employees, with an estimated value of $176 billion (Kotler and Andreasen, 1996, p. 275). Many nonprofit organizations rely heavily on volunteers to build community goodwill, provide support services to staff and clients, and reduce organization expenses. In addition, volunteers have the satisfaction of contributing to a worthy organization.

Museums make considerable use of volunteers to operate information desks; serve as docents; work in gift shops; support curators and researchers; staff public affairs, education, and development units; and even work in security roles. Some small U.S. museums are managed entirely by volunteers. The Smithsonian Institution in 1994 had 5,300 people serving as volunteers in its museums and research institutes, and they contributed an estimated 574,800 hours of service. That same year the Smithsonian employed some 7,000 staff and spent over $400 million for their salaries and benefits (Conaway, 1995, p. 28). By the end of the 1980s, U.S. museums had attracted the services of 377,000 volunteers, more than 2.5 times the size of the total paid staff. Most volunteers work part time, although nearly 10 percent work thirty-five hours or more per week (American Association of Museums, 1994, p. 81). Clearly, museums would be far worse off if they had to forgo volunteer support.

Fortunately, in both urban and rural areas, museums can find adults and retired persons with education and skills that support museum programs and operations. Museum volunteers are likely to be former teachers, scientists, accountants, lawyers, and other professionals. Yet some museum managers believe that competent paid staff are ultimately more desirable than unpaid volunteers. Museums recognize that although volunteers seem to be "cost-free," there are costs involved in recruiting, training, and supporting volunteers. Museums with large volunteer groups count on volunteers' reliability; their failure to show up at information booths, for example, can cause disruptions. Museums have to evaluate volunteers' performance to ensure that volunteers in important front-line roles are serving visitors well.

The proper way to attract and motivate volunteers is to treat them as a distinct market segment, with particular needs and expectations. Years ago, volunteers sought mainly the gratification of helping other people. Today increasing numbers of volunteers are motivated by a desire for personal benefits as well. They may seek skills or status through their involvement in a museum. They may value the opportunity to be invited to special events. They may seek interpersonal and social opportunities.

Museums should have a systematic procedure for attracting volunteers. The normal method is to ask current volunteers to nominate friends and associates. If this method produces too few new volunteers, museums can advertise. To be sure, not all volunteers are acceptable or can be assigned to the activities they want to perform. Volunteer training should cover not only the specific tasks to which volunteers are assigned but also knowledge of museum organization and its history and development. Many volunteers will also need training in communication techniques, information retrieval, working with computers, and responding to visitors who have diverse learning and communication styles.

In return, museums have to give their volunteers recognition and challenge. Recognition can take the form of acknowledgment in a museum's newsletter or magazine, at annual recognition and awards receptions, and in personal letters of appreciation from management. Volunteers also appreciate the training they receive, and it can be a factor in their willingness to continue to volunteer. Volunteers also appreciate benefits that may be attached to their roles. The Field Museum offers its nearly four hundred volunteers an array of benefits, including discounts in the restaurants and shops, discounts on continuing education courses, insurance coverage while working on the museum premises, free or discounted parking, opportunities to assist on field trips and travel tours, and invitations to volunteer recognition dinners.

Retaining volunteers presents a challenge. Volunteers are sensitive to slights from management and staff, such as being ordered around or being asked to work extra hours. Supervisors have to be sensitive to the needs and feelings of volunteers; management and staff should be friendly, show appreciation, and be open to volunteers' comments, suggestions, and complaints. Volunteer managers need to develop a motivating benefit package for volunteers, work hard to retain them, and not take their services for granted.

ATTRACTING AND MOTIVATING DONORS

A major resource challenge for museums is to attract money and other material resources needed to carry on their activities. This goes by various names: fundraising, development, donor marketing. The art of *fundraising* has passed through several stages of evolution. Its earliest form amounted to *begging:* institutions would implore fortunate people for money and donated materials. The next stage consisted of *collections:* organizations (churches, for example) gathered annual and special contributions from a willing and defined group of members and supporters. Collections has the advantage of being done on a regular basis. In recent times, *campaigning* has emerged as a concept: an organization appoints a specific person or staff to solicit money from various sources by means of a planned fundraising campaign, such as an endowment campaign or a capital campaign to cover infrastructure costs. Most recently, fundraising has been repositioned as *development:* a museum systematically builds up various classes of loyal donors who give consistently and who receive benefits in the process.

As fundraising organizations, museums typically pass through three stages in their thinking about fundraising: the *product stage,* the *sales stage,* and the *marketing stage.* In the product stage, the prevailing idea is, "We are a worthwhile institution; people ought to support us." The art collection or the museum facility itself is regarded as the principal value, rather than visitors, the general public, or the outcomes of the museum's programs. Money is raised primarily by the founders or board members through an "old-boy network," and a few loyal donors supply most of the funds. The museum relies on volunteers to raise additional funds.

In the sales stage, the prevailing idea is, "There are a lot of people out there who might give us money, and we must find them." The museum appoints a development director who hires a staff. The staff raises money from all possible sources, sometimes with a hard-sell approach. In this stage, funds are often raised helter-skelter; long-term development is subordinated to short-term opportunities, and the museum improvises and relies on external circumstances. Further, the development office has little influence over museum policies and strategies because its job is to raise money, not help develop offerings or museum strategy. A majority of museums operate in this stage.

In the marketing stage, the prevailing idea is, "We have to analyze our position in the marketplace, concentrate on different donor sources whose interests parallel the museum's, and design a continuous solicitation program that supplies appropriate satisfactions to each donor group." This approach involves carefully segmenting the donor markets, measuring the giving potential of each market, using research and communications to develop each market, and developing a plan and budget for each market, based on its potential. A distinctive feature of this approach is generating offerings and benefits that appeal to prospective donors. This goes beyond depending on external circumstances not under the organization's control. A small but growing number of large museums have advanced to this stage.

Analyzing Donor Markets

Museums can distinguish four major donor markets: *individual givers, foundations, corporations,* and *governments.* Donor markets are separate from the revenues museums derive from earned-income sources, such as admission fees, royalties, publications, program fees, fees from traveling exhibitions, gift shop sales, food services, parking, and facility rental. The American Association of Museums (1994, pp. 83–89) estimates, on the basis of late 1980s data, that U.S. museums derived their total operational income as follows: 39.2 percent from government and public-sector sources; 30.4 percent from earned-income sources; 18.9 percent from private sources including individual, corporate, and foundation giving; and 11.5 percent from endowment and investment income. Small museums, however, are generally not recipients of public-sector funds and tend to be financially dependent on community support, membership, gifts, and earned income.

Individual Giving

Individuals are the major source of charitable giving. In 1992, individual giving accounted for 81 percent of the total in charitable money, or $102.55 billion. The remainder came from bequests ($8.54 billion), foundations ($9.21 billion), and corporations ($5.92 billion). That same year, religious organizations raised the highest proportion of charitable money ($57.15 billion, or 45.3 percent), followed by educational institutions ($15.07 billion), human service organizations ($12.47 billion), health-related organizations ($10.83 billion), and arts and cultural organizations, including museums ($9.57 billion). Environmental and wildlife organizations that year raised $3.19 billion and international affairs organizations $1.86 billion (Independent Sector, 1992).

Almost everyone in the nation contributes money to one or more organizations each year, the amount varying with the giver's income, age, education, sex, ethnic and racial background, and other characteristics. High-income people, people in their middle years, and highly educated people, contribute a disproportionately large amount. At the same time, giving levels vary considerably within each group. In relation to their income, some wealthy individuals give little and some low-income individuals give a great deal. Among affluent professionals, for example, physicians tend to give less than lawyers.

Why do individuals give to charitable causes? The best working hypothesis is that individuals *give* in order to *get* something back. Donations generally should not be viewed as a transfer but as a transaction. The question then arises, What does the donor expect to derive in terms of satisfaction, advantages, and benefits? Let us look at some of the motives underlying individuals' giving behavior.

- The *self-esteem giver* gains self-esteem and boosts self-image through giving.

- The *recognition giver* gains social status and enhances prestige and often has a strong need to belong.

- The *habit giver* gives out of a habit of giving and also does not want to be embarrassed by being identified as a nongiver.

- The *nuisance giver* gives to get rid of a gift solicitor and to avoid further solicitations.

- The *required giver* gives in the workplace due to pressure from peers to donate.

- The *people-to-people giver* gives out of a sense of solidarity with other people and often gives to help out specific individuals.

- The *ethical giver* feels a moral, often a religious, obligation to contribute to the well-being of other people and, by extension, institutions.

Is there such a thing as giving without expecting to get something in return? In many cases, charitable activity can be viewed as a mixture of self-interested and public-regarding behaviors, in varying combinations. Yet most givers do have expectations of some kind. They expect the recipient organization to use the money efficiently. They often expect a show of gratitude from the fundraiser. Even anonymous givers receive something in return: a private feeling of self-worth for undertaking a meritorious action.

Giving motives are clues for fundraisers. Harold Seymour (1966) suggested that in many mass donor markets, one-third of the givers are *responsible* and donate without being solicited, one-third are *responsive* and donate when asked, and one-third react to *compulsion* and pressure. Each of these groups can be differentiated further into specific motive segments. For example, one group might give in response to a museum out of pride, yet another might respond to a competitive appeal ("let's catch up to the other museum"). Too many museums ask people to give because the museum is needy rather than to support a promising program or activity. The latter is more effective. People respond to what they sense as the relevance, importance, and urgency of a giving opportunity. Seymour argues that the case for giving has to catch the eye, warm the heart, and stir the imagination.

Fundraisers differentiate between small, medium, and large donors. Many fundraisers prefer to concentrate most of their effort on large potential donors, feeling that attracting a few large gifts produces more funds than many small gifts. Fundraisers use a five-step approach to the large potential donor:

Identification → Introduction → Cultivation → Solicitation → Appreciation

Fundraisers first *identify* wealthy individuals who could conceivably have a strong interest in the museum. Then they arrange for an *introduction*. Next, they *cultivate* the potential donor's interest without asking for any money. By asking too early, they may get less than is possible. Eventually, they undertake *solicitation*. After receiving the donation, they express *appreciation*.

Large individual gift fundraising is most effective when the museum has developed a wish list of exciting projects that it can show to prospective donors. Large art museums, for example, classify their wished-for gifts in several financial sizes, ranging from the purchase of a small work of art for, say, under $10,000 to the purchase of a masterpiece costing millions. The list might also include renovating a particular gallery, improving the library, adding a wing to the building, and so on. One of the most powerful appeals is to offer to identify donors by name as supporters of a gallery, wing, theater, or other museum facility.

Museums also organize fundraising campaigns that can last for several months and that aim to raise funds for a variety of purposes. A *capital campaign* seeks to raise funds for building additions, infrastructure modernization such as lighting, heating, and air-conditioning, and other needed investments in physical plant and equipment. An *endowment campaign* seeks to raise funds for a museum's endowment, capital, and long-term financial stability, funds that can be used both for long- and short-term needs. Endowment campaigns finance programs and services rather than physical plant and equipment and operating costs. Museums also run *annual fundraising drives,* in which funds are raised for specific and special needs or perhaps for critical and emergency needs. Often museum members and patrons are asked to contribute to annual fundraising drives in addition to paying their annual membership dues.

Fundraisers can facilitate giving by accepting gifts in all forms: membership fees; cash donations in the form of annual or unrestricted giving; cash donations in the form of restricted giving, earmarked for particular programs and uses; in-kind services such as gifts of computers and gifts of business development and marketing expertise; gifts of collections, stock, and other assets; matching gifts;

gifts for sponsoring special events; and deferred gifts and bequests. Many museums have worked up a variety of gift plans that can be tailored to the needs of individuals ranging from middle-class members to wealthy donors. A major source of giving is a museum's board of trustees. In some museums, board members are asked to contribute a fixed amount each year or are expected to provide occasional gifts. However, museums are also coming to recognize the crucial expertise and services board members can provide in the areas of marketing, accounting, business development, and management. Accordingly, museums are recruiting board members not simply for their monetary contributions but equally for the in-kind contributions they can render. (The Model Museum Practice at the end of this chapter illustrates the forms of member and donor marketing used at the Art Institute of Chicago.)

Foundation Giving

Currently, there are over sixty-five thousand foundations in the United States, all set up to contribute money to worthwhile causes. They fall into the following groups:

Family foundations. Set up by wealthy individuals to support a limited number of activities of interest, family foundations typically do not have permanent officers or full-time staff members. Decisions tend to be made by family members or counsel.

General foundations. Set up to support a wide range of causes and usually run by professional staff, general foundations range from extremely large organizations that give to many different recipients, such as the Ford and Rockefeller Foundations, to organizations that focus their money in specialized areas, such as health (Robert Wood Johnson Foundation), education (Carnegie Endowment), or the arts (Pew Charitable Trusts, Lila Wallace–Reader's Digest Fund).

Corporate foundations. Set up by business corporations, these foundations may donate up to 5 percent of a corporation's adjusted gross income.

Community foundations. Set up by groups of small foundations in particular geographical areas, community foundations often pool small foundation funds for maximum impact and focus their activities on specific towns, cities, and metropolitan regions.

Fundraisers must be skilled at identifying the foundations most likely to support a given project or museum. Fortunately, there are many resources for researching foundations and their giving patterns. The best single source is the Foundation Center, a nonprofit organization with research centers in New York City, Washington, D.C., and Chicago, which serves as an information clearinghouse. In addition, many libraries carry materials describing foundations, such as the *Foundation Grants Index,* the *Foundation Directory, Foundation News,* and *Fund Raising Management.* The key concept in identifying likely foundation givers is *matching.* A museum should search for foundations matched to its interests and scale of operation. A small museum may send a proposal to the Ford Foundation; however, the Ford Foundation accepts about one out of every one hundred proposals and may be less disposed toward helping a small museum requesting a small grant. The small museum should instead target local, regional, or specialized foundations. Corporate foundations often target their giving to communities in which their headquarters, manufacturing, and distribution facilities are located. Corporate foundations can also be responsive to organizations that offer important services to their employees, and museums do play that role in raising the quality of life in communities.

After identifying a few likely foundations, a museum should determine each foundation's level of interest before investing a lot of time in grant preparation. Most foundations respond to letters of inquiry, telephone calls, or personal visits. The foundation officer may be very encouraging or discouraging. If the former, the museum can then invest time in preparing a strong proposal.

Writing successful grant proposals has become a special art, with many guides currently available to help the grant seeker (see Flanagan, 1991; Edles, 1993; Panas, 1984). Grant proposals should include

1. A *cover letter*, describing the background and nature of the proposal

2. The *proposal*, describing the project, its uniqueness, and its importance and value

3. The *budget* for the project (the price tag normally includes the estimated cost of achieving the grant proposal objective and some coverage of the museum's operating and fixed expenses as well)

4. The *personnel* working on the project and their credentials

Grant proposals should be brief, well organized, and readable. The grant writer should know the *buying criteria* that the target foundation uses to select among the many proposals it receives. Many foundations describe their criteria in their annual reports. Criteria may also be learned by talking to knowledgeable people or inferred from recent proposals the foundation funded. Here are some of the most common criteria foundations use when making grants:

- The importance and quality of the project, including the number of people who would benefit from it

- The organization's neediness and worthwhileness

- The organization's ability to use the funds effectively and efficiently

- The importance of satisfying the individuals who are making the proposal

- The degree of benefit the foundation will derive from supporting the proposal

Understanding the relative importance of each criterion can also help the museum select the proposal features to emphasize. For example, if a foundation is highly influenced by who presents the proposal, the museum should send its highest ranking officials. However, if the foundation attaches the most importance to the number of people who would benefit from the proposal, the museum should try to specify the impact its proposal will have and emphasize statistics and other quantifiable measures of impact.

Museums generally try to cultivate a handful of appropriate foundations in advance of making specific proposals, a technique referred to as *relationship marketing,* or *building bridges.* The museum's development officer arranges for various curators to meet their foundation counterparts. Then, when the curator has a proposal to submit, he or she knows to whom to present it. Furthermore, the foundation is more likely to be favorably disposed toward a museum with which it has a long-standing relationship. Knowing foundation staff also enables fundraisers to do a better job of tracking the proposal's progress.

As public-sector funding has declined, foundations have been under increasing pressure to support museums and other cultural and educational organizations. Yet these expectations have led to foundation uncertainty. A large portion of foundation support in recent years has been tied to matching or supplementary grants from federal, state, and local public-sector agencies. The decline in these sources can jeopardize foundation-giving activities. Moreover, even under the best of circumstances, foundation-giving levels are limited, and the scope of grants tends to be highly specific and defined ("Hard Money," 1995).

Corporate Giving

Business organizations represent another distinct source of support for museums. Corporations have been supportive of such causes as higher education, health services, civic and community causes, cultural organizations, and social services. In 1992, U.S. businesses contributed $5.92 billion of the $126.22 billion received in total charity, though this amounted to less than 1 percent of businesses' pre-tax income and thus less than the allowable limits on corporate giving. Since 1992, however, corporate giving has increased—to $8.5 billion in 1996, according to the *Chronicle of Philanthropy* (June 12, 1997)—but considerable potential still exists. In terms of the major forms of giving to arts and humanities organizations, corporate giving is lagging. Based on 1994 data, charitable contributions to the arts and humanities in the United States came from these sources: corporations (7 percent), foundations (13 percent), and individuals (80 percent) (President's Committee on the Arts and the Humanities, 1997, pp. 18–21).

Corporate giving undergoes fluctuations that mirror business conditions. There has been a trend among some corporate givers to move from support of cultural organizations to support of local-community social and urban services and human resources. Another factor in the 1990s is the shift in corporate attitudes from philanthropic giving to giving as a strategic investment. Businesses are looking to support organizations to which contributing can yield financial or marketing returns (Jahnke, 1993, p. 51).

Nevertheless, today's museum leaders have recognized that corporate sponsorships and partnerships are a vital means of support, as costs increase and government funding declines. The experience of the secretary of the Smithsonian Institution, I. Michael Heyman (1996), is instructive. Heyman reflected on the choices and decisions he had to make to support the Smithsonian's traveling 150th anniversary exhibition.

> I had to address the problem of costs . . . [and how to] expand our usefulness to the American people in a time of reduced budgets and rising costs. . . . So I approved a strategy that breaks new ground . . . the inauguration of a corporate partnership program, akin to that which provides support for the Olympics and similar events. In the last few years of economic reordering and political transformation the very conditions under which we and our society operate have changed. For the Smithsonian, public funding is still available to support our core activities—in that, we are luckier than most; but even the optimists among us know that we face a future of fewer available public resources. If we find funds nowhere else, we are doomed, at best, to a static future and, at worst, to one of continuing erosion. Where then to turn? Donations by individuals will always be crucial. . . . We in the non-profit world [also] find ourselves turning to corporate support more and more as one vital potential source.

In fact, corporate support of museums extends back before World War II, when leading corporations (Westinghouse, General Electric, Bell Telephone, Union Carbide, and International Harvester, among others) sponsored exhibitions and entire galleries at Chicago's Museum of Science & Industry—probably the first U.S. museum to solicit corporate support on a large scale. These corporations teamed up with the museum to show off their technologies and project a sense of technological progress and achievement (Jahnke, 1993). Later, other science museums, such as the Franklin Institute in Philadelphia and Boston's Museum of Science, followed Chicago's lead. According to David Ellis, director of Boston's Museum of Science (quoted in Jahnke, 1993), the relationship of corporations and museums is closer today than in the past, but there are also more and clearer guidelines governing what is permitted and what is not. "It was not uncommon for corporate sponsors in years past," Ellis observes, "to place their products in an exhibition. That is far less common today. . . . We are in the business of education. We are not an exhibit hall for hire. . . . There is a line that museums must take great care not to cross."

Corporate Expectations. Clearly, corporate giving differs from foundation giving in a number of important ways. Corporations have wider scope in the gifts they can give and the conditions of giving. A firm can give money, securities, in-kind services and goods, and use of facilities. A museum can solicit office equipment, professional marketing and advertising know-how, legal services, and so on, either free or at cost. Corporations regard gift giving as a minor or ancillary activity in their overall operations, in contrast to foundations, for which it is the major activity. Corporations will vary their giving level with the level of their current and expected income. They have to be responsive to the attitudes of stockholders, to whom they have the first financial obligation. Corporations are more likely than foundations to avoid supporting controversial causes.

Corporations pay more attention than foundations to the benefits that any grant of theirs will return to them. Contributions that can be shown to increase community corporate goodwill, reach a targeted consumer group with a favorable image, or train needed manpower is more likely to be acceptable to boards of directors and stockholders. In a national survey conducted by the Business Committee for the Arts in 1994, U.S. firms and corporations gave the following reasons for supporting the arts: demonstrating good corporate citizenship (74 percent); enhancing quality of life in their community (66 percent); boosting their image and reputation (46 percent), strengthening employee relations (22 percent), and increasing sales (19 percent). In exchange for their support, companies may be looking for increased visibility for their products, associations with organizations that can strengthen their image, employee amenities such as free tickets and invitations to exhibition opening events, and the use of the museum's elegant and high-profile facilities. Corporations often seek to locate headquarters in areas that offer cultural amenities such as museums, and the same corporations will support museums and other cultural organizations in order to maintain a good quality of life for their employees.

Forms of Corporate-Museum Partnerships. G. Donald Adams, former external relations officer at the Henry Ford Museum and marketing director at the Automotive Hall of Fame in Dearborn, Michigan (interviewed May 5, 1996), has observed that the Henry Ford Museum in the mid-1990s was deriving revenues from corporate sponsorships and partnerships at a time when corporations were spending increasing funds on sponsorships of events (Olympics, tennis and golf tournaments, car races, museum exhibitions) relative to conventional advertising. According to Adams, museum visitors are good sales prospects who are otherwise hard to reach. A corporation sponsors an event at a museum because it brings together the kind of people the company wants to reach—an educated constituency, an organization and audiences well placed in the community, targeted segments.

What are today's museums offering corporations? The Dallas Museum of Art in the early 1990s contracted with companies for *seasonal sponsorships.* In exchange for a $50,000 quarterly or semiannual contribution, a company could have its corporate logo prominently displayed, make use of museum facilities for corporate events, and provide museum benefits to its employees. The Henry Ford Museum & Greenfield Village in the mid-1990s created several types of corporate sponsorships and partnerships. A company could take out a full-year sponsorship for $100,000 or shorter sponsorships for varying lesser amounts. Companies were invited to sponsor special events and weekend activities. In return, the museum prominently displayed their corporate logos in its facilities and publications.

Several types of corporate-museum collaborations and partnerships have emerged. They vary in duration and intensity. At one end of the range, sometimes supported by a company foundation, is sponsorship of a museum exhibition or program, in which the sponsor receives recognition and acknowledgment in a listing of supporters at a museum entrance, in printed materials, and at Web sites. A corporate sponsor will also be invited to an opening night event and be given benefits for employees. This type of relationship does not carry any hint of affiliation between a museum and a company or any endorsement of a product or a company.

In the intermediate range, a museum and a corporation can form a partnership in which the company's products are shown in the museum—if not in the exhibits, then in related programs and events (for example, a fashion show). The Victoria and Albert Museum, in London, regularly establishes corporate marketing partnerships that permit the corporate partner to show a company or product logo and communicate corporate messages in exchange for a financial contribution. In other forms of joint activity, the company can communicate its identity, image, and message (including product information) by means of public relations and advertising. Corporate sponsors might distribute products at museum events. Corporate sponsors of the Smithsonian's 150th anniversary celebration in 1996 produced television commercials associating their corporate image and products with the Smithsonian and its celebration. Corporate sponsors received acknowledgments in the Smithsonian's public relations and promotional activities. The sponsors were allowed to organize corporate exhibitions alongside the Smithsonian traveling exhibition at each tour venue.

Longer-term relationships have arisen between museums and companies. These permit companies to invest in museums over an extended period in order to reap future benefits. One example is corporate investments in the films shown in IMAX or Omnimax theaters. Another form of relationship is *transaction-based marketing activity*. A corporation donates a specific amount of cash or equipment or in-kind transfers in direct proportion to sales and product revenues. In 1997, the Smithsonian Institution entered into a transaction-based marketing relationship with the Novus Corporation, the parent company of Discover Card. Novus will market an affinity credit card bearing the Smithsonian logo to individuals who particularly identify with the Smithsonian Institution and wish to support it and who will have the satisfaction of contributing support each time they make purchases with the card.

Yet another type of long-term marketing relationship is *cause marketing*, sometimes known as the *joint issue promotion.* A corporation teams up with a museum to jointly tackle a social problem. Money may or may not pass between the corporation and the museum, but the company and the museum will be promoted together. An example is the three-way partnership that developed in the mid-1990s among the Smithsonian Institutions's Traveling Exhibition Service (SITES), the National Geographic Society, and the Nissan Motor Corporation U.S.A. The partnership has effectively promoted geography literacy at thousands of schools by means of traveling exhibitions, educational materials, and production and distribution of geography learning games. National Geographic and the Smithsonian have received financial support in the partnership.

Another type of business relationship involves the licensing to companies, for a fee or a percentage of revenues, of proprietary images held by museums. Such partnerships with manufacturing companies permit the companies to market products bearing images from museum collections as virtually brand products. Products range from silk ties and coffee mugs to furniture reproductions of museum originals. The company and the museum share in the revenues (Andreasen, 1996).

In each of these marketing relationships, there is considerable reciprocity. Museums are indirectly endorsing the sponsoring company and its products. They are allowing corporate images and messages to be communicated directly in museums or in association with museums. Companies can bask in the goodwill and the high regard museums enjoy in their communities. In return, museums receive financial support and in-kind services and contributions they need to carry out their missions.

Museums can derive from partnerships particular benefits that can prove useful in the museums' own marketing activities. Sponsoring companies often conduct research to ascertain what impact their sponsorships have had on visitors and on the local community. Museums might allow corporation sponsors to include a few marketing questions in museum visitor surveys. The Henry Ford Museum, for example, has found that a significant number of visitors can recall a corporate sponsorship and that they express a high degree of approval (G. Donald Adams, interviewed May 5, 1996). Corporate sponsors can take encouragement from a 1993 opinion survey of nearly two thousand American men and women aged eighteen and over. Thirty-one percent of respondents indicated that when price and quality are equal, a company's business practices, including sponsorships, influence their purchases. Moreover, 54 percent of respondents in that survey said they would pay a premium for a product that supports a cause they care about.

Selecting Corporate Prospects and Managing Risk. Museums need to know how to identify good corporate prospects. Of the millions of business enterprises, relatively few are appropriate to any specific museum, and a museum ordinarily does not have the resources to cultivate more than a handful of corporate givers. The best prospects for corporate giving and marketing partnerships will have a number of the following characteristics:

- *Proximity.* Corporations find it hard to refuse to support worthwhile organizations in the cities and regions where they operate.

- *Kindred activities.* Corporations prefer to support museums with some area of shared interest. Thus a science museum might focus its fundraising efforts on high-tech companies or manufacturers of scientific instruments.

- *Declared areas of support.* Some corporations have a particular area of interest in making contributions. Thus a contemporary art museum might approach the Borg-Warner Corporation, in Chicago, because of the latter's active purchase of contemporary art.

- *History of large gifts.* Some large corporations have a record of generous giving practices. Museums, however, have to realize that these corporations receive a great many requests.

- *Personal relationships and contacts.* Museums should review their corporate contacts and direct staff, officers, and patrons with personal contacts with corporations to pursue good relations and solicit support. For example, a museum's board of trustees will consist of influential individuals who can open many corporate doors. Corporations tend to respond to peer influence.

- *Specific capability.* Some corporations may have a unique resource needed by a museum. Thus a museum might solicit a paint manufacturer to donate paint to refurbish its galleries or solicit a computer company if it needs computers. A corporate product in a museum can have a marketing advantage for that company.

As corporate sponsorships and partnerships with museums multiply, some ambiguity and tension may arise in these relationships, which may lead into uncharted territory. Many corporations are not yet clear how they can use museums as partners. Many museums, conversely, are not clear how to attract corporate support and what a fair exchange involves.

Thus there are risks for museums in corporate sponsorships and partnerships, and these risks have to be anticipated and managed. Any partnership can involve substantial research, communication, and transactions that may distract a museum's limited development and marketing staff from other important work. Relationships with businesses can convey to individual supporters their support is no longer necessary or a priority, a perception that can lead to reductions in gifts and individual support. Some studies have found, however, that a well-managed museum-corporate partnership can raise a museum's visibility and lead to increased private contributions. Museums have to guard against affiliations with companies that have tarnished images or questionable practices. Museums have to be firm in protecting their control of content and the professional standards of their employees while negotiating a sponsor's claims. The way to protect against risks is to rigorously research the backgrounds of prospective partners, negotiate clearly over expectations and goals, assert professional standards, develop marketing skills commensurate with the sponsoring company's skills, and revisit the relationship periodically to ensure that it is productive and not counterproductive.

The development strategy of a hypothetical big science museum illustrates some of the issues we have been discussing. The museum sought to raise several million dollars to build a new exhibition on computers. Its existing exhibition was wholly inadequate for attracting students and families. The museum was willing to name the new exhibition after a major corporate donor that would supply at least 60 percent of the money sought. This donor would take the lead in attracting additional corporate and individual donors.

The museum needed to identify one or more major corporations to approach. The fundraisers recognized that these corporate prospects would have to be large, affluent companies that had an interest in the project. The fundraisers developed the matrix shown in Figure 11.1 to classify corporate givers by their giving potential and their interest potential. The museum found that computer companies fell in the upper left cell. Computer companies have excellent profits *(high giving potential)* and good reason to be interested in museum computer exhibits *(high interest potential)*. These companies also have an interest in good causes and in obtaining public goodwill. The museum decided that approaching a computer company would make good sense.

But which computer company to approach? Now the museum introduced additional criteria. One company had already given a major donation to this museum for another project; it was ruled out. However, when the museum considered whether it had any good contacts with other computer companies, it found that an important member of the museum's board of trustees was an old friend of the chairman of a major computer company in the West. A *prospect solicitation plan* was prepared. As a start, museum fundraisers researched the computer company's sales, profits, major officers, charitable record, and other characteristics. This information was useful in deciding whom to approach at the computer corporation, how much to ask for, what benefits to offer, and so on. A decision was made to approach the corporation's president, ask for $3 million, and offer to name the museum's computer exhibition after the corporation.

The final step was *plan implementation.* The museum board member arranged to visit his friend, the computer company's chairman. He was accompanied by the museum president and also the vice president for development.

Figure 11.1. Classifying Corporate Donors by Level of Interest and Giving Potential.

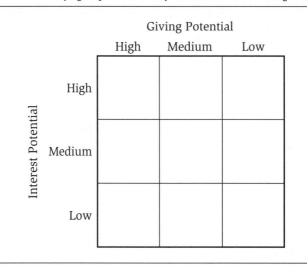

They made their presentation to the chairman and the computer company's foundation director, and received an assurance that the proposal would be given careful consideration. A subsequent meeting took place at the museum. Ultimately, the computer company funded the project.

Linda Hardwick, director of development at the Indianapolis Museum of Art (interviewed May 12, 1997), observes that even companies that are not in the habit of supporting museums or entering marketing partnerships with them may still be available for some type of affiliation. Museum marketing and development staff therefore have to make companies aware of the range of opportunities and benefits that can flow from museum affiliations. Companies may lack an idea of the choices available for sponsorship, the different levels of support they can offer, and the benefits they can derive from even a modest relationship with a museum. Hardwick says the job she and her staff face is to "sell" the museum, find and cultivate prospects, figure out the gift (or sponsorship) interests of potential individual and corporate donors, match museum programs and activities with donor interests, and "be quick on your feet, carry a Rolodex in your head, and always be ready to seize opportunities." Here are some of the ways, according to Hardwick, a corporation can support a museum and derive benefits from the support it provides.

- In exchange for an annual corporate contribution, the museum can offer discounted memberships to the corporation's employees or a special free day for employees and their families, credited to the corporation. Or, the human resources department of a corporation may wish to make the "payment" to purchase this employee benefit outright.

- A company may wish to direct its annual operating gift to a special event, such as a members' exhibition opening, a major donor reception, a regularly scheduled educational program such as the school tour program, or a weekend free family day, and, in return, receive prominent public recognition.

- If the museum needs volunteers for a corporate-sponsored program, the company itself can ask its employees to volunteer as a way to further involve them and demonstrate the company's commitment to the community. These opportunities also can fulfill the corporation's commitment to employee volunteerism.

- The marketing departments of companies frequently rent museum space for business meetings, staff retreats, social events with clients, and employee recognition events. If the company is a regular contributor to the museum, the rental fees can be waived or discounted.

- A corporation can make in-kind gifts to museums (computer or telecommunications hardware, printed materials, donations of expertise, such as a corporate marketing leader working with the museum on a marketing issue, and so on). Such gifts are important in relieving pressure on museum budgets, and corporations often find them easier to make than monetary gifts.

Government Giving

Arts and cultural organizations in the United States receive various types of support from government agencies: federal agencies such as the National Endowment for the Arts, the National Endowment for the Humanities, and the Institute of Museum and Library Services; state government agencies such as humanities and arts councils; and local agencies such as county and municipal governments. Large museums normally have staff to oversee government grants. This requires monitoring announcements of government grant opportunities as well as spending time at agencies to get to know granting officials. Government agencies require detailed paperwork in proposals, placing major weight on the proposal's probable contribution to the public good. They tend to pay less attention to agency benefit and to personal relations with the soliciting organization.

Government giving as a source of support for museums has been curtailed. Governments have been under pressure to make tougher spending choices than in the past, and social services agencies are increasingly being given precedence over arts and cultural organizations. There is, however, one countervailing trend to public-sector cuts in support for museums and other cultural organizations: local and regional government agencies, particularly in central cities and urban centers, are coming to recognize the value of museums as tourist destinations and as generators of local jobs and income. For example, the Philadelphia Museum of Art's 1996 Cézanne exhibition generated thirty-seven thousand room-nights, and visitors from outside Philadelphia—approximately 90 percent of the exhibition's visitors—spent an average of $402 each. The blockbuster exhibition contributed an estimated $86.5 million to the area's economy (Cable News Network, Sept. 6, 1996). Some museum leaders contend that museums have not been sufficiently vigorous in justifying their value to the community or in seeking public-sector support. Local governments are becoming more receptive to providing support, and the travel and hospitality industries are becoming more interested in participating in marketing partnerships.

A variety of mechanisms for support already exist at the local and state levels. Several states have authorized cultural tax districts in which portions of real estate or sales taxes are dedicated to support local cultural organizations. In the Denver metropolitan area, six counties have established a special district known as the Scientific and Cultural Facilities District. The district receives one-tenth of 1 percent of the counties' combined sales taxes to allocate to museums and cultural and educational institutions. Funds are allocated according to institution size, and a portion is set aside for competitive grants. The city of Chicago has another form of governmental support for its museums. Several of the city's museums that are situated on public parkland, including the Art Institute of Chicago, the Field Museum, and the Museum of Science & Industry, receive appropriations annually from the Chicago Park District, a city agency. Representatives of the Park District sit on the museums' boards of directors.

A large number of state governments in the United States provide annual appropriations to support arts and cultural organizations, including museums. Fund are often channeled through state and local arts and humanities councils. In 1995, state governments appropriated $259.5 million to state arts councils, although in sixteen states, the level of support was lower than the year before. State governments have a variety of ways to finance museums and other cultural organizations, including bond issues, revenues derived from automobile license plate fees, income tax return checkoffs, revenues from corporate filing fees, culture tax districts, and revenues derived from state lotteries (Rafool and Loyacono, 1995).

Bond issues are increasingly used for museum support. The Art Institute of Chicago was one of the first U.S. museums to borrow funds in the tax-exempt bond market, convincing the market that its assets (exclusive of collections and real estate), as well as its revenue streams, were sufficient to offset risks. The bonds were issued under the auspices of the state of Illinois.

Fundraising Goals and Strategy

Given their major donor sources, museums must set annual and long-range goals for fundraising. One large museum set the following goals:

- Increase contributions received each year by an average of 10 percent
- Keep fundraising expenses-to-contributions ratio below 20 percent

- Increase the median size of contributions by 10 percent
- Increase foundation grants by 15 percent, corporate grants by 10 percent, and government grants by 5 percent

Presumably, these goals would be checked for consistency and prioritized in terms of importance.

Setting annual goals for contributions allows a museum to know how much to budget for fundraising, motivate staff and volunteers to make a strong effort, and measure fundraising effectiveness. Organizations can take several approaches to setting fundraising goals:

- *Incremental approach.* The museum takes last year's revenue, increases it to cover inflation, and then modifies it up or down, depending on the expected economic climate. Thus a museum may decide to raise about 10 percent more than it did in the preceding year.
- *Need approach.* The museum forecasts its financial needs and sets a goal based on these needs. Thus a museum will estimate its future building costs, staff salaries, energy costs, and other expenditures and set its targets accordingly.
- *Opportunity approach.* The museum makes a fresh estimate of how much money it could raise from each donor group with differing levels of fundraising effort. It sets a goal of maximizing the net difference between donations and costs.

The opportunity approach is the most sound. The development officer analyzes the potential of each donor group. If the proposed goal is accepted, he or she then knows how much staff effort to allocate to each group.

Figure 11.2 shows the relationship between donations, expenditures, and surplus. The donation response function shows the donations that are likely to be raised with different levels of fundraising expenditure. Nonfundraising expenditures can be subtracted to reveal the gross surplus before expenditures. The 45-degree line shows the fundraising expenditures. The vertical distance between the last two curves shows the net surplus associated with various fundraising expenditures. The highest point on the surplus curve shows the fundraising expenditure level that will maximize net surplus.

Fundraising Tactics

Fundraising strategy sets the overall parameters for the fundraising effort. The development officer must implement the strategy with specific actions. Table 11.2 lists the major tactics that are effective in four donor markets: the mass anonymous small-gift market, members and their friends market, affluent citizen market, and wealthy donor market.

The *mass anonymous small-gift market* consists of all citizens who might be induced to contribute a small sum to a museum. The key idea is to use low-cost

Figure 11.2. Relationship Between Donations, Marketing Expenditures, and Surplus.

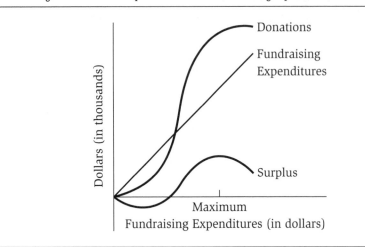

methods of fundraising, because the contributions from noninvolved individuals can be expected to be low. Direct mail has become one of the major fundraising tools for this market.

The *members and their friends market* consists of the people who already belong to the museum and people who are similar but do not yet belong. This market can be tapped for donations in a number of ways. Art museums, for example, raise money from this market through memberships and offering events and dinners. Each fundraising method requires careful planning to maximize its potential revenue.

The *affluent citizens market* consists of persons whose income and interest in the museum could lead them to give anywhere from fifty to several hundred dollars as a donation. This market is worth pursuing with more than direct mail. One highly effective technique is to issue invitations for special dinners and events. Another method is letter writing and telephone calling from museum supporters to their affluent friends, asking for donations.

The *wealthy donors market* consists of persons whose wealth and potential interest is such that they might be induced to contribute anywhere from one thousand to several million dollars. These individuals are usually well known in their communities, and they are solicited by many organizations. Many set up foundations to handle these solicitations, so that they do not have to be personally involved. Some fundraisers spend considerable amounts of time with these individuals in the hope of attracting a major gift. One museum fundraiser spent five years cultivating the friendship of a wealthy widow before receiving a gift.

All the various fundraising tactics can be carried on under the auspices of a *campaign,* which we define as *an organized and time-sequenced set of activities and events for raising a given sum of money within a particular time period.*

Table 11.2. Fundraising Methods.

Market	Method
Mass anonymous small gift	Direct mail
	TV and radio
	Thrift shops
	Raffles
	Tours
	Marathons, walkathons
Members and their friends	Anniversary celebrations
	Art shows
	Auctions
	Benefits
	Book sales
	Fashion shows
	Dances
	Dinners, luncheons, breakfasts
	Fairs
	Telethons
	Parties in unusual places
Affluent citizens	Dinners and testimonials
	Telephone calls from high-status people
	Letters from high-status people
Wealthy donors	Bequests, memorials
	Cultivation and grooming
	Testimonials

When planning capital campaigns, museums should follow these guidelines:

- Do not run capital campaigns too often; they can lose their special quality in the minds of donors.

- Set an achievable goal; there is nothing more embarrassing than failing to reach a capital campaign goal.

- Do not allow the campaign to last too long; it eventually will lose its momentum.

- Arrange a matching feature so that wealthy donors or organizations promise to give amounts equal to a set sum raised by general fundraising. Fundraisers have to cultivate challenge grants early in the planning.

- Prepare an attractive booklet describing the cause behind the campaign and showing what the contributions will make possible in terms of new or improved programs, services, and facilities.

- Solicit board members for large gifts before the campaign begins; next, solicit wealthy donors. These steps will show others that the campaign is generating considerable support and enthusiasm and will thus encourage others to give.

A perennial issue is whether potential donors should be coached in how much to give or whether this should be left to their own judgment. There are three possibilities: do not specify any amount; propose a specific dollar amount on the low side; and propose a specific dollar amount on the high side. The first approach is the most common. People differ in what they can give, and the amount may be best left to individual judgments. Proposing a specific amount on the low side is viewed as accomplishing two things. It helps prospects know what is considered a proper amount to give, and it allows the less experienced donors to get into the habit of giving. This is why it is called a *foot-in-the-door* approach. The problem is that many people who might have given more will take this as an adequate amount to give. Proposing a high amount to give works on the theory of *door-in-the-face*. It stretches people's ideas of what they should give, and it can be hoped that donors will give that much or something close to it. High suggested amounts can induce givers to give more than they otherwise would.

Evaluating Fundraising Effectiveness

A museum must make a continuous effort to evaluate the effectiveness of its various fundraising efforts. It can make evaluations in several ways.

Percentage of goal reached. The first thing to look at is how close the museum came to achieving its annual goal. This may also require judging whether the goal was set high or low in the first place. Every museum wants to achieve its goal or better. So the development officer may have proposed a low goal to make that goal more reachable. However, the museum's senior management may want to set a high goal to motivate more effort by the development office.

Number of donors. Museums hope to increase the number of donors annually. They should estimate the number of actual donors in relation to the potential number of donors. Many museums will find they have disappointing penetration in a given donor market.

Average gift size. Museums also want to increase the average gift size. The development officer should estimate the potential number of gifts that might be obtained in each gift-size class against the current number to determine the size classes that deserve targeted effort in the next fundraising period.

Expenses-to-contributions ratio. A museum is ultimately interested in its net contributions, not gross fundraising revenue. An expenses-to-contributions ratio in the neighborhood of 10 to 20 percent is a respectable sign. Many large donors look at this key ratio before they decide whether to offer support to an organization.

Staff member effectiveness. The museum also has to evaluate the effectiveness of individual members of the development staff according to these indicators: number of leads developed, number of proposals written, average value of proposal, number of proposals closed, percentage of proposals closed, average value closed, average cost per proposal closed, cost per dollar raised. Those staff members who are not performing may require additional training or may have to be replaced.

SUMMARY

Museums have traditionally relied on public-sector support of one kind or another—support from agencies of the national, state, regional, and local governments. Many museums in recent years have also built notable earned-income programs. Yet a major source of support for museums of all types has been and will continue to be individual, foundation, and corporate giving. Individual giving can take the form of membership dues, contributions to capital campaigns, gifts, and bequests. U.S. foundations are a significant source of programmatic support for museums. Corporate giving can take the form of philanthropy, particularly when a company has a corporate foundation arm, or marketing sponsorships and partnerships, through which companies expect to derive revenue, goodwill, and other benefits from their support of museums. Government agencies continue to provide support, although the levels are declining. Not all museums have the staff and resources to devote to fundraising and development, yet even small museums have development opportunities that may be overlooked—for example, cultivating members of their communities who can contribute valuable in-kind services, companies that can contribute equipment, and affluent individuals who might, if asked, take a more active and supportive role. For fundraising and development to work, museums have to build professional staffs. Because development work is staff-intensive and costly, museums have to monitor progress and evaluate staff proficiencies and the ratio of funds raised to costs incurred in the development work.

O

MODEL MUSEUM PRACTICE

Audience and Membership Development
at the Art Institute of Chicago

"Well into the 1980s," Robert E. Mars, executive vice president for administrative affairs at the Art Institute of Chicago (interviewed Aug. 14, 1996), observes, "the belief was common in the museum world that if you exhibited great objects in attractive, intelligent ways, people would flock to your museum. That belief no longer holds. Today, we recognize that a museum has to be focused on the people it serves or wishes to serve, as well as on the objects it acquires."

The Art Institute of Chicago (AIC) devoted considerable attention in the early 1990s to satisfying and retaining audiences and building support. Several factors converged to shape audience development as a priority. The museum recognized that critical segments of the community (African Americans, families with young children, young professionals) were underserved by existing programs and operations. AIC's membership was aging. The mid-1990s membership base of approximately ninety thousand had remained at the same level for several years. The museum's base level (that is without the impact that popular special exhibitions might have when they occur) visitorship level (1.2 million) had not moved higher. Concern was expressed that without further growth, AIC would lack the financial wherewithal to sustain high-quality programming.

The museum launched a strategic planning process, part of which focused on the types of people served, their satisfaction levels, and the segments that were inactive or underrepresented. Diversifying AIC's audience was a critical goal. The strategic focus on audience and membership development unearthed several lines of inquiry: finding new museum visitors among target segments; making the museum-going experience of high enough value to convert newcomers into regular visitors and then into members; moving members up the ladder, converting members in low-end categories into high-end ones and then converting members into donors; and shaping an appealing museum image and then launching a promotion and communication campaign that included use of media and public relations along with advertising to reinforce the image.

The concept of a membership ladder reflects a key reality: museums, like symphony orchestras and theater groups, cannot depend on occasional visitors to sustain themselves; each needs a subscription and membership base—an ongoing relationship with the community that generates continuing, predictable, expanding participation and support.

Focusing on audiences and membership has taken a variety of forms at the Art Institute of Chicago. Recognizing that the young professional segment of the community was fast growing, affluent, and influential, AIC organized in May 1995 a monthly evening program to reach young professionals employed in downtown Chicago who were available after working hours for museum events. The After Hours program is held on Thursday evenings and draws between twelve hundred and fifteen hundred guests, on the average. Activities include a bar and light refreshments, jazz performances, lectures and guided gallery tours, and gift shop visits. The evening also provides a high-quality social experience— the opportunity to mingle and meet with other young professionals in a relaxed, elegant, and distinctive setting. An average of one hundred new memberships are generated each month. Downtown restaurants have recognized the value; several offer discounts to After Hours participants. An After Hours radio advertising spot tells listeners: "Think you know the place to go this Thursday night? Think again. Because now there's a new place, where the jazz is hot, the conversation is lively, and the art just amazing. It's a place to meet friends. Wind down. Catch up. Grab a bite. And dive into an atmosphere that's full of possibilities. . . ."

After Hours developed out of a specialized membership group, known as the Evening Associates. Composed largely of young professionals, the group and its board assumed responsibility for building membership among the young professional community, generating attractive programming, and soliciting financial support for AIC's activities. The group's membership stood at over one thousand in the mid-1990s. The After Hours program experience demonstrates the value of giving support groups a voice in developing programs and raising funds.

AIC is in close proximity to thousands of downtown business firms, corporations, and associations and their employees. In the early 1990s, the museum created ArtExpress, a program in which museum curators and educators travel to a company's headquarters, usually during the noon hour, to share over a brown-bag lunch with company employees museum offerings (through reproductions, objects, and slide shows) and to answer questions. Participants receive free-admission passes to the museum, copies of the member magazine, discounts at the museum's restaurants and shops, and a special membership offer.

AIC has invested considerable resources in attracting underserved segments of the community. The museum is focusing on Chicago's African American community, with the support of a grant from the Lila Wallace–Reader's Digest Fund. It also is giving priority attention to three city neighborhoods with target segments and to families with young children, for whom AIC has developed a range of educational programs. The museum also is giving emphasis to high-end supporters. A series of collection-based affiliated groups (prints and drawings, American Art, African and American Indian art, Asian art, European art) bring collectors, connoisseurs, and patrons together around the development of a particular collection area. Members meet with curators, attend lectures, join tours to museums in the United States and abroad, and give advice and support for new acquisitions.

The strategic planning framework at AIC evolved over a period of several years. An active board member provided funds for an audience development initiative. A trustee committee on marketing and business development was broadened to include audience development. Alongside the trustee committee, a management committee was formed to deal with audience development, consisting of the director, the deputy director, and two other top museum leaders. The committee initially examined two areas: building audiences and membership and improving the quality of the museum-going experience, including orientation, services, and evaluation. It then added a third area: examining the effects of organizational roles and structure on visitor behavior and identifying improvements in structures and staff training and other incentives to provide a high-quality visitor experience.

In 1996 and 1997, a further step was taken at AIC to join the marketing and audience focus together with the work of planning and designing exhibits and related programming. The museum hosted three small-scale exhibitions in 1997 and organized a "strategic marketing group" to coordinate development, promotion, and management in tandem with museum marketing, audience development, visitor relations, and curatorial staff. In the past each exhibit would have been promoted separately and, if it was small, would not have generated a lot of public interest. The goal here was to raise the profile of even small-scale exhibitions, build relationships and synergies among them, and find ways to add value to the experience of visiting these shows. The museum's strategic planning structure is shown in Exhibit 11.1.

AIC's methods for reaching new audiences and building membership and donorship have evolved. The Monet exhibition in 1995 boosted visitorship, membership, and sales. One effect was to raise membership from 90,000 to 150,000. The goal is to establish a new base level of membership somewhere in between these two numbers and then attempt to build from this higher base. Initial results from this effort have been encouraging as evidenced by the fact

○○○○○

Exhibit 11.1. AIC Strategic Planning.

Strategic Planning

Marketing and Audience Development Committee
(Trustees and Managers)

Audience Development Committee
(Management)

- Visitor acquisition
- Visitor experience
- Visitor services
- Membership retention
- Staff training

Strategic Marketing Group
(Staff)

- Coordinating exhibition development with visitorship and membership
- Building value for audiences
- Designing exhibitions to reinforce one another
- Exhibition and program promotion
- Building value for particular audience/membership segments

Source: Art Institute of Chicago.

○○○○○

that membership stood at 140,000 as of June 1997. Large-scale exhibitions will have a role but growing emphasis is placed on the interrelationships of exhibits and achieving balance, reach, and synergy of the whole.

Several lessons have been learned. There is no single pathway, program, or structure for building audience and membership goals; rather this requires multiple programs, continual monitoring, high-quality in programs and services, and flexibility in shifting emphases and resources as circumstances require. High-level management support is crucial. A particular value that museums can offer is sociability in relaxed, safe, and elegant settings—occasions and events in which people can mingle and meet with one another and share enjoyable recreational experiences. Museums also have to build relationships with their communities and selected segments thereof, which then become the basis for recruiting volunteers, members, and lifelong supporters. Finally, museum supporters often want a voice in the support activities they engage in and a sense of ownership.

Christine O'Neill, AIC vice president for development (interviewed Sept. 17, 1996), says the Art Institute of Chicago is taking time to learn about the people whom it is serving and to find ways to connect audiences to the exhibitions and programs offered. "Museums have to offer value as museums—value built around collections, exhibitions, and visual experiences—rather than as entertainment centers. The museum-going experience is multifaceted, and each facet has to be satisfied and integrated into the whole experience."

CHAPTER TWELVE

Developing the Marketing Organization

Plans, Budgets, Implementation, and Control

*A second fundamental expectation is connectedness. The successful museum
of the next century must be connected to the community . . . the museum
must be a listener. . . . Key to the listening process is, to whom do we listen?
What questions do we ask? And most important, what are we willing
to do about changing as a result of the listening?*
—Harold K. Skramstad Jr.

To carry out a consumer-oriented, market-responsive strategy, a museum must develop an effective marketing organization and efficient procedures for planning, budgeting, implementing, and controlling its marketing activities. Some marketing professionals argue that marketing should infuse all departments, goals, and strategies of an organization. Others take a more limited view of marketing as but a single managerial function. This chapter will examine both views. We will consider these marketing components and the role they play in generating a vital and accessible museum. The chapter concludes with a comprehensive marketing audit, the instrument museums can use to assess their marketing activities in relation to internal and external environments, goals and resources, and their strategies and plans.

MARKETING'S ROLE IN THE MUSEUM

Every museum faces markets and publics with which it develops relationships. Indeed, it can be argued that museums, especially large ones, are among the most complex and variegated of organizations, embracing many constituencies and audiences to which managers have to respond. The multiplicity of constituencies alone suggests the importance of marketing applications in museums.

Must a museum establish formal marketing positions and responsibilities to conduct its marketing activities effectively? There are three positions on this issue. The first is that no special positions are needed because the museum's managers themselves possess sufficient sensitivity to the needs of the various publics and audiences. The director, curators, development officer, and public relations manager have enough awareness of the needs of patrons, visitors, scholars, and connoisseurs that they do not have to set up the additional position of marketing manager. Furthermore, museum managers can always hire outside marketing skills and services as needed. They can hire a marketing research firm, advertising agency or public relations firm, fundraising specialists, and so on. The second view is that a museum, if it is large enough and has varied offerings and deals with diverse markets, can benefit from establishing a marketing department from which various museum managers can draw assistance. This marketing department might consist of a marketing director, a marketing researcher, an advertising and communications manager, and a customer service manager.

The third view is that a large museum can benefit from establishing a senior-level marketing officer, in addition to its marketing specialists. This officer will have four primary tasks: (1) provide other museum managers with information about the market environment and trends; (2) participate in setting annual goals and resource-acquisition strategies; (3) serve as a marketing conscience for the museum, defining marketing's role in strategic planning, program development, and customer service and countering the tendency of other managers to get so engrossed in their operations as to lose sight of market forces and customer relationships; and (4) be responsible for coordinating various marketing services.

Most museums in the United States and overseas are relatively small. Their staffs are small; their endowments are small or nonexistent; their operating revenues are limited. Although small size does not obviate the need to plan for and respond to different markets, it does limit a museum's opportunities to undertake formal marketing services. Rather than hiring a manager, small museums may have access to marketing talent from volunteers in the community or board members. The critical issue, however, is whether or not the museum's managers recognize the importance of being market and customer centered and are motivated to acquire the information and skills needed to serve their markets adequately.

Characteristics of a Consumer-Centered Museum

As previous chapters have shown, museum visitors, members, and patrons can be viewed as *consumers*. A consumer-oriented museum will have the following characteristics:

- It will factor in consumer interests in planning museum exhibitions, programs, and activities.
- It will rely heavily on research to learn about customer needs, perceptions, and preferences.

- It will identify market segments with different needs and interests and arrange programs and experiences to satisfy each target segment.
- It will define competition broadly to include all other leisure-time activities and recreational options that might compete with visiting a museum.
- Its market strategy will use a variety of marketing tools, not merely advertising and public relations.

How Far to Go in Adopting a Consumer Orientation

We have argued that marketing can be successful only if it tailors the organization's offerings to the needs, wants, and preferences of target consumer publics. We have defined marketing as *a social and managerial process by which individuals and groups obtain what they want through creating, offering, and exchanging products and services of value with others.*

Marketing at its core is an exchange process. In the museum context, visitors arrive with a variety of needs, interests, and preferences and seek to satisfy these through museum experiences and activities. Many professionals in nonprofit organizations, however, fear that such an approach, taken to an extreme, will mean that anything goes to please the masses. They fear the museum's basic mission will be compromised; their professional judgments replaced or supplanted by marketing judgments.

Some concerns are warranted. As in every field, there is good practice and bad. Marketing's role has to be seen as one of supporting a museum's objectives. Marketing does not define the museum's objectives. Marketing is a set of tools and a process wrapped in a philosophy that assists an organization in achieving its objectives. In museums the marketing staff work with directors, curators, exhibition designers, education specialists, and other professionals to implement the latter's vision and decisions. Marketing staff may have an advisory role when professional staff formulate program offerings. In the areas of designing communications, promoting offerings, and communicating with audiences, marketing staff have more weight in the decision-making process.

Organizational Design and Structure

Several factors influence an organization's design and structure and the place of marketing in that structure. Among them are the organization's size and scale, its strategic objectives, and its product offerings.

Size, Scale, and Structure. Using budget size as an indicator, the great majority of U.S. museums are small, with annual incomes of less than $100,000. Four out of five U.S. museums can thus be classified as small, 12 percent are medium-sized, and 7.3 percent are large museums, with annual budgets in excess of $1 million (Institute of Museum and Library Services, 1992, pp. 3–10; American Association of Museums, 1994, pp. 32, 80–81).

In a small organization with two or three employees, an organization chart and formal structure are not necessary. One person might do all the marketing work, including research, sales, advertising, customer service, and other activities. As the organization expands, a marketing department emerges to plan and carry out these activities. In large organizations the marketing department contains some specialists—marketing researcher, product specialist, communications specialist, pricing specialist, and so on. In their study of successful business organizations, Peters and Waterman (1982) found certain common characteristics that can apply to museum organizations. Successful organizations tended to have significant areas of informal behavior (such as Hewlett-Packard's *management by wandering around,* IBM's *open-door policy,* or 3M's *clubs* that encourage small-group interaction). Their structures tended to be decentralized, with small, independent divisions or groups to encourage innovation. The structures were also simple and lean, allowing for flexible adaptation to changing conditions.

Strategy. An organization's strategy in many cases will define its structure. A small museum developing new offerings and services in a fast-changing environment might need a flexible structure that encourages individual and small-group action—a decentralized structure with ample informal communication. A larger, more established museum that operates in relatively stable markets might need a structure providing greater integration—a more centralized structure with well-defined roles and communication through established channels.

Product Offerings. Organizational structures also are influenced by the type and range of products and services that an organization provides. A well-established museum is likely to have large collections to preserve, exhibitions to produce, and educational materials and programs to generate for students in local schools and for adults. For its multiple collections the museum will employ curators, who are responsible for acquiring, conserving, researching, and displaying their collections. Curators are the equivalent of *product managers* in business organizations. In the marketing environment, curators must attend to the audiences for the exhibitions they mount as well as to their collections and professional concerns. Curators increasingly work closely with a staff of exhibition designers, educators, and other specialists (sometimes including marketing staff) to present and draw attention to their collections, research, and exhibitions.

Human Resources

At all levels, a museum has to fill its structure with people who have the needed skills, motivation, and personal characteristics. Personnel have to be recruited, assigned, trained, and supported. The selection and development of managers is particularly important. Different strategic aims are likely to shape the types of managers recruited. New venture strategies, for example, require managers with entrepreneurial skills, whereas maintenance strategies require managers with firm administrative skills. In recent years, museums have begun to recognize the importance of personnel planning. Systematic, long-term human resource planning can give a museum a strong competitive advantage in all its functions, including marketing (see Mills, 1985).

DEVELOPING MARKETING PLANS

Museums need to develop effective marketing plans that spell out marketing projects, activities, and costs (one of the stages in the strategic market planning process discussed in Chapter Three). The strategic plan describes the organization's overall mission and objectives, while marketing plans deal with each business, functional, or program unit and plans, as seen from the viewpoint of consumers and markets. A written marketing plan serves several purposes (Gumpert, 1994). First, when a plan is written down, inconsistencies, unknowns, gaps, and implausibilities can be readily identified. Second, the plan helps focus management on new market conditions and key marketing issues. Third, it develops a set of performance goals. Fourth, it leads to an implementation timetable for undertaking tasks and achieving goals.

Formulating Marketing Plans

Marketing plans typically have most, if not all, of the following sections:

Executive summary. This brief opening summary highlights the main goals and recommendations to be found in the body of the plan. It permits senior management and board members to grasp quickly the major thrust of the plan. A table of contents should follow the executive summary.

Current marketing situation. This section presents relevant background data on the market, product offerings, and competition and also legal, political, and economic developments.

Opportunity and issue analysis. This section identifies the current marketing situation: the major opportunities and threats, strengths and weaknesses, and the issues the museum will face during the time frame of the plan.

Goals. This section describes the two types of goals that will have been set by the museum in light of the opportunities and issues analysis: marketing goals (regaining lapsed members, building up an underserved audience segment, refurbishing the museum's image, and the like) and financial goals (revenue maximization, full cost recovery, and so on).

Marketing strategy. This section describes the marketing strategy, general positioning, and initiatives the museum will pursue.

Action programs. This section is an action plan that spells out specific programs and steps to be taken by specific staff members in specific time periods.

Each element of the marketing strategy is elaborated to answer these questions: *What* will be done? *When* will it be done? *Who* will do it? *How much* will it cost? *What kind* of benefit and *how much* benefit will it generate for the museum?

Budget. This section spells out the amount of money needed to carry out the plan.

Controls. This section describes the information that will be collected and evaluated to measure the progress toward achieving the plan's goals each quarter and the corrective actions that might be taken if required. A contingency plan is sometimes included, which outlines the steps that management would implement in response to specific adverse developments that might occur, steps such as offering reduced admission charges or other benefits. The purpose of contingency planning is to encourage managers to give prior thought to difficulties that might lie ahead.

A Marketing Plan in Action

The Memorial Art Gallery (MAG) of the University of Rochester, in upstate New York, faced a considerable challenge in the early 1990s: to reverse a decline in membership and audience size and make the museum accessible to a more diversified public. MAG operates both as a university art museum and as a city museum. It is located in downtown Rochester, at a distance from the main university campus.

MAG managers in the early 1990s began to recognize changes taking place in the museum's environment that threatened to impair the museum's ability to attract visitors and supporters. Its base of patrons was shrinking as a result of an aging patron population and the departure of some patrons to the warm Southern states. The urban populace was changing, with a growing population of ethnic minorities that had little connection with the museum. MAG was not attracting enough families with children, young professionals, and members of minority groups. And not of least importance, the museum's funding support from the university was declining, and public-sector support overall was modest and static. Recognition of the changing environment led MAG in the mid-1990s to develop a marketing plan, the chief objectives of which were membership and audience expansion and diversification and the development of new private support.

Museum staff, along with the museum's board, developed a marketing plan to tackle the following challenges:

- Transforming the staff and museum culture from a product-driven, top-down culture to an audience-driven culture; resolving doubts about marketing's role and achieving a threshold for trying new things, including marketing tools; and building internal consensus toward a set of agreed-on marketing planning goals

- Convening marketing task forces to undertake elements of the marketing plan and engage staff, volunteers, supporters, and board members in the ongoing planning process

- Obtaining various forms of expertise needed by the museum from board members, staff, volunteers, and supporters (including in-kind donations of equipment and of marketing, communications, and public relations services)

- Generating a body of research to examine audience and membership perceptions, preferences, and satisfaction levels

- Identifying target segments, establishing planning goals, and relating museum offerings to these target segments

- Creating a communications strategy and programs to reach the target segments and the broader public

- Creating membership retention and acquisition strategies and programs, including offering new program benefits as well as adding value to existing programs

By the late 1990s, MAG's marketing planning had begun to pay off in increased visitorship and membership and successful programs for attracting the target segments (Deborah Rothman, public relations manager, Memorial Art Gallery, interviewed Oct. 10, 1996).

DEVELOPING MARKETING BUDGETS

Marketing planning involves budget planning. Marketing activities involve objectives and goals, incur costs, and require monitoring and evaluation. A budget is an organization's plan of action expressed in monetary terms. It is not merely blueprints indicating expenses and revenues. A budget indicates priorities, the level of investment of resources in particular program areas. Budgets are monitoring tools and sets of benchmarks for measuring performance in relation to objectives. While focusing on shorter-term factors, budgets are indispensable instruments for achieving longer-term marketing and strategic objectives.

Budgeting has three basic functions. First, a budget records the museum's financial objectives for the coming year or years. Second, it serves as a tool to monitor the museum's financial activities throughout the year, providing a benchmark with which managers and the board can determine whether financial goals are being met. Third, it requires the museum to predict the effects of marketing strategies and tactics over a period of years and to measure performance.

The budgeting process is integral to the program planning process. On the policy level, a budget defines in detail how the museum's financial resources will be used to accomplish the strategic plan. Budget planning is also influenced by questions of cost-effectiveness and efficiency: How much will each program cost? How much money must be raised? How much can be earned? What will be the schedule of disbursements and income over the life of each program? (Bryce, 1992).

Common Budgeting Problems

Budgeting in museums can be characterized as a balancing act of meeting the museum's objectives to the fullest possible extent within the limits of its financial capacity. But as they attempt to maximize the use of their limited resources, museum managers can make certain mistakes in carrying out the budgeting process.

Emphasis on New Programs. A common budgeting problem in museums involves attitudes toward existing and new programs. Existing programs are assumed to be a fundamental part of the museum's operations and therefore are accepted virtually unexamined. In contrast, proposed new programs, often modest in comparison to existing programs, are subject to close scrutiny and negotiated endlessly by staff and the board. New programs have to find budgetary room within the confines of the museum's total resources, most likely already stretched to capacity. Furthermore, managers can fail to examine the productivity of existing programs—the resources and expenses involved in generating program earnings. The tendency is to institutionalize existing programs. To ensure that knowledgeable resource allocations are made, both existing and new program activities should be assessed equally in the budgeting process.

Incremental and Decremental Budgeting Policy. Normally, the budgeting process begins with an estimate of revenues. For example, a museum's financial officer estimates that because of decreased grant support and because the current year's revenue did not meet projections, the total funds available next year will be 10 percent under the current level. As a result all attention is focused on how to cut 10 percent from expenses. A common response is that the 10 percent reduction (or 10 percent increase in good times!) should be equally shared by all budgetary units in the museum. This approach to budgeting is flawed, however, because it assumes that all items in the budget are equally worthwhile. A focus on the decrement or the increment, rather than on the needs and importance of each budgeted function, is distorting and likely to undermine the museum's strategic vision and goals. The notion of equal cuts can also foster mediocrity.

Late Preparation. Budgets are often prepared at about the time of the new fiscal year, long after key decisions such as committing to next season's shows or hiring new staff are made. To use the budget merely to record actions already taken is to obtain only a portion of the benefits that can be derived from the budgeting process. Budgets should be prepared and approved by the board as early as new programming decisions are being made.

Lack of Participation. Frequently, budgets are prepared by one member of the professional staff, usually the business officer or the director. Discussion of program needs and changing priorities is limited, and as a result, decisions are made without full information. Instead, all key staff and board members should participate in the budgeting process to ensure that the budget accurately reflects short-terms goals and plans. Full participation also encourages commitment to accomplishing those plans.

Key Variables Not Taken into Account. When preparing budgets, museums often fail to plan for the impact of variables both within and outside their control. Although some factors will be uncontrollable, a good rule of thumb is to scan as many environmental variables as possible with a view toward anticipating contingencies. For example, an exhibition planner may have cut expenses in preparing a major exhibition. The budgeters must consider whether this means that fewer visitors are likely to come and revenue will consequently be less than originally anticipated. Environmental factors such as a rainy season or a deep recession are also contingencies that can negatively affect the budget.

Lack of Consistency and Direction. At some museums, budgetary practices and procedures are not clearly defined. Budget forms and instructions should be standardized and understood by all who have responsibility for budget items. Once budgets are submitted, they should be reviewed by the museum director, the business manager, and appropriate board members. Meetings should be held between the budget reviewers and submitters to discuss and explain any necessary adjustments. Sometimes program managers set revenue budgets lower than expected to avoid the appearance of failure. They also set expense budgets high to attract more resources. It is up to the director and the board to create an environment in which all program managers will be motivated to project budgets as accurately as possible.

No Periodic Review. In some museums the budget is put to rest once it is completed and approved by the board. However, the budget should be used regularly, often monthly, as a tool to review how well the museum is doing in relation to the budgeted plan. By comparing actual expenses and revenues on a monthly or quarterly basis with those projected in the budget, the museum can determine possible trouble areas before they get out of hand.

Perceived Inflexibility. Budgets should not be considered as carved in stone. They have to be viewed as changeable because they must be adjusted periodically to take account of changing circumstances. Although a plan is of no value unless it has consistency and stability, change is a built-in factor. For example, an art museum's marketing manager will normally plan an advertising budget for the entire season, attributing certain costs to each exhibition planned for the year. Assume that one exhibition becomes an unexpected hit and its run is extended three extra weeks. The marketing manager may want to increase the advertising budget for that show to get the word out about its great success and its extended run. The cost for additional advertising can be allocated to the additional revenues it will help generate. It is this kind of flexibility in shifting resources as opportunities arise that should be built in, although shifts in particular areas must also be considered in relation to other areas and to the whole.

Types of Budgets

A museum may use one or more types of budgets, the most common of which are the *traditional (line-item) budget* and the *program budget.*

The Traditional (Line-Item) Budget. The line-item budget lists all expenses by their object or source: salaries, benefits, travel, supplies, phone, rent, postage, printing, and so on. Revenues are treated similarly and are listed in such categories as admission fees, membership dues, gift shop sales, and grants. The line-item budget is flawed in that it does not indicate which expenses created which revenues so that the real productivity of each function or program could be clearly known.

The Program Budget. The program, or project, budget distributes revenue and expenses across the museum's functional areas and programs, such as research, exhibitions, care of collections, promotion, and fundraising. This budget gives managers much more information than the line-item budget. For example, it may show that the lecture series is operating at a deficit but special events are operating at a surplus. Or it may show that fundraising expenses are too high for the amount of revenue they generate. Such information can lead to a reprioritization of various activities and programs and an analysis of how to increase the cost effectiveness of various projects.

In the program budget, a portion of staff salaries, office rent, utilities, and the like is allocated to each of the museum's main programs. For example, staff members must estimate the percentage of time spent on each program so that salary costs and a percentage of the space taken up by each activity can be allocated to a given program. Care must be taken, however, not to overdo the monitoring of each telephone call and postage stamp, as this causes frustration and wastes time. Close monitoring may be useful for short periods of time to get a rough approximation of what percentage of certain costs should be applied to each program. The expenses that cannot be reasonably applied to specific programs should be placed in a general administration category. Table 12.1 shows how a line-item budget and a program budget may be combined, displaying the distribution of costs among various items for each program.

The Budget as a Control Tool

In order for a budget to be a useful control mechanism, it must be broken down into periodic increments corresponding to the financial statements. Comparisons should then be made throughout the year between the budget and the financial statements. Most museums do not have resources to fall back on when it is determined that budgeted revenues have not been met or that expenses have been excessive. So the board and staff must be prepared to take action when the financial statements indicate a significant deviation from the budget. If the board and staff fail to take aggressive corrective action, the board is shirking its responsibility, and the budget has become a meaningless formality.

Budgeting Principles

There are several principles that should guide managers in formulating budgets.

Balanced Budget. As a nonprofit public service organization, a museum needs at least a *balanced budget* in order to operate and to remain solvent. A balanced budget means that the total budgeted revenue equals the amount budgeted for expenses. Managers may knowingly choose to operate certain programs at a financial loss. But when they do so, they must plan for other programs to compensate for expected shortfalls so that the overall budget is in balance.

Table 12.1. Example of a Program Budget and Line-Item Budget Combined.

	Salaries and Benefits	Rent and Utilities	Supplies and Materials	Travel	Printing and Postage	Total
Research						
Exhibit Design and Development						
Education						
Fundraising						
Total						

Budgeting a Deficit. Many museums incorporate a deficit—where total expenses exceed total revenues—into the budget. In such cases, funds for operations are provided by some form of indebtedness: loans, slowly paid bills, or "borrowing" from restricted funds. These are all obligations that the museum will eventually have to meet. Because the budget reflects the museum's goals, operating under a deficit means that the goals are not being fully realized.

Some museums create a deficit as a strategy for raising funds. They intentionally overspend and create a crisis that they hope will attract the needed financial support. Although this strategy may have been effective in the past, in the current era of accountability where good planning and fiscal prudence are highly valued, even long-standing loyal donors are no longer sympathetic to this approach.

Contingency, or Reserve, Fund. A contingency, or reserve, fund should be included in the budget plan. It has been recommended that between 5 and 10 percent of the museum's budget should be set aside for this account. The size of the contingency fund will vary according to the following factors:

- The size of the budget (larger museums can allocate a smaller percentage of revenues to the fund)
- The predictability of levels and sources of income (the less predictable the income, the larger the fund should be)
- The stability of the museum (the more unstable, the larger the fund should be)
- The extent to which expenditures are fixed in advance (the more flexibility, the less the fund can be)
- The experience of the current management (the less the experience, the greater the fund should be)

The reserve fund can be used in two ways. First, it can compensate for costly contingencies: the huge snowstorm the night of a major event that reduces ticket sales far below projected revenue, the unexpected legal expenses, the cash flow problem of bills to pay before income has come in. Second, at the end of the fiscal year, any money remaining in the fund becomes a reserve to be invested for future growth and to help carry the museum through future tough times.

Determining Costs. There are two common methods for determining program and activity costs. The first approach, *incremental budgeting*, is used for activities the museum has carried out in the past. It relies heavily on previous years' information about actual expenses and income. The manager investigates changes in the line items for each program, such as printing and paper costs, postage, advertising fees, and so on. If administrative costs are built into program budgets, salary and rent increases should also be included. Then a percentage is added to reflect the expected inflation in costs. Similarly, costs may be reduced incrementally. For example, a museum may choose to switch from a four-color brochure to a two-color brochure to save money. The second approach, *zero-based budgeting,* requires that each line item of the budget be established from scratch. This is always necessary for new projects, but it is also useful for reevaluating ongoing expenses. With a zero-based budget, staff members start with a budget of zero and must justify each amount they request.

The most effective method to determine costs is a combination of these two approaches. Previous expenses are extremely useful in planning the upcoming budget. Yet each budget item should be carefully examined to see if it can be reduced or if anticipated benefits can be achieved more efficiently some other way. Budgeters find it is most realistic to estimate costs on the high side. It is also important to account for the fact that new programs and activities will add to administrative costs such as staff, space, and equipment (Wolf, 1990).

Budgeters must also take into account both their fixed and variable expenses. Because variable costs are more adaptable than fixed costs, managers often balance their budgets by varying costs per production, service, or program. However, museums must not fail to recognize the interdependence between the income and expense sides of the variable budget. Suppose the first draft of a budget for a major fundraising event shows a deficit and so a decision is made to cut $100,000 from the expenses by replacing a major celebrity speaker with a someone less well known. When the original budget was planned, the ticket sales were predicated on the appearance of the celebrity speaker. Replacing this speaker with John Doe will certainly result in lower ticket income. However, in the revised budget, no reduction is made in projected ticket sales income. At year's end everyone is shocked that ticket sales did not meet projections, yet this could have been predicted by examining revenue and cost linkages. The most accurate and revealing method of budgeting variable costs is to compare them to projected income on a precise event-by-event basis (Fogel, 1988).

MARKETING IMPLEMENTATION

Sound budgeting and a brilliant strategic marketing plan count for little if they are not implemented properly. While strategy addresses the *what* and *why* of marketing activities, implementation addresses the *who, where, when,* and *how.* We define *marketing implementation* as *the process that turns marketing plans into action assignments and ensures that such assignments are executed in a manner that accomplishes the plan's stated objectives.* In the following sections we examine the diagnostic and implementation skills related to the effective implementation of marketing programs.

Diagnostic Skills

Many best-laid plans fail to see the light of day. Plans to innovate may fizzle out when management or board members are reluctant to commit funds to recommended projects. Plans to improve quality may get no further than some airy rhetoric. Without successful implementation a strategy represents merely lost time and frustration to those who develop and support it.

A major implication of this is that a strategy is not well conceived if it is not implementable. Therefore the factors that allow for successful implementation must be considered during the formulation process itself. A strategist must be able to look ahead and ask, Is this strategy workable? Can I make it happen? If this assessment yields an answer of no, or "only at an unacceptable risk," then the planning process must continue.

Marketing Implementation Skills

A set of skills must be practiced throughout the organization's functions, programs, and policies to achieve effective implementation. Managers must have *allocation skills,* which are used in budgeting resources (time, money, and personnel) to various functions and programs according to standards of efficiency and effectiveness. *Monitoring skills* are used in managing a system of controls to evaluate the results of marketing actions. *Organizing skills* are used in developing an effective working organization. Understanding the informal as well as formal organization is important to carrying out effective implementation. *Interacting skills* are used by managers to get things done by influencing others. This includes applying effective behavior patterns during the implementation process and effectively using the organization's power structure and leadership.

Behavior Patterns for Effective Implementation. A plan is a commitment to action—a commitment by people with their own ideas, attitudes, preferences, concerns, and needs. Steps must be taken to lend a sense of realism, motivation, and confidence that the new direction can be achieved. People must see the strategy's relevance, feel they are capable of implementing it, understand the required behaviors, know whether they have achieved the objective, and be rewarded for doing so. Hambrick and Cannella (1989) have identified several patterns of behavior for effective plan implementation (see Exhibit 12.1).

Internal and External Marketing Implementation. The Mint Museum of Art, in Charlotte, North Carolina, founded in 1936, is a highly respected museum with European and American paintings and world-class collections in European and English ceramics, pre-Columbian art, Andean ceramics, Spanish colonial paintings and decorative arts, and traditional North Carolina crafts and folk art. Until the early 1990s, the museum functioned in a relatively narrow, inward-looking way. It focused largely on art collectors, socially prominent families, patrons, and

○○○○○

Exhibit 12.1. Steps for Effective Implementation.

Obtain broad-based inputs and participation at the formulation stage. Widespread participation helps to secure intellectual and social commitment to the new course of action and to highlight the major issues expected to arise during implementation.

Carefully assess the obstacles to implementation. There are both internal and external obstacles to consider:

- *Internal obstacles.* The success of a strategy depends on the material and human resources within the organization. The organization may have the wrong configurations of systems and procedures, or inadequate human resources or financial backing. Equally important, there may be political resistance from those who stand to lose something of value if the new strategy is implemented, ideological resistance from those who believe the new strategy violates deeply held values, or blind resistance from those who are intolerant or afraid of change itself.

- *External obstacles.* Management must also consider the possibility of external resistance from contributors, government agencies, audience segments, competitors, suppliers, or other parties. Opposition from any of these groups may limit or undermine the expected benefits of the strategy.

Make early moves across the full array of implementation levers—resource commitments, policies and programs, structure, rewards, and people.

- *Resource commitments.* The commitment of resources is crucial to the success of any new strategy, for it signals true commitment to the strategy. Many strategies fail because resources are not decisively allocated to support the strategy.

- *Policies and programs.* The strategy must be translated into concrete action plans and assignments within the organization's various departments. Within the marketing area, the strategy should be converted into discrete plans and policies in the areas of product development, pricing, promotion, distribution, and service.

- *Structure.* The new strategy will often entail developing new groups and relationships. New information systems may also be required to improve decision making and maximize the likelihood of successful implementation.

- *Rewards.* The impact of incentives and rewards must be factored in. Rewards can be formal, such as incentive schemes, promotions, or commissions; or informal, such as private or public pats on the back, a sense of pride, and enthusiasm. People often work in nonprofit organizations for the intangible rewards they receive; if these are missing, motivation may be lacking.

- *People.* Some plans require special skills for their implementation. Additions to the team, training and development programs, personal coaching and counseling, and replacement of individuals are among the options available. Additionally, all persons involved in implementing the strategy must have the personal characteristics of being able to deal with messy problems, willingness to work hard, creativity, flexibility, and tolerance for ambiguity.

Sell, sell, sell the strategy to everyone who matters—upward, downward, and outward. Managers, staff, and board executives must be sold on the merits and viability of a strategy. External stakeholders such as membership groups, business sponsors, the media, and regulatory agencies must also be sold on supporting the plan. These external parties are no different from insiders in their potential for skepticism and anxiety about the new strategy. By keeping these parties well informed, unfavorable reaction can be greatly reduced or eliminated.

Fine-tune, adjust, and respond as events and trends arise. Be prepared to adjust the strategy for changes in the environment or behavior of affected individuals or groups. Because all contingencies and eventualities cannot be envisioned at the outset, a strategy should come with broad guidance systems but should allow for spontaneity and responsiveness as well.

Source: Hambrick and Cannella, 1989.

○○○○○

individuals active in the arts. The museum was less attentive to the general public and its visitors. It had little connection with the surrounding urban and suburban communities—in fact, its entrance was on a sheltered street in an affluent neighborhood, and many people perceived it as inaccessible. Building a new museum wing in the 1980s, however, led to creating a new entrance that opened on a broad, well-traveled street.

On July 1, 1992, the Mint Museum transformed itself from a department of the city government into a private, nonprofit association. This change in governance was just one part of a complex and thorough-going modernization. In 1993, the museum engaged in a far-reaching and intensive planning process that culminated in board approval of a five-year strategic plan. The Mint Museum had committed itself to a transformation that was to take place in a relatively short span of time and required several parallel initiatives and planning processes: redefining the museum's mission, reconfiguring its internal organization and culture, reaching out to its community, developing its membership, reinstalling its permanent collections and redeploying its programs, altering its image and communications programs, and building partnerships with schools, businesses, and other community organizations (interview with Bruce Evans, Feb. 23, 1996).

The Mint Museum's transformation is a good example of the special characteristics of strategic planning and marketing in the context of museums: the close connection between external marketing (to citizens in the community, museum visitors and members, political and business leaders, donors, and sponsors) and internal marketing (to staff, management, board of directors, and volunteers) and, indeed, the need to reshape to one degree or another the internal culture as a condition for reaching external publics effectively. Before the museum could launch the planning, management had to engage staff, the board, and volunteers in a concept of change and transformation and the process involved and get them invested at each step along the way. Evans, director and CEO of the Mint Museum of Art since 1991, observed that "[A]s the new director, the one thing I didn't want to do was to come in and say, 'Here's my agenda.' I told the staff that I wasn't going to articulate a vision for the museum until it was ours. . . . We co-created a vision, but I had no idea that's what it was all about. Change for us was inevitable. It was simply a question of whether it was managed, positive change or negative, reactionary change" (quoted in American Association of Museums, Part 2, *Perspectives,* 1995, p. 3).

The Mint Museum's internal and external marketing planning is proceeding with considerable commitment, energy, and achievement. The early signs of accomplishment are positive: by the mid-1990s, the museum had received a $1.25 million grant from the Lila Wallace–Reader's Digest Fund to support the museum's community outreach. The museum has experienced major membership growth and now has the third-largest volunteer group of any U.S. art museum. It has obtained a significant increase in corporate sponsorship, established a community advisory committee, and conducted an image-building program that won media praise.

Power Relationships in Organizations

Any consideration of implementing plans and fitting them to organizations has to take into account the element of power and power relationships in organizations. The effective marketing organization acknowledges power and leadership and deploys them effectively to achieve its ends. An influential factor in all organizations, power can be defined as the ability to get another individual, group, or entire organization to do something that might not be done otherwise (Stern and El-Ansary, 1992). Power is often associated with negative concepts, such as strong-arm tactics or political clout. However, it has a much broader meaning. Power is the result of possessing and controlling resources valued by another party. A has power over B to the extent that A controls a resource valued by B. Conversely, interdependence occurs when each controls a resource that is valued by the other. Power is not entirely determined by a person's formal position in the organization's hierarchy. Several types of resource-based power can be distinguished in museums and other organizations.

Reward power is based on a person's ability to provide valued resources in the form of rewards, material incentives, promotions, or recognition in exchange for a desired action.

Coercive power is based on the threat to punish if a party did not take a desired action. Coercive power should be viewed as a last resort; it generally produces poorer results in the long run than other types of power.

Expert power is held by those who possess valued information, knowledge, or ability. Outside consultants and other specialists are called on from time to time for expert power.

Authoritative power is held by those empowered to make decisions by an organizational or a social system. A museum's director, for example, has the power to hire and fire employees, and a board of trustees has the power to hire and fire the director.

Referent power is held by persons and organizations when they are highly respected and admired. Referent power in museums resides in a variety of individuals: members, the board of trustees, the chair of a fundraising campaign, the head of the membership group. Individuals with referent power help museums strengthen their connections with the community, government agencies, and businesses.

Leadership

Effective leadership requires an understanding of all these sources of power and the levels at which they are operating in a given situation. A leader of a museum has two primary tasks: *external leadership* (the ability to translate external needs into an internal vision) and *internal leadership* (the ability to translate vision into employee action). The leader must understand employees, motivate them, and point the way to accomplishing the organization's goals.

Leadership is not just a responsibility of top managers. Every employee must *be* empowered and *feel* empowered to think and behave as a leader within his or her domain. To be empowered, an employee needs a full understanding of the museum's mission, goals, and constraints and must also be given freedom for a certain amount of independent decision making and room for a certain amount of learning-process error. The museum will then reflect the qualities of leadership in all departments and at all levels. In other words, the museum's leadership capability is the sum of all its individual leaders' capabilities.

An important characteristic of good leadership is the capacity for change. Managers must show a capacity to learn from past experiences, the ability for self-assessment, and the ability to engage in continual learning. Strong leaders supply a vision, change or reinforce the organization's culture, have the determination to chart new directions and devote resources to new projects and services, and have the courage to take risks and abandon failing initiatives and programs. A leader knows that good ideas are meaningless unless they can be translated into action.

MARKETING CONTROL

Performance is the ultimate test of any organization. The Peter F. Drucker Foundation for Nonprofit Management (1993, p. 39) says, "The discipline of thinking through what results will be demanded of the nonprofit institution can protect it from squandering its resources." This final step in marketing planning, measurement, evaluation of performance, and adjustment of strategy and tactics, should be kept in mind throughout the process. When museum managers embark on various strategies, their information is necessarily limited. As experience and further knowledge are gained, strategies and tactics should be evaluated in light of new information. Frequent monitoring, evaluation, and control will validate the current approach, stimulate modification of the approach or its goals, or encourage its abandonment altogether.

An organization should establish three levels of performance control or evaluation: *short-range,* or *periodic, control* to assess progress and effectiveness of operational marketing plans on a daily, weekly, monthly, or quarterly basis; *midrange control,* usually conducted annually; and *long-range,* or *strategic, control,* usually every three to five years.

Periodic and Annual Control

The control process for each program should be driven by a *management by objectives* approach. Four steps are involved. First, management sets monthly or quarterly goals. Second, it monitors marketplace performance. Third, it determines the causes of serious performance deviations. Fourth, it takes corrective action to close the gaps between goals and performance: changing the action program or the goals or even dropping the program. Too often, management drains human and financial resources from productive efforts in an attempt to salvage an ineffective project. It is far better to abandon an ineffective strategy early than to continue it unproductively. The time and expenses already invested are *sunk costs,* that is, they are historical, *not* recoverable, and should *not* be considered when evaluating the best course of action.

Management starts the control process by developing aggregate goals for the planning period—for example, increasing the number of museum memberships or raising corporate donations to the museum. It is then up to the marketing manager to determine meaningful criteria for measuring achievement as well as the conditions for success. For example, the membership department may have specific renewal and new member goals. During the relevant period, managers check the reports of results against the goals, and if necessary, take corrective actions.

Control Tools

Three common quantitative control tools used by management to evaluate results are sales and revenue analysis, expense analysis, and ratio analysis. Two useful qualitative measures are customer satisfaction tracking and a marketing effectiveness-efficiency review.

Sales and Revenue Analysis. Sales and revenue analysis measures and evaluates actual sales and revenue achieved in relation to goals (set by season, specific exhibition, target audience, and so on). For example, the marketing manager might wish to determine if early membership renewals are meeting current goals and how the current figures compare to those of the previous season. If the goals are not being met, the manager might decide to increase direct-mail or telemarketing efforts to the target group.

Expense Analysis. The budget can help managers to determine if the organization is setting reasonable expense targets and to track actual spending and receipts against planned targets. For example, suppose a museum categorizes its membership drive expenses into the following categories:

Category	Cost	Number of Members	Cost per Member
Early renewal	$10,952	3,400	$3.22
Official renewal	10,593	4,200	2.67
Telemarketing	61,391	3,157	19.45
New members	54,771	1,483	36.93

Note that new members are the most costly to acquire. But if they renew each year for several years, the initial recruitment cost is well worth it.

All variances between actual and budgeted performance are signals that demand attention. Positive variance, with actual spending lower than planned, may result from poor performance in program implementation or from lower than anticipated expenditures. Negative variance may result from cost overruns or from lower-than-expected revenues. Either of these variances, positive or negative, can signal problems that need to be dealt with in a timely manner to avoid serious financial problems.

Ratio Analysis. A museum needs to analyze various ratios to compare monthly, quarterly, or yearly progress and determine relative effectiveness and efficiency. For example, a museum can analyze the *ratio of admissions revenue to total revenue and contributed support* to see whether admissions revenue for the year increased or decreased as a percentage of total combined earned revenue and contributed support. A key ratio to watch is *marketing expense to sales.* For example, a marketing manager might track separately ratios of telemarketing expense to sales, advertising expense to sales, marketing research expense to sales, and promotions expense to sales. A museum might also wish to compare the *expenses and revenues of various programs to total museum expenses and revenues* to determine whether programs are receiving a growing or dwindling budget share.

Consumer Satisfaction Tracking. The preceding control measures are largely financial and quantitative. They are important but not sufficient. Also needed are qualitative measures that monitor changing levels of consumer preference and satisfaction so that management can take action before problems arise. The main customer satisfaction tracking systems are the following:

Complaint and suggestion systems. Market-oriented organizations record, analyze, and respond to all written and oral complaints that come from consumers. The complaints are tabulated, and management attempts to correct whatever is causing the most frequent types of complaints. If the complaints are program related, this information is shared with the relevant decision makers. Market-oriented organizations try to maximize the opportunities for consumer complaining so that management can get a more complete picture of customer reactions to the products and services. Systems should be developed so that individuals who have regular contact with customers, such as front desk personnel, guards, and telemarketers, will record and report all complaints and suggestions.

Member panels. Some organizations organize panels of consumers who agree to communicate their attitudes periodically via telephone calls or mail questionnaires. These panels are more representative of the range of consumer attitudes than the complaint and suggestion systems.

Mystery shoppers (ghost shoppers). Museums can hire an individual to pose as a visitor in various areas of the museum and report on favorable and unfavorable experiences with services. Reports can extend to all aspects of the museum organization, including orientation services, security guards, exhibition design, rest rooms, gift shops, and parking facilities.

Customer satisfaction surveys. Museums can mail periodic surveys to a large sample of visitors, asking them to evaluate friendliness, service, quality, and other aspects of interest. This system allows management to identify weaknesses in customer service and motivate employees to provide better service.

Marketing Efficiency and Effectiveness Review. The final step in the annual control process is to evaluate how effectively and efficiently the museum has accomplished its goals. Marketing effectiveness is not necessarily revealed by current visitation levels and revenue performance. Good results might be due to being in the right place at the right time rather than to having effective marketing management. Marketing improvements might boost results from good to excellent. Conversely, a marketing department might have poor results in spite of excellent marketing planning due to unforeseen external factors.

The Peter F. Drucker Foundation for Nonprofit Management (1993) recommends that organizations evaluate *effectiveness* by having managers ask the following questions:

- If we weren't already doing this, if we were not already committed to this, would we start doing it now?
- Are we working in the right areas? Do we need to change our focus?
- What have we learned and what do we recommend?
- What, if anything, should we do differently?

In evaluating the *efficiency* of specific projects, managers should raise such specific questions as these:

- Are higher revenue projections achievable?
- What additional sources of revenue are possible: raising fees, exerting extra efforts on existing activities, initiating new programs, providing new services?
- Can expenditures be reduced by cutting certain costs?
- Can alternative approaches be used to improve efficiency and thereby lower costs without affecting quality?

In evaluating one program activity against another, the museum board and the staff should be careful in applying the criterion of cost effectiveness. It might be useful for evaluating and comparing methods (direct mail versus print advertising, for example), yet from a larger perspective, the museum's mission might dictate that managers should carry on activities and programs that are *not* cost effective in themselves—educational programs, conservation projects, and so on. The primary criterion should relate to the museum's mission, purposes, and goals (Wolf, 1990).

STRATEGIC CONTROL

From time to time, museums need to undertake a critical review of their overall marketing effectiveness. Marketing is an area where rapid obsolescence of objectives, policies, strategies, and programs is a constant possibility. Each museum should periodically reassess its overall approach to the marketplace. An important tool for this process is the marketing audit.

The Marketing Audit

The marketing audit assists managers in assessing and improving organizational performance. We define it as *a comprehensive, systematic, independent, and periodic examination of an organization's marketing environment, objectives, strategies, and activities with a view of determining problem areas and opportunities and recommending a plan of action to improve the organization's strategic marketing performance.* A marketing audit has four main characteristics.

Comprehensive. The marketing audit covers all the marketing issues facing an organization, not just one or two prejudged trouble spots. It can shed critical light on the relationships of the parts to one another and to the whole. The value of a truly comprehensive audit becomes apparent when it identifies unanticipated strengths or weaknesses, often to the surprise of management.

Systematic. The marketing audit involves an orderly sequence of diagnostic steps covering the organization's marketing environment and specific marketing activities. It is structured to start with the issues that are broadest and have the most general organizational impact and then proceeds to cover the parts of organizations and program and functional areas. Most important, the diagnosis is followed by a corrective action plan with both short- and long-run proposals to improve marketing effectiveness.

Independent. The marketing audit is normally conducted by an outside consultant or an inside party who has sufficient experience, credibility, and independence to attain top management's confidence and the needed objectivity. Many museums, however, tend to have little or no budget for outside consultants and also tend to have small staffs who work closely together and leave little room for an independent insider. In such a situation, separate audits can be undertaken by well-informed members of management and the board of directors. Their combined information can be analyzed and discussed in a committee of the whole, with a primary goal of maintaining honesty and objectivity.

Periodic. The marketing audit should be carried out periodically, not only when there is a crisis. Regular audits allow the museum not only to react effectively to pressing problems but also to be proactive and show continual improvements. Ironically, some organizations face crises partly because they failed to review their marketing operation during good times.

A marketing audit may be requested by a funding agency or a governing body but is most often requested by a museum's management. Because the audit is like a photograph and represents the museum at a particular point in time, some audit processes should be ongoing (for a series of photographs), and others should be repeated as situations change or new information becomes available.

Marketing Audit Components

The marketing audit has the following six major components:

- *Marketing environment audit.* Analyzes major macroenvironmental forces and trends affecting the key elements of the museum's task environment: visitors, donors, members, competitors, and other constituencies.

- *Marketing strategy audit.* Reviews the museum's marketing objectives and marketing strategy to appraise how well they are adapted to the current and forecasted marketing environment.

- *Marketing organization audit.* Evaluates the capability of the marketing department or museum management as a whole for implementing the necessary strategy for the forecasted environment.

- *Marketing systems audit.* Assesses the quality of the museum's various systems for gathering information, planning, and control.

- *Marketing productivity audit.* Examines the profitability of different marketing units within the museum and the cost effectiveness of different marketing programs.

- *Marketing function audit.* Makes in-depth evaluations of major marketing-mix components: products (exhibitions, educational programs), prices (admission fees, membership dues), distribution (ease of access to the museum facility, quality of museum materials used in classrooms, quality and scope of the museum's Web site), advertising, sales promotion, and public relations.

Exhibit 12.2 shows the features, sections, and questions used in a marketing audit.

OOOOO

Exhibit 12.2. Marketing Audit Guide.

Part I: Marketing Environment Audit
Macroenvironment

A. Demographic
1. What major demographic developments and trends pose opportunities or threats for this museum?
2. What actions, if any, has the museum taken in response to these developments?

B. Economic
1. What major developments and trends in income, prices, savings, and interest rates are affecting the museum?
2. What major changes are taking place in the sources and amounts of contributed income (that is, from individuals, corporations, foundations), grant income (that is, from public authorities and agencies), and earned income?
3. What actions has the museum taken in response to these trends and developments?

C. Political
1. What recent legislation and regulatory rules have affected this museum?
2. What federal, state, and local agencies should be monitored for future actions?
3. What actions has the museum taken in response to these developments?

D. Cultural
1. What changes are occurring in consumer lifestyles, tastes, values, leisure-time activities, and so on that might affect this museum?
2. What changes are occurring in ethnic and cultural communities that can affect this museum?
3. What actions has the museum taken in response to these developments?

Task Environment

A. Consumers, funders, and other constituencies
1. What is happening to overall market size, growth, and geographical distribution? Have the audience base and the membership base been growing, shrinking, or staying the same over the past several years?
2. How do the visitor base and the membership base compare to the local and national averages for similar museums?
3. What are the major market segments? What are their expected rates of growth? Which are high-opportunity and low-opportunity segments?
4. How much of the visitor's volume is repeat versus first-time? What percent of consumers can be classified as light, moderate, or heavy users of this museum's services?
5. How do current consumers and potential consumers rate this museum and how do they rate the competitors, particularly with respect to reputation, program quality, service, cost, and personnel?
6. How do different segments of consumers make their leisure-time activity decisions?
7. How do consumers find out about and decide to try this museum's offerings?
8. What new values, benefits, and satisfactions are being sought by consumers in this museum's market? Can you prioritize these consumer needs?
9. What actions have been taken by this museum to meet these consumer needs and preferences? What benefits does this museum offer to each segment? To private and public donors and benefactors? To volunteers?

Exhibit 12.2. Marketing Audit Guide, Cont'd.

10. What publics (for example, constituencies, media, government, corporations, and so on) represent particular opportunities or problems for this museum?
11. What steps has the museum taken to fully benefit from public opportunities and to avert potential crises?

B. Competitors
   1. Who are the direct and indirect competitors of this museum?
   2. What are the objectives and strategies of each major competitor? What are their strengths and weaknesses?
   3. What trends can be foreseen in future competition and in substitutes for the products and programs that this museum offers?

Part II: Marketing Objectives and Strategy Audit

A. Museum objectives
   1. Is the museum's mission clearly stated in market-oriented terms? Is the mission feasible in terms of the museum's resources and capabilities? How well is the mission understood by the museum members? Are there major changes needed in this museum's mission in the next five years?
   2. What are this museum's strengths and weaknesses?
   3. Are the marketing objectives and goals appropriate, given the museum's competitive position, resources, and opportunities?
   4. Are the marketing objectives clear-cut?

B. Marketing Strategy
   1. What is the core marketing strategy? Is it a sound strategy?
   2. Has the museum established both short-term and long-term goals?
   3. Are adequate resources budgeted to accomplish the marketing goals?
   4. Are the museum's marketing resources allocated optimally to prime market segments, geographical areas, and the museum's major offerings?
   5. Are the marketing resources allocated optimally to the major elements of the marketing mix, including quality, service, marketing staff, communications, promotion, public relations, pricing decisions, and distribution channels?
   6. Does the museum carry out periodic reviews of the efficacy of its operations and evaluations of its resource allocation decisions? How and with what results?

Part III: Marketing Organization Audit

1. Is there a high-level marketing officer in the museum with sufficient responsibility and authority over those museum activities that affect consumers and markets?
2. Are there good communications and working relations between marketing and other key functional areas?
3. Are there any personnel carrying out marketing tasks who need more training, motivation, supervision, or evaluation? How much and what kind of outside consultation and training in marketing does the staff get?

Part IV: Marketing Systems Audit

A. Marketing information system
   1. What types of information does the museum possess about its markets, consumers, and other publics?
   2. Is marketing research being adequately used by managers? Do managers understand the types and capabilities of various market research techniques? Do managers have the skills to develop and evaluate market research functions in house? If not, are they aware of the resources available for contracting out this function?

Exhibit 12.2. Marketing Audit Guide, Cont'd.

3. Is the marketing information system producing accurate, sufficient, and timely information about market developments?
B. Marketing planning system
   1. Is the marketing planning system well conceived and effective?
   2. Is market forecasting and market-potential measurement soundly carried out?
C. Marketing control system
   1. Are the control procedures (monthly, quarterly, seasonally, and so on) adequate to ensure that annual plan goals are being achieved?
   2. Is provision made to analyze periodically the potential of different products, markets, and geographical areas?
   3. Is provision made to periodically examine and validate various marketing costs?
   4. What quality control procedures does the museum have?

Part V: Marketing Productivity Audit

A. Revenue-potential analysis
   1. What is the revenue potential of the museum's various products (that is, memberships, ticket purchases, special events and programs, food service, site rental fees, gift shop sales, and so on)?
   2. What is the revenue potential of various target markets?
B. Cost-effectiveness analysis
   1. Do any marketing activities appear to have excessive costs? Has a cost-benefit analysis been made for each type of marketing expenditure? Are expenditures tracked regularly? Can cost-reducing steps be taken? Can certain money be better spent in other areas?
   2. What are the museum's sources of contributed income? What are the sources of grant income? Earned income? How have the percentages of support from the various sources changed over recent years? How much time and effort does the marketing function expend for each of these sources? Are these expenses justified in terms of the return?

Part VI: Marketing Function Audit

A. Product
   1. What are the product line objectives? Are these objectives sound? Is the current product line meeting these objectives?
   2. Are there particular products or services that should be phased out?
   3. Are there new products or services that are worth adding?
   4. Are any products able to benefit from quality, feature, or style improvement?
B. Price
   1. What are the pricing objectives, policies, strategies, and procedures? To what extent are prices set on sound cost, demand, and competitive criteria? What are the procedures for establishing and reviewing pricing policy?
   2. Is pricing demand oriented? Are there variations by market segments, time of use, number of exhibitions and programs attended?
   3. What discounts to the basic fee structure are offered and with what rationale? What discounts are offered by competitors?
   4. Are there joint pricing arrangements with other museums and with educational and cultural organizations in the area? What are the results of these joint pricing arrangements in terms of audience, revenue flows, and so on?

Exhibit 12.2. Marketing Audit Guide, Cont'd.

---

5. Do the consumers see the museum's prices as being in line with the perceived value of its offerings?
6. What short-term promotional pricing policies are used and with what effect?

C. Distribution
1. Are the museum's public spaces the best locations for its various exhibits? Are current venues adequate and appropriate for the type of product the museum is offering?
2. How can the current space be improved in terms of creating ambience and comfort for consumers? What steps have been taken in this regard? What feedback is received from consumers regarding deficits and improvements?
3. List the museum's objectives in terms of physical facility improvements, both in the short term and long term, and comparing costs to expected benefits.
4. Should the museum extend the locations in which it reaches consumers? Should there be other locations for its core exhibitions and public programs? Other locations for auxiliary services such as gift shops and restaurants?
5. How effective is the distribution of offerings to schools? How cost-effective are electronic and digital channels?
6. Are information, ticket reservations, and payment decentralized and convenient to target audiences?
7. What other resources are available to the museum for developing earned income through distribution (for example, royalty fees for exhibitions, print and electronic publications, educational materials, tangible products, and so on)?

D. Advertising, sales promotion, public relations, and database marketing
1. What are the museum's advertising objectives? Are they sound? Feasible?
2. Is the right amount of resources being spent on advertising? How is the advertising budget determined? Is cost effectiveness tracked on a regular basis?
3. Are the ad themes and copy effective? What do consumers and the public think about the advertising? Does it generate interest? Motivation? Visits?
4. Are the advertising media well chosen? Are media results monitored and reviewed on a regular basis?
5. Does the museum have a paid or volunteer advertising agency? What functions does the ad agency perform for the museum?
6. Is promotion used effectively? Are a variety of promotional tactics being used, such as direct mail, telemarketing, cooperative efforts, and so on? Is promotion designed for and directed to different target markets?
7. Is there a sound public relations program? Are public relations opportunities regularly and frequently taken into consideration?
8. Does the organization gather rich information about visitors, members, and donors that can be used to customize programs and communications to specific individuals and groups?
9. What system is used to handle consumer inquiries resulting from advertising and promotion? What follow-up is done? Does the museum engage in internal marketing to encourage staff and volunteers to be responsive to inquiries, public concerns, and other issues?
0. What is done about negative feedback from consumers? How are complaints dealt with? What kind of follow-up is undertaken?

○○○○○

SUMMARY

Museums that strive to be consumer oriented and market responsive have to have organizational structures and cultures that support the consumer point of view and marketing principles and methods. Some marketing professionals regard marketing as infusing the entire organization, which is assumed to reflect the consumer perspective; others take a more limited view of marketing as a single management function, although they might concede that consumer and marketing perspectives should have some effect on all programs and operations. Many museums lack the resources to create a marketing staff or hire an outside marketing expert. Yet even these smaller museums can train their managers and staff in marketing principles and methods, and nothing stands in the way of any museum embracing the points of view of visitors and members. A museum's marketing plan will examine the existing market situation; analyze trends, opportunities, and threats in the surrounding environment; formulate goals and strategies; define action programs and budgets to carry out goals and plans; and establish monitoring and evaluation systems to determine whether marketing goals and strategies are being achieved and, if not, what corrective actions can be taken. Marketing audits are the means for museums to ascertain systematically and comprehensively whether marketing plans are appropriate and are being implemented successfully.

Securing the Future of Museums

*Marketing is so basic that it cannot be considered a separate function.
It is the whole business seen from the point of view of its final result,
that is, from the customer's point of view.*
—Peter F. Drucker

*The fourth floor of the American Museum of Natural History
was the shrine, the principal magic place, the sanctum sanctorum
of my youth. I first visited with my father at age five and
decided right then to dedicate my life to paleontology.*
—Stephen Jay Gould

Museums are precious institutions that define, record, and sustain civilization. Without museums, humankind would hardly understand its past, cope with its present, advance in its future, and enjoy and learn from transcendent experiences of beauty, history, nature, and the universe. Yet museums are not guaranteed an existence. Some museums have had to close their doors, and others are likely to face this prospect in the future. The hard fact is that if a museum cannot demonstrate its value to its patrons and the public, it is not likely to garner the resources to survive.

This concluding chapter reviews directions for museums in the future and proposals for action. Some proposals are managerial: controlling costs and seeking collaborations and partnerships. Others involve marketing. We will review the role of marketing for museums and make the case for collaborations, alliances, and partnerships. Nothing in these proposals poses a threat to museum missions, professional standards, or autonomy.

Museums operate in a particular fiduciary and legal framework. Unlike performing arts and other cultural organizations (but akin to libraries), museums re responsible for collecting objects—art, artifacts, specimens, and other ms—that collectively represent a record of the natural world; or the heritage people, a nation, or a community; or the expression of art and creativity as iced across the span of human history. Museums are obliged to preserve s so that future generations can enjoy and learn from them and under-here they came from. The distinctive museum enterprise of maintaining, preserving, interpreting, and exhibiting collections is a costly undertaking, in many cases requiring both government subsidy and private support. Museums are primarily mission driven, although they are finding synergy and reinforcement in drawing on the ideas, experiences, and solutions that marketing offers. Because the museum mission, broadly speaking, is educational and public service oriented, museum operations and programs aim for inclusiveness, accessibility, and use by a broad and diverse range of people.

One more observation is germane. Museums come in many different forms and sizes and have many different missions. They are singular rather than uniform. They share certain obligations, purposes, and goals, yet each institution is a distinctive organization, reflecting specific historical developments, circumstances, audiences, and resources.

MUSEUMS AND MARKETING

We have defined marketing as a process in which individuals and groups obtain what they need and desire through creating and exchanging products, services, experiences, and ultimately value with others (Kotler, 1997, p. 15). Every manner of organization is involved in marketing because it is involved in persuading others of its value and exchanging things of value with others.

Once a museum determines that marketing principles and tools have applicability for their missions and goals, staff responsible for a museum's plan for marketing will plan for marketing in one or more of the categories discussed throughout this book: existing product marketing, new product marketing, distribution marketing, service marketing, sales and promotion marketing, price and donor marketing, and brand marketing. Marketing managers, depending on the museum's objectives and strategies, will shape the "marketing mix," the best combination of tools available that can bring in visitors, members, and donors.

Museums must manage their existing offerings—their collections, exhibitions, educational programs, and services—in ways that maintain quality and appeal. Museum offerings, like commercial products, can decline in quality or grow stale over time. Audience expectations for exhibit design or interpretation can change over time. There are instances of museum exhibitions that have sat unchanged for thirty or forty years and visitors to them become apathetic, bored, or hostile.

Museums compete with other organizations in terms of quality, availability, and price, and so they must continually add value to their offerings. Members and active visitors expect new programs and new exhibits, and these are incentives to return frequently. Visitors expect new features and services periodically, such as seating areas for relaxation and better parking lot lighting or even valet parking. Added benefits are also enhancements for which certain visitor segments are willing to pay a higher price. The Museum Campus, in Chicago, slated to open in June 1998, has to work very hard at positioning itself and adding value in relation to competitors, including a similar "campus" at Navy Pier and in Grant Park along the lakefront.

Staff also have to find the distribution channels that will make the museum's offerings more accessible and convenient for different groups. Museums not only work to attract students to their buildings, for example; they also send staff to visit schools, sponsor off-site nature camps and retreats, and display collections over the Internet because distributed offerings reach more·of the public outside the museum and can then bring more of the public into the museum.

As museums build membership and attract newcomers, they will want to redouble their efforts at service marketing as well as at developing new programs and strengthening existing ones.

As museums tackle fundraising and revenue raising, they will have to increase their skills in sales and promotion marketing. Staff will need to know how to use advertising, direct mail, and telemarketing; how to make persuasive presentations to interested groups; and how to use mass and specialized media for reaching targeted audiences. Museums also have to determine how to price their many varied offerings, from setting appropriate admission fees to establishing membership fee levels and benefits to pricing gift shop sales. And museums have to set a price and value for donations, gifts, and other support from corporations and individuals.

Finally, museums will strive to develop a distinctive and attractive image and identity. Brand names and images are the strongest identities of all, and brands can serve museums just as well as they serve companies and commercial products. Once established, the image behind a brand name will communicate qualities that people respect and value and will want to turn to often. In some cases, a museum's brand identity is the incentive for people to enter the museum and experience its offerings. Brands are promises; for museums, they serve as invitations. Brands enable people to act quickly with little need for additional information or analysis.

These various areas of marketing represent a set of principles and tools, a framework for planning and development, that museum professionals can employ in building a secure future for their museums.

FUTURE DIRECTIONS FOR MUSEUMS

they face the future, museums can consider several possible directions and can pursue a certain path in response to challenges, threats, crises, or op- ities. One direction involves organizational changes of one kind or an- second involves modifications or additions, particularly in relation to programming, within an existing organizational framework. Organizational change for some museums has involved downsizing and reducing operations as a means to deal with financial pressures. Other museums, like the Guggenheim, in New York City, have gone international, establishing museums in several countries. Yet other museums have changed their governance and legal status, moving from public to private or vice versa. The Dutch National Museums were transformed between 1989 and 1995 from government-owned institutions into quasi-private organizations. A growing number of museums, including the San Jose Museum of Art and the Whitney Museum of American Art, are establishing partnerships—sharing resources, pursuing joint marketing activities, undertaking joint purchasing arrangements, and so on. Some museums are merging, as the Laguna Art Museum and the Newport Harbor Art Museum did in forming the Orange County Museum of Art, in California. Some museums have substantially changed their mission, collections, organizational structure, or corporate culture, such as the Parrish Museum, in Southampton, Long Island, New York.

Museums are also making changes within their existing organizations. First, they can move toward broadening their offerings and building appeal to a wider public, as the Johnson County Museums, in Shawnee, Kansas, have done. Second, museums can move in the direction of building the strongest possible links to their surrounding communities; the Corcoran Gallery of Art, in Washington, D.C., is a good example. With such support, museums are in a position to grow; without it, their prospects are limited. Another direction, distinct from the community direction though not exclusive from it, is for a museum to become a destination for tourists. Cleveland's Rock and Roll Museum and Hall of Fame has attracted tourists and also boosted the appeal of other attractions in the Cleveland area. Museums that have succeeded in building community support are in a position to turn to the community for added support when it is needed. A case in point is the successful 1988 action by the Missouri Historical Society, in St. Louis, to win citizen support in an election to include the museum in the local cultural tax district. Similarly, Durham, North Carolina, citizens in the mid-1990s approved a $3.5 million city bond issue to help support expansion at the North Carolina Museum of Life and Science.

Museums are also recognizing the importance of upgrading their facilities and services, improving comfort and user-friendliness. The Oregon Museum of Science & Industry, in Portland, for example, created areas for families to sit in and for grandparents to relax in. Other museums, in broadening their image, mission, and audience, are moving in the direction of becoming centers of contemporary thinking and problem solving, relating their collections to present-day concerns and future aspirations. The Missouri Historical Society is a leading example of a U.S. museum seeking to make itself relevant to its urban publics now and in the evolving future. The museum's exhibits and programs focus on the neighborhoods and reflect diverse ethnic, religious, generational, and social class perspectives.

COLLABORATING WITH OTHER INSTITUTIONS

Museums are discovering the value of engaging in collaborations and partnerships with a variety of other organizations—museums and other cultural organizations, educational institutions, businesses, foundations, and government agencies.

Partnering with Museums and Other Cultural Organizations

On January 24, 1997, the *New York Times* ran a quarter-page ad announcing the debut of *See China in Philadelphia,* scheduled to run for three months in Philadelphia. The exhibition was a collaboration of three Philadelphia museums to celebrate Chinese art. The Franklin Institute offered daily demonstrations of ancient Chinese craft techniques by contemporary artisans invited to Philadelphia from the People's Republic of China. The Philadelphia Museum of Art offered its extensive collection of Chinese porcelain and other ancient Chinese art. The University of Pennsylvania's Museum of Archaeology and Anthropology offered its majestic rotunda and its collection of Chinese art. In addition, the three museums partnered with two participating hotels, USAir, Amtrak, and National Car Rental to cosponsor this event. Similarly, in 1996, a group of Indianapolis museums, led by the Indianapolis Art Center and the Children's Museum of Indianapolis, created a critical mass of programming devoted to the theme of creativity in individual lives and in societies. Their collaboration transformed discrete museum programs into a citywide set of sought-after programs, events, and experiences.

Museum collaborations and partnerships are occurring more frequently. When a joint activity is well conceived, visitors, museums, business firms, and the community all benefit. By working together, participating organizations can attract more attention from audiences and the media; by combining resources, they can lower their costs. Museums are benefiting from partnerships in the following areas.

Sharing Exhibits and Programs. It is a long-standing practice for large museums to collaborate in organizing large-scale exhibitions. Such sharing makes it easier to assemble exhibit objects, manage traveling exhibition costs, and build revenues from larger audiences. For example, *Jewels of the Romanovs: Treasures of the Russian Imperial Court* opened in 1997 at the Corcoran Gallery of Art and subsequently traveled to Houston's Museum of Fine Arts, the San Diego Museum of Art, and the Brooks Museum in Memphis. It is quite common for one museum to lead in curating a shared exhibit, although exhibit design and occasionally the objects can vary from one site to another. Some museums are forming ongoing partnerships. In the early 1990s, a group of eight U.S. science museums and science and technology centers organized a consortium known as the Science Museum Exhibit Collaborative. The purpose was to improve the quality of museum exhibits and educational programs and create quality programming for the member organizations. Each member produced two exhibits over a two-year period, and these exhibits circulated at cost among consortium members and on a fee basis to outside museums.

Art museums, to a greater extent than in the past, are collaborating in a variety of ways. The partnership that is sending artworks from New York's Whitney Museum of American Art to the San Jose Museum of Art, the foundation-museum partnership, the Museum Loan Network, that is helping smaller art museums acquire loans and exhibits from larger museums, and the Smithsonian Institution Traveling Exhibition Service (SITES) are all taking museum collections to larger audiences and making the participating museums better known to and appreciated by the public.

Museums and libraries are increasingly collaborating. The American Library Association, for example, has a partnership with SITES to distribute exhibits to U.S. rural libraries. The Art Institute of Chicago has organized a program with the Chicago Public Library to distribute free passes to the museum to library users. The goal is to reach young people and low- and moderate-income Chicagoans, who are more likely to use public libraries than to visit the museum. The newly reorganized Institute of Museum and Library Services (combining two federal agencies) is planning programs with incentives for museums and libraries to share their respective resources more actively.

Sharing Facilities, Personnel, and Expertise. Major museums typically possess expert resources they can share. They might arrange for an exhibit or conservation specialist to assist staff at smaller museums in the area, either free or at cost. The Smithsonian's Center for Museum Studies trains museum employees at small rural, ethnic, and community museums across the United States. Such sharing of expertise diffuses best museum practices across the museum world. Sometimes a museum becomes so proficient at a certain activity that it becomes a major outsourcer of this activity. It can take over the management function of this activity at other museums in the same way that a hotel chain contracts to manage hotels it does not own. The Walt Disney Company, for example, has contracted with several museum organizations to design their halls and exhibitions. Disney is collaborating with the Port Discovery Children's Museum, in Baltimore, scheduled to open by the end of the 1990s. Zoos typically share animals for breeding and occasionally also share their staffs' expertise in captive breeding, genetic research, and veterinary medicine. Museums are also finding ways to share purchasing and contracts and thus reduce costs. The Western Museums Association, for example, a regional U.S. museum association based in Medford, Oregon, has established a purchasing cooperative for member museums, resulting in discounts on supplies and contracts.

Sharing Promotion and Marketing. Local and regional museum consortia have emerged to pool resources in order to build more effective promotion, advertising, and marketing campaigns. An example is a public relations and promotion consortium of large and small museums in southeastern Pennsylvania and northern Delaware that includes the Longwood Gardens, Brandywine River Museum, Winterthur Museum and Gardens, Delaware Museum of Natural History, Hagley Museum, Delaware Art Museum, Nemours Mansion and Gardens, Rockwood Museum, and the Historical Society of Delaware. What began as a group of public relations staff getting together to share concerns and interests evolved into a joint advertising and marketing consortium aimed at the tourist markets just to the north in Philadelphia and New York and to the south in Baltimore and Washington, D.C. Another regional association, the Museum Educators of Southern California, jointly publicizes and promotes the offerings of twenty-five member museums, ranging from the Cabrillo Marine Aquarium and the Autry Museum of Western Heritage to the J. Paul Getty Museum, the Los Angeles Zoo, and the Los Angeles Museum of Contemporary Art. The association's attractive illustrated brochure, "One Year of Museums Around Los Angeles," is widely distributed to convention bureaus, tourist information offices, tour operators, hotels, restaurants, airlines, railroads, and bus companies.

The unique partnership among three geographically adjacent museums in Chicago, the Museum Campus, is illustrated on p. 355. Museums in a given region can form partnerships to advertise and promote themselves to each other's publics. The marketing alliance between the Minnesota Historical Society, in St. Paul, and the Field Museum, in Chicago, is an example. Each museum is readily accessible by air, rail, and bus to residents living in the other city, and each market is large. Museums collaborating on exhibits or advertising can also collaborate in fundraising in conjunction with corporate and foundation sponsors that support multicity traveling exhibitions.

Alliances are of particular value to small and medium-sized museums, many of which are located in rural areas and small towns at a distance from population centers and tourist destinations. Such museums can build public relations and marketing partnerships with other small museums in the area. They can jointly promote themselves with local and state agencies and with the tourist, travel, and hospitality industry to raise their visibility; they might even seek to attract busloads of tourists whose itinerary would include stops at several museums. They can encourage companies to support a cluster of museums in adjacent areas so

Field Museum, Chicago, one of three museums being united in the Museum Campus, designed by Teng & Associates, Inc., for the Chicago Department of Transportation.

Source: Teng & Associates, Inc.

as to create a critical mass of cultural, educational, and leisure resources. Regional museum consortia contribute to the quality of life for residents and employees and attract tourist spending, advantages that businesses are likely to appreciate and support. Small museums in the United States have established a national marketing and communications presence in the form of the Small Museums Administrators' Committee (SMAC), a standing professional committee of the American Association of Museums. SMAC's newsletter, *The Cornerstone,* is an information clearinghouse that promotes collaboration and partnership.

Partnering with the Business Community

The Smithsonian Institution and the Bethlehem Steel Corporation announced in February 1997 a joint project in Bethlehem, Pennsylvania, that will lead to the establishment of a new and independent National Museum of Industrial History. The museum, to be housed in converted former steel plants owned by the corporation, will also be supported by the local and county governments and the regional economic redevelopment authority. Long-term loans from the Smithsonian and Bethlehem Steel collections will combine to form one of the largest collections of U.S. industrial history in the nation. The Smithsonian will also provide limited curatorial and technical support. The Smithsonian benefits in sharing its resources with other communities and in reducing storage and conservation costs for the loaned objects. Bethlehem Steel benefits by converting unused facilities into useful ones, celebrating its corporate history and raising its visibility, and strengthening the community where its headquarters are located. The city of Bethlehem benefits by converting unproductive property into a tourist destination and gaining an anchor that will form the core of a redeveloped area of the city.

Business and corporate partnerships represent important opportunities for museums. These partnerships can provide museums with financial support and noncash contributions (equipment; office and other services; management, marketing, and legal expertise; and other in-kind contributions). Businesses gain a reputation for good citizenship, add polish to and promote their images, enhance a community's quality of life, and retain highly skilled and talented employees who appreciate the values of cultural organizations. Museums have to clearly communicate the benefits corporations will derive from supporting them.

Museums are finding a variety of ways to partner with corporations. Colonial Williamsburg partners with the manufacturers who produce its licensed commercial products sold in on-site and off-site stores. The Whitney Museum of American Art has formed partnerships with clothing design firms: it hosts fashion events and licenses designs from its collections, receives corporate support for exhibitions, and undertakes joint advertising and promotion with its business partners. The Tate Gallery and the Victoria and Albert Museum, among other British museums, have actively pursued corporate partnerships. The scale of these partnerships is shown in statistics offered by the Association for Business Sponsorship of the Arts. When the association began in the 1970s, overall corporate support for the arts amounted to roughly £600,000 annually; by 1995, a greater number of companies were contributing an estimated £582 million (Thorncroft, 1996). Finally, an increasing number of multisided marketing partnerships, centered on blockbuster exhibitions, are being formed by museums, hotels, and travel and tour operators in large urban centers. The museums gain visibility and audiences, the hospitality industry gains bookings and clients, tourists receive the convenience of package deals and earn discounts, and cities derive jobs, revenues, and tax receipts.

Partnering with Foundations

Foundations that support museums tend to focus on helping museums build stronger organizations and firmer support systems. Foundations, in addition, prefer to support programs that will achieve definable goals in a limited period of time. An example is the multimillion-dollar program financed by the Lila Wallace–Reader's Digest Fund to assist urban museums in reaching wider audiences, particularly underserved groups. Another example is the Museum Loan Network, the joint program of the Pew Charitable Trusts and the Knight Foundation that assists smaller art museums in obtaining loans from large ones and thereby improving their offerings and public appeal.

Foundations generally have more limited funds than corporations but larger numbers of applicants seeking support. For this reason, a foundation is likely to limit its partnering to local organizations or to classes of organizations and programs that it has a mission to support.

Partnering with Governments

Local and regional governments increasingly recognize the value of museums as destination points for tourists, as anchors for redeveloped areas, as generators of income and jobs for local residents, and as contributors to the quality of life in a community. Consequently, a growing number of them are investing in new and expanded museums, often financing this investment with sales or hotel and restaurant tax receipts, cultural tax districts, tax-exempt municipal bonds, and lottery earnings. Local, state, and regional government bodies in the United States and in Great Britain also support museums with appropriations and grants.

Partnerships for museums, in the final analysis, can overcome a variety of shortcomings and resource constraints that have interfered with the ability of small and medium-sized museums, in particular, to build attractive offerings, promote themselves, and reach larger audiences. These and even larger museums are justified in being concerned about increasing competition from information and entertainment conglomerates (Disney/ABC, Time Warner, Sony,

Paramount/Viacom, and others) that seek to capture and dominate consumers' time, energy, and spending by means of resorts, retail shops, restaurants, theme parks, and other destinations, as well as through the media. Can museum alliances and partnerships, off-site electronic services, satellites, and even franchises effectively serve the image-building, promotion, marketing, and distribution needs of museums as effectively as the far larger budgets, variegated product lines, and multiple distribution channels of the entertainment conglomerates serve theirs?

DEVELOPING A LARGER NUMBER OF MUSEUM-GOERS

Museums have to cultivate a large number of museum-goers. If we define museum-goers as people who visit one or more museums a year, it is estimated that fewer than one person in three in any given city or urban area is a museum-goer. Levels of museum visitation, though increasing in some sectors and among certain groups, are still lower than is desirable and feasible. Museums add value to people's lives and to the collective good of society. They are therefore justified in taking a more aggressive stance toward building audiences. To the extent that museums believe their offerings are better than competitive leisure-time offerings—mind-numbing television programs, slick theme parks, endless spectator sports—they have a right to take on a missionary view of audience attraction and conversion.

The ability of museums to reach the largest audience possible and make museum resources available to the greatest number of people is ultimately one of the most crucial objectives that museums can achieve. Expanding the museum-going population comprises three related tasks:

- Getting children to enjoy museums
- Getting adult non-museum-goers to become museum-goers
- Getting museum-goers to visit museums more frequently

Getting Children to Enjoy Museums

A society can almost read its future by observing what its children are doing, thinking, and caring about. If children grow up so interested in rap music, video games, and sports that they find museums and libraries stuffy and boring, then museums, and society itself, will face a dismal future. There are at least three disturbing developments that threaten to dissuade young people from visiting museums:

- Public schools are cutting down on arts programs. Today, only an estimated 39 percent of the high schools in the United States have an arts program. Many school districts offer relatively few history courses. Many science classes are taught by unqualified teachers.

- A growing proportion of children are coming from poorer, less-educated households where parents are not museum-goers and therefore their children are less likely to visit museums.

- Children grow up today with an entertainment mind-set. Their attention is wedded to television programs, video games, and other fast-action, noncognitive, and nonintellectual diversions. Museums have to take this into account as they compete for the attention of children.

Museum staff have to become more creative in making museums engaging to the young visitors who come on school outings or with their parents. Although museums have incorporated education into their offerings, they may have to change their styles of presentation and interpretation to engage the interests of the new generation. They do have to monitor more intensively the outcomes of the educational programs they organize.

- Exhibits should be interesting and enjoyable to children. That typically means balancing instructional elements with entertaining and attention-getting ones. Electronic and computer-based media and interactive machines as adjuncts to exhibitions have great appeal for young people and can help them learn. Some critics are concerned about "too much entertainment." Ed Rothstein, cultural editor for the *New York Times,* has observed that "one risk of the new approach to arts education is that the museum may be turned into just a fun place . . . studded with gift shops and decorated with banners" (1995). Museums, of course, have to strike the right balance.

- Docents should be carefully selected for their empathy with young people and their focus on the children's emotional and personal responses, not on simply conveying facts. Docents should keep the session short and make it as interactive as possible, not a one-way monologue.

- Schools need to prepare young people for the museum visit with assignments, guides, and thought-provoking exercises so that students have a goal in mind and museum-based learning becomes better integrated with school-based learning.

Several museums are pioneering ways to work jointly with school systems to define learning objectives in which the museum's resources can be of special value. Let us look at three exemplary cases.

The Metropolitan Museum of Art spends $2 million a year on programs for young children; about 191,500 schoolchildren participate annually, almost two out of every ten children in New York City's public school system. The Met also trains about 4,110 school teachers a year, and it operates The Met Goes to School, a program reaching 7,500 students in classrooms in their last school year.

The Brooklyn Museum devotes about $800,000 to children's programs. In 1988, it began the Adopt-a-School program, which provides teacher training and classroom activities. The museum has also assisted the public school system in creating a middle school centered on museum and object-based learning. Today, fifteen schools are partners with the Brooklyn Museum. (See also the Model Museum Practice in Chapter Seven, which examines The Newark Museum's outreach to children and youth.)

The Science Museum of Minnesota (SMM), in St. Paul, has organized successful programs for attracting teenagers that are worth review by other museums. SMM encourages teenagers to participate in museum activities as laboratory assistants, interns, and volunteers. It organized the Projects Club for high school students, which allows students to do their own research, work on museum projects, and participate in social events. The result is that young people feel comfortable and welcome at SMM; participants also spread positive word of mouth. It is common to see teenagers at the museum in the evening lining up for Omnimax films and strolling through the galleries.

Converting Non-Museum-Goers into Museum-Goers

Most museums can assume that one or more untapped segments in their communities could be recruited as visitors if approached in the right way. Museums are experimenting with a variety of ways to attract these nonvisitors. Some are organizing family-centered and community-oriented holiday celebrations, ethnic heritage events, musical and theatrical performances, family workshops, and other popular events that have proved effective at enticing nonvisitors to come to museums. Some are organizing new types of collections and exhibits to appeal to wider audiences. Still others are devoting resources to promotion and community relations goals and building wider audiences as a result. Museums in large urban centers in particular are successfully employing marketing principles and tools to reach target groups, rather than expending resources in scattershot fashion. Some observers believe that the ultimate solution for underserved groups is to follow the lead of specialized museums and to build ethnic and community-oriented museums that will appeal directly to underserved ethnic and minority groups. Museums of this type have assumed a positive role, particularly in large urban centers, although they are typically underfunded and have difficulty raising the support they need over the long run.

Getting Museum-Goers to Visit More Frequently

If a museum fails to change its exhibits and offer new programs periodically, people have little reason to visit regularly. Again, as with all things affecting museums, museum leaders have to strike a balance: in this case, a balance between permanent exhibits featuring celebrated collections that have appeal to tourists and out-of-towners and new programming that appeals to local residents. There are several initiatives a museum can take to secure a more continuous flow of visitors. First, the museum can refresh its exhibits and add new ones more frequently. In this way, it projects a more dynamic and engaging image that in turn energizes potential audiences and supporters. Second, a museum can add variety and mix to its programming, offering programs that appeal to a broad range of audiences. Third, a museum can build a stronger membership program, attracting a higher level of regular participation. Fourth, a museum can better allocate audience usage, smoothing out peak usage and drawing larger audiences to times of slack demand. Ticketing and pricing are two means to distribute usage. Another is targeting different groups of visitors for different times, developing programs that attract older citizens and tourists on weekdays, families with young children on weekends, adult couples and single people in the evenings.

Museums in the past underpromoted themselves and rested content with serving relatively narrow audiences. Museums in the future are likely to promote themselves vigorously, demonstrate creatively the variety of value and benefits they offer, and seek different targeted publics for different types of programs. Museums offer people opportunities for great and fulfilling experiences that they cannot find anywhere else. Maintaining and enlarging audiences through effective planning, promotion, and marketing approaches should be a goal museums will readily pursue.

Finally, it may be worthwhile to speculate on the prospects of museums as a new century opens. Museums offer the public rich, multidimensional sensory experiences with rare, authentic objects, along with the research, knowledge, and interpretation behind them—these are things only museums provide. Is it realistic to think that museums in the future will attract increasing numbers of people who feel oversaturated with the mass media and the destinations operated by the entertainment conglomerates, the simple and ersatz experiences and escapist ideas and imagery they offer? That people who seek safe public spaces for recreation, learning, and sociability for their children and themselves will come to museums in ever-greater numbers? That people who seek to fill more of their lives with intellectual, aesthetic, spiritual delights and enchanting, celebrative, and transforming experiences will think first of museums? This book is an effort to make it happen.

This essay, written in 1981, is published here for the first time. It explores the bases for making choices of what museums acquire and how they build collections. It refers to art museum collections specifically, but the principles involved apply to all museums. The essay goes to the core of museum operations—the collections and their appeal.

TWENTY-ONE WAYS TO BUY ART

Stephen E. Weil

You are the director of a municipally funded museum of twentieth century art in a small mid-western city. Your board of trustees has asked that you draft a brief policy statement providing guidance as to how the museum's acquisition funds might best be spent over the next several years. These funds are projected at approximately $75,000 annually, roughly two-thirds of which are appropriated by the city council with the balance raised privately.

The museum's existing collection consists of some 900 paintings and sculpture plus a scattering of prints and drawings. While the quality is generally high, the collection is extremely uneven in its representation of major twentieth century movements, that is, there are strong holdings in such areas as American abstract expressionism, German expressionism, and Italian futurism but virtually no examples at all of cubism, photo-realism, surrealism, neo-plasticism, constructivism, or color field painting.

You have asked your staff for their individual recommendations as to what the chief focus of the policy statement should be. Their responses follow. Choose the one (or, if more than one, not more than three that can be harmoniously combined) that you will use as the basis for this document.

1. "This collection has tremendous gaps. If we have the slightest pretense to being a place where people can learn about the art of our time, then the highest priority must be given to filling those gaps. As things stand, we're giving our visitors a completely distorted picture.

Let's concentrate on cubist painting first—that's the most critical lack—and go on from there. As a long-range goal, it's essential that we represent the full spectrum of twentieth century art."

2. "If this museum is popular for anything, it's our docent program. And the docents have told us time and again how badly they need paintings and sculpture that lend themselves to vivid explanation. We are, after all, an educational institution and it seems to me that our front-line educators—the people who must face the public every day in the galleries—are the ones who best know what kind of raw material they need in order to build an effective presentation."

3. "We must never forget that museums are the last surviving heirs of the great royal and ecclesiastical patrons of the Renaissance. If art is to retain its vigor, then the young and deserving artist will always need a helping hand at an early stage of his or her career. What better use could we make of our limited acquisition funds than to nurture the roots of creativity by concentrating our purchases on the work of emerging artists?"

4. "It seems to me that we should simply hold out for the very finest objects that we can possibly afford. I'd rather accumulate our acquisition funds for ten years and buy a single masterpiece of the highest aesthetic quality for $750,000—or more, if we could put our cash into a money market fund—than fritter it away every year on things that may never amount to anything. The Louvre has its Mona Lisa. Why should we not aspire to have ours?"

5. "To me the most salient thing is that we're entering a period of great social and economic turbulence. I think we must seek to acquire works of art that have strong positive (or even, if you will, edifying) qualities, works that can speak affirmatively to a public sorely in need of uplift. Art no longer deserves to be a central concern of society when it abandons its moral role. Then it becomes merely decoration or self-indulgence. If this museum cannot be a strong force for good, what would justify its continued existence?"

6. "To me, an art museum is first and foremost a history museum, a museum of art history. Central to our collecting should be objects that reflect significant moments in the development of contemporary art. You may object that such objects often lack the finish of later work—something that seems to dazzle the public—or even appear crude or ungainly. No matter—our duty is to preserve that first moment of inspiration, innovation, or invention so that future generations can read the unsullied record clear."

7. "Since it's the city council that votes to give us most of our acquisition funds, it seems to me that *they* ought be consulted. I wouldn't expect them to tell us exactly what to buy, but it makes good sense to get some kind of indication of what they'd like to see us collect. They're not exactly a bunch of dummies, though we sometimes treat them that way. We can't afford to get so lost in our precious, aesthetic fog that we start forgetting that basic truth about he who pays the piper calling the tune."

8. "If the museum is to attract more support, it must first itself be attractive. Those four empty sculpture niches in front of the building have become a public joke. There was even a cartoon about them last week. Ever since I've been here, we've been hoping that 'something would turn up' to fill them. Nothing ever does, and something else always takes priority. We should now be using our acquisition money to commission a good sculptor to fill those niches. Then we can go on to other things, but let's get our own house in order first."

9. "From any century, only a handful of artists will prove worthy of remembrance. If we are to carry out our obligation to future generations, then it's critical that we identify the great artists of our period and concentrate our collecting activities around them. The rest will sooner or later be largely forgotten, and—if our funds are short—then we have to be tough-minded enough to be the ones to forget them sooner."

10. "Given such a skimpy budget, it's clear that the only way we can continue building the collection over the near-term will be through gifts. That should be our chief effort—to identity those works of art in the hands of potential donors that we can reasonably anticipate to be given one day. To duplicate those with purchases would simply be a waste. Once we know, then we'll have a better idea of how to work around them in what we buy. The big thing for now is not to rush until we know what the future promises."

11. "Most of our recent acquisitions lack any flair. That's a problem. What we really need to buy now are things that can attract some attention, things that may have a glamorous background (a Marilyn Monroe or Patty Hearst collection, for example) or a rousing story to tell. Without enough money to buy great things, at least we can buy things that would get some media coverage. That way we can build a following. I've never understood why someone from our public affairs office doesn't sit on the acquisitions committee."

12. "We have two choices: merely to be a mirror of the times (and thus the slaves of fashion) or to take leadership and—through our purchases— put our endorsement on the art that is theoretically and ideologically

correct for this particular time. By that I mean advanced art that is
purged of biography, personality, anecdote, or anything extrinsic to
the means of its making. The latter is the only responsible way to go,
and it doesn't require expensive 'brand-name' artists to do it. We
can do just as well with young people who follow the proper critical
imperatives."

13. "It's largely the taxpayers of this city who pay for our acquisitions.
    Why don't we ask *them* what they'd like to see us acquire? We are—
    in every sense—a public institution, and the public is entitled to have
    a say. We should set up a citizen's advisory council—and include some
    of the people who never come here because there's never been any-
    thing here that they wanted to see."

14. "Realistically, $75,000 a year is not going to buy much quality in the
    way of painting and sculpture. But just think of what we could do if
    we decided to beef up our print department and also began to collect
    photography—in my view the most exciting development in contempo-
    rary art. Also (crass as this may sound) it's something of a bargain. We
    have an obligation to make the best use possible of our resources, and
    this would be the wisest and most prudent way to go."

15. "Now is a good time to come to grips with our obligation to local
    artists. If *we* aren't going to see to it that examples of their work are
    properly preserved and assure them that their careers are worthy of
    study, then who ever will? Certainly not the New York or Chicago mu-
    seums. Their prices would fit our budget admirably, and we'd be in
    position to buy their very top works. As a community-based museum,
    I don't see how we can avoid such an obligation."

16. "Until we can break past a level of $75,000, we're really out of the art
    market and that will increasingly be the case with every passing year.
    I would urge that we suspend collecting in any conventional sense and
    turn our energies toward the greater study of our collection. With the
    funds available, we should be able to buy the kind of documentation—
    preparatory sketches, scrapbooks, manuscripts, and the like—that
    would make us a center for scholarship in those fields where we're
    strongest. A museum, after all, isn't just things—it's also information
    about things."

17. "To me, how we buy is just as important as what we buy. If this city is
    ever to have an active art scene—an absolute essential if this museum
    is to flourish—then it will need a stronger group of dealers than it has
    today. If we don't patronize the local galleries, who will? What we
    should be doing is making our wants known and letting them do the
    leg work of tracking things down. Buying art is something with more

than one dimension, and it's high time we became sensitive to the wider implications of what we do."

18. "The question of acquisitions is inseparable from the general budgetary constraints that the museum will face in the next few years. I think particularly of our shrinking funds for conservation and security. Surely, there must be fine works of art available that are too bulky for pilfering and could appropriately be shown behind heavy plexiglass or otherwise made of damage-resistant materials. Stuff like that could even save us money on handicap compliance. Someone has to remember that the *true* cost of any object is not just the purchase price—it also includes the ongoing expenses of safeguarding and preserving it."

19. "We all know that women and minority artists are seriously underrepresented in this collection. The least we can do is to use our acquisition funds to try to correct this imbalance. No loss of quality need be involved, and if the museum can't go about its collecting business in a fair, just, and socially constructive way, then it simply doesn't deserve continued public support."

20. "It's time to face the facts: we will never have the resources to be a miniature museum of modern art with representative examples of every contemporary style. Given our budget, we could only fill the gaps—cubism, for example—with second-rate material or worse. What we can and should do is to build on what we have already and acquire further examples in those fields where we're strongest. It's the only way we'll ever build a national reputation. It's like that military maxim: to try to be strong everywhere is to be weak everywhere."

21. "What's been forgotten is that there's scarcely an important work in this collection that was important when we bought it. In the old days, the curators just went to the great cities of the world and gambled on what looked new and fresh and exciting. Sure, there were some mistakes and they clutter up our storage, but we would never have gotten our Pollocks or Beckmanns or futurist things if we waited until art history had stamped them as important. We should keep that up: guts, instinct, and the willingness to make some mistakes. Buy broad, buy big, and let the masterpieces fall as they will."

REFERENCES

Adams, G. D. *Museum Public Relations.* Nashville, Tenn.: American Association for State and Local History, 1983.

Adams, G. D. "Cultural Tourism: The Arrival of the Intelligent Traveler." *Museum News,* Nov.–Dec. 1995, pp. 32–37.

Adams, G. D., and Boatright, J. "The Selling of the Museum, 1986." *Museum News,* Apr. 1986, p. 16.

Agustin, L. "Science Centers Foster Parent Involvement." *ASTC Newsletter,* Jan.–Feb. 1997, pp. 1, 9.

Alexander, E. P. *Museums in Motion: An Introduction to the History and Functions of Museums.* Nashville, Tenn.: American Association for State and Local History, 1979.

Alreck, P. L., and Settle, R. B. *The Survey Research Handbook.* Burr Ridge, Ill.: Irwin, 1985.

American Association of Art Museum Directors. *Statistical Survey of the American Association of Art Museum Directors.* New York: American Association of Art Museum Directors, 1997.

American Association of Museums. *America's Museums: The Belmont Report.* A report to the Federal Council on the Arts and the Humanities. Washington, D.C.: American Association of Museums, 1969.

American Association of Museums. *Excellence and Equity: Education and the Public Dimension of Museums.* Washington, D.C.: American Association of Museums, 1992.

American Association of Museums. *Museums Count: A Report by the American Association of Museums.* Washington, D.C.: American Association of Museums, 1994.

American Association of Museums. *New Visions: Tools for Change in Museums.* Washington, D.C.: American Association of Museums, 1995.

Anderson, M. L. "CyberMuse: Perils and Pleasures of the Virtual Museum." *Museum News,* Nov.–Dec. 1994, p. 37.

Anderson, P., and Roe, B. C. *The Museum Impact and Evaluation Study.* 3 vols. Chicago: Museum of Science & Industry, 1993.

Andreasen, A. R. "Cost-Conscious Marketing Research." *Harvard Business Review,* July–Aug. 1983, p. 74.

Andreasen, A. R. "Profits for Nonprofits: Find a Corporate Partner." *Harvard Business Review,* Nov.–Dec. 1996, p. 5.

Association of Art Museum Directors. *Museums in Recessions.* A. T. Kearney Museum Survey. New York: American Association of Museum Directors, 1991.

Association of Performing Arts Presenters. *Profile of Member Organizations.* Washington, D.C.: Association of Performing Arts Presenters, 1991–1992.

Bay, A. P. *A Kid's Guide to the Smithsonian.* Washington, D.C.: Smithsonian Institution Press, 1996.

The BCA Report. "National Survey: Business Support to the Arts." New York: Business Committee for the Arts, 1994.

Bello, M. *A World of Discovery: An Exploration of Behind-the-Scenes Research in the Arts, Sciences and Humanities.* Washington, D.C.: Smithsonian Institution Press, 1993.

Belth, S. Personal communication. Authors express appreciation for providing background information used in Chapter Nine.

Bickford, A., Pekarik, A. J., Doering, Z. D., and Yalowitz, S. S. *Ocean Views: A Study of Visitors to the Ocean Planet Exhibition at the National Museum of Natural History.* Report No. 96–5. Washington, D.C.: Institutional Studies Office, Smithsonian Institution, 1996.

Bissell, D. *Marketing Promotions Guide.* Chicago: League of Chicago Theatres, 1985.

Bitgood, S., and Tisdal, C. "Does Lobby Orientation Influence Visitor Satisfaction?" *Visitor Behavior,* Fall 1996, pp. 13–15.

Bond, C. "An Art Museum That Can Go Wherever the Railroads Run." *Smithsonian,* Aug. 1996, pp. 76–80.

Boorstin, D. *The Image.* New York: Vintage Books, 1992.

Borun, M., Chambers, M., and Cleghorn, A. "Family Learning in Four Science Museums." *Current Trends,* 1995, pp. 116–124.

Borun, M., Chambers, M., and Cleghorn, A. "Families Are Learning in Science Museums." *Curator: The Museum Jourfal,* 1996, *39*(2), 123–138.

Boston Museum of Fine Arts. "Nagoya/Boston Museum of Fine Arts Contract Signed on December 15, 1995" (press release), Boston Museum of Fine Arts, Dec. 18, 1995.

Boyd, W. L. "Wanted: An Effective Director." *Curator: The Museum Journal,* 1995, *38*(3), 177.

Boyer, B. H. *The Natural History of the Field Museum: Exploring the Earth and Its People.* Chicago: Field Museum of Natural History, 1993.

Brigham, D. *Public Culture in the Early Republic.* Washington, D.C.: Smithsonian Institution Press, 1995.

Britz, K. "Memory, Meaning, and Small Museums." *History News,* 1995, *50*(4), 15–18.

Bryce, H. *Financial and Strategic Management for Nonprofit Organizations.* (2nd ed.) Upper Saddle River, N.J.: Prentice Hall, 1992.

Canadian Congress of Advertising. *The Art Gallery of Ontario—Barnes Exhibit: Gold, Government & Advocacy.* Toronto: Canadian Congress of Advertising, 1995.

Chreiber, E. G. "Promoting the Performing Arts." In D. McElwee, M. Stein-Le Feber, R. White, and A. Gurein, *Media Resource Guide.* (5th ed.) Los Angeles: Foundation for American Communications, 1987a.

Chreiber, E. G. "Rhoda Weiss's Public Relations Tips for Nonprofit Organizations." In D. McElwee, M. Stein-Le Feber, R. White, and A. Gurein, *Media Resource Guide.* (5th ed.) Los Angeles: Foundation for American Communications, 1987b.

Claritas, Inc. "PRIZM: The Next Generation." Seminar series, 1994.

Cohen, D. "The Newark Museum, Flower of the Garden State, the Place Where Shangri-La and New Jersey Meet." *Smithsonian,* June 1991, pp. 92–101.

Commission on Museums for a New Century. *Museums for a New Century: A Report of the Commission on Museums for a New Century.* Washington, D.C.: American Association of Museums, 1984.

Commission on the Future of the Smithsonian Institution. *E Pluribus Unum: The Divine Paradox.* Washington, D.C.: Smithsonian Institution, 1995.

Conaway, J. *The Smithsonian: 150 Years of Adventure, Discovery, and Wonder.* Washington, D.C.: Smithsonian Books/Knopf, 1995.

Costello, T. M. "The People Say 'Yes' to Museums: In St. Louis, the Voters Back Public Funding." *Museum News,* Apr. 1985, pp. 30–35.

Csikszentmihalyi, M. "Notes on Art Museum Experiences." In A. Walsh (ed.), *Insights: Museums, Visitors, Attitudes, Expectations: A Focus Group Experiment.* Santa Monica, Calif.: Getty Center for Education in the Arts and J. Paul Getty Museum, 1991.

Dana, J. C. "The New Museum." *The Museologist,* 1988, *51*(178), 8–15. (Originally published 1917)

Danvers, R. W. *National Needs Assessment of Small, Emerging, Minority and Rural Museums in the United States.* Washington, D.C.: Institute of Museum Services, 1992.

D'Arcy, D. "The Job (Almost) Nobody Wanted." *ARTnews,* Jan. 1995, pp. 128–133.

Davies, S. *By Popular Demand: A Strategic Analysis of the Market Potential for Museums and Art Galleries in the UK.* London: Museums & Galleries Commission, 1994.

Davis, J. *The Museum Book: A Report on the Work of Project Muse.* Cambridge, Mass.: Harvard Graduate School of Education, 1996.

De Salvo, D. (ed.). *Past Imperfect: A Museum Looks at Itself.* Southampton, N.Y.: Parrish Art Museum/New Press, 1993.

Debus, M. *Handbook for Excellence in Focus Group Research.* Washington, D.C.: Academy for Educational Development, n.d.

Diggle, K. *Guide to Arts Marketing.* London: Rhinegold, 1984.

Diggle, K. "Charging Ahead." *Museums Journal,* Apr. 1995, pp. 32–33.

DiMaggio, P., and Useem, M. "Decentralized Policy Research: The Case of Arts Organizations." Unpublished manuscript, Center for the Study of Public Policy, Cambridge, Mass., n.d.

Doering, Z. D. *Who Attends Our Cultural Institutions: A Progress Report Based on the Smithsonian Institution Marketing Study.* Research Note 95–5. Washington, D.C.: Office of Institutional Studies, Smithsonian Institution, 1995.

Doering, Z. D., and Bickford, A. *Visits and Visitors to the Smithsonian Institution: A Summary of Studies.* Washington, D.C.: Office of Institutional Studies, Smithsonian Institution, 1994.

Doering, Z. D., and Pekarik, A. J. "Visitors to the National Museums: A View from the Smithsonian Institution." Paper presented at "Museums and Their Visitors: Challenges for the Future," held at Haus der Geschichte, Bonn, Nov. 23, 1995.

Doering, Z. D., and Pekarik, A. J. "Assessment of Informal Education in Holocaust Museums." Unpublished manuscript, Office of Institutional Studies, Smithsonian Institution, Washington, D.C., n.d.

Drucker, P. F. *The Five Most Important Questions You Will Ever Ask About Your Nonprofit Organization.* San Francisco: Jossey-Bass, 1993.

Drucker, P. F. *Management: Tasks, Responsibilities, Practices.* New York: HarperCollins, 1974.

Dunn, S. "Telemarketing Power." *Arts Reach,* Premier Issue, 1992, p. 16.

Edles, L. P. *Fundraising: Hands-On Tactics for Nonprofit Groups.* New York: McGraw-Hill, 1993.

Falconer, H. "More Than Just a Job." *Museums Journal,* Sept. 1995, pp. 21–23.

Falk, J. H. *Leisure Decisions Influencing African American Use of Museums.* Professional Practice Series. Washington, D.C.: American Association of Museums, 1993.

Falk, J. H., and Dierking, L. D. *The Museum Experience.* Washington, D.C.: Whalesback Books, 1992.

Feldstein, M. (ed.). *The Economics of Art Museums.* Chicago: University of Chicago Press, 1991.

Festinger, L. *A Theory of Cognitive Dissonance.* Stanford, Calif.: Stanford University Press, 1957.

Festinger, L., and Branch, D. "Reactions of Humans to Cognitive Dissonance." In A. J. Bachrach (ed.), *Experimental Foundations of Clinical Psychology.* New York: Basic Books, 1962.

Finke, G. D. "Brand Awareness, Museum-Style: Boston's Museum of Science Uses Branding to Boost the Bottom Line." *Visual Merchandising and Store Design,* Oct. 1996, pp. 138–142.

Flanagan, J. *Successful Fundraising: A Complete Handbook for Volunteers and Professionals.* Chicago: Contemporary Books, 1991.

Fogel, H. "When Bad Things Happen to Good Orchestras." *Symphony,* Apr.–May 1988.

Garfield, D. "Inspiring Change: Post-Heroic Management: An Interview with Harold Skramstad and Steve Hamp at the Henry Ford Museum." *Museum News,* Jan.–Feb. 1995, pp. 32–34, 47, 49, 51–56.

Goedert, P. C. *UBIT Update: The IRS Re-Emphasizes the Rules.* Denver, Colo.: Museum Store Association, 1996.

Gould, S. J. "Evolution by Walking." *Natural History Magazine,* 1995, *104*(3), 10–15.

Gray, S. "Americans' Gifts Top $150 Billion." *Chronicle of Philanthropy,* June 12, 1997, pp. 39–42.

Gumpert, D. E. "How to Really Create a Successful Marketing Plan." *Inc.,* 1994, pp. 42–43.

Gurian, E. H. "Noodling Around with Exhibition Opportunities." In I. Karp and S. D. Lavine (eds.), *Exhibiting Cultures: The Poetics and Politics of Museum Display.* Washington, D.C.: Smithsonian Institution Press, 1991.

Gurian, E. H. (ed.). *Institutional Trauma: Major Change in Museums and Its Effect on Staff.* Washington, D.C.: American Association of Museums, 1995.

Hales, L. "At the Getty: Views on Architecture, Views of Los Angeles." *Washington Post,* Feb. 6, 1997, p. 15.

Hambrick, D. C., and Cannella, A. A., Jr. "Strategy Implementation as Substance and Selling." *Academy of Management Executive,* 1989, *3*(4), 278–285.

"Hard Money." *Museum News,* Sept.–Oct. 1995, pp. 32–62.

Harris, T. L. *The Marketer's Guide to Public Relations.* New York: Wiley, 1991.

Hatzenstein, H., and Sachs, W. S. *Direct Marketing.* New York: Macmillian, 1992.

Henderson, A., and Kaeppler, A. *Exhibiting Dilemmas: Issues of Representation at the Smithsonian.* Washington, D.C. and London: Smithsonian Institution Press, 1997.

Heyman, I. M. Speech made to the National Press Club, Washington, D.C., Dec. 17, 1996.

Hood, M. G. "Staying Away: Why People Choose Not to Visit Museums." *Museum News,* Apr. 1983, pp. 50–57.

Huizinga, J. *Homo Ludens: A Study of the Play Element in Culture.* New York: Routledge, 1949.

Independent Sector. *Giving and Volunteering in the United States.* Washington, D.C.: Independent Sector, 1992.

Institute of Museum and Library Services. *National Needs Assessment of Small, Emerging, Minority and Rural Museums in the United States: A Report to Congress.* Washington, D.C.: Institute of Museum Services, 1992.

Jackson, R., and Wang, P. *Strategic Database Marketing.* Lincolnwood, Ill.: NTC, 1994.

Jahnke, A. "Losing the Win-Win Game?" *Museum News,* Sept.–Oct. 1993, p. 51.

Janes, R. R. *Museums and the Paradox of Change: A Case Study in Urgent Adaptation.* Calgary, Alberta: Glenbow Museum, 1995.

Kino, C. "Traveling Collections." *Atlantic Monthly,* Nov. 1995, pp. 122–126.

Kotler, P. "Atmospherics as a Marketing Tool." *Journal of Retailing,* Winter 1973–1974, pp. 48–64.

Kotler, P. *Marketing for Nonprofit Organizations.* (2nd ed.) Upper Saddle River, N.J.: Prentice Hall, 1982.

Kotler, P. *Marketing Management: Analysis, Planning, Implementation, and Control.* (8th ed.) Upper Saddle River, N.J.: Prentice Hall, 1994.

Kotler, P. *Marketing Management: Analysis, Planning, Implementation, and Control.* (9th ed.) Upper Saddle River, N.J.: Prentice Hall, 1997.

Kotler, P., and Andreasen, A. R. *Strategic Marketing for Nonprofit Organizations.* (4th ed.) Upper Saddle River, N.J.: Prentice Hall, 1991.

Kotler, P., and Andreasen, A. R. *Strategic Marketing for Nonprofit Organizations.* (5th ed.) Upper Saddle River, N.J.: Prentice Hall, 1996.

Kotler, P., and Scheff, J. *Standing Room Only: Strategies for Marketing the Performing Arts.* Boston: Harvard Business School Press, 1997.

Kroenert, R. "The High Museum of Art." Case study of research at the High Museum of Art, Goizueta Business School, Emory University, 1995.

Krugman, H. E. "What Makes Advertising Effective?" *Harvard Business Review,* Mar.–Apr. 1975, p. 98.

Labyak, J. "The Membership Challenge: Responding Responsibly to Reduced Budgets." *ICOM News,* 1995, *48*(1), 14–15.

Lankford, S., Bitgood, S., and Cota, A. (eds.). *Visitor Behavior.* 1995, *10*(2) (entire issue).

Leavitt, T. W. "Permanent Problem?" *Museum News,* May–June 1991, pp. 58–59.

Lee, S. "Blockbuster Exhibitions: Hype or Hope for Museums?" *Cultural Post,* 1979, *25*(1), 8–9.

Levitt, T. *The Marketing Imagination.* New York: Free Press, 1986.

Manners, T. "TV Talk Show Tour Extends Marketing Reach." *Marketing News,* Aug. 16, 1985, p. 1.

Maple, T. L., and Archibald, E. F. *Zoo Man: Inside the Zoo Revolution.* Atlanta, Ga.: Longstreet Press, 1993.

Marketing the Arts in Cleveland: An In-Depth Survey. Commissioned by the Cleveland Foundation. Cleveland, Ohio: Ziff Marketing/Clark, Martire & Bartolomeo, 1985.

Martin, D. "The Art of Collecting Crowds: Brooklyn Museum's New Chief Seeks Diverse Audience." *New York Times,* Apr. 24, 1997, pp. B1, B6.

Maslow, A. H. *Motivation and Personality.* New York: HarperCollins, 1954.

Melillo, J. (ed.). *Market the Arts.* New York: FEDAPT, 1983.

Mensch, P. van. "The Extension of Museum Concept." *Museumvisie,* 1989, *13,* 20–24.

Mensch, P. van. "Toward Museums for a New Century." In A. Rovatsou (ed.), *Symposium: Museums, Space and Power.* Icofom Study Series 22. Athens, Greece: Icomhellenic National Committee, May 1993.

Middleton, V. "Vision, Strategy, and Corporate Planning: An Overview." In R. Harrison (ed.), *Manual of Heritage Management.* London: Butterworth-Heinemann, 1994.

Miles, R. S. "Museum Audiences." *International Journal of Museum Management and Curatorship,* 1986, *5*(1), 73–80.

Mills, D. Q. "Planning with People in Mind." *Harvard Business Review,* July–Aug. 1985, pp. 97–105.

Mokwa, M., Dawson, W., and Prieve, E. (eds.). *Marketing the Arts.* New York: Praeger, 1980.

Moore, K. *Museums and Popular Culture.* London: Cassell, 1997.

Moss, W. W. "An Archival View." In *Office of the Smithsonian Institution Archives Annual Report for FY 1993.* Washington, D.C.: Smithsonian Institution, 1993.

Museums & Galleries Commission. *Museums Matter.* London: Museums & Galleries Commission, 1992.

Museums for the New Millennium: A Symposium for the Museum Community. Washington, D.C.: Smithsonian Institution/American Association of Museums, 1997.

National Portrait Gallery. *1846: Portrait of the Nation.* Washington, D.C.: Smithsonian Institution Press, 1996.

National Trust for Historic Preservation. *Preserving Our Past, Building Our Future* (videotape). Washington, D.C.: National Trust for Historic Preservation, 1994.

"New Visions Basics: A Process of Inquiry That Invigorates Your Museum." *Excellence and Equity,* Winter 1996.

Newman, D. *Subscribe Now!* New York: Theatre Communications Group, 1983.

Newsom, B. Y., and Silver, A. Z. (eds.). *The Art Museum as Educator: A Collection of Studies as Guides to Practice and Policy.* Berkeley: University of California Press, 1978.

O'Connor, T. "Training for Change." *Museums Journal,* Sept. 1995, p. 22.

O'Donnell, S. C. "The New York City Museum School: Learning Process." *Museum News,* May–June 1995, pp. 39–40.

Ohta, R. J. "My Eyes Have Seen the Glory: Visitor Experience at a Controversial Flag Exhibition." Unpublished manuscript, Phoenix, Ariz., 1996.

Osgood, C. E., Suci, G. J., and Tannenbaum, P. H. *The Measurement of Meaning.* Urbana: University of Illinois Press, 1957.

Panas, J. *Megagifts: Who Gives Them, Who Gets Them.* Chicago: Pluribus Press, 1984.

Parkhurst, C. "America's Museums: Prices and Priorities." *Cultural Affairs,* 1969, *7,* 12.

"Perfect Site: Museums on the World Wide Web." *Museum News,* Jan.–Feb. 1997, pp. 34–40.

Perrot, P. N. "Summary of Remarks Presented by Paul N. Perrot to the Smithsonian Council, Saturday, November 11, 1972." Unpublished document. Records of the Smithsonian Council, #81–009, Office of the Smithsonian Institution Archives, Washington, D.C.

The Peter F. Drucker Foundation for Nonprofit Management. *The Drucker Foundation Self-Assessment Tool for Nonprofit Organizations: Participant's Workbook.* San Francisco: Jossey-Bass, 1993.

Peters, T. J., and Waterman, R. H., Jr. *In Search of Excellence: Lessons from America's Best-Run Companies.* New York: HarperCollins, 1982.

Popcorn, F. *The Popcorn Report.* New York: HarperCollins, 1992.

Popcorn, F. *Clicking.* New York: HarperCollins, 1996.

Positioning for the Future: A Detailed Review of Constituency-Based Research. Report to the Atlanta History Center, July 26, 1994. Atlanta: Performance Marketing, 1994.

President's Committee on the Arts and the Humanities. *Creative America: A Report to the President by the President's Committee on the Arts and the Humanities.* Washington, D.C.: U.S. Government Printing Office, 1997.

Rafool, M., and Loyacono, L. *Creative Solutions for Funding the Arts.* Denver, Colo.: National Conference of State Legislatures, 1995.

Ray, M. L. *Advertising and Communication Management.* Upper Saddle River, N.J.: Prentice Hall, 1982.

Reinhardt, C. "Workshop: How to Handle a Crisis." *Public Relations Journal,* Nov. 1987, pp. 43–44.

Ripley, S. D. *The Sacred Grove: Essays on Museums.* New York: Simon & Schuster, 1969.

Ripley, S. D. *The Sacred Grove: Essays on Museums.* Washington, D.C.: Smithsonian Institution Press, 1978 (paperback).

Robbins, J. E., and Robbins, S. S. "Segmentation for 'Fine Arts' Marketing: Is King Tut Classless as Well as Ageless?" In N. Beckwith and others (eds.), *1979 Educators' Conference Proceedings.* Chicago: American Marketing Association, 1979.

Robinson, F. W. "The Moral Dilemma of American Art Museums." *Museum News,* Mar.–Apr. 1995, pp. 42–43.

Roman, E. *Integrated Direct Marketing: The Cutting Edge Strategy for Synchronizing Advertising, Direct Mail, Telemarketing, and Field Sales.* Lincolnwood, Ill.: NTC, 1995.

Rothstein, E. "Playing to Tomorrow's Audience." *New York Times,* Dec. 24, 1995, sec. 2, p. 1.

Runyard, S. *Museums and Tourism: Mutual Benefit.* London: Museums & Galleries Commission, 1993.

Runyard, S. "A Brit in Boston." *Museums Journal,* Oct. 1995, p. 21.

Schor, J. B. *The Overworked American: The Unexpected Decline of Leisure.* New York: Basic Books, 1991.

Schuster, J.M.D. *The Audience for American Art Museums.* Research Division Report No. 23 for the National Endowment for the Arts. Washington, D.C.: Seven Locks Press, 1991.

Seaman, B. "Bridging the Gap." *Museums Journal,* Sept. 1995, pp. 28–29.

Serrell, B. "Learning Styles and Museum Visitors." *ILVS Review,* 1991, *2*(1), 137–139.

Serrell, B. "The Question of Visitor Styles." *Visitor Studies,* 1993, *6,* 48–53.

Serrell, B. *Exhibit Labels: An Interpretive Approach.* Walnut Creek, Calif.: Altamira Press, 1996.

Seymour, H. *Designs for Fund Raising: Principles, Patterns, Techniques.* New York: McGraw-Hill, 1966.

Smithsonian Institution. *Smithsonian Institution Collection Statistics.* Washington, D.C.: Smithsonian Institution, 1995.

SOMARC Practical Guide Series: Practical Advertising—Media Planning. Washington, D.C.: The Futures Group Intl, 1995.

Spalding, J. "Building Audiences and Winning Support." In T. Ambrose (ed.), *Money, Money, Money, and Museums.* Edinburgh: Scottish Museums Council, 1991.

Spalding, J. "Interpretation? No, Communication." *Muse,* 1993, *11*(3), 10–14.

Stern, L. W., and El-Ansary, A. I. *Marketing Channels.* (4th ed.) Upper Saddle River, N.J.: Prentice Hall, 1992.

Stone, B. *Successful Direct Marketing Methods.* Lincolnwood, Ill.: NTC/Crain Books, 1979, 1988.

Sullivan, R. Remarks at the Smithsonian Dialogue II Conference "What About Diffusion?" Amazonia Science Gallery, National Zoological Park, Washington, D.C., Mar. 18, 1997.

Thorncroft, A. "Arts Face a Harsh Set of Realities." *Financial Times Survey,* July 4, 1996, p. 2.

Ullberg, A. D., with Ullberg, P. *Museum Trusteeship.* Washington, D.C.: American Association of Museums, 1981.

U.S. Census Bureau. *Report on Parks, Recreation, and Travel Statistics,* no. 419 ("Attendance Rates for Various Art Activities, 1992") and no. 411 ("Participation in Various Leisure Activities, 1992").

Virginia Museum of Fine Arts. *Annual Report, 1994–95.* Richmond: Virginia Museum of Fine Arts, 1995.

Vsgele, S. *Handbook of Direct Mail.* London: Prentice Hall International, 1992.

Wade, C. "Prospect Cards Boost Bottom Line." *Arts Reach,* Dec. 1992, pp. 8–10.

Walsh, A. (ed.). *Insights: Museums, Visitors, Attitudes, Expectations: A Focus Group Experiment.* Santa Monica, Calif.: Getty Center for Education in the Arts and J. Paul Getty Museum, 1991.

Walshe, P. *Pricing in the Arts Report 1990.* Arts Council of Great Britain and the Scottish Arts Council. Millard Brown International: Great Britain, Feb. 1991. *See also,*

P. Walshe, quoted in Chris Blamires, "What Price Entertainment?" *Journal of the Market Research Society,* 1992, *34*(4), 378–379.

Watson, S. "Striking a Bargain." *Museums Journal,* Sept. 1995, p. 22.

Waxman, S. "A Peek into the Nation's Attic: Smithsonian Traveling Show Awes Visitors in Los Angeles." *Washington Post,* Feb. 10, 1996, pp. C1, C6.

Webb, E. *Nonreactive Measures in the Social Sciences.* (2nd ed.) Boston: Houghton Mifflin, 1981.

"A Weekend in the Life of Washington," *Washington Post,* July 3, 1992, p. 8.

Weil, S. E. "Creampuffs and Hardball: Are You Really Worth What You Cost?" *Museum News,* Sept.–Oct. 1994, pp. 42–43, 60, 62.

Weil, S. E. *A Cabinet of Curiosities: Inquiries into Museums and Their Prospects.* Washington, D.C.: Smithsonian Institution Press, 1995.

Weiss, M. J. *The Clustering of America.* New York: HarperCollins, 1988.

White, J. "When 'No' Doesn't Mean 'No' in Telephone Fundraising." *Arts Reach,* Apr.–May 1994, p. 10.

Wilson, D. M. "What Do We Need Money For?" In T. Ambrose (ed.), *Money, Money, Money, and Museums.* Edinburgh: Scottish Museums Council, 1991.

Witteborg, L. P. *Good Show! A Practical Guide for Temporary Exhibitions.* Washington, D.C.: Smithsonian Institution Traveling Exhibition Service, 1981.

Wolf, T. *Managing a Nonprofit Organization.* New York: Fireside/Simon & Schuster, 1990.

Wolfe, D. *Marketing to Boomers and Beyond.* New York: McGraw-Hill, 1993.

Woods, R. (ed.). *Leisure Futures.* London: Henley Centre for Forecasting, 1994.

Yale, D. R. *The Publicity Handbook.* Lincolnwood, Ill.: NTC, 1991.

Zarco, L. R. "Radio: The Cinderella Medium." *Arts Reach,* Feb.–Mar. 1993, pp. 10–12.

Ziebarth, E. K., Smith, S. J., Doering, Z. D., and Pekarik, A. J. *Air and Space Encounters: A Report Based on the 1994 National Air and Space Museum Visitor Survey.* Report No. 95–4. Washington, D.C.: Office of Institutional Studies, Smithsonian Institution, May 1995.

INDEX

Chapter Six: The epigraph on p. 147 is from a personal interview with B. Serrell on January 2, 1997. The quotations in this chapter attributed to B. Serrell derive from personal interviews on January 2, 1997, and April 29, 1997. Used with permission.

Chapter Seven: The epigraph on p. 174 is reprinted with permission from the J. Paul Getty Museum.

The quotations attributed to R. Sullivan derive from a personal interview on October 1, 1997. Used with permission.

Mission statement from the Missouri Historical Society is used with permission.

Model museum practice is reprinted with permission from the Newark Museum.

Chapter Eight: Model museum practice is used with permission from the Virginia Museum of Fine Arts.

Chapter Nine: Model museum practice is used with permission from Boston's Museum of Science.

Chapter Ten: The epigraph on p. 264 is from a personal interview with D. Nimer on September 15, 1997. Used with permission.

Model museum practice is used with permission from the Genesee Country Village & Museum.

Chapter Eleven: The epigraph on p. 287 is reprinted with permission from *Museum News,* Mar./Apr. 1995. Copyright 1995, the American Association of Museums. All rights reserved.

The quotations attributed to L. Hardwick derive from a personal interview on May 12, 1997. Used with permission.

Excerpts of M. Heyman's speech to the National Press Club on December 17, 1996, are used with permission.

Model musum practice is used with permission from the Art Institute of Chicago.

Conclusion: The epigraph on p. 348 is from *Management: Tasks, Responsibilities, Practices.* Copyright © 1973, 1974 by Peter F. Drucker. Reprinted by permission of HarperCollins Publishers, Inc.

the male file

Even if your sexual desire is high, chances are the amount of sex you are having is low. Just 8 percent of 1,422 men surveyed in a national sex poll said they had sex four or more times a week. The average was seven times a month. The typical encounter lasted 15 minutes to an hour.

drives. Actually, it doesn't take much to brighten up your sexual appetite. Russell J. Reiter, Dr. Med., Ph.D., professor of neuroendocrinology at the University of Texas Health Science Center in San Antonio, advises that you try to get at least 30 minutes of exposure each day—particularly during the winter months.

Plan ahead. It may not sound romantic, but in today's high-speed, 24-hour society, couples who wait for the perfect moment to have sex will find themselves going without it. "A lot of the time sex is just a leftover at the end of the day, and even if you warm a leftover up, it just isn't the same," says Dr. Birch. Rather than waiting until the last minute, he suggests, make a "sex date." Put it on your calendar just as you would an important meeting. "This way you can have sex when you're refreshed, when you're not dead tired."

Remember why you're together. As our lives get more and more hectic—with children, careers and various other accoutrements of adulthood—it's easy to forget that the person we're with is more than a friend, partner and helpmate. She's also a lover, and will appreciate being treated like one. "Tell her how sexy she looks, or how nice her breasts are," says Dr. Birch. "It doesn't have to end with intercourse. You just want to be comfortable playing."

Insomnia

Taking Your Place in the Land of Nod

Even smart guys can't agree on how much sleep is enough. Thomas Edison only needed four or five hours of shut-eye a night to keep the lightbulb in his brain burning bright. But Albert Einstein had to rack up at least ten hours of Zzzs before E could equal MC^2. Now, if these two geniuses couldn't agree on a magic formula, what chance do the rest of us have?

Pretty good, if we listen to our bodies. You don't have to be a brainiac to know that each of us needs different amounts of sleep to feel properly rested. Most of us fall somewhere between Edison and Einstein—at least when it comes to sleeping. But one in three of us—up to 60 million Americans—suffer regular bouts of insomnia, meaning we either can't fall asleep easily or can't stay asleep through the night. And about a third of those call the problem severe.

In many cases, getting less shut-eye is just a natural part of getting older. By the time you turn 40, you don't sleep as soundly as you once did. You wake up more frequently and stay awake longer. And if you happen to have grown more sedentary and put on a few pounds, the odds of getting a good night's sleep decrease even further, says James Perl, Ph.D., author of *Sleep Right in Five Nights*.

More is at stake than just a little drowsiness. The National Highway Transportation Safety Administration estimates that up to 600,000 automobile accidents a year involve sleepiness, and up to 12,000 highway deaths annually could be sleep related. Studies show that one in five drivers has fallen asleep behind the wheel.

Mention the disastrous Exxon Valdez oil spill that fouled Prince William Sound in 1989 and the first thing people remember is the captain's drinking. But federal investigators determined that the prime cause was the third mate's fatigue from lack of sleep. Even the near meltdown at Three Mile Island nuclear power plant in Pennsylvania was linked to workers who were too tired to notice a mechanical failure.

"Not getting enough sleep can lead to tremendous impairment in productivity on the job," says Karl Doghramji, M.D., associate professor of psychiatry and director of the Sleep Disorders Center at Thomas Jefferson University Hospital in Philadelphia. "Someone with insomnia may have difficulty with memory loss. He may have difficulty with falling asleep inappropriately and he may have difficulty in

Rest in a Pill

Experts agree that when life's turbulence starts interfering with sound sleep, it's critical to focus on the underlying problem and not just look for a quick fix. Only in a very small number of extreme insomnia cases—following the death of a loved one, for example—will sleeping pills be necessary.

A prescription drug like alprazolam (Xanax) works by reducing activity inside the brain. This can help you fall asleep—and stay asleep—more readily than you might otherwise. But only use under a doctor's close supervision, says James D. Frost, M.D., a sleep specialist and professor of neurology at Baylor College of Medicine in Houston.

Sleeping pills, including both over-the-counter preparations and prescription drugs, often cause side effects and, more importantly, their use may lead to dependency. "Most people can solve their sleeping problems in many ways other than resorting to the use of drugs," says Dr. Frost.

interpersonal relationships because he's always fatigued and therefore, withdrawn, less involved and irritable."

Sleepless Nights, Tired Days

We all have occasional bad nights when the numbers on the clock seem frozen in place. We toss and turn, curse the darkness and impatiently wait for morning. For some guys, however, insomnia isn't so short-lived—or harmless. They may have chronic insomnia for months, years or even decades. Starved for sleep, they lurch around like extras from *Night of the Living Dead*. They're always forgetting names and phone numbers. On their days off they're too wiped out to do anything fun. Desperate for sleep, they may begin reaching for the bottle—or worse. "About 40 percent of people with insomnia medicate themselves, either with over-the-counter medications or with alcohol," says Dr. Doghramji. "It can be very dangerous."

Although there are a number of physical problems that can lead to insomnia—kidney disease and chronic pain, to name just two—it's caused by emotional factors such as worry and stress in more than half of all cases. Trouble at work will often keep you awake at night. So will relationship problems or worries about the kids. And for some guys, insomnia becomes the thing they worry about: They can't sleep because they're afraid they won't sleep.

Put Insomnia to Bed

In most cases your normally restful sleep will return once the underlying stress has been resolved. But if weeks or months go by and you're still not getting enough shut-eye, then it's time for a checkup, says Dr. Doghramji. There may be something physically wrong that's thrown you into exile from the land of nod. More likely, all you'll really need are some minor adjustments to your night life. Here's what the sleep experts recommend.

Keep regular hours. Men who adopt the Warren Zevon song "I'll Sleep When I'm Dead" as their personal anthem may wind up sleeping sooner than they'd like. The National Commission on Sleep Disorders Research found that individuals who slept fewer than six hours a night had a 70 percent higher mortality rate than those who slept seven or eight hours nightly.

To break the insomnia cycle, it's critical to go to bed and get up at the same times every day, says James D. Frost, M.D., a sleep specialist and professor of neurology at Baylor College of Medicine in Houston. This forces the body's internal clock to stay in synch with your daily schedule. There's nothing wrong with occasionally staying up late, experts say. Just be sure to get up at the usual time the next morning to prevent one sleepless night from turning into many.

Don't nap to catch up. While there's nothing wrong with the occasional siesta, using naps to make up for lost sleep will only throw off the body's internal clock. "You may develop an inability to sleep at the desired time and subsequently have difficulty remaining awake during your usual waking time," says Dr. Frost.

Don't cheat on weekends. If you change your sleeping patterns on the weekend, you may find yourself suffering from Sunday night insomnia—which is nowhere near as much fun as Monday Night Football.

"Generally, the time we're sleepy at night is strongly influenced by the time we get up in the morning," Dr. Perl says. "If you usually get up at 6:00 A.M. during the week but get up on Saturday at 7:00 A.M. and Sunday at 8:00 A.M., your body's clock is two hours behind. So you won't be sleepy until two hours past your normal bedtime Sunday night."

If you do stay up an extra hour or so, the best solution is to get up at your usual time the next morning, advises Dr. Perl. You may feel drowsy, but at least your body's internal clock will still be ticking and on time.

Make time for workouts. Studies have shown that getting 20 to 30 minutes of vigorous exercise causes the metabolism first to speed up then slow down to sleep-inducing levels. The slowdown usually occurs about six hours after exercising, so it's best to workout in the afternoon or evening, says Dr. Frost. "It's not a good idea to

FAST FACTS

How common: One in three adults suffer regular bouts of sleeplessness, with about one-third of those calling the problem severe.

Risk factors: Stress, anxiety, poor sleep habits, kidney disease, chronic pain and medical problems.

Age group affected: By the time we hit age 40, the amount of deep sleep we get has diminished considerably. Since our sleep is shallower, we wake up more frequently and for longer periods of time.

Gender gap: Women are about twice as likely to experience sleep problems as men.

Who to see: Internist, neurologist, psychologist, sleep specialist.

exercise just before bedtime because that will only speed you up," he says.

Soak away sleeplessness. Even if you miss your workout, you can get the same sleep benefit by soaking in a hot bath about two to four hours before bedtime. This is because hot water, like exercise, raises your body temperature. Then, two to four hours later, your temperature will drop, easing the way to sleep.

Save the bedroom for sleeping. We often use our bedrooms for watching movies, doing office work and discussing—or, worse, arguing about—family matters. "Many people fall into the trap of making the bedroom a place of stimulation rather than a place of winding down," says Dr. Frost. Unless you're sleeping, making love or preparing for sleep, do it somewhere else, experts advise.

Don't struggle. On those nights when you just can't get to sleep, don't lie there getting frustrated. Get out of bed for a while, suggests Dr. Doghramji. Get a light snack, watch TV or read a book for a while. Do whatever it is you normally do to unwind. Then go back to bed when you're feeling drowsy.

Check your worries at the bedroom door. It's no mystery that going to bed when you're tense or upset virtually guarantees you won't sleep. "Stress seems to be the biggest contributor to insomnia," says Dr. Perl. Sleep experts often advise men to write down their worries—and some possible solutions—before they get into bed. This won't make the problems disappear, but the act of identifying solutions often has a calming effect. "Probably the single biggest cause of insomnia is worrying about insomnia," says Dr. Frost.

Don't booze or you'll lose. Having a nightcap is a time-honored way to end the evening. It also may begin the next day much grumpier than you'd prefer. Although alcohol can make you drowsy, it disrupts normal sleep quality so you'll probably wake up more tired than you otherwise would, says Dr. Doghramji. If you want, enjoy a drink with supper, then call it quits, he advises.

Steer clear of caffeine. Caffeine stimulates the central nervous system, so avoid beverages such as tea, colas or cocoa before bedtime, says Dr. Frost. If you normally drink coffee after dinner, switch to decaf instead.

Have a nighttime snack. You may feel too old for milk and cookies, but experts agree that having a light snack at bedtime can help you fall asleep more easily. Just having something in your stomach will make you feel more comfortable, says Dr. Doghramji. In addition, milk and other protein-rich foods such as cheese, eggs, beans, meat and poultry contain a naturally occurring amino acid called trypto-phan, which triggers the release of soothing hormones into the bloodstream.

Mine some minerals. Calcium and magnesium are natural sedatives that help some people relax and sleep better, Dr. Perl says. He recommends taking a tablet containing one gram of calcium and 500 milligrams of magnesium before bedtime. Ask your doctor or pharmacist which mineral supplement may be right for you.

Don't watch the clock. Some men are well-rested after five hours of sleep, while others need ten. So don't worry what the clock says. Ask yourself how you feel. If you're consistently waking up tired, says Dr. Doghramji, then you probably need to get more sleep. Conversely, if you wake up with your spirits as high as the rising sun, then you're clearly doing something right.

Take the CURE

Experts agree that in order to sleep better you may need to spend less time in bed. While this may sound like one of those mystical paradoxes from *Kung Fu*, it's actually a behavioral approach Dr. Perl refers to as CURE. It stands for:

*C*ut down on your time in bed.

*U*se your time awake at night as newfound time.

*R*elax about sleeping less because it won't hurt your health.

*E*very day get out of bed at the same time.

The basic idea of CURE is to train your body to sleep more efficiently so you get deeper, more restorative sleep.

Here's how it works. Figure out how much sleep you actually get each night— not how long you lie in bed, but how many hours you actually sleep. If you normally sleep six hours, for example, that's how long you'll spend in bed. Even if it takes you a few hours to fall asleep, you can only stay in bed those six hours. At first you may be tired, but eventually you'll find yourself falling asleep faster, sleeping more deeply and waking up less often, says Dr. Perl.

Irritable Bowel Syndrome

Controlling a Spastic Colon

Physicians tend to define irritable bowel syndrome (IBS) the way the U.S. Supreme Court views pornography. They can't really tell you what it is, but they know it when they see it.

An estimated 15 percent of people in the United States have IBS, although few ever consult a physician. Among those who do see a doctor for gastrointestinal disorders, IBS is the leading culprit. That's hardly surprising since it is basically a catchall diagnosis that includes constipation, diarrhea and stomach pain or cramping. But the discomfort isn't confined to your plumbing system. Those suffering from IBS often have headaches, backaches and fatigue as well. When there is no physical or organic cause for the symptoms, it's usually labeled IBS.

At times, it goes by aliases, with spastic colon and nervous diarrhea being the two most common. The adjectives used to describe the problem—irritable, spastic and nervous—are apt because that's precisely what is happening in your stomach. For reasons that are often unclear, your digestive system has turned irritable or angry, becoming nervous and unpredictable.

"IBS is a disorder in which the gastroenterological system is not infected or inflamed but simply doesn't work in a normal manner," says Edward Feldman, M.D., clinical professor of medicine at the University of California, Los Angeles, School of Medicine.

Often, a diagnosis of IBS is arrived at by process of elimination. "The problem with IBS is that you can't see it under the microscope like cancer," says Robert S. Sandler, M.D., associate professor of medicine at the University of North Carolina School of Medicine in Chapel Hill. "It has been historically difficult to make a diagnosis, and typically it has been made by exclusion: `Well, it's not cancer, it's not infection, it must be irritable bowel.'"

What separates IBS from simple constipation or diarrhea is that both symptoms are usually present, often alternating. "People who just have constipation don't have IBS," says Dr. Sandler. "It's when you swing back and forth between different kinds of stools." Also, he says, the constipation or diarrhea is often accompanied by abdominal pain or cramping.

Stress and Distress

One of the more irritating traits of IBS is that it tends to strike at the worst possible time. Like right before an important job interview. Or when you're scheduled to make a presentation at a big meeting. Chances are, it's no coincidence. If you're feeling nervous and shaky, your digestive system probably is, too.

"Irritable bowel is often triggered by stress," says Stephen Hanauer, M.D., professor of medicine and clinical pharmacology at the University of Chicago Medical Center. "So learning how to cope with stress would greatly help the problem."

Any of the proven stress reduction techniques—meditation, self-hypnosis or biofeedback—should make your bowels, not to mention the rest of you, less irritable.

IBS usually doesn't lead to more serious intestinal problems, but it certainly can be annoying. If you have a sudden change in your bowel habits or experience bleeding, fever, weight loss or symptoms that awaken you at night, see your doctor. Here are some ways you can avoid an unpleasant bout with bothersome bowels.

Feed on fiber, forswear fat. Experts say you need 20 to 35 grams of fiber daily, but the average American consumes less than half that amount. Adding bran, grains, fruits, vegetables, beans and other legumes to your diet is the best way to maintain regular bowel movements. In addition, some physicians believe fiber helps ease the abdominal cramping that accompanies irritable bowel syndrome. The additional fiber, however, may increase intestinal gas or cause you to feel bloated, so you need to make the boost very gradually. You also should avoid fatty foods such as cheese, ice cream and almost anything fried, which can make your bowels irritable.

Drink water. As you increase the amount of fiber in your diet, be sure to drink more water—six to eight eight-ounce glasses a day. Otherwise, the added fiber may actually clog your system instead of cleaning it out.

Exercise. Regular exercise helps keep you regular. It also is one of the most effective ways to reduce IBS-inducing stress.

Plan ahead. If you know a stressful situation is coming up, Dr. Hanauer advises, avoid heavy meals and try to eat at least two to three hours beforehand.

Avoid drinking problems. If you take milk in your coffee or tea, you may be asking for trouble. Milk and caffeinated beverages such as coffee can aggravate IBS, for different reasons. If you're lactose intolerant, as some people with IBS are, milk will give your digestive system fits. Coffee and other caffeinated drinks speed the rate at which stools move through the bowels—a real problem if you have diarrhea.

Skip dessert. Sugars and artificial sweeteners such as sorbitol are hard to digest and can irritate the bowels. So if you suffer from IBS, avoid sugar-free chewing gum and candy. If your sweet tooth is acting up, eat fruit. As an added bonus, pears, figs, oranges and peaches are all good sources of fiber.

FAST FACTS

How common: Experts estimate that 15 percent of people in the United States have irritable bowel syndrome (IBS).

Risk factors: Not enough fiber and water in the diet, lack of regular exercise, and stress.

Age group affected: Primarily a problem for those between the ages of 20 and 60. Few elderly people have IBS.

Gender gap: Men and women are at equal risk for irritable bowel syndrome. Women, however, seek a doctor's help more often than men.

Who to see: Family doctor, gastroenterologist.

Use this as a last measure. In severe cases, when patients don't respond to treatment, Dr. Hanauer says low doses of tricyclic antidepressants can be helpful in alleviating the symptoms by reducing the overstimulated movement of the bowels and inhibiting pain impulses.

Jet Lag

Avoiding a Crash Landing

Tony Bennett may have left his heart in San Francisco, but anyone who has flown coast-to-coast for an early morning business meeting knows that he got off easy.

Crossing time zones crosses up your natural biological rhythms. Your body may be in New York, but your stomach, mind and muscles feel like they're still on a cable car that was mistakenly switched onto roller-coaster tracks back in the city by the bay. Fatigue, diarrhea, insomnia and other highly unpleasant symptoms can make the skies anything but friendly for frequent fliers and first-time air travelers alike.

Jet lag is a distinctly modern malady. The pioneers never had to worry about time zones and internal body clocks as they headed west by covered wagon—although that would help explain the way Gabby Hayes talked in those old westerns.

The problem is really quite simple: It's not nice to fool Mother Nature.

"When you suddenly move yourself to a new time zone, your internal clock has not had time to be reset," says James D. Frost, M.D., a jet lag specialist and professor of neurology at Baylor College of Medicine in Houston. "It takes time for you to get in synch with the outside world."

A Long Day's Journey into Night

Jet lag is rarely serious, although it can make you feel as though you've lost a night's sleep—which, on long journeys, you probably have, says David N. Neubauer, M.D., a psychiatrist and associate director of the Johns Hopkins Sleep Disorders Center in Baltimore. Whatever the hour at your new destination, your internal clock is still on home time. It takes time for the various clocks—both internal and external—to be fully synchronized.

For most men, jet lag will last about one day for every time zone crossed, says Dr. Neubauer. A businessman flying from Chicago to New York, for example, will "lose" one hour and will probably be somewhat tired the next day—similar to the way most of us feel on the spring morning each year when daylight savings time kicks in. Now, imagine setting your clock ahead six hours. That's what passengers flying from New York to Europe face—daylight savings time, with a vengeance. It can take a full week to recover after an Atlantic crossing.

Your natural body clock may determine how badly you feel after a long flight. It seems the early bird catches the jet lag. "People who are early birds tend to be more likely to run into difficulties with jet lag than somebody who's a night owl," Dr. Neubauer says.

Timely Tips

Travel light. When flying east across time zones, it's best to fly early so you can enjoy at least a few hours of daylight after landing. "The body's clock responds most to environmental lighting. That's the stimulus it uses the most," says Walter Tapp, Ph.D., a neuroscientist with the Veteran's Administration Hospital in East Orange, New Jersey, and the University of Medicine and Dentistry of New Jersey–New Jersey Medical School in Newark. If you want to reset your body's internal clock, you first must see the light.

If you arrive in New York at 10:00 P.M. from the West Coast, your body's clock will still be set on 7:00 P.M. New York may be the city that never sleeps, but chances are you need to—but won't for a while. So the result of the late-day flight is likely to be insomnia that night and exhaustion the next day.

Fly by night. When heading west across time zones, it's best to fly later in the day. And this is no fly-by-night theory. Taking that same cross-country flight in the opposite direction, you arrive on the West Coast at 7:00 P.M., but your body is telling you it's 10:00 P.M. Your day just got three hours longer. This shouldn't be too much of a problem because the body naturally prefers a longer day, says Dr. Neubauer. It's important, however, to gear your activities around the new schedule. In this case, that means staying awake until the clock on the wall—and not your body's clock—says it's bedtime. After a day or two you should be back on track.

Set your watch before you leave. As soon as you're on the plane, set your watch to the time zone of your destination, says Dr. Frost. "You want to start thinking in terms of the new environment as soon as possible," he says.

Tank up on water. Airplane cabins are notoriously dry, which is why airplane travelers often come to ground feeling dry and dehydrated. Drink several glasses of water before boarding and while you're in the air, says Dr. Neubauer.

Pass on the cocktails. Drinking alcohol when you fly will only worsen dehydration, Dr. Neubauer says. Booze also disturbs sleep, which will make it harder to recover from jet lag once you arrive. As a rule, drink lightly or not at all while flying and for at least a day or two after arriving, he advises. "Some of the symptoms described as jet lag are more consistent with a hangover," Dr. Neubauer says.

Stick with decaf. Like alcohol, caffeine-laden beverages such as coffee, tea and cola can ruin normal sleep. They also make it easier to ignore fatigue, which will make the jet lag worse later on. "They tend to delay the synchronization of the internal clock with the outside world," says Dr. Frost. You don't have to give up caffeine entirely, he adds. Just don't overdo it, either in the air or while you're adjusting to the new schedule on the ground.

Feast and fast. Charles Ehret, Ph.D., senior scientist emeritus of Argonne National Laboratory and president of General Chronobionics in Hinsdale, Illinois, has developed an anti-jet lag program that involves a four-day sequence alternating between feasting and fasting prior to the day of arrival. Under Dr. Ehret's plan, feasting means eating as much as you want, while fasting means cutting your usual calorie count in half.

Four days before your departure, eat high protein foods at breakfast and lunch, and plan meals rich in complex carbohydrates for dinner, says Dr. Ehret. Sticking to your regular eating schedule will help prevent the jet lag blues, too.

Here are sample menus for a fasting day.

Protein breakfast—1 egg, any style; ½ piece of lightly buttered toast

Protein lunch—1 chicken breast, skin removed; 1 cup bouillon; ½ cup low-fat pot cheese or cottage cheese

Complex-carbohydrate supper—1 small bowl of pasta, lightly buttered; 1 piece of bread, lightly buttered; 1 cup cooked vegetables

Don't crash early. Even if you want nothing more than to hit the sheets for a few hours after your trip, taking a long nap is going to disturb your sleep later on, making it that much harder to adjust to your new time zone, says Dr. Frost. If you simply can't stay awake, limit your nap to about one hour. Then get up and stay up until bedtime.

Make time for exercise. In one study, Canadian researchers simulated jet lag in two groups of hamsters. Animals in one group were left to adjust on their own, while those in the other were set loose on exercise wheels. The active hamsters needed only about 1½ days to adjust to the new schedule, while their idle mates needed more than 11 days. "You don't want to overdo it on the first day, but exercise clearly helps some people feel better," says Dr. Frost.

Check out melatonin. Researchers have found that taking small amounts of a hormone called melatonin, which is naturally secreted by the brain during sleep, helps reset your internal clock. Commonly available at health food stores, melatonin may "fool" the brain into thinking it's bedtime, even when your internal clock says it's not. Research continues, and the Food and Drug Administration has not yet approved melatonin for use to combat jet lag.

FAST FACTS

How common: Nearly everyone who travels across time zones may experience some amount of jet lag. Figure on one day of recovery for every time zone crossed.

Risk factors: Flying east late in the day, caffeine and alcohol consumption, not getting enough sleep.

Age group affected: Jet lag can occur at all ages. May be more of a problem as you get older.

Gender gap: Men and women apparently suffer the same symptoms from jet lag and are equally prone to getting them.

Who to see: Jet lag rarely requires a doctor's visit. But if you travel often and are truly suffering, consult your family doctor. He might refer you to a neurologist or sleep specialist.

"It looks pretty certain that melatonin, in relatively small doses, can change the phase of the body's clock—kind of the local time it's set to," Dr. Tapp says. But while it appears promising, more research is needed to make sure melatonin doesn't adversely affect performance, Dr. Tapp adds. "It seems to be very effective," says Dr. Neubauer. "I don't think there's enough evidence to strongly recommend it, but it definitely warrants more research."

If you do decide to give it a try, do not exceed the dosage recommended on the label.

Jock Itch

How to Keep the Jewels Clean

It's not something you write home to Mom about. Heck, you don't even tell Dad about it. And letting friends know?

Not in *this* lifetime.

"Jock itch is clearly an embarrassing problem for a lot of men," says Paul Lazar, M.D., professor of clinical dermatology at Northwestern University Medical School in Chicago. "They just don't like to talk about it," he says. "A lot of these 'groin pulls' you hear about that allegedly sideline major athletes are really just bad cases of jock itch."

Frequently, jock itch is caused by the same fungus that causes athlete's foot, says Dr. Lazar. The symptoms are also similar: redness, peeling and a fiery itch that can make you feel like you're being burned at the stake. "Involvement is typically concentrated in the groin area close to the genitals," says Dr. Lazar.

A Fungal Frenzy

How do these little scourges get into your crotch? "Pulling your underwear up and over infected feet can transfer the same organisms causing your athlete's foot to your groin," says Keith Schulze, M.D., a dermatologist in private practice in Wharton, Texas. But, he adds, because the organisms that cause jock itch are so common in the environment, they are impossible to avoid entirely. Just like retired in-laws—if you offer them a pleasant place to move in, they will. The good news is that jock itch is a problem you can both prevent and cure fairly easily.

"It's been my experience that, even in a bad case, response to treatment is generally much faster than with a bad case of athlete's foot," says William Dvorine, M.D., chief of dermatology at St. Agnes Hospital in Baltimore. "What might take months in athlete's foot can generally be handled in a matter of weeks with jock itch."

The chief reason: It's generally easier to deny the groin guerrillas the sort of environment that makes curing the same problem on your feet so difficult. That is, since you don't wear shoes on your groin, there should be no big problem keeping out the heat and moisture. Which leads us to the logical next step in our discussion—engaging the enemy in combat, and killing him.

FAST FACTS

How common: Very common, affecting up to 70 percent of the population at some point in their lives.

Risk factors: Moisture in and around the groin, synthetic underwear, tight underwear (including athletic supporters), dirty groin and excess weight.

Age group affected: All age groups are affected, but it rarely develops before adolescence. That's when increased hair growth and an active lifestyle can mean more friction and perspiration.

Gender gap: A woman with itching in the groin is somewhat more likely to have a yeast infection. The causes are different and so are the cures.

Who to see: Most cases of jock itch can be tackled without a doctor's involvement. Particularly nasty cases should be seen by a dermatologist.

Groin Warfare

Winning the war against jock itch requires, above all, a full-scale attack on moisture. The more your groin resembles a greenhouse, the more likely you are to develop jock itch. "Fungi are plants; like all plants, they like greenhouses," Dr. Lazar says.

Wear boxer shorts. Loose-fitting underwear promotes drier skin by letting air circulate more freely, Dr. Dvorine says. Jock itch gets its name from the fact that more "jocks" get it. How come? Because they sweat a lot and wear jockstraps—constrictive, tightly-fitted articles of clothing that trap moisture and the plants that love it against your skin.

Watch what you wear for underwear. Cotton is highly recommended, but the newer synthetics that pull moisture away from the skin—Coolmax, for example—should help you stay dry also, says Dr. Schulze. Avoid older synthetics, like polyester, that absorb no water but instead actually hold it against your skin.

Powder yourself. A broad range of drying powders—from plain old talcum to more sophisticated offerings incorporating antifungal medications—are available commercially. What works for athlete's foot generally works better for jock itch, says Dr. Dvorine, so don't shy away from medicated powders containing tolnaftate (Tinactin Powder Aerosol), miconazole (Micatin) or undecylenic acid (Desenex) just because your local drugstore stacks them under a sign that says athlete's foot.

One warning: Stay away from products containing cornstarch. Since yeast organisms may also be involved in causing jock itch, and yeast thrives on cornstarch, applying it to your groin is like throwing ammunition to the enemy.

Wash frequently. But remember to dry your groin thoroughly each time. Soap helps kill the organisms that cause jock itch, and scrubbing helps remove the dead skin they like to eat. Use a clean towel to dry—an old one might have infected skin on it. Briefly use a hair dryer on a low setting for even more thorough drying.

Change your underwear often. The more you're sweating, the more often you should change, Dr. Schulze says. It's a simple way of staying dry—fresh underwear is by definition dry underwear. Changing into freshly laundered underwear also ensures that you're putting on Skivvies that have little, if any, dead—and possibly infected—skin attached to them.

If you insist on wearing an athletic supporter, get out of it immediately after working out instead of sitting there slinging the bull with your buddies.

Put your socks on first. Since the organisms that cause jock itch—as well as athlete's foot—are everywhere, it's hard to keep them off your feet. But it is possible to keep them off your groin, says Dr. Schulze. Since pulling your underwear up and over infected feet can transfer the same organisms causing your athlete's foot to your groin, you should put a clean pair of socks on before you pull on your underwear.

Shed a few pounds. Folds in flabby skin are perfect places for fungus and bacteria to set up shop. If you're overweight and experience frequent jock itch, there is probably a connection between the two.

Visit your dermatologist. If all else fails, or before, consult your dermatologist. He is far more likely than you are to make an accurate diagnosis, which in the long run may save you an enormous amount of painful self-discipline in elevators. He can also provide prescription medications that may be necessary to deal with tough cases. They include oral antifungals, like griseofulvin (Grisactin), for most cases and broad-spectrum antibiotics for extreme cases.

But note: These drugs have been known to interact with others and do produce unpleasant side effects in some, so ask your dermatologist about possible drug interactions with medications you're taking.

Kidney Stones

Bypassing the Ultimate Pain

It's the 50th time your wife has told "The Story." In graphic detail she relates the agonizing moments of her ten-hour labor. It's a harrowing tale. Her badge of honor. Childbirth, she says, is an experience in pain that mere men could never relate to.

Not so fast.

Imagine, if you must, a pea-sized rock traveling ever so slowly through your kidney and then down the tube connecting your kidney to your bladder. Each time the pebble makes any progress, the tube—called the ureter—gets gouged, resulting in a sharp, excruciating, widespread ache. All the while, your urine is backing up.

Not in a sweat yet? Then picture the stone slowly pushing its way down your urethra—yes, the tube that goes through you-know-what—until it is finally, and this could be a whole month later, shot from your body during urination. Now that's pain—pain that can cause nausea and vomiting.

This instrument of torture is called a kidney stone, and about 15 percent of men will get one at some point in their lives. They are, unquestionably, the kingpins of internal ache, says Gary Curhan, M.D., chief of clinical nephrology at West Roxbury Veterans Affairs Medical Center in West Roxbury, Massachusetts.

"It's the worst pain a man can have. Women who've had them say they'd rather go through natural childbirth again than have another kidney stone. It feels like a knife that's being twisted inside you," says Dr. Curhan.

Just a Spoonful of Sugar

The main culprits behind about two-thirds of kidney stones are the minerals calcium oxalate and calcium phosphate. If you have too much of these substances in your urine, they can accumulate to form a crystal, which then grows into a stone.

"It's like if you're having coffee and put in two teaspoons of sugar, they'll dissolve," Dr. Curhan explains. "But if you put ten teaspoons in, they'll stay at the bottom of the cup." There isn't enough fluid to dilute the mineral buildup.

Doctors have no definitive answers why some people get stones and others

Kidney Infections

Despite their propensity for getting stones, men did luck out in one area. They rarely suffer from kidney infections, also known as pyelonephritis.

Mainly, that's because of anatomy. Infectious organisms have to make the trip up the urinary tract before they can get to the kidneys. Men's urethras are much longer than women's and aren't as close to the anus, which is home to bacteria that can cause such infections. Also, the prostate, which secretes antibacterial agents, acts as a barrier against infection-causers.

"It's really a non-issue for men," says Howard Trachtman, M.D., chief of the Division of Nephrology at Schneider Children's Hospital at the Long Island campus of Albert Einstein College of Medicine in New Hyde Park, New York. "Boys and girls have an equal incidence of urinary tract infections up to about age two months, then women get 90 percent of them."

When men start suffering from prostate troubles in their sixties and seventies, however, the infections become just as big a problem to men as women, Dr. Trachtman notes.

The symptoms of pyelonephritis are hard to ignore. Severe chills, high fever and pain in the joints and muscles are a sure sign. The urge to urinate, which is common in bladder infections, isn't usually an indication of kidney infection. Instead, you'll need to touch the kidney area for signs of tenderness.

Treatment includes antibiotics, complete bed rest until the symptoms go away and an increase in liquid intake, which will ensure frequent urination.

---

don't. But they know the first episode usually occurs between ages 20 and 40, and diet and heredity play key roles.

Kidney stones hurt, but they're often not serious. As long as there isn't an infection, you can wait weeks or even months for a small stone to pass on its own. But beware: Dr. Curhan says about 50 percent of people with stones will form a second stone in eight to ten years.

Still, the odds are high that every first-time stone sufferer will make a desperate call to their doc, says Jack McAninch, M.D., professor of urology and vice-chairman of the Department of Urology at the University of California, San Francisco. "Most stones require calling the doctor because of the intense pain they cause," Dr. McAninch says.

FAST FACTS

How common: Roughly one in seven men will develop a kidney stone in their lifetimes. Annually, just over a million people develop kidney stones.

Risk factors: Insufficient water intake, excessive salt intake, lots of meat in the diet, heredity. Also, chances are 50-50 that if you've had a kidney stone, you might develop another.

Age group affected: A first stone usually occurs between the ages of 20 and 40.

Gender gap: Affects men three times more often than women.

Who to see: Urologist or nephrologist.

Heading Off Pain at the Pass

Here's the important part: Kidney stones are easily prevented. Here are some steps that could stop a stone from developing.

Drink your troubles away. The more liquid you chug, the more urine you'll produce, which means stone-forming substances won't have as great a chance to build up in the first place.

"The most straightforward thing is to drink more, which will make your urine more diluted," says Howard Trachtman, M.D., chief of the Division of Nephrology at Schneider Children's Hospital at the Long Island campus of Albert Einstein College of Medicine in New Hyde Park, New York. Dr. Trachtman suggests drinking six to eight glasses of water a day: two at each meal and one in-between.

Cut back on meat. Many guys don't consider it a real meal until they've sunk their teeth into a juicy rib eye or sirloin. But men who eat more animal protein, which includes lower-fat meats, like chicken, are at greater risk of forming stones. "Animal protein does three things," says Dr. Curhan. "It increases urinary calcium secretion and increases uric acid secretion, both of which contribute to stones. And it lowers urinary citrate, which inhibits stone formation." The recommended daily meat intake is 2½ to 3 ounces of cooked lean meat, poultry or fish.

Pass on the salt. "Modest salt restriction is helpful," says Dr. Trachtman. "The kidney handles salt and calcium in parallel. If it's motivated to excrete high amounts of salt, that will be paralleled with high amounts of calcium in the urine."

Peel some bananas. Potassium, a nutrient found in fruits, like bananas, cantaloupe and apricots, and in vegetables, like lima beans and potatoes, has been linked with a lower incidence of kidney stones, says Dr. Curhan. On the other hand, you want to avoid foods with stone-forming oxalates, which include beets, spinach,

Gallstones: Eradicating the Pain in the Gut

The gallbladder is little more than a reservoir for bile, a fluid produced by the liver to aid in the digestion of fats. Day in, day out, it fills and empties in a boring, predictable way.

Sometimes, however, the chemicals that make up bile—most often cholesterol but sometimes calcium-containing pigments—crystallize into solid particles: gallstones. If a gallstone blocks the passageway from the gallbladder to the intestine, bile backs up, pressure builds up and pain develops. Severe pain.

A gallstone attack is disabling, and often excruciating. It's typically sudden, sharp and focused on the upper right portion of your abdomen. Nothing will make it go away before it's ready, a half-hour to a few hours later.

To make things worse, a gallstone attack can scare you half to death. "Sometimes it extends to the shoulder or upper back, or it may appear under the breastbone," says R. Thomas Holzbach, M.D., head of the Gastrointestinal Research Unit at the Cleveland Clinic Foundation. "It can be mistaken for a heart attack."

Like so many other unpleasant things, gallstones become more common with age. By the time you reach age 75, the odds are about one in five that you'll have one. Although women are even more likely to develop stones, the gender gap closes with age, and seems to be narrowing in general.

Genetics and regional lifestyles play a role: Gallstones are unheard of among the Masai of East Africa, while they're rampant among Pima Indians. Scandinavians and Chileans get many, while Asians get few. White men are more likely to have gallstones than black men.

You can't do much about your ethnicity, but you do have some control over another gallstone risk factor: weight. The more corpulent you are, it seems, the higher your chance of gallstones.

peanuts and chocolate. Some studies suggest vitamin B_6, which is found in kidney beans and sunflower seeds, could have anti-stone effects, but the jury is still out.

Drink your milk. In the past, doctors have directed men with stones to restrict their calcium intake. They argued that since most stones are calcium based, dietary calcium could only make matters worse. But a Harvard-based study that Dr. Curhan and three other physicians completed in 1993 shows just the opposite might be true. In a four-year study of 45,000 men ages 40 to 75, Dr. Curhan's team

Ironically, shedding pounds quickly puts you at far greater risk of a gallstone attack than remaining hefty. "The rapid loss of weight is clearly associated with the development of gallstones," says Dr. Everhart. Three to four pounds per week—the fast-track slimming promised by liquid formula diets—means major risk.

The gallbladder is a body part you can live very nicely without, and the standard treatment for gallstone attacks is to remove the offending organ. There are alternatives: Drugs and chemicals to dissolve the stones.

But let's not be too hasty about this. Only about 10 percent of men who develop gallstones actually have symptoms that are associated with them, according to Dr. Holzbach. Many discover their gallstones in the course of x-rays or ultrasounds taken for other reasons.

In this situation, the medical consensus seems pretty clear: Let them be.

If you have gallstones without any symptoms or pain, that might change someday. But then again, it might not. It's been estimated that 1 to 2 percent of "silent" stones act up in the ten years after diagnosis. And the longer they sit there quietly, the less likely they'll ever bring you grief.

Surgery, if you choose to have it, is a lot simpler than it used to be. With a slender tube, or laparoscope, the surgeon can remove the gallbladder through a series of small slits in the abdominal wall, rather than slicing your abdomen open. You're out of the hospital in about a day or two and may be up to speed in a week depending on your age and general health condition.

The nonsurgical approach—drugs or chemicals to dissolve the stone—can work for relatively small stones. They're likely to come back later, however, particularly if there are multiple stones, which frequently is the case, and this won't happen if your gallbladder is gone.

found that men who consumed more than four glasses of milk a day had a nearly 50 percent lower risk of developing kidney stones during the next four years than men who consumed less than two glasses a day worth of calcium.

"I wouldn't recommend restricting calcium," says Dr. Curhan. "About three glasses a day, or 800 milligrams, is fine." But he stresses not going overboard—consuming four times the recommended daily allowance won't provide four times the kidney stone protection.

If the Stone Won't Roll

For the most part, treatment of stones is limited to a regimen of medication, fluids and diet. Once the stone is passed, a day's collection of urine can be tested for mineral makeup, and based on the results, a doctor can prescribe a medication in some cases.

But in about 10 percent of cases, doctors have to intervene and break up a stubborn kidney stone when it just can't be passed. The most common method is non-invasive lithotripsy, in which sound waves are used to do the deed. With this procedure, you're partially submerged in water while a machine sends shock waves through the water that pulverize the stones. A more recent development is a lithotriptor that doesn't require immersion in water.

In a small number of cases, stones are just too hard or bulky to crush with sound waves. Only 1 percent of all doctor-intervened cases involves open surgery.

Lactose Intolerance

Coping with a Common Dairy Dilemma

Ever have a big, cool glass of moo juice or an ice-cream bar and feel shortly after like a percolator turned on in your intestines?

Then it's a good bet that you have lactose intolerance. Lactose is a sugar found in dairy products, like milk, ice cream or yogurt, and in products that contain milk, like pizza dough. To digest lactose, your body needs to produce an enzyme, lactase. With no lactase your body just passes the lactose along to the intestines. The sugar then "gets into the colon, where bacteria chew it up and break it down into small molecules that draw fluid into the colon," explains Robert S. Sandler, M.D., associate professor of medicine at the University of North Carolina School of Medicine in Chapel Hill.

In other words, the lactose "ferments," causing a nasty bloated feeling, cramps, gas and, more likely than not, diarrhea.

The Older You Get . . .

Lactose intolerance is so common, and often so benign, that it's hard to call it a disorder. "A lot of people say, 'I don't drink milk,'" says Sheah Rarback, R.D., spokeswoman for the American Dietetic Association in Miami. "It made them feel sick once, they got gas and bloated and stopped eating that food."

Babies usually produce loads of lactase. But as our bodies grow they stop producing it. An estimated 70 percent of the world's adult population has lost some or all of its ability to produce the enzyme. In the United States lactose intolerance is common among African Americans (an estimated 45 to 80 percent suffer from it), Mexican Americans (47 to 74 percent) and Asians (65 to 100 percent). The problem occurs in only 6 to 25 percent of American Whites.

Coping with the Curdling

Lactose intolerance can play small havoc on a guy's eating patterns. Men like a cold glass of milk from time to time, and nothing tops a meal like a bowl of ice cream. If you think slim, you probably relish yogurt and share the common view that it is one of nature's most perfect foods. Yogurt got its great reputation when, in

1907, the Russian-born scientist Elie Metchnikoff, a Nobel Prize winner in physiology and medicine, wrote a best seller entitled *The Prolongation of Life* in which he concluded that yogurt was associated with the extraordinary longevity of Bulgarians who happened to eat quite a lot of it. Metchnikoff was partially wrong: Yogurt's great but no miracle food. But it does seem strange that nature would deny adults easy access to this and other seemingly beneficial food products.

Here are some steps to deal with the problem.

Get tested. While millions experience lactose intolerance, not everybody has it equally bad. If you are uncertain what you have, an easy way to find out is to stop consuming dairy products for a week. If the symptoms go away, you are probably one of those millions.

Or you can seek out a doctor specializing in gastrointestinal disorders for a breath hydrogen test. With this procedure, you drink a lactose solution on an empty tummy and then get your breath sampled over an eight-hour period. The doctor will be watching for an increase in hydrogen.

Skip it. There's no "cure" for lactose intolerance, so the simplest way to avoid the problem is to skip it. Cut out milk, cheese, yogurt—the works. The good news is that if your calcium intake is adequate, "Milk is not a necessary ingredient in the diet for adults," and eliminating the food is "not a problem," Rarback says.

Cut back. Total avoidance of dairy products might be overkill. From 30 to 95 percent of those who are lactose intolerant can stand a single eight-ounce glass of milk or its equal, and any extra undigested lactose will just pass through without discomfort.

Some milk products are lower in lactose than others. Hard or aged cheeses, for example, have little lactose. So head for naturally aged Swiss or Cheddar. Emmenthal, Roquefort and Camembert cheeses are also low in lactose. Avoid cottage cheese. Butter's okay. Avoid ice cream. A little whipped cream is okay although you should abstain from sour cream. Sweetened condensed milk is a no-no and that's what they put in pies, so watch out. Many of the people with lactose intolerance can handle acidophilus milk.

The idea here is: Find your level, and then don't overdo it.

Fill in the gaps. Dairy products provide large doses of calcium and other vitamins and minerals. Calcium plays a key—although as yet not fully understood—role in building strong bones and preventing osteoporosis in old age. Cut out dairy products and you're possibly writing yourself down for eventual bone problems. So monitor your diet to be sure you're getting enough calcium and vitamins, and consider supplements if you are concerned.

Eat the enzyme. Lactose intolerance has been termed the hot disorder of the

FAST FACTS

How common: Very common. As much as 70 percent of the world's adult population, including as many as 50 million Americans report discomfort from consuming milk products.

Risk factors: There's no particular risk factors since there's no good explanation as to why it happens. As the body ages it loses the ability to digest lactose.

Age group affected: More common the older a man gets.

Gender gap: Both sexes are equally affected.

Who to see: Family doctor. If you think you're lactose intolerant and want to find out but don't want to experiment on your own, there are tests that can be performed.

1990s, and medical companies have poured millions into the development of enzyme supplements such as Dairy Ease and Lactaid.

Dairy Ease, Lactaid and similar products provide the lactase your body doesn't provide. They essentially predigest for you. There are no negative side effects associated with these products, but they come in a variety of forms: pills, tablets or liquid. Be sure to follow directions; the drops, for example, need to be added to milk as much as 24 hours prior to consumption in order for it to be easily digestible. Tablets, on the other hand, are taken right along with the food.

Go alternative. Soy milk is the best alternative for those craving something like a glass of moo juice, although it's not as rich in vitamins. Delete ice cream from your diet and go for fruits instead. Tofu can be interchanged for cheese. Be creative in finding alternatives to dairy products.

Walk it off. If your insides are rumbling from a misbegotten bowl of ice cream, take a walk. Strolling helps push food through the intestines and could help cause the release of a hormone that encourages bowel activity. Herbal teas also help relieve gas, as do over-the-counter medications containing simethicone.

Laryngitis

Speak Softly and Keep a Strong Voice

After a season of towering home runs, magnificent pitching and come-from-behind wins, the Milwaukee Brewers strode triumphantly into the World Series for the first time a few years back. From the ballpark to neighborhood bars, guys gathered to wildly scream and yell for their beloved team.

But when the cheering stopped, the Brewers had lost the Series, and some of the team's most enthusiastic fans had lost something more precious: their voices.

"We didn't see a large increase in the number of patients with voice problems after that series, but we did see a few more. However, voice misuse like that is a very typical cause of laryngitis," says Bruce Campbell, M.D., an otolaryngologist at the Medical College of Wisconsin in Milwaukee.

In fact, laryngitis, an inflammation of the vocal cords, is a common disorder that can strike men at any age, says Greg Grillone, M.D., an otolaryngologist and director of the Voice Center at Boston University Medical Center.

"Virtually every man at some time during his life will experience a bout of laryngitis, ranging from mild hoarseness to total loss of voice," Dr. Grillone says.

The Voice Stops Here

When the larynx, also known as the voice box, is in tip-top condition, air passes through it and vibrates a tensed pair of flaps called the vocal cords. These vibrations produce sounds that are shaped into words by the mouth and tongue.

But when the vocal cords swell up, they don't vibrate as well, making it difficult to speak. Nasty bacterial infections, colds and flus are the most common reasons for your voice box to swell. You also can lose your voice if you overstrain it by howling at an umpire's lousy calls or by singing all night, Dr. Campbell says. Smoke, allergies, chemical fumes, dry air and alcohol can compound the problem.

Usually laryngitis fades in three or four days. If it persists or if you have a temperature of 101°F or higher or if you cough up any blood, see your doctor, says Hinda Greene, D.O., an internal medicine and emergency medicine physician at the Cleveland Clinic Hospital in Fort Lauderdale, Florida.

FAST FACTS

How common: Any guy is susceptible to laryngitis, and virtually all will suffer from it at some point.

Risk factors: Smoking, recent colds or flu, exposure to harsh chemicals, allergies, excessive yelling, screaming or singing.

Age group affected: Possible at any age.

Gender gap: Men and women are equally likely to get laryngitis.

Who to see: Family doctor or otolaryngologist.

Keeping in Sound Shape

Fortunately, laryngitis often can be prevented. Here's how.

Pace yourself. "The more yelling and screaming you do, the greater the chance that you'll be hoarse for a few days," says Bradley M. Block, M.D., a family doctor in private practice in Winter Park, Florida. Try to keep the volume of your voice down. Use amplification if you're talking to a large group. Avoid screaming or trying to talk over loud noises. If you talk nonstop during the day, rearrange your schedule so you can give your voice a ten-minute rest every couple of hours, Dr. Block suggests.

Nub the butts. Smoking can chronically inflame the vocal cords. So if you smoke, quit, suggests Eric G. Anderson, M.D., a family physician in La Jolla, California. If you're a nonsmoker, avoid passive smoke—common in nightclubs and some restaurants—since it also can trigger laryngitis.

Go easy on the booze. Excessive amounts of beer, wine and other alcoholic beverages can dilate blood vessels and cause swelling of the larynx (a structure in your throat that contains the vocal cords), Dr. Grillone says. If you do imbibe, limit yourself to no more than one or two drinks a day.

Stop clearing your throat. Habitually rumbling your throat can irritate the voice box. "It's a mannerism that certainly could cause trouble," Dr. Anderson says. To break this habit, take a sip of water whenever you feel the urge to do it.

Mask out harmful fumes. Wear a respiratory mask if you're working around harsh chemicals or paints that can harm your voice, Dr. Block says. Make sure your work area is well-ventilated and take a five- to ten-minute break for some fresh air at least once an hour.

Get a grip on postnasal drip. Nasal congestion caused by flus, colds and allergies can ooze down into the throat and irritate the vocal cords, Dr. Campbell says. Break up any mucus with an over-the-counter expectorant that contains guaifenesin, like Robitussin-PE.

Pump up the humidity. Regular use of air conditioners or heating systems can strip humidity from the air and can dry out your vocal cords, Dr. Block says. Crack open a window occasionally in warm weather or use a humidifier to replenish moisture in your home during cold weather.

When Words Fail You

If, despite these precautions, you wake up one morning sounding like Marlon Brando or Joe Cocker, don't panic. There are plenty of other homegrown solutions that will help you get your voice back pronto.

"For laryngitis many of the old remedies suggested by your grandmother still hold true," Dr. Anderson says. Here's a sampling.

Keep quiet. "You should rest your voice completely," Dr. Greene says. "Whispering isn't as bad as talking, but you're still using your vocal cords. It's like walking on a sprained ankle. You wouldn't do that if you wanted your ankle to get well. It's the same thing with your voice. If you need to communicate with someone, write notes. I know it's tough to do that, but that's how your vocal cords are going to heal the fastest," she says.

Get plenty of snooze time. Don't play "modern warrior" and march off to work or the gym in the belief that you can fight through the hurt. Allow yourself the luxury of being a couch potato for a couple of days so your body's natural defenses can help you fight off the problem, Dr. Greene says.

Steam it away. Sometimes standing in a steaming hot shower for 10 to 15 minutes will help your throat feel better when you have laryngitis, Dr. Greene says. You also might try pouring boiling hot water into a basin containing a dab of mentholated rub. Then drape a towel over your head, lean over and breathe in the fumes for two or three minutes, Dr. Anderson says. Do that three times a day for two or three days. Using a humidifier also may help.

Calm it with honey. A teaspoon of honey swallowed slowly may bathe the area around your vocal cords in a soothing liquid, Dr. Anderson suggests.

Drink plenty of fluids. Drinking at least one eight-ounce glass of water every hour while you're awake will help refresh your dry throat and reduce the swelling of your vocal cords, says Dr. Greene.

Lung Cancer

Easy to Avoid, Hard to Cure

It's a grim accolade: Of all man-killing cancers, lung cancer is tops. In fact, more than twice as many men die from lung cancer than from its next closest rival, prostate cancer. That's the bad news. The good news is that lung cancer is unique in that we know what causes it. Approximately 80 to 90 percent of cases are caused by outside contaminants, or carcinogens, particularly tobacco smoke, which generally are easy to sidestep.

It's no wonder that medical specialists like the folks at the American Lung Association (ALA) always stress prevention when talking about this disease. But there's another reason as well: "Lung cancer may be one of the most preventable cancers, but it's also one of the least curable," says Alfred Munzer, M.D., co-director of pulmonary medicine at Washington Adventist Hospital in Takoma Park, Maryland, and past president of the ALA. The average five-year survival rate for lung cancer is only 13 percent.

The main reason for this is that lung cancer is difficult to detect: Symptoms such as coughing and shortness of breath don't show up until the cancer is already well-advanced—and difficult to treat. Even the diagnostic tools most commonly used in hopes of finding it early—chest x-rays and sputum analysis—have trouble picking up tumors in time to significantly improve a patient's life span. What to do?

The Big Three

A number of factors play a role in the onset of lung cancer, but three preventive steps stand out.

Stop smoking. "By far the most important thing you can do is to not smoke," says Dr. Munzer. Overall, smokers are ten times more likely to die from lung cancer than nonsmokers. Once you stop, however, the lungs immediately begin to nurture themselves back to health, slowly but surely. Ten years after quitting, a smoker's risk of lung cancer drops to 30 to 50 percent that of other smokers who continued their habit. After 15 to 20 years risk becomes similar to that of someone who never smoked at all. By one estimate, taking the "Don't smoke" advice saves 434,000 lives a year.

Don't get it secondhand. Studies have consistently found that breathing other people's smoke is almost as bad as smoking yourself, which is why smokers are increasingly being booted out of public buildings, offices, restaurants and shopping malls. In 1993 the Environmental Protection Agency (EPA) declared secondhand smoke a cancer-causing substance and held it responsible for 3,000 lung cancer deaths in nonsmokers each year. By some estimates, having close contact with a smoker raises your risk of lung cancer by 30 to 70 percent, depending on how heavily the other person smokes. In short, if you don't smoke, other people who do smoke provide a major risk factor for lung cancer.

Vent the cellar. It comes from beneath the earth, undetectable by smell, sight, taste or touch. It's radon, a natural radioactive gas formed by the breakdown of uranium in rocks and soil. In the open air it's harmless, but when trapped in airtight houses, it can build to dangerous levels. According to the EPA, radon is the leading cause of lung cancer after smoking. It's a controversial point: Many studies have failed to find strong links between radon exposure and lung cancer, but many others have, including long-term studies in Sweden that find high exposures over time boost the risk of lung cancer by 30 to 80 percent, depending on the amount of radon exposure. Smoking multiplies the danger.

To get rid of radon, first get a test kit from your local hardware store to determine household levels. If they're high, one solution is to have a contractor install a simple system of venting pipes and fans to suck air from beneath your basement and release it above the house. In the meantime open a window: Even a small draft can cut radon concentration by half or more.

The Carrot Defense and Other Tactics

That's not the end of the story when it comes to prevention, however. There's a new area of research called chemoprevention, which has nothing to do with dangerous drugs and everything to do with healthy eating. "In study after study, people who choose to eat more fruits and vegetables tend to have lower rates of lung cancer," says Susan Mayne, Ph.D., associate director for Cancer Prevention and Control Research at Yale Cancer Center. Studies have found that people who ate few fruits and vegetables had twice the rate of lung cancer as people who ate a lot.

One of the specific nutrients that may have anticancer effects is beta-carotene, a nutrient that's plentiful in dark green leafy vegetables such as spinach, and orange-colored fruits and vegetables such as apricots and carrots. Another is vitamin E, which is found in many vegetable oils. The jury is still out on whether supplements of these nutrients will stave off lung cancer. For example, two large studies during 1994 came to conflicting conclusions about their effects.

Bottom line: Forget supplementing your diet with any nutrient in particular and

FAST FACTS

How common: Lung cancer kills 94,000 men a year—roughly one per 1,000—in the United States, more than any other form of cancer.

Risk factors: Cigarette smoke is responsible for 90 percent of lung cancer in men. Radon exposure may also play a role, especially in smokers. Family history of the disease also puts you at slightly higher risk.

Age group affected: Chances of getting lung cancer are greatest in men after age 60.

Gender gap: 35,000 more men die of lung cancer each year than women, probably because men have smoked longer than women.

Who to see: Oncologist.

focus on eating more produce in general. "Fruits and vegetables are very complex mixtures of literally hundreds of different chemical compounds," says Dr. Mayne. "Most of them we know little about, but preliminary data suggests that several compounds in fruits and vegetables may have cancer-inhibiting properties." The National Cancer Institute (NCI) recommends getting at least five helpings of fruits and vegetables daily. Beyond that, a diet rich in fruits and vegetables will also be proportionately lower in fat, which some research suggests may also be a risk factor for lung cancer.

Breathing Easier

If lung cancer strikes you, the basic treatment plan is to surgically remove the tumor, which generally means taking out either a lobe of one lung or the whole lung. Essentially, you could be left with only half of your lung power, and if you've been a smoker, you may be further plagued by emphysema or bronchitis. If surgery is not appropriate (because, for example, there's another respiratory problem, such as pneumonia, or the cancer has spread to other parts of the body), doctors may instead prescribe radiation or chemotherapy.

New technology may make treatment less drastic, especially for tumors that are still small. One particularly promising treatment being tested is called photodynamic therapy. In it, patients are injected with a drug that tumor cells soak up. A laser device that's moved to the site through the airway then emits a specific wavelength of light, which activates the drug and kills the cancer cells. "The benefit is that there's not much toxicity involved and it hopefully eliminates the need for a major operation," says Harvey I. Pass, M.D., head of the thoracic oncology section of the NCI's surgery branch.

Even more exciting are vital improvements in diagnosis, which is particularly crucial for smokers, people with a family history of the disease and others at high risk. Among them:

Shining a light: With the help of a light/camera device in the airway, computers analyze light reflected off of cells, identifying patterns that are distinctive to tumors.

Cellular bloodhounds: Antibodies that are highly sensitive to cell changes are put into spit samples; the antibodies home in on abnormal or cancerous cells and flag them with a red stain.

Gene forecasting: DNA obtained from spit samples is artificially mutated *Jurassic Park*-like to find evidence of cancer-making cell changes.

"These techniques may even allow us to detect abnormalities *before* they become cancer, which helps determine which patients to keep an eye on, and where to look for problems," says Dr. Pass.

Lyme Disease

Don't Let Ticks Bug You

Lyme disease is the country's most common bugborne ailment. But don't let that number one rating fool you: Lyme disease doesn't rack up meganumbers. The Centers for Disease Control and Prevention (CDC) in Atlanta reports about 9,000 cases annually. And that figure has been stable for five years.

So a guy's chance of actually contracting Lyme disease is low. You have to be in the wrong place at the wrong time with the wrong bug, bearing the wrong bacteria, and it has to bite you. That's a lot of wrongs.

Learning about Lyme

The wrong bug goes by the formal name *Ixodes dammini* but most men know it as the deer tick. The ones to worry about are usually in the nymphal stage of their growth, meaning they're just tiny enough—poppy-seed size—that you don't notice them. They hook onto your body, sink their mouth parts into your skin and start sucking blood—usually without you knowing.

Nasty as that notion is, you won't get Lyme unless your bloodsucker is infected with the bacteria that causes it—*Borrelia burgdorferi*. Even then, in most cases, Lyme sends up a red flag—a distinctive, round, radiating rash.

"It looks like a red blotch. And it can start smaller than a quarter and spread to three inches or more," describes Durland Fish, Ph.D., associate research scientist in the Department of Epidemiology and Public Health at Yale University School of Medicine.

About 70 percent of the men nipped by an infected tick develop that telltale rash. The other 30 percent will come down with different, flulike signs: fever, chills, headache, stiff neck, fatigue, muscle aches, joint pain. Being men, we may not call the doctor until the faux flu beats us down—usually by persisting longer than a normal flu or by making repeat appearances.

Occasionally, an infected man gets more exotic symptoms: irregular heartbeat or shortness of breath, Bell's palsy, which is a facial paralysis, and loss of memory or concentration.

And infected men who ignore the disease for too long may be sentencing them-selves to a form of arthritis that can last a lifetime. This intermittent arthritis—typ-ically in the knees—has been dubbed Lyme arthritis.

In reality, though, most men bitten by ticks won't develop so much as an itch. Even in those parts of the country that are rich in sick ticks, fewer than 2 percent of all tick bites lead to Lyme disease. "And in many places, you're at absolutely no risk of Lyme disease," says Dr. Fish. "If you do live or recreate in a tick-infested area, though, you should institute some sort of bite protection," he adds.

Scouting the Enemy

Man is part of the problem with infectious ticks—successful man. We like to build handsome homes on the fringes of forests. We love a lawn that backs up to the woods. "And it's at the edge of the forest where risk lies," says Andrew Spielman, Sc.D., professor of tropical health at the Harvard School of Public Health. "Ticks like the low woody vegetation at the edge of the forest," he says.

But the Lyme bomb doesn't tick in all woods.

Phone home. "It's important to determine what your risk of acquiring Lyme disease really is," says Dr. Fish.

A call to your local health department will help you evaluate risk. Another likely source is your local agricultural extension service. Your state health department and the CDC can also answer questions.

"The risk is geographically very specific," explains Roy Campbell, M.D., medical epidemiologist for the CDC's Division of Vector-Borne Infectious Disease in Fort Collins, Colorado. "There are three hot spots—the Northeast, the upper Midwest and northern California. But even there, risk varies from place to place. You can't get Lyme disease standing on a slab of concrete in New York City. But the region around Lyme (Connecticut, where the disease was first identified and named in the mid-1970s) reports one case per 100 people—a very high rate for any disease."

Tackle the yard. If you do live on the edge of the woods in a hot spot, you can make it less hot by keeping the lawn mowed and by removing leaf and wood piles that attract tick hosts—mice and chipmunks. Bird feeders host tick parties, too.

A ten-foot high fence can keep out the deer on which ticks breed, reducing risk by 80 percent, Dr. Fish found. A single late-spring spraying of insecticide on your lawn can drop risk another 90 percent, he says.

Think vacation. Say you live in the South, where Lyme disease is rare. But it's summer and you've always wanted to cool off in a place like Martha's Vineyard or Nantucket. Both Massachusetts islands are havens for infected ticks. "But that's not in any tourist brochures," says Dr. Fish. So, in addition to taking the tick pulse of your home environs, check out your vacation choice, too.

FAST FACTS

How common: The Centers for Disease Control and Prevention in Atlanta reports about 9,000 cases of Lyme disease annually.

Risk factors: Exposure to infected ticks. That's more likely to occur from May through October, with early summer the riskiest time. The most likely sites of infection are in Connecticut, Delaware, Maryland, Massachusetts, Minnesota, New Jersey, New York, Pennsylvania, Rhode Island and Wisconsin. In those places forestry workers, telephone linemen, construction workers, railroad workers and outdoorsmen are at highest risk.

Age group affected: Fifty-five percent of cases hit children ages 19 and younger; 30 percent hit adults ages 20 to 49; the remaining 15 percent hit adults ages 50 and older.

Gender gap: Equally divided between men and women.

Who to see: Family doctor, infectious disease specialist or rheumatologist.

Entering the Woods

Few men will avoid the woods just because of fear of Lyme disease, but that doesn't mean we should be reckless out there either. Here are precautions for playing in tick hot spots.

Don't get naked. Wear white painter's pants or light khakis, not shorts, advises Dr. Spielman. Stuff your pant legs in your socks. And wear long-sleeved shirts. You can spot dark ticks better on light-colored clothes. And you can impede them by covering up bare skin. "Look down now and then to see if anything's traveling north. If it is, then knock it off," adds Dr. Spielman.

Pump it out. To make your clothing even less congenial to bugs, spritz them with a repellent that contains permethrin (Perma-Kill 4-Week Tick Killer), says Dr. Fish. A few outdoor-gear retailers, travel health clinics and catalogs sell permethrin in aerosol cans, but it's not easy to find. Do not use it on the skin, however. If you do wear short sleeves or shorts, cover exposed bare skin with a repellent that contains 35 percent DEET (diethyltoluamide), says Dr. Campbell.

Walk the straight and narrow. One way to avoid ticks is by avoiding the deep brush and high grasses of suspect woodlands. "Stay in the middle of trails," advises Dr. Campbell.

Hunting the Wild Tick

The tick check is important as well to avoiding Lyme disease, say epidemiologists. If you nab the parasite right away, even if it's infected, your risk of disease drops like a stone. Ticks are the slow feeders of the fauna world. It takes them at least 24 hours and probably closer to 48 to pass *Borrelia b.* into your blood, Dr. Campbell says.

Groom the gorilla. Ticks love hairy places. That's why you need a hat in infected territory. And why you especially need to check for ticks in other hairy areas, like the groin.

Tiny nymphal ticks can hide without fear on your hairy head, where you can't see them. So if you don't wear a hat, ask your wife or girlfriend to help you tick hunt there. (*And* on your back—another hiding place.) Then return the favor.

Pick ticks. If you do bag a tick, remove it carefully. Use a pair of tweezers with a fine tip—or even forceps—to grasp its body as close to its mouth parts as possible. Slowly and gently pull the tick straight out using steady pressure. Don't twist or squeeze it—or tainted saliva may squirt into the bite. After you remove the tick, disinfect the spot and wash your hands with soap and water. (It's a good idea to save the tick in a glass jar for identification.)

Call Doctor Lyme. Okay, your surgical skills were a mite sloppy. A few days after removal you notice a round red blotch where the tick was. Then it spreads and you feel like you have the flu. Pick up the phone and call your family doctor. He won't have any trouble with a Lyme diagnosis once he sees that rash.

If you're one of the 30 percent who doesn't develop the rash, it's a tougher call for the family doctor and he may refer you to a rheumatologist.

And if you are diagnosed with Lyme, a course of antibiotics should wipe it out. Antibiotics cure 95 percent of all Lyme cases.

Malaria

How to Skip the Tropical Punch

It's a disease of explorers, adventurers and patriotic tough guys, right? Malaria: Endured by Hemingways on African safaris, Marines in Asian rice paddies, Indiana Jones on bad days in Borneo. An exotic infection, a manly mark, a red bite of courage. That's malaria.

Don't be fooled. Catching a deadly disease from a mosquito is hardly exotic or adventurous. According to statistics from the Centers for Disease Control and Prevention (CDC) in Atlanta, the mosquitoborne infectious disease continues to devastate the tropical Third World, striking over 120 million people every year and causing more than a million deaths.

Malaria isn't common in this country because public health measures wiped it out almost 50 years ago. The CDC tallies an average 1,000 cases annually, with roughly two-thirds of those among men. Between 1980 and 1992 only 45 unfortunates lost their lives to the disease here.

Tropical travelers can't ignore malaria, though. The CDC predicts risk to increase as more Americans visit countries where malaria is endemic—and as the parasite that causes it becomes more resistant to available drugs.

Basic Vampirology

Four species of a one-celled organism called *Plasmodium* can cause malaria. But it takes an infected female of the anopheline mosquito to transport any of the *Plasmodium* parasites to humans.

The anopheles is like the tiniest vampire. It alights on a hunk of flesh, sinks in a stinger and partakes of a blood meal. We get infected by the drool of the ghoul: *Plasmodium* slides out of the mosquito's salivary glands and into our bloodstreams. Eventually, our tainted blood cells burst, spewing more infection into our bloodstreams, downriver to our livers.

That explosion is what starts malaria's classic signs: shuddering chills, raging fever and drenching sweats. Other symptoms can show up, too: joint pain, backache and headache, diarrhea, nausea and vomiting. If malaria is allowed to progress, delirium, coma and death usually follow.

"So we have to prevent being bitten," says Stephen Bezruchka, M.D., author of *The Pocket Doctor* and *Trekking in Nepal: A Travelers Guide* and a faculty member in the international health program at the University of Washington in Seattle.

Foiling the Bloodsucker

Travelers have to use two different kinds of prevention, says Monica E. Parise, M.D., epidemic intelligence service officer of the CDC's malaria section.

The first is preventive medication. In the movies the preventive drug of choice was always quinine. Today, the drugs most commonly used are different: mefloquine (Lariam), the antibiotic doxycycline (Vibramycin) and chloroquine (Aralen).

The other preventive is personal protection—proper clothes, insect repellent and so on.

But first things first.

Bone up. Before you go swinging on vines in jungles—or even climbing ruins in southern Mexico, call the CDC's 24-hour hot line. The call will get you the latest details about disease risk at your destination—and the most up-to-date preventive medication. The telephone number is (404) 332-4555.

Much of tropical and subtropical countries are malarious, including parts of Mexico and the rest of Central and South America, the Middle East and parts of Asia, the lands of the central and south Pacific and sub-Saharan Africa. Cities and tourist spots are generally safe, but Africa is an exception. The continent is home to the *Plasmodium* species from hell, *P. falciparum*, which is most associated with death. Eighty percent of the deaths reported to the CDC start with sting from an African mosquito.

Phone early. Don't wait until the day before departure to call the CDC. If you're going to an area infected with malaria, you'll need time to call your family doctor to get a preventive prescription. Or seek out a travel clinic where a knowledgeable doctor or nurse can advise you on the right medication to take. The medication is based on the activities you will undertake, your level of risk assumption and the types and habits of the mosquitoes and parasites where you will be.

Many of the antimalarials should be started one to two weeks before takeoff. Although side effects are minor (some nausea, diarrhea, dizziness or sleep disturbances have been reported), a two-week head start will point out any problems. In order to be effective, take the medication as prescribed and then always continue the medication for four weeks following your trip.

Men may hate to take pills, especially healthy men, but just think about the last batch of American troops who went to Africa—270 of them ignored their meds, landed in Somalia and soon started sweating malaria bullets.

FAST FACTS

How common: Malaria does not occur in the United States—an average of 1,000 cases, which are imported by travelers, are reported annually to the Centers for Disease Control and Prevention (CDC) in Atlanta.

Risk factors: Travelers going to rural areas of malarious countries are at highest risk. Campers in tents are at greater risk than businessmen in air-conditioned hotel rooms. Rainy seasons, which breed mosquitoes, are riskier than dry seasons.

Age group affected: Most cases of malaria occur in Americans ages 20 to 39—not coincidentally, the years of greatest travel. Mortality increases with increasing age among American travelers. The greatest death toll worldwide, however, is among children under age five.

Gender gap: About 65 percent of the cases reported to the CDC occur in men.

Who to see: Malaria doesn't give you much time. See your family doctor if he's familiar with the disease. Many emergency-care doctors have treated cases, too. And tropical medicine specialists would know malaria best of all.

Body Armor

"Even if you take the medication correctly, you won't lower your risk to zero," warns Dr. Parise. In addition to preventive drugs, you also have to raise some walls between yourself and the evil anopheles. Here's how:

Buy a bednet. If you're roughing it in the tropics, a bednet is essential, say malariologists. If possible, soak or spray it with an insecticide containing permethrin. One way to do this is with a product called Perma-Kill 4-Week Tick Killer, says Dr. Bezruchka. One container is enough to spray four sets of clothes and a bednet. The company that makes it also supplies the military. A few outdoor-gear retailers, travel health clinics and catalogs also sell permethrin in aerosol cans, but it's not easy to find.

Soak and spray. Other items besides your bednet need to be treated with permethrin, too. Make sure you spray your clothes. Or soak them in the liquid form of the insecticide and let them dry. Permethrin is not for use on the skin, however. For protecting bare skin, use an insect repellent that contains about 35 percent DEET (diethyltoluamide), says Dr. Parise.

Wear lights or whites. "Mosquitoes like colorful clothing," says Dr. Bezruchka. And they like naked muscle even more. That's why your khakis should be long-sleeved and full-legged.

"If you cover up your skin, the mosquito won't be able to find a place to feed," Dr. Bezruchka adds. Consider using a mosquito head net as well. They are available from surplus or camping supply stores.

Sweat in the sun. Avoid exercise at night, says Dr. Bezruchka. "Those are the times mosquitoes are the most active. And they like sweat, too," he says. In fact, experts advise staying inside a screened room or netted tent from dusk to dawn in risky places. "That's one of the main things I do when I travel," he says.

Pack a doctor's bag. If you're leaving civilization and medical care far behind—in Borneo or along the Zambezi River, for instance—Dr. Parise advises taking medication to treat malaria with you, just in case. That drug is usually pyrimethamine/sulfadoxine (Fansidar). It will help you fight the disease until you can reach a doctor.

In Case of Fever

If you take your medication and keep your body covered, the risk of malaria lowers to near nil, says Jane Zucker, M.D., an epidemiologist at CDC. But if you do start to run a fever within six days of exposure or even several months after coming home, don't wait around to see if it gets better or worse. And don't even consider toughing it out. Since symptoms of malaria are so common—remember, they include headache, chills, sweats, back pain, nausea, diarrhea and cough—malaria can be misdiagnosed.

Get to a doctor. At the first sign of a fever pick up the telephone and call your family doctor. If he's not available, call an emergency room. "Malaria, especially from *falciparum*, can progress rapidly," says Dr. Bezruchka.

Tell the doc right away that you've been in a malarial country. Diagnosis can be done from a blood smear. Treatment often is antibiotics or quinine.

Malaria may be deadly, but death is preventable. "Malaria is a completely treatable disease," says Dr. Zucker, "if diagnosed and treated promptly."

Memory Loss

Keeping Tabs on the Car Keys

What's going on here? Your boss asks you a detail about that meeting in Chicago last week and you can't remember. You have an important lunch date this afternoon and you forgot to make a restaurant reservation. Walking down the street, you run into a new client; his name totally escapes you. To cap it off, you spend the afternoon in a sales conference listening to that punk from marketing rattle off facts and figures like he had a computer chip installed in his 22-year-old brain.

Even for the most self-confident among us, on days like this a twinge of doubt is bound to creep in. Am I losing my edge?

The answer is both yes and no. Experts agree that certain parts of our memories do indeed fade with age. The good news is that the decline is probably not as severe as you think, and you can learn plenty of countermeasures to make up for what you've lost. Even better, experts believe some memory skills actually improve as we get older, providing men in their thirties and forties with mental advantages those smart-aleck kids can't begin to match.

The Facts of Life

Just as our time in the 100-yard dash is probably slower now than it was ten years ago, so some of our memory functions—those requiring speedy thinking, by and large—aren't what they used to be. "The slowing in memory is tied to the biological deterioration of the nervous system," says Michael Pressley, Ph.D., professor of educational psychology and statistics at the State University of New York at Albany. "You function more slowly as you get older."

According to a report published by Harvard Medical School, some memory functions, such as the ability to recognize faces and the ability to memorize new materials, start slowing down as early as our twenties. By your midthirties you can expect to have more trouble than you used to remembering names, and words may be getting stuck on the tip of your tongue a little more often. These changes continue over the course of a lifetime, but they're so slight and so gradual that they shouldn't cause significant problems, if they ever do, until you're well into your seventies or eighties. Severe memory loss before then is cause to see a doctor.

When it comes to the run-of-the-mill memory glitches that annoy and sometimes embarrass, your lifestyle is almost certainly the culprit, not your wiring. Experts agree that stress, lack of sleep and the overwhelming number of distractions competing for our attention in the modern world are much more often the causes of forgetfulness than any physical decline.

The busier you are—and in midlife, responsibilities and distractions are at their peak—the more likely you are to start missing some of the fine print along the way. "If the demands on your memory are heavier, you're probably making more errors," says Dr. Pressley.

Take That, Young Whippersnappers

Despite their loss of focus and speed, men in their thirties and forties have at least two qualities of memory that younger men can't hope to match: experience and perspective. With time we develop what the English neurobiologist Steven Rose, author of *The Making of Memory*, calls "better strategies to cope with and manipulate information." This is a skill that used to be known, Rose says, as "wisdom."

According to Anderson D. Smith, Ph.D., director of the School of Psychology at the Georgia Institute of Technology in Atlanta, older men tend to focus on details less effectively than younger men, but that's partly because of the fact that they're busy looking at the bigger picture.

One form of memory that remains strong into one's sixties or seventies—and may even improve with age—is what Dr. Smith calls semantic memory, which includes conceptual knowledge about the world as well as general vocabulary skills. Semantic memory helps us add knowledge based on what we already know. "Most people think of memory as a warehouse," Dr. Smith says, "but that's probably not the best metaphor. A better one would be a scaffolding. The larger it is, the more places you have to add more features."

Pay Attention!

How to make the most of the memory you have? The first rule to remember is concentration. You can't lock something in your mind that hasn't entered it in the first place. Therefore, do anything you can that will help your mind to focus.

One of the best ways to keep the brain capable of concentration is to take care of yourself. Like any body organ, the brain, and hence the memory, benefits from proper care. Numerous studies suggest that regular exercise and a balanced diet help the brain to function at peak efficiency. "Anything that promotes health and well-

FAST FACTS

How common: Some degree of memory decline with aging is virtually universal.

Risk factors: Aging is unavoidable, but good health, an active lifestyle and mental stimulation can offset most age-related memory loss.

Age group affected: Some forms of memory, such as the ability to remember names and memorize new information, start declining as early as our twenties and continue declining gradually over a lifetime. Other forms of memory show no signs of deterioration and may grow even stronger with age.

Gender gap: Researchers have found no difference in the rate or types of normal age-related memory loss between the sexes. There's some evidence that men are slightly less likely to get Alzheimer's disease than women, possibly because testosterone may provide men's brains with some protection.

Who to see: Neurologist, mental health expert. Some hospitals have memory assessment clinics.

being is going to promote the thinking process," Dr. Smith says. "We all know that if we feel better, we perform better."

Here are some specific areas to watch.

Chill out. Growing evidence confirms what most of us would intuitively suspect: The more frantic you are, the worse your memory's likely to be. A five-year study with 130 volunteers at McGill University in Montreal found that people with high levels of a stress hormone called cortisol in their blood retained new information less efficiently than people who didn't.

Keep your blood pressure down. Various studies have suggested a link between high blood pressure and memory problems. One, at Duke University Medical Center in Durham, North Carolina, found that people with high blood pressure had lower-than-average scores on learning tests. Those findings were reinforced by a study at the National Institute on Aging in Bethesda, Maryland, in which researchers used magnetic resonance imaging to compare the brains of (otherwise healthy) men with high blood pressure and those without. The result: Men with high blood pressure had lost more brain tissue.

Sleep to remember, remember to sleep. People who are well-rested and alert remember more than people who are tired and distracted. Dreams help, too. During a test at the Weizmann Institute of Science in Israel some sleepers were awakened while in the midst of rapid eye movement sleep, when dreams are deepest. Others were allowed to sleep undisturbed. The latter group performed newly learned tasks faster and better the next morning. In addition, tests show that your chances of remembering something are better if you go to sleep immediately after absorbing it. Going out for a nightcap before hitting the sack will only muddle the issue.

Just say no. Alcohol—and marijuana and cocaine for that matter—can muddle the brain in more ways than one. Experts say the evidence is overwhelming that these drugs fog memory. Chronic alcohol abuse can lead to one of the most devastating memory diseases, Korsakoff's syndrome, which causes the brain to shrink.

In one interesting circumstance, though, alcohol actually benefits memory. According to Dr. Pressley, if you have an experience while you're drunk and then forget it when you sober up, you're more likely to be able to recall the experience by getting drunk again. This points up the importance of context in memory: re-creating the mental state in which the original experience occurred. Drunkenness in this case acts as a mental cue.

Cut the coffee, stub the butt. Other drugs to avoid if you're concerned about mental sharpness are caffeine and nicotine. Both are stimulants, and what goes up must come down. The inevitable crash from a coffee or cigarette high can interfere with concentration, and therefore affect memory.

Mind your medications. Concentration can also be affected by any number of products in your medicine cabinet. Antihistamines, for example, can cause grogginess. So can ibuprofen, for some people. Add various high blood pressure medications to the list, along with any cough suppressants that contain codeine, alcohol, dextromethorphan. All can be fuzzmakers and memory breakers.

Calisthenics and Cheating

If your memory's getting a little flabby, memory experts have plenty of exercises to suggest for helping it stay in shape. The experts can also recommend techniques that will help you take some of the pressure off your memory by learning how to cheat on its behalf. Forest R. Scogin, Ph.D., professor of psychology at the University of Alabama in Tuscaloosa, readily admits that most of these suggestions aren't stunningly original. "My colleagues make fun of me when I tell them they can improve their memories by writing things down," he says. "They tell me, 'It must have taken you years to figure that one out!' But the fact is it works."

Here are a few of the experts' favorite memory enhancers.

Write it down. Okay, so the idea of writing down something you want to remember isn't exactly the sort of insight you're paying good money for. Here's a free bonus: Tying a piece of string around your finger can help remind you of something, too.

Of Potions and Pills

Are "smart drugs" available that will improve your memory?

In a word, no, according to experts, although there are some products that claim they will. Thomas H. Crook, Ph.D., a clinical psychologist and president of Memory Assessment Clinics in Bethesda, Maryland, has analyzed many of those products, and he found "absolutely no evidence" that they have any direct impact on memory. There is a chance that some supplements could actually hurt memory by upsetting the neurological balance in the brain.

It's possible that an effective memory drug could be developed in the future. The pharmaceutical companies are spending millions trying to find one, but once again, Dr. Crook and his colleagues are skeptical. "We've all had the experience of working with compounds that seemed tremendously encouraging but that turned out to be disappointing," he says. There are "flickers of hope" that certain drugs may benefit those with memory disorders such as age-associated memory impairment and Alzheimer's disease, he says, and one of them has even been approved by the Food and Drug Administration. There's no evidence, however, to indicate these drugs will do anything to improve the memory of healthy people with normal memories.

Create a file system. One way you can help your mind to encode the information you're ingesting is to give yourself some mental markers that will put that information into context. "Anything we can do to better organize information, the more efficiently we'll be able to retrieve it," says Dr. Scogin.

People with good memory skills are those who surround new information with images, details and organizing cues. Useful markers can range from comparisons ("That's almost exactly the amount of money I paid for those Knicks tickets last month") to literal landmarks, such as taking a moment to notice the tree under which you've parked your bike. Having a specific place for keeping things, like keys, also cuts the mental strain of trying to remember where you put them each time you go out the door.

Play games with yourself. Games like bridge and gin rummy are good memory workouts, Dr. Scogin says. Practice memorizing names and faces by watching game shows on TV and try to remember the names of the guests, says Douglas Herrmann, Ph.D., author of *Super Memory*.

Relax. If you still can't pry that elusive word loose, don't push it. Anxiety blocks memory performance, according to Dr. Pressley. The word you're looking for may pop into your mind as soon as you stop looking for it.

Free-associate. Make up rhymes or mental images that will give structure to information you want to hold on to, recommends Dr. Scogin. "What's her name, I think it's Jane," for example. If you want to remember the name of a guy named Frank Taylor, picture him altering a suit for Frank Sinatra.

Cram. When all else fails, going over something again and again does work, boring though it may be.

Is It Alzheimer's?

The chances that those annoying memory lapses you're experiencing represent the early stages of Alzheimer's disease are extremely remote.

Alzheimer's is a brain disease characterized by progressive deterioration of brain tissue. It causes memory loss that's debilitating and often bizarre. As a report from the Mayo Clinic puts it, if someone can't remember where he put his eyeglasses, that's forgetfulness; an Alzheimer's patient might forget he wears eyeglasses altogether.

The odds of Alzheimer's occurring in anyone under age 65 are as low as 1 or 2 in 100,000, reports Zaven Khachaturian, Ph.D., director of the Office of Alzheimer's Disease Research at the National Institute on Aging. The incidence balloons dramatically much later in life, in the seventies and eighties.

You needn't worry unduly if your mother or father or grandparents have been diagnosed with Alzheimer's disease, adds Dr. Khachaturian. Genetic predisposition is indeed a risk factor for Alzheimer's, he says, but it increases your chance of contracting the disease by perhaps 5 to 10 percent. Other risk factors haven't been conclusively identified as yet—head trauma and exposure to aluminum are suspected but not proved—but the presence of several is assumed to be necessary to provoke onset of the disease.

Is there anything you should be doing today to minimize your risk of developing Alzheimer's disease in the future? "You can select the right parents," Dr. Khachaturian says. "That's about as much as we know right now."

Midlife Crisis

An Opportunity in Disguise

In the movie *City Slickers* the character played by Billy Crystal hits his 39th birthday and finds himself in a slump. His boss tries to find out what's the matter, but Crystal's character just sits there, staring glumly ahead. Finally, he looks up with a pained expression.

"Did you ever reach a point in your life," he asks, "where you say to yourself, 'This is the best I'm ever going to look, the best I'm ever going to feel, the best I'm ever going to do? And it ain't that great?'"

That's as good a description as any of what a midlife crisis is all about. Of course, Billy Crystal's alter ego is far from the only hombre to ride nervously past the buzzards of Midlife Gulch. Ulysses, Dante and Michelangelo have been there. So have Sigmund Freud and Carl Jung. In his late thirties Shakespeare switched from writing comedies to tragedies, producing in the process *King Lear*, *Macbeth*, *Hamlet* and *Othello*—all tales of men who discover too late that their lives have gone seriously awry.

A Vague, Uncomfortable Feeling

What, exactly, constitutes a midlife crisis? Experts agree there's no single definition, although a pervasive sense of disappointment and a nagging feeling that time's running out would be among the major coordinates. Larry Bumpass, Ph.D., a sociologist at the University of Wisconsin in Madison who directs the National Survey of Families and Households, says there's "an array" of at least 40 events that commonly occur at midlife, from losing a job to the death of a parent, a flagging libido, divorce or illness.

Midlife for men today is tougher than it's ever been, says Ronald Levant, Ed.D., a psychologist who teaches at Harvard Medical School. The *Ozzie and Harriet* model of family life no longer prevails, he says, and new demands on men can exacerbate the confusion of midlife transition. "It's more of a crisis now than it might have been for our fathers because of the dynamic changes in the role of women and the structure of the American family," Dr. Levant says. "Midlife men are now living with role expectations that are vastly different from when they grew up. The traditional masculine code has been broken."

Panic Not Required

Many experts believe the word "crisis" overstates the degree of angst most mid-dle-age men experience. These same experts also say that many of the stereotypes about men at midlife—such as their burning desire to hold onto youth by latching onto a younger woman—aren't necessarily true. "Sure, we all know somebody who left his wife for his secretary when he was 45. But men leave their wives when they're younger, too," says Dr. Bumpass.

In fact, Dr. Bumpass's research demonstrates quite clearly that the risk of di-vorce actually declines the longer people are married. Another study, conducted at the New England Research Institute in Watertown, Massachusetts, by John B. McKinlay, Ph.D., a psychologist at the institute, showed that only 2 percent of over 1,700 middle-age and older men surveyed reported having more than one current sexual partner, a far lower rate than the stereotypes would have us believe.

The word "crisis" applies more to how midlife transitions are handled than to the fact that transitions are taking place, says Leonard Felder, Ph.D., a psychologist in private practice in Los Angeles and an expert on midlife and career issues. "Most people between the ages of 30 and 50 go through some major shifts in the way they see themselves and the way they feel about their lives," he says. "That's normal. It's a crisis if men act impulsively during it. If they throw away their wives, kids, friends, then it's a crisis. If they carefully think this through, it's a fascinating transition."

Taking Stock of Your Life

That midlife regrets can serve as a potent catalyst for personal growth is a theme sounded repeatedly by experts from many disciplines. "I would go so far as to call it a midlife opportunity," says Marsha Sinetar, Ph.D., an organizational psychologist and the author of *Do What You Love the Money Will Follow.* "It's time to look at questions like, Who am I? What do I believe? What do I really need? Those are issues worth examining. This means taking yourself seriously, perhaps for the first time."

The first recommended step for getting the most out of your midlife agonies is to listen to them. Therapists say there's a strong temptation to deny the questions that come up at midlife because the answers are sometimes threatening. "Accept what's happening," says Dr. Sinetar. "Try to relax into the chaos. Trust that you're going to find something wonderful in it."

Here are some ways to help that happen.

Goof off. Probably the most pleasant technique for tapping into the subcon-scious is to hop off the roller coaster for a while. "We need to find spaces for privacy and silence, time for reflection and creative, leisurely engagements," Dr. Sinetar says. She recommends making a point to spend some quiet time alone every day, reading inspiring verse or surrounded by nature, if possible. A more extended prayer and meditation retreat also may prove invaluable.

During those quiet times, Dr. Sinetar advises disengaging the intellect as much as possible; the point is to daydream, to renew, to muse. "The mind does not want to change," she says. "New insights, new ideas, new optimism surface as you give yourself room to breathe."

Write your story. The art of journaling—in essence writing an autobiography—is a key part of the midlife workshops given by Janice Brewi, S.T.D., co-director of a consulting firm called Mid-Life Directions in Newark, New Jersey. "Taking a good look at your life re-energizes you," she says. "There's a need to make peace, a need to remember the good things, a need to learn perspective."

Tell the truth. Now is the time to start being honest about who you really are, Dr. Sinetar says. In that pursuit, it's important to find somebody trustworthy and competent to practice telling your truth to—that way you'll hear it yourself. Friends can help, but many men haven't developed the facility for intimate discussion that women have. Better late than never. Robert Simmons, Ph.D., a clinical psychologist in private practice in Alexandria, Virginia, says there are men's groups in many cities specifically geared toward exploring these sorts of issues.

Finding a therapist is another option. If you do look for professional help, Dr. Sinetar strongly recommends choosing someone who will help you work through the process of rediscovery rather than stunt it by defining your crisis as something to be gotten through as quickly and as "neatly" as possible. The same goes for friends, says Dr. Felder. When choosing your "cabinet of advisers," he says, always remember that you're the president, and "don't pick people who are trying to sell you on what *they* did."

Uncover yourself. Carl Jung observed, and subsequent studies have borne out, a tendency in midlife to undergo what Jung called a "contra-sexual transition," in which men become more nurturing, needy and reflective while women become more independent and aggressive. "Unlived parts of our personalities can begin to make themselves known in midlife," says Dr. Brewi.

Encouraging those unlived parts of ourselves to emerge can provide an exhilarating sense of discovery—and help relieve the sense of loss that often accompanies midlife transition. Many men become involved in community affairs: coaching their son's soccer team, perhaps, or volunteering at the local soup kitchen.

Career Considerations

One of the most difficult aspects of middle age for men is dealing with disappointments in their careers. In his book *The Male Ego*, Willard Gaylin, M.D., says that when men in our culture commit suicide (which they do almost eight times as frequently as women), in most cases the reason is "perceived social humiliation" related to business failure.

A "reorganization of life goals" is one of midlife's principal tasks, says Gilbert Brim, Ph.D., a social psychologist who heads the John D. and Catherine T. MacArthur Foundation Research Network on Successful Mid-Life Development in Vero Beach, Florida. For anyone who feels frustrated by his professional progress so far, Dr. Brim recommends in his book *Ambition: How We Manage Success and Failure throughout Our Lives* a three-step process of career re-evaluation.

Extend the deadline. Many of us set arbitrary deadlines for ourselves, Dr. Brim says, then grow despondent when we've failed to meet them in the time allotted. The simple solution is to grant yourself an extension. "You can tell yourself, 'Okay, I didn't get rich this year. I'll make it next year,'" says Dr. Brim.

Lower your aspiration. This is another instance of relieving self-induced pressure. Shoot for making a hundred thousand dollars instead of ten million, Dr. Brim says, or buy a cozy cottage on the beach instead of that 12-room Victorian you've always dreamed of. One of the signs of midlife maturity is accepting limitations.

Abandon the goal. When all else fails, Dr. Brim says, give up on a goal that's not achievable. Again, an ability to accept reality is key to successful midlife transitions. The goal is peace of mind, not winning some sweepstakes you've created for yourself. Similar exercises work, Dr. Brim adds, for those who have achieved their goals

The Male Menopause Myth

Furious debate has swirled about the existence of a so-called male menopause. The idea is that, beginning in middle age, men may experience a reduction in testosterone that is roughly equivalent to the decrease in estrogen that occurs at a similar midlife period in women. It has been proposed that this hormone is associated with a reduction in general energy level, muscular strength and sex drive. Not surprisingly, various hormone replacement therapies have hit the market that some say will put the spring back in a man's step, among other places.

These treatments are highly controversial and unproven. Laurence A. Levine, M.D., director of the Male Sexual Health Program at Rush-Presbyterian-St. Luke's Medical Center in Chicago, says testosterone replacement therapy presents a risk of accelerating benign and malignant prostate growth.

Considerable doubt exists, too, that healthy men need a testosterone boost in the first place. "Almost always when a testosterone deficiency occurs, disease can be found as the cause," says William Hazzard, M.D., chairman of the Department of Internal Medicine at the Bowman Gray School of Medicine at Wake Forest University in Winston-Salem, North Carolina. Where disease is not present, he adds, the decline in testosterone levels over a lifetime is so gradual as to be "almost unmeasurable."

Where does this leave the idea of male menopause? Nowhere, according to Dr. Hazzard and others. Men experiencing mood changes or loss of sexual desire can almost certainly blame their psyches, not their testes.

and still feel dissatisfied—a group that is a lot larger than you probably think. In this case the first alternative would be finding a new, more ambitious goal to achieve; alternative two would be switching to a new pursuit entirely. "Linus Pauling is a perfect example of that," Dr. Brim says. "After winning the Nobel Prize in chemistry, he switched to being a world-peace leader."

Motion Sickness

Calming the Queasies

Forget the thrill of fighting Earth's gravity in a rocket-powered space shuttle. The only g-force most astronauts feel is the gag force—the urge to blow galactic regurgitation throughout the universe.

Motion sickness leaves about two-thirds of all astronauts feeling like their Tang breakfasts are about to take flight. In fact, astronauts carry little airline sickness bags on board for just this reason.

"The bags are a little different from airplane bags in that you can shut them closed. Your crewmates appreciate that," says Eileen Hawley, a NASA spokeswoman from Johnson Space Center in Houston.

Even though motion sickness in space differs physiologically from the kind you get on Earth, it goes to show that we're all prone to turbulent tummies, whether we're taking a road trip or exploring the final frontier.

"We're not born on roller coasters and most people aren't born on ships. We're born on stationary land. When we're transported to a moving environment, we need to adjust," says Christopher Linstrom, M.D. director of otology, neurotology and skull base surgery at the New York Eye and Ear Infirmary in New York City.

The Ins and Outs of Motion Sickness

There are two sorts of people, Dr. Linstrom says. Those who adjust and those who don't. Only a rare few can claim never having been afflicted with the nausea, queasiness, vomiting, cold sweat and urge to urinate that accompany motion sickness. And that's probably because they haven't been given the right quality and quantity of provocative stimulation.

Despite its prevalence, motion sickness in many ways remains a mystery. Doctors aren't sure why some people suffer more and longer than others (particularly women), why some people seem naturally less prone to suffer motion sickness and why others find their tendencies to get motion sickness diminishes with age.

Motion sickness occurs when your body fails to properly adjust to unfamiliar movement.

"People get motion sickness because of a maladjustment, usually in the inner

FAST FACTS

How common: Motion sickness afflicts up to 90 percent of people.

Risk factors: Unfamiliar, sustained movement triggers motion sickness.

Age group affected: All men are prone, but in general, motion sickness diminishes with age.

Gender gap: Doctors believe women suffer more than men, but the evidence is anecdotal. No studies have been done to prove it.

Who to see: Motion sickness rarely requires a doctor—the problem usually starts when the movement starts and ends when you become stationary. But if you are prone to motion sickness and want to take preventive steps, see your family doctor for a possible prescription.

ear," says Dr. Linstrom. Your inner ear contains a sensitive network of fluid-filled canals and sacs called the vestibular system. This system keeps track of your body's motion, helps you maintain balance and tells your brain where your head is—or where it should be.

Generally, your inner ear is a lot smarter than your brain when it comes to motion—that's why so many people get sick reading in a car. Focusing on a stationary page, rather than the slowly moving horizon, provokes an argument between your inner ear and your eyes. Both send conflicting messages to the brain. These mixed signals end up making you especially nauseous if you're also hearing traffic, feeling bumps on the road and smelling fumes from other cars.

To make matters worse, anxiety may exacerbate motion sickness. So don't take a first date on a fast-moving ride, like a flight simulator or high-speed boat.

But even if you find yourself and your belly on the Spiral of Death roller coaster with no graceful way of backing out, just relax. Nobody ever died of motion sickness, though many have wanted to.

Keeping Nausea at Bay

Besides relaxing, you can take a few other measures before leaving home to help avoid motion sickness. Doing so might even prevent the syndrome altogether. Dr. Linstrom and others suggest trying these commonsense preventive measures.

Minimize your motion. Choosing the right seat is paramount in avoiding motion sickness. Pick the most stable seat. In a car this means sitting up front, while looking ahead. Better yet, offer to drive. Drivers are less prone to motion sickness than passengers. On a bus sit two seats behind the front door. On a plane, train or boat sit in the center, where the rocking motion is minimized.

Focus on the horizon. Look at a distant object and fixate on it. By staring straight ahead, the brain perceives less movement. Avoid looking out side windows. Watching telephone poles and trees whizzing by at high speeds will make you feel like you're in a top-fuel dragster taking a hairpin turn at 200 miles per hour.

Stick to freeways. Take the most direct route. The rocking of stop-and-go traffic and rutted roads moves your head about, which provokes nausea.

No reading allowed. Reading in a moving vehicle will send you reaching so quickly for the motion sickness bag you'd probably outdraw Jesse James. Ponder your retirement instead. Or think about how you can make the world a better place.

Get plenty of fresh air. Stay on deck. Open the car windows. Turn on the fan. Any unpleasant odor—especially tobacco—can trigger motion sickness. "Nobody really knows why," says Daniel Mowrey, Ph.D., a motion sickness expert with the American Phytotherapy Research Laboratory in Salt Lake City. "There's a lot of association that goes on between taste, smell and the stimulation of the stomach."

Eat first. Eat a small, low-fat meal before the journey and avoid an empty stomach throughout. "Mostly you don't want to eat a big meal and throw up," Dr. Linstrom says. "Eat a little. It's just common sense."

No drinking or smoking. Alcohol and nicotine make the dizziness worse and can cause an upset stomach.

Think positive thoughts. Anxiety can worsen motion sickness, says Dr. Linstrom. For many, even thinking about motion sickness makes them sick. Try easing your distress by reminding yourself that "the worse that can happen is a knockdown vomiting session," he says.

You can't think yourself out of motion sickness once it starts. But you can lower anxiety before nausea hits. So think about happy things: Design a new workshop in your head, make weekend plans, listen to soothing music on earphones. But don't start playing air guitar like you're Eric Clapton at the Rose Bowl, because moving your head will only make you feel worse.

Try gingerroot. Medicinal gingerroot for motion sickness has been around as long as doctors have been disagreeing about its effectiveness. Dr. Mowrey swears by it; in fact, he rarely encourages patients to follow any other preventive measures. "If people follow directions with gingerroot, there's usually no need to do anything else," he says. Dr. Mowrey tells patients to take 1,500 to 5,000 milligrams 10 to 20 minutes before leaving. At the first sign of queasiness take anywhere from two to six more capsules. "It really doesn't matter how many you take," he says. "It can't hurt you."

Sample motion potions. If you've tried the nondrug remedies to no avail, you might want to pull out the big guns. Dramamine (its generic name is dimenhydrinate) is an over-the-counter (OTC) antihistamine that stops your inner ear from sending a chemical message to your brain that orders you to vomit. Take the prescribed dosage a half-hour to an hour before you leave. As with most antihistamines, it can make you drowsy, so avoid driving or operating heavy machinery after taking a dose. Another safe bet is Bonine (meclizine hydrochloride). For some people it's better, since it tends to produce less drowsiness.

If the OTCs aren't making your nausea go away, then try the prescription drug scopolamine. More commonly known as the skin patch, scopolamine depresses the central nervous system. In patch form it releases a slow, steady dose of the drug into your bloodstream for up to several days. Most people put the patch behind their ears, but "you can put it on your belly button if you want—anywhere is fine," Dr. Linstrom says.

Patients are told by Dr. Linstrom to begin wearing the patch a half-day or day before their trips. He also suggests cutting the patch in half. "Most people are very sensitive to it," he said. In full dose the drug's common side effects include delayed ejaculation, blurred vision and dry mouth. Still, Dr. Linstrom prefers the patch to other drugs. "I usually recommend it first," he says. "The other drugs for motion sickness have sedative side effects. Scopolamine doesn't dull a person's alertness."

Use cruise control. Particularly after an ocean cruise, you may feel as though you're still moving. Rarely, and for reasons unknown, this syndrome can last for months or years. To help combat this, try the following exercise after your trip to help re-establish your sense of balance, suggests Dr. Linstrom. Do the exercise in bed or sitting in a chair with arms. Never do it in the office or on the subway, and never do it to the point of nausea. And be forewarned. "You may feel worse before you feel better," Dr. Linstrom says.

Here's what to do: Bend your head forward and backward, first slowly, then quickly, 20 times, with your eyes open. Then, turn your head from side to side slowly, then quickly, 20 times, with your eyes open. As dizziness subsides, repeat the exercise with your eyes closed. Stop immediately if you feel like you're losing your balance or are getting sick. Done properly, this exercise should help your body re-adjust its internal balancing mechanism.

Muscle Aches and Pains

Avoiding Weekend-Warrior Wipeout

All excuses have failed you and for the first time in years you are actually cleaning your garage. One of two things happens next.

(a) You successfully spend the day rearranging cinder blocks, woodpiles, boxes, old tires and paint cans. The next morning, you're barely able to get out of bed because of the soreness in your arms, back and legs.

(b) You lift a box of wood scraps and a muscle in your back rips, sending you, the box and all pride tumbling. Your wife and the neighbors have to carry you to the couch.

The Damage Men Do

Those two scenarios sketch out the range of possible damage, from a simple strain to a serious tear, you can do to yourself by asking too much of your muscles when you're out of shape.

A muscle is made to stretch, but if you stretch it farther than it's accustomed to, it strains and eventually tears. Actually, a strain is technically a tear, since on a microscopic level the muscle fibers have begun to pull apart. As the strain gets more severe, the muscle fibers separate wider. The more separation there is, the greater the damage and the longer the recovery.

Up to a point, straining your muscles isn't a bad thing: Our muscle tissues actually strengthen themselves by healing those tiny rips, which is why a little soreness is the price we pay for getting into shape. But when the damage to the muscle fibers is more serious, the muscles can swell or turn stiff.

The worst tears are so sudden and sharp they make a sound like gunfire. "You can hear a distinct pop," says Ronald Lawrence, M.D., a professor at the University of California, Los Angeles, School of Medicine and president of the American Medical Athletic Association. "A lot of runners actually think they've been shot."

It's not hard to figure out how much damage you've done. If you're hurting immediately, you probably have a tear. Muscle strain takes at least a couple of hours to show up, which is how the weekend warriors among us can so blithely get in way over our heads.

FAST FACTS

How common: All men get sore muscles from time to time, be it from holding baby for too long, pulling out dead bushes from the yard or playing basketball a bit too intensely.

Risk factors: Poor conditioning, overdoing exercise.

Age group affected: Everyone beyond the age of about ten experiences muscle pain. Once into your twenties, your muscles begin to lose elasticity, making them more susceptible to strains.

Gender gap: Men in general have more muscle problems than women because they exercise more vigorously and because they tend to be less patient in letting muscle injuries heal.

Who to see: Most muscle injuries don't require medical care, but if there's substantial swelling and bruising and a significant amount of pain, you should have it checked. See your family doctor or an orthopedic specialist with a background in sports medicine.

Another way to tell the difference between a tear, strain or general soreness is to take the two-finger test. "A muscle tear is very specific," says Marjorie Albohm, director of sports medicine at the Center for Hip and Knee Surgery in Mooresville, Indiana. "You can pinpoint it with two fingers: 'It hurts right there.' Muscle soreness is a more generalized stiffness and aching: 'My legs are sore.'"

Avoid the Agony

The best way to avoid injury to your muscles is to stay in shape through a regular program of physical exercise. "Activity in and of itself will help keep the muscles sound," says Alan Mikesky, Ph.D., an exercise physiologist at Indiana University-Purdue University at Indianapolis.

Here are a few basics.

Start slowly. The single most important rule when starting your task—be it gardening, basketball or box stacking—is to warm your muscles up gradually. Dr. Mikesky recommends a short period of light general activity, which can include anything from walking to light jogging or bike riding. "Do just enough exercise to elevate the heart rate to the point where you can feel yourself getting warm," he says. "When you start thinking you might want to take your shirt off, that's about right."

Stretch—or don't. Opinions differ over whether stretching is appropriate before exercising. Some doctors now believe it isn't. Even if you do stretch before exercising, understand that that is not the same thing as warming up. "Warming up refers to literally warming the muscle up by engaging in activity that moves blood into the muscle," says Dr. Mikesky.

Where doctors agree is that stretching is often better after exercising than before and that whenever you do it, be careful not to do aggressive, "ballistic" type stretches (bouncing, especially) that have the potential to strain the muscle by forcing it past the point that it's ready to go.

Cool down. Giving your muscles time to gradually recover from exercise is as important as giving them time to warm up. Slowing your activity down gradually keeps blood circulating through strained muscle fibers, says Frederick C. Hagerman, Ph.D., professor of exercise physiology at Ohio University in Athens and a consultant to the U.S. Olympic rowing team. That allows muscles to absorb lactic acid (a chemical by-product the muscle cells produce during exercise) more efficiently and to return gradually to their normal elasticity without stiffness setting in. Walking for five or ten minutes is a good way to cool down, he says, or simply continue your workout activity at a slower pace for a few minutes.

Flush yourself. Muscles need water, especially when they're being put through some serious paces. "Muscles are about 75 percent water," says Wayne Westcott, Ph.D., a strength training consultant for the YMCA. "So during training, the most important thing a person can do is to stay hydrated." He recommends downing a couple of glasses of water before and after a workout, and "ad-libbing" a cup or two during the workout if possible. Dr. Westcott also suggests avoiding diuretic beverages such as coffee, tea and alcohol before working out.

Take precautions. A study at the University of Texas in Austin found that taking 400 milligrams of ibuprofen four hours before strenuous exercise, followed by two more doses at equal intervals after the exercise, helps prevent muscle soreness. While the results were preliminary, popping two ibuprofen prior to the muscle-straining exercise might offer some relief afterward. But doctors also question using drugs for preventive purposes, so ask your doctor first, and never exceed the recommended dosages on the bottle.

Consider antioxidants. For more consistent muscle protection consider putting yourself on an antioxidant regimen. Antioxidants—vitamins C, E and beta-carotene, primarily—combat the free radical molecules that can damage muscles, among other tissues. Kenneth Cooper, M.D., president of the Cooper Clinic in Dallas and author of *Antioxidant Revolution*, suggests that men between the ages of 22 and 50 who follow a light exercise regimen take a daily antioxidant "cocktail" consisting of 400 international units (IU) of vitamin E (he recommends "natural" E, as opposed to synthetic), 1,500 milligrams of vitamin C (750 milligrams taken twice during the day) and 25,000 IU (that's equal to 15 milligrams) of beta-carotene.

Muscles normally account for 40 percent of a human's body weight. There are 639 named muscles in body, the bulkiest of which is the gluteus maximus, or buttock. Of all the muscles, the one with the longest name is the *levator labii superioris alaeque nasi*. It runs down your face, with part connecting to your upper lip and part connecting to your nostril. It's the muscle immortalized by the famous Elvis Presley and Billy Idol sneer.

Dealing with the Aftermath

Okay, so you've overdone it. What can you do to minimize the price your muscles are going to pay? There's an easy mnemonic recipe to follow called RICE, which stands for rest, ice, compress and elevate. Here's a review of each ingredient in that recipe, plus a couple of tips for what to do after the immediate damage has been contained.

Rest and elevate. The first thing you want to do is to get off the injured muscle so that healing can begin. How long you stay off it depends on how severe the injury is, Dr. Mikesky says: It could range from a couple of hours to a full day or even two. Elevating the injured area keeps blood flowing away from the muscle instead of toward it, thereby reducing swelling. According to Brian Halpern, M.D., clinical instructor of sports medicine at the Hospital for Special Surgery in New York City, swelling increases both your pain and your stiffness, so keeping swelling down is a good first step toward recovery. Taking some ibuprofen will also help keep the swelling down.

Ice. Putting ice on an injured muscle will immediately help reduce swelling by limiting circulation to the injured tissues. Keep an ice pack, a plastic bag filled with ice or even a package of frozen peas or corn on the area for 20 to 30 minutes, Dr. Mikesky says. Repeat three or four times a day for two to four days.

Compress. You can give an injured muscle some support, and help it heal more quickly, by lightly wrapping it in an elastic bandage or similar binding. The slight compression caused by the bandage decreases the swelling of the injured area.

Heat it. Once swelling has subsided, many experts believe applying heat to the injured area will hasten a complete recovery. Moist heat can penetrate the muscle, Dr. Lawrence says, restoring circulation, which will help flush the injured area. A steam bath, a hot towel or the hot wet packs sold in drugstores are good sources of wet heat, he says. Dr. Lawrence cautions that dry heat, such as that given off by heating pads, will retard healing by drawing blood away from the muscle.

Be patient. The main requirement for healing injured muscles is time.

How much time? "The best rule of thumb is overkill," says Dr. Bryant Stamford, Ph.D., director of the Health Promotion and Wellness Center at the University of Louisville. "Whenever it comes to an injury there is a tendency toward underkill—people who are active don't want to be inactive." Albohm cautions that even minor muscle strains can take up to eight weeks to heal, and strenuously exercising them before they heal can cause more damage.

To determine when a muscle has healed enough, Dr. Stamford suggests monitoring your symptoms closely. When the swelling goes down, that's the first step toward healing; the second step is when you can use the injured muscle without pain. "Stop at the slightest indication of pain," he says. "Treat the injury with respect."

See also Sports Injuries

Nail Problems

Maintaining a Good Clip

Fingernails are wondrous things. They scratch your itch. They itch your scratch. They remove gunk from frying pans that sponges just won't remove. They make impatient noises when drummed on a desk; the message is clear.

And toenails. Excellent at collecting lint from socks, the sharp edges of these nerve-dead plates also can wreak havoc on the calves of unsuspecting bed partners in need of discipline.

It's nice that whatever spiritual or natural force designed the human body decided to build in protective shields for the tips of digits. Nails are so self-supporting that for most men, there is only one thing to worry about: How to keep them clipped and neat. Nails grow an average of 1½ inches a year, a growth most men find neither practical nor beautiful.

Every now and then, however, bad things occur to your nails: fungus sprouts, cuticles split, corners dig into your skin. Here's what to do in those rare cases when nails turn from protectors into aggressors.

Ingrown Nails: Removing the Edge

They say that clothes make the man. Wearing the wrong clothes, however, can also break him. Take those lizard-skin boots with toes so sharp they could pick a lock. Seen from the inside—where the big toe is getting speared by its own nail—things aren't so pretty.

Ingrown nails often are caused by tight shoes, says Diana Bihova, M.D., clinical assistant professor of dermatology at New York University School of Medicine/Medical Center in New York City. Badly trimmed or gnawed nails can also "train" the sharp edge of the nail to grow down and into the skin rather than safely out over the edge.

"Some men also have an inherited tendency to get ingrown toenails," adds Ralph C. Daniel III, M.D., clinical professor of dermatology at the University of Mississippi Medical Center in Jackson. "And people with wide feet get them more often."

Once ingrown nails get a toehold, you may need a doctor to get them out again.

In most cases, however, you can prevent them from getting started in the first place. Here's what doctors recommend.

Bigger is better. Look for shoes with a half-inch between the tip of your big toe and the end of the shoe. And make sure your toes can wiggle freely without being crushed against the sides. "Running shoes and walking shoes are good," says Dr. Daniel. During the warm months open-toed sandals can also help.

Cut carefully. Perhaps the easiest way to prevent ingrown nails is to cut your toenails straight across when they reach the end of the toe, advises Paul Kechijian, M.D., clinical associate professor of dermatology and chief of the nail section at New York University School of Medicine/Medical Center. Angling the corners or cutting nails too short can encourage them to grow into the skin rather than outward over the edge.

It's also a good idea to trim your nails after a shower or bath, when the nail is softest.

Try an uplifting technique. Once a nail has penetrated the skin, you need to encourage it to grow outward. Soak the toe in warm water (to which you've added a teaspoon of salt) for 10 to 15 minutes, advises Dr. Daniel. "Then put a wisp of cotton under the side of the nail that's ingrowing," he says. "The cotton will help lift the nail off the skin as it grows out."

If there's pus or reddish streaks on the toe or if you have a fever or a great deal of swelling, don't try to treat it yourself, he adds. Get to a doctor right away.

Fungus: Fighting the Funk

Given the ugly nature of this condition, it's fortunate that 80 to 90 percent of nail fungus infections occur on toenails rather than in plain sight on the fingers. What isn't so fortunate, however, is that the fungus can be difficult to avoid.

Coaches have long advised young athletes—on pain of permanent foot death—never to walk barefoot on locker-room floors. But researchers now know that foot fungus—which can cause nails to thicken and turn ugly shades of yellow or white—isn't so easily fooled. It's everywhere—in bathrooms and on floors and walls—so wearing sandals at the pool or gym probably won't make much of a difference in the long term, says Dr. Kechijian.

What makes one guy vulnerable and another resistant probably boils down to heredity. "We know that a person who develops fungus has a genetic tendency not to fight it off well," explains Dr. Daniel. "Usually one of your parents has the condition as well."

While there's no sure way to prevent nail fungus, there are some ways to help keep it away—or at least shorten its stay.

FAST FACTS

How common: Dermatologists estimate that between 2 and 13 percent of Americans have foot fungus. Hangnails and ingrown toenails are extremely common, as is blood under the nails, particularly in athletes.

Risk factors: Nail problems are typically caused by such things as tight shoes or improper trimming and sweaty feet. In addition, stop-and-start sports, dry skin or family history can raise the risks.

Age group affected: Ingrown toenails affect all ages, while fungal infections are more common in older people. Blood under the nails typically occurs in active people ages 20 to 50, and hangnails usually occur after age 30.

Gender gap: While more men than women get foot fungus, other nail problems occur equally in both sexes.

Who to see: Dermatologist, podiatrist.

Step out in style. Since foot fungus thrives in damp conditions, putting down a thick, thirsty mat—preferably one made from cotton, which is better at absorbing moisture than synthetic materials—outside the tub or shower will help keep your feet dry and the fungus away, says Dr. Bihova.

Blow it away. Some experts recommend blow-drying your feet after showers or baths to make them as fungus-*unfriendly* as possible. Set the dryer on cool and blow-dry under, around and between the toes after bathing. Make sure your toenails are dry, too, says Dr. Bihova.

Dust it away. Once your feet are dry, sprinkling them with an over-the-counter antifungal powder containing the ingredients miconazole (Micatin) or tolnaftate (Tinactin) can help keep them dry and prevent the fungus from spreading, Dr. Daniel says.

Help your feet breathe. One of the best ways to prevent fungus growth is to give your feet plenty of fresh air. Wearing sandals can help. During the colder months wear shoes made from leather or canvas—materials that allow moisture to escape and your feet to breathe, says Dr. Bihova.

Ask for prescription help. When you're ready to get tough on nail fungus, two of the oral prescription drugs, itraconazole (Sporanox) and fluconazole (Diflucan), often will help clear it up. The bad news is that the drugs are typically taken until the entire toenail grows out—usually a year to 18 months. In addition, the "cure" isn't always permanent. "The recurrence rate may be as high as 75 percent for toenails and 25 percent for fingernails," says Dr. Bihova.

Black Nail: How to Strike Back

You strip off your tennis socks only to find a matched pair of black toenails. Your weekend's woodworking has left you with two black thumbs. With all those dinged digits you finally understand what "hitting the nail on the head" really means.

Blackened nails occur when blood vessels rupture under the nailplate, a condition doctors refer to as a hematoma. Weekend carpentry is one common cause of blackened nails. Running, tennis and other stop-and-start sports, which put tremendous pressure on toes, can also be responsible. "Hematomas are hard to prevent," says Dr. Daniel.

If the pain is extreme, your doctor may remove the nail or cut a hole through it to drain the blood and relieve the pressure. In most cases, however, "you can just leave the toe alone," says Dr. Kechijian. "The black nail will grow out and fall off."

In addition, there are a few ways to sidestep the problem and minimize the hurt.

Ice it. If you've just given your nail a good whack, get it into ice water as soon as possible, says Dr. Bihova. "If you can get close to ice water the moment you're injured, you can actually prevent the swelling," she says.

Make sure the shoe fits. When buying shoes, make sure your toes have plenty of room in which to wiggle. "You have to have shoes that fit well," says Dr. Daniel.

Get professional advice. When you've just whacked your thumb with a hammer, the cause of black nail seems pretty obvious. But sometimes you're not sure what's behind the change of hues. "A melanoma can sometimes show up as a black line under a nail," warns Dr. Kechijian. "It's not common, but if the black area doesn't change for three or four months and if you don't remember banging it, you'd better get it checked out."

Hangnails: When the Tips Want to Split

A tiny sliver of skin splits off from around your fingernail. And there it hangs— a little piece of pain just waiting to happen. And happen it does—when it hangs up on your sweater, for example, or gets snagged in your sweetheart's hair.

A hangnail—which has nothing to do with the nail—occurs when the skin around the nail (the cuticle) dries up, dies and peels off, leaving behind a lifeless tatter. The hangnail itself isn't the problem. Trouble occurs when it pulls away from the surrounding skin, which can cause bleeding, throbbing or infection.

While hangnails can be annoying, they're generally easier to avoid. Here's what skin-care experts recommend.

Touch them not. The less you push and bang on your cuticles, the less likely it

Shridhar Chillal of Pune, Maharashtra, India, in 1993 grabbed the world record for the longest fingernails. The five nails on his left hand measured a total of 205 inches—he last cut them 41 years prior, in 1952.

is that hangnails will form, says Dr. Kechijian. "Their function is to keep out bacteria, so you shouldn't push them down or try to get rid of them," he says.

Snip *in extremis.* "If you do have a hangnail, cut it off with cuticle scissors so it doesn't get torn anymore," advises Dr. Kechijian. "Don't try to bite it or chew it or tear it off," he adds. "It will only get infected."

Moisturize. Regularly applying moisturizer to your hands will help keep cuticles moist and intact. "Every time you wash your hands or take a shower, rub moisturizer in around your cuticles and nails," advises Dr. Bihova. "Do it while your hands are still moist. It increases the moisturizer's penetration."

Experts agree that most moisturizers, whether they cost $2 or $85, do pretty much the same job. So experiment until you find one you like. Then use it regularly.

Nausea and Vomiting

Taming a Belly That's a Beast

You awake at 2:00 A.M. and your stomach feels like a sack of angry snakes. Maybe it was that greasy, double-pepperoni pizza. Or the six-pack. Or the stogie you had with a nightcap. You realize, woefully, that you don't have to work at Mario's to toss pizza.

Just what is it that causes your belly to turn on you? In the scenario above it's pretty obvious: Your digestive tract is revolting against the beating you gave it. But too much food or drink is just one cause of a tumultuous tummy. A bad reaction to medicine, illnesses such as stomach flu or too much motion are also common triggers. So are migraine headaches, emotional stress, food poisoning and bad odors.

And in a few cases nausea coupled with other symptoms—severe stomach pain, for instance—could mean something more serious, like colitis, ulcers or gallstones, requiring a look by a doctor.

Everyday Gut Reactions

Your digestive tract is a sophisticated but sensitive machine. It chops up food, grinds it and mixes it with juices that break the food down further. The body absorbs what it needs and shoves the waste out the back door. It's a complex process regulated by a swirl of communication involving nerves, muscles and hormones. When bodily sensors pick up a problem—or just *think* there's a problem—you feel distress signals—nausea—in your gut.

But it's not always easy pinpointing the culprit. The nauseating effect of medicine or tainted food, for example, can be difficult to trace, says Duane T. Smoot, M.D., a gastroenterologist at Howard University in Washington, D.C. Medicines can affect the body differently depending on what food—if any—is in the stomach.

And the timing of food poisoning can be deceptive. "Depending on the type of food poisoning, it could come within an hour of a meal or it could be the day after the meal," Dr. Smoot says.

Here are some remedies for the everyday belly in rebellion.

Distract yourself. Agonizing over your nausea can make matters worse. William H. Redd, Ph.D., a psychologist at Memorial Sloan-Kettering Cancer Center

FAST FACTS

How common: Every man, no matter how cautious, gets nauseous at least a few times in his life.

Risk factors: Medicines; overindulgence in food; various illnesses; air, sea and automobile travel.

Age group affected: All ages suffer nausea.

Gender gap: Nausea is a basic body function that men and women share alike. But because of lifestyle and physiological differences, the causes can differ between the sexes.

Who to see: In extreme cases call your family doctor. He might refer you to a gastroenterologist.

in New York City, showed in a study that chemotherapy patients can become nauseated just by imagining their treatment. When they imagined a pastoral setting or a medical procedure unrelated to cancer, they did not get nauseated.

So take some deep breaths and relax. Deep breathing can go a long way toward settling a queasy stomach.

Also, absorb yourself in a mentally engaging activity, says Dr. Redd. "Some people who are very good with music can put on a set of headphones and focus in on music and get benefit," he says. "But the average person may have to do something where they are more cognitively engaged. Do video games or find ways in which your attention is focused on something other than your symptom, and then the severity of your symptom diminishes."

Have a snack. Odd as it may seem, eating something can help settle a queasy stomach. Try something bland and starchy—crackers and dry toast are good—but avoid fatty foods such as butter.

Break the habit. Take a sober look at your lifestyle. Smoking, alcohol and caffeine irritate the digestive system and fatty foods slow down the digestive process. Any could be behind your queasiness.

Mix a drink. No, guys, alcohol could be what got you here in the first place. Here are a couple of stomach-soothing concoctions.

— Mix your Maalox with a few drops of spirits of peppermint and a quart of distilled water. Take a few sips and set the rest aside in case you need it later.

— Sip a carbonated soft drink that's gone flat or suck on some ice chips. You can also try the flat syrup of Coca-Cola over cracked ice.

Just don't overload your stomach with fluids too fast, because that could make you feel worse, says Sally Van Boheemen, R.N., manager of marine medical services for Seattle-based Holland America Line/Windstar Cruises.

The Old Heave-Ho

If your stomach won't hold its lunch no matter what you do, get out of that crowded elevator, find the men's room and just heave-ho. "You often feel better, and often times you have no choice anyway," says Kenneth L. Koch, M.D., professor of medicine and director of the Motility Laboratory at Pennsylvania State University's Milton S. Hershey Medical Center in Hershey.

When your brain's vomit center activates, it puts the stomach's propulsion into reverse. You have little control over this extremely complex action, but you can make the experience a little less, well, wretched.

Give it a rest. If you've just launched lunch, this concept will probably come naturally: Don't put anything into your stomach for at least an hour.

Go liquid. Tossing your liquids creates the danger of dehydration. If you're feeling light-headed or dizzy, particularly when you stand up or sit down, you might need to replenish. Wait until your nausea has subsided, then sip clear liquids, which your stomach will find easier to take. Sports drinks such as Gatorade are ideal. "The nice thing about those sports drinks is that they have sodium and potassium—electrolytes," says Thomas P. Gage, M.D., of South Potomac Gastroenterological Associates in Fort Washington, Maryland. "They'll help treat dehydration more readily than just having water or soda."

Beware the tear. Severe vomiting episodes can actually injure the esophageal or stomach walls, so you might need a doctor's help in bringing it under control with antinausea drugs. "It's not uncommon at all, and it may cause bleeding," says Dr. Gage. "What often happens is that somebody vomits a couple of times and then will vomit up blood, and that's because they've had a tear."

Be a man of the cloth. Keep a wet washcloth handy for cleanup and to help get that nasty taste out of your mouth.

Consider medication. For particularly severe nausea and vomiting talk to your doctor fast. He may recommend one of several varieties of drugs that help reduce nausea.

"If symptoms persist or if you have a fever or chills, or if you are concerned about the severity of these symptoms, you should see your doctor or go to the emergency room," says Dr. Koch. "Men must be aware that occasionally a heart attack can feel like indigestion or queasiness."

See also Food Poisoning, Motion Sickness

Neck and Shoulder Pain

Take the World off Your Shoulders

Yes, pain in the neck is a pain in the neck, but look at it from your neck's perspective: If you had to hold up the equivalent of a 16-pound bowling ball all day, you'd grumble, too.

All right, that's like blaming a bad cough on the fact that you have lungs. In fact, neck pains come in all shapes and sizes and from a myriad of causes beyond having a big skull.

If you're a man who spends his workdays behind a desk, bad posture, stress and head fatigue—possibly computer related—may be the top causes of your neck pains. If you load trucks, build bridges or do other blue-collar work, it may be strain caused by unnatural arm and shoulder use.

If sports or working out is your passion, it may be unexpected jerks and jolts coupled with improper muscle conditioning. And for all of us the possibilities include sleeping at an odd angle or having our car hit from behind in the evening commute.

According to Wayne Westcott, Ph.D., a strength training consultant for the YMCA, "Most men, even if they're athletic, don't do any neck exercises, so their neck loses strength—strength that's critically important. If, at the end of the day, they engage in a game of golf or some other activity, or if they get nudged by the car behind them on the drive home, they're very susceptible to injury because they're in a weakened state."

Sharing the Pain

What's more, neck pain can easily become shoulder pain. Our necks act as major conduits for nerves that branch out from the spinal cord to the shoulders, arms and hands. As we twist, turn and nod our heads or slump, shrug and scrunch our shoulders, the nerves that are threaded past the discs and through the vertebrae in our necks get squeezed and pinched. Suddenly, for no discernible reason we're feeling pain in distant parts of our bodies.

"A lot of times neck problems will 'refer' pain to the shoulder," says Todd Edelson, a physical therapist in Montclair, New Jersey. "So unless a patient has a clear-cut shoulder injury, like a rotator cuff or a muscle tear, I look to the neck. If it's a vague complaint or if the onset occurs for no apparent reason, the neck is the most likely source of the pain."

Whiplash—when the head is wrenched violently forward and backward, usually during car accidents—remains a major cause of head and shoulder injuries. Less dramatic but just as pervasive, according to Robert S. Kunkel, M.D., an internist and member of the Headache Center, specializing in neck and head pain, at the Cleveland Clinic, is tension. "If someone gets tense, they tighten up their neck and shoulder muscles," he says. "Or they clench their teeth, which tightens muscles in the neck. That leads to muscle spasms in the neck and down into the shoulders."

Stopping Neck Neglect

More often than not, neck and shoulder problems are the result of neglecting the muscles there. That means most troubles can be easily avoided with a little preventive maintenance. Here's how.

Stay loose. Keeping your neck and shoulders limber helps keep neck problems at bay, according to Douglas Einstadter, M.D., assistant professor of medicine at Case Western Reserve University in Cleveland. He recommends performing some simple neck-stretching exercises several times a day, including rolling your head around slowly in a circular motion and slowly bending your head down to touch your chin on either shoulder. "The idea is not to push it," he says, "but you want to keep your neck in use so that it doesn't have a chance to get stiff."

Work out. As Dr. Westcott has pointed out, strength as well as flexibility helps prevent neck injuries. A study of jet fighter pilots confirms that assessment. Because neck pain is a common problem for pilots, the study examined 27 student fighter pilots at the Finnish Air Force Academy. Those who developed neck pain and those who didn't differed in only one respect: The group that had no neck pain participated in muscle endurance training.

The pilots in this study didn't specifically exercise their neck muscles—their superior upper body strength was apparently enough to do the trick—but that doesn't mean you can't. Most gyms where football players work out have a four-way neck machine, and Dr. Westcott recommends using one. In the absence of that, he suggests following a simple resistance regimen at home.

Lower your chin to your chest with your hands clasped behind your head. Raise your chin slowly all the way back, using your hands to provide enough resistance to stimulate your neck muscles. Then reverse the exercise, holding your hands on your forehead. Dr. Westcott recommends five repetitions of these exercises three times a week.

FAST FACTS

How common: Complaints of neck and shoulder pain are exceeded only by complaints of back pain and headache. It's estimated that 45 percent of working men have had at least one attack of stiff neck, 23 percent have had at least one attack of pain in the shoulder and upper arm and 51 percent have had both of these symptoms.

Risk factors: Bad posture, poorly designed office furniture, poor sleeping habits, car accident.

Age group affected: Men of all ages can have neck and shoulder pain, but we're less flexible and, as a result, more prone to injury as we get into our forties.

Gender gap: Evidence suggests that the incidence of neck and shoulder pain is about equal for both sexes.

Who to see: Most neck pain is treatable by your family doctor. Treatment by a physical therapist or a chiropractor may also be effective. For persistent, serious pain consult an orthopedic surgeon or a neurosurgeon.

Watch yourself. Take some time to observe the contortions you put your body through, especially at work. If you're straining on a regular basis, you need to make some changes. "There are simple ways you can alter your position or the way your job is designed," says James Kramer, M.D., co-director of the sports medicine fellowship at the Moses H. Cone Memorial Hospital in Greensboro, North Carolina. "A lot of it is common sense."

Put a mirror beside your desk or workstation to better observe your postural habits, suggests Emil Pascarelli, M.D., professor of clinical medicine, specializing in cumulative trauma disorders at Columbia-Presbyterian Medical Center/Eastside in New York City, and co-author of the book *Repetitive Strain Injury: A Computer User's Guide*. He cautions, however, that changing bad posture habits takes time and diligence because our ligaments literally mold themselves into the positions with which they're consistently held.

Listen to yourself. Men tend to ignore neck and shoulder pain, thinking the problem will go away on its own, according to Jerel Glassman, D.O., a rehabilitation medicine physician at St. Mary's Spine Center in San Francisco. "Often they've reached the end of their ropes before seeking treatment," he says. Problem is, failing to treat some neck and shoulder strains will only make them worse, Dr. Glassman says.

Snub the butts. Smoking has been shown to cause the discs in the lower back to deteriorate, according to Augustus A. White III, M.D., professor of orthopedic surgery at Harvard Medical School, and it's assumed the same happens to the discs in the neck. The exact cause isn't clear, he says, but it's likely that by impeding circulation, cigarettes prevent the discs from getting adequate nutrition.

Remember your headrest. Not enough people use the headrests in their cars, says Edward J. Resnick, M.D., professor of orthopedic surgery at the Temple University School of Medicine in Philadelphia. To get the best protection, make sure that the middle of your headrest is adjusted so that it's comfortably supporting the middle of the back of your head.

Sitting Pretty

Desk jobs used to be women's jobs. No more. With the advent of computers and the "information age," more and more men, from stockbrokers and journalists to graphic designers and architects, are working at desks all day—and risking neck and shoulder pain as they do. The good news is that bad posture is another problem that can be corrected with a little preventive maintenance. Here are some specifics to watch out for.

Keep your head up. You don't want to sit like a rigid stick figure, but you do want to sit up straight. "We see so many people with rounded shoulders and a forward sloping head and neck," says Dr. Kunkel. "That posture can cause pressure on a nerve, sending pain down the arm."

The key to good posture is staying in balance, stresses Scott W. Donkin, D.C., author of the book *Sitting on the Job*. Three of the most common bad postural habits to avoid, he says, are consistently leaning forward, backward, sideways or twisting; consistently looking downward with your chin tucked against your chest, and slouching with your butt on the forward edge of your chair for long periods of time.

And if you work with a computer, make sure you can look straight ahead at the monitor. "A monitor that's too high is a disaster for the neck and shoulders," says Chris Grant, Ph.D., a research fellow with the Center for Ergonomics at the University of Michigan in Ann Arbor. This is especially true if you wear reading glasses.

Get some support. Sitting in a chair that properly supports your back and your neck is one of the most effective ways to prevent neck and shoulder problems, according to Dr. Grant. Ideally, your chair should provide you with solid back support without being too rigid, allowing you to sit comfortably with the head balanced over the shoulders. Some chairs come with a support for the lower back built in. If your chair doesn't have one, Edelson says, you can buy a cylindrical support pillow at a medical supply store, or simply roll up a towel and wedge it behind the small of your back.

Since the body loathes being forced into one static position all day, Dr. Grant recommends an adjustable chair so that you can easily change its height and the angle of its backrest and seat. "It's essential that a work chair permit posture changes," she says. "In fact, some experts believe that freedom to move around is the single most important consideration in chairs designed for computer workstations."

Stop the scrunch. Holding a telephone receiver between your shoulder and ear is another ticket to Neck Pain Boulevard. Get yourself a headset—or better yet, two headsets, recommends Dr. Pascarelli. "Use them both at home and at the office."

Avoid the draft. Cold air blowing from an air-conditioning vent or open car window can cause your neck muscles to contract. That creates tension in those muscles, and eventually pain.

Take a break. Frequent breaks are a crucial necksaver for anyone working long hours in a static position. Schedule several "microbreaks" a day, suggests Dr. Donkin, both sitting and standing. Take a minute to stretch your arms and legs, breathe deeply, wiggle your toes and fingers, throw your chest out and up, roll your shoulders, look up, look down, look sideways and—he swears this is helpful—smile.

Sleep right. Posture while you're sleeping counts, too. Dr. Donkin recommends a thin pillow that will keep your neck level with the bed. The best sleeping positions, he says, are on your back or on your side. And try not to hold your arms over your head—that puts a strain on your shoulders.

Fight the Pain

If you've already developed neck pain or shoulder pain that's referred from the neck, you're experiencing a genuine medical mystery. A study that Dr. Einstadter helped conduct found wide variations both in the reasons doctors performed surgery for neck pain and the frequency with which they performed it. That indicates, he says, how little we know for certain about curing neck pain. "It's a common problem, but it hasn't been put to much scientific study."

For that reason, he says, unless your doctor suspects nerve damage, a ruptured disc or some similarly serious neurologic problem, you're more likely to end up with limited medical intervention.

Here are some contributions you can make to your own treatment.

Medicate moderately. Don't hesitate to treat yourself with aspirin or ibuprofen when neck pain first begins, Dr. White says. Use as indicated on the bottle—most likely, two pills three or four times a day. If the pain persists for more than a couple of weeks, see a doctor.

Cool it, heat it. Many doctors suggest treating neck and shoulder pain with either moist heat or ice. Unfortunately, there's widespread disagreement as to which works best. Dr. Kunkel takes a middle road. "I tell my patients to try both techniques and to stick with the one they prefer," he says.

For heat Dr. Kunkel recommends standing under a hot shower or buying a hot moist pack at a drugstore. These should be applied for 15 to 20 minutes prior to doing any exercising of the neck and shoulders, he says. For those taking the ice route (which probably is the correct approach if muscles are swollen) Edelson recommends holding an ice pack or a bag of frozen peas or corn on the neck for 10 to 15 minutes several times a day.

Search for clues. Give some thought to your physical history before you seek treatment. A neck problem now may have started with an injury you sustained years ago, according to Dr. Donkin. Any leads you can provide for your doctor or therapist may help pinpoint your problem and lead to the most effective treatment.

Nosebleeds

Messy, but Easy to Control

Once upon a time soothsayers attached all sorts of meanings to nosebleeds. They interpreted them as signs of amorousness, good fortune or, hedging their bets, grave foreboding.

As it turns out, things aren't quite so complicated. Most nosebleeds occur when tender tissues inside the nose get dry and irritated—or when you accidentally put your nose somewhere you shouldn't, like in the path of a boxing glove.

Nosebleeds are more common in men than women, if only because men are more likely to have their noses in the line of fire, says Graham Boyce, M.D., assistant professor of otolaryngology-head and neck surgery at Louisiana State University School of Medicine in New Orleans.

Tough Outside, Sensitive Inside

Although the outer portions of your nose are comprised of tough cartilage, the inside is packed with fragile blood vessels and lined with a mucous layer. It doesn't take much of a scrape or smack to get the blood flowing, says Dr. Boyce.

In most cases the blood comes from a network of small capillaries in the front part of your nasal septum. That's the ridge of bone and cartilage that divides your nose in half. Doctors call these bleeds anterior nosebleeds because the vessels in question are up front. Injury is a common cause of anterior nosebleeds. So is dry air, which can cause the membrane lining your septum to crack and bleed.

"For some the problem is aggravated during the winter," says Jerome C. Goldstein, M.D., visiting professor of otolaryngology-head and neck surgery at Johns Hopkins University in Baltimore and Georgetown University in Washington, D.C. "When the heat comes on in the house, many homes get drier than the Sahara desert. The Sahara is 26 percent relative humidity. Some homes, where humidifiers are not used when the heat is on, fall below that."

In addition, men with deviated or crooked septums are prone to bleeds. "A piece of the septum can stick out in the airway—stick out in the breeze, so to speak—and be more prone to getting dried out," explains C. Thomas Yarington,

M.D., clinical professor of otolaryngology at the University of Washington and head of the Mason Clinic, both in Seattle.

Smoking also dries out the membranes and increases the risk of nosebleeds. More rarely, serious conditions such as high blood pressure, leukemia or tumors may be to blame. So if you're getting a nosebleed every other month or so and can't figure out why, it's probably a good idea to see a doctor, Dr. Goldstein says.

But the vast majority of nosebleeds aren't anything to worry about. Even the amount of blood, which can resemble a veritable torrent, rarely amounts to more than four ounces, or about half a cup. Still, even a minor nosebleed can be scary and uncomfortable. There's also the laundry bill to consider.

Preventing the Flow

So rather than trying to turn off the taps after the bleeding starts, here are a few ways to prevent it from occurring.

Crank up the humidity. Since dry nasal membranes are perhaps the most common cause of nosebleeds, putting extra moisture in the air will help keep them moist and protected. Electric humidifiers work well. Or you can make your own humidifier. "Set a pie tin filled with a half-inch of water in each room," suggests John A. Henderson, M.D., assistant professor of ear, nose and throat surgery at the University of California at San Diego. As the water evaporates and goes airborne, it becomes an effective and inexpensive source of lubrication for parched noses.

Humidify from the inside out. Another way to pump up the moisture is by drinking eight eight-ounce glasses of water every day. This will help moisten and protect mucous membranes throughout your body, including in the nose, Dr. Yarington says.

Have a schnozz spritz. Sniffing a saline solution is perhaps the fastest way to put soothing moisture directly where it counts. You can buy a ready-made solution in drugstores. Or make your own by mixing a quarter-teaspoon of table salt in eight ounces of warm water.

Rub on protection. When you first notice the inside of your nose getting dry and crackly, try lubricating it with a small dab of antibiotic ointment, like Bacitracin or Polysporin, suggests Lloyd M. Loft, M.D., professor of otolaryngology at New York Medical College in Valhalla. Although petroleum jelly is also a lubricant, it should be avoided because it can damage cilia, tiny hairs inside the nose that help trap grit and grime, he says.

Build up the B. In order to produce free-flowing and protective mucus, your body needs an ample supply of B vitamins. At a minimum, you should be getting five servings a day of fruits and vegetables. Other foods high in B vitamins include lean meats, legumes, whole grains and low-fat or nonfat dairy products. If you're not sure you're getting enough or if you simply want extra insurance, ask your doctor which multivitamin might be right for you.

Lay off the hooch. When Scottish researchers studied the drinking habits of 140 hospital patients admitted with nosebleeds, they found they were almost twice as likely to drink regularly as people admitted for other nose or throat problems. The study concluded that high alcohol consumption can cause more nosebleeds.

Stop smoking. Giving up cigarettes will help give your poor, dried-out nose a chance to recover its natural lubrication, says Lee Eisenberg, M.D., assistant professor of otolaryngology at Columbia University in New York City.

Check your blood pressure. Since having high blood pressure puts additional stress on delicate blood vessels inside the nose, it may result in nosebleeds. So if you've been having nosebleeds and don't know why, see your doctor for advice, says Dr. Loft.

Ask about surgery. In some cases guys who have repeated nosebleeds have a "malfunctioning" stretch of blood vessel. If that's happening to you, your doctor may advise that you have it cauterized—sealed off to prevent future bleeds, says Dr. Goldstein. In addition, surgery may be required when nosebleeds are caused by a deviated septum, says Dr. Yarington. The procedure is usually straightforward, and your doctor may be able to straighten out the problem on an outpatient basis, using only a local anesthetic.

First-Aid Basics

Until they design a nose that's lined with Teflon and swaddled in titanium, you'll never be able to prevent all nosebleeds from occurring. But when you do get one, here are some easy ways to slow the flow.

Give a pinch. As soon as the bleeding starts, gently pinch the soft parts of your nose together between your thumb and two fingers while at the same time pressing inward toward your face. This will help seal off leaky blood vessels. Hold the position for at least five minutes.

To make sure gravity works for you instead of against you, be sure to stand or sit up so your head is higher than the level of your heart.

Blow gently. Once the bleeding is under control, blow your nose gently to expel blood clots that may have formed. "Clots will eventually break down and be a source of a secondary bleed," Dr. Henderson explains. After you've blown your nose, pinch your nose shut and hold it for an extra ten minutes, he adds.

When Bleeding Won't Stop

While most nosebleeds are minor, occasionally the blood just keeps flowing. When that happens, chances are you have a posterior nosebleed in which large blood vessels at the back of the nose have been damaged. "You can bleed a pint in 20 minutes unless it's controlled," warns Dr. Yarington.

Fortunately, posterior bleeds are rare, affecting no more than about 1 percent of the population during a lifetime. People with high blood pressure are among those at risk, as are the elderly, whose blood vessels are more brittle and prone to injury. A hard blow to the head—from a car accident, for example—can also cause posterior bleeds.

Since the blood vessels that cause this type of nosebleed are out of reach at the back of your nose, you can't treat them yourself. So if you have heavy bleeding that doesn't stop after 15 minutes or the blood is flowing down the back of your throat, head for your doctor's office or the emergency room right away.

A doctor can stanch the bleeding by packing the back of your nose with gauze. Or he may put internal pressure on the blood vessels by inserting a balloon in your nose and then inflating it with air or water.

Since this type of nosebleed can be quite serious, your doctor may ask you to stay in the hospital until the packing comes out and a scab forms—usually after two to three days.

Oily Skin

How to Avoid the Sheen

Experts call it the T zone—the stretch of skin that starts at the chin, goes up across the nose and gets topped by the horizontal stretch of the forehead. For all the oil this expanse of skin can generate, the T might as well stand for Texas.

"Oily skin is just overactive glands. And it's common in men because they have larger oil glands than women," says Hillard H. Pearlstein, M.D., assistant clinical professor of dermatology at Mount Sinai School of Medicine of the City University of New York in New York City.

Not only do men have larger oil glands, but male hormones direct both male and female versions of those cells. "The oil glands are under the strict control of male hormones. Women don't produce so much oil because estrogen blocks most of the male hormone they put out," says Alan R. Shalita, M.D., chairman of the Department of Dermatology at the State University of New York Health Science Center in Brooklyn.

Who gets oily skin? So many men that no statistician has ever tracked it. One issue is genetics. If oily skin runs in your family, chances are you have it, too, says Dr. Pearlstein. But it's not true that any one ethnic group is more or less prone to oily skin, he adds.

In general, it's mostly a function of the body you are born with. Some people have it and others don't, and outside triggers don't make much difference. "Oily skin is pure anatomy," notes Guy Webster, M.D., Ph.D., associate professor of dermatology and director of the Center for Cutaneous Pharmacology at Jefferson Medical College of Thomas Jefferson University in Philadelphia.

In other words, you can't prevent oily skin, says Dr. Pearlstein. "It's like preventing yourself from being short," he says.

Cleaning Lessons

There *are* some good things about oily skin. For one, it protects you better from the tracks of age than normal or dry skin. And as it did for your Stone Age cousins, oily skin helps protect you from harsh weather. And if you like getting noticed, light bounces nicely off your forehead.

But if oily skin bothers you, the first line of defense is proper cleaning.

Take control of your soap. "You fix oily skin by washing your face," says Dr. Webster. "But you have to wash your face more judiciously, and avoid irritating cleansers," he adds.

A judicious wash starts with the proper soap. You're probably used to soaping up with whatever bar is lying around the bathroom. Your wife bought it. Or maybe your girlfriend gave it to you for Christmas. Or it was on special at the supermarket.

But you need to choose soap specifically for oily skin if you want to improve the state of your face. You don't want the same soap that your dry-skinned partner uses. Avoid soaps labeled moisturizing—you want to dry up that grease, not moisturize it. Instead, look for soaps made for oily skin.

Try something new. Your washing product doesn't even have to be a bar of soap. Cleansing lotions can be at least as effective.

One deep-cleaning ingredient to look for on labels is salicylic acid, says Ronald R. Brancaccio, M.D., clinical associate professor of dermatology at New York University Medical Center in New York City. He also recommends Oxy and Neutrogena "washes," which are liquid, and Neutrogena soap for acne-prone skin.

Opt for cleansing products from the beauty giants, like Clearasil, Clinique, Avon and L'Oreal, because they have research departments at least as huge as their hype, suggests Dr. Shalita. "So they generally have something to back up their claims," he says. Some of the big cosmetics companies have lines specifically for men, too.

Sneak in a cleaning. If you've changed your soap and your skin is still bothering you, don't overclean, but wipe instead. An easy way to do that is to keep a jar of cleansing pads (such as Oxy or Neutrogena) nearby, says Lia Schorr, author of *Lia Schorr's Skin Care Guide for Men* and owner of the Lia Schorr Skin Care Salon in New York City. You can find them in most drugstores. "If you keep a bottle of pads at the office, you can clean your face conveniently during the day," she says. Or try oil control blotting papers to get rid of oil without wetness.

After Mastering Soap

You've braved the bath aisles of the megasized pharmacies. You've toughed out the cosmetics counters in your local department stores. Don't stop yet. Here are more products to consider that get beyond routine cleaning.

Slap on astringent. On one of your skin-product safaris get a bottle of astringent or clarifying lotion that's labeled for oily skin (such as Johnson's Clean and Clear astringent). After you've washed your face, anoint your skin with the astringent. Both products contain alcohol and help to remove soap residue, oil and dead skin cells. "Oily skin care is a mopping-up procedure," says Dr. Pearlstein.

FAST FACTS

How common: Most men have oily foreheads, noses and skin from hormones and overactive glands.

Risk factors: Genetics.

Age group affected: Puberty turns on the oil glands. Oil production decreases by your late sixties or seventies.

Gender gap: Male hormones stimulate the oil glands, so men produce more oil than women.

Who to see: If you can't conquer oily skin on your own but it's just a cosmetic issue, consider seeing a cosmetician who specializes in skin care. For bigger problems see your family doctor. You might be referred to a dermatologist.

Make a mud pie. Facial masks absorb excess oil. Masks are usually creams with particles of clay in them. Generally, the darker the color of the mask, the more oil it will sop up. Yes, these are the 1990s—men can have a facial without losing face.

Sun carefully. Sunscreen is an item you routinely use on your skin (or should). Look for screeners that have an alcohol or gel base (such as PreSun Active 15). They'll help de-grease your skin, too.

Beyond Cleaning

If your skin is uncomfortably oily, there are things to avoid as well as acquire.

Screen your food. Certain foods sometimes grease up the skin of susceptible men, says Dr. Pearlstein. "Chocolate can stimulate oil production. So can anything with iodine—seafood, iodized salt. Sometimes cola drinks and nuts will do it. And sharp cheeses can contribute to oily skin," he says.

Wash off your workout. "Men often perceive their skin as being oily because it feels that way when they sweat. They rub their hands on their faces and get an oil slick. But it's really more sweat than oil," says Dr. Webster.

If that sounds familiar, what you want to do is shower right after a workout, says Schorr. Don't sit around shooting the bull in your briefs or hoisting a brew in your sweats. Run the hot water and de-grease.

Osteoporosis

Preventing the Snap

An affliction most associated with elderly women, osteoporosis is a thinning of bone mass that makes bones frail and susceptible to breaking.

For women the trouble comes from the loss of estrogen, a key hormone that among other things helps maintain bone mass. Menopause causes estrogen levels to drop, leading to accelerated bone degeneration.

But before you snap your jockstrap and say "no problemo for me," realize that millions of men suffer from frail bones, too. No one knows exactly what causes osteoporosis in men, but heredity, low testosterone levels, physical inactivity, smoking, alcohol and eating habits may all play a role.

Keeping the Jelly

Bones have three main layers. The outermost part is hard, dense bone called cortical bone. At the center of the bone, like the jelly part of a jelly doughnut, is the marrow. Between them is trabecular bone, sometimes called spongy bone, not because it's soft but because it contains little hollow spaces like those in a sponge.

This middle tissue, made up of proteins and minerals, naturally thins as we age. The loss begins at about age 35; most men can expect to lose 15 to 45 percent of their trabecular bone during their lifetime.

This only becomes a problem, however, if that loss leads to a bone mass that is below the fracture threshold, explains Michael Holick, M.D., a specialist in osteoporosis at Boston University Medical Center. Then, you have severe osteoporosis: Your bones do not have enough support to prevent them from breaking.

Trouble is, there are no symptoms associated with osteoporosis. Only when a bone actually fractures is the severity of bone-mass loss discovered.

But once you have it, watch out. A minor fall that would cause nothing more than a bruise when you're playing touch football at age 21 could mean a major fracture of the hip that requires hip replacement to the same person 30 years later.

Or consider that bone degeneration could mean an easy snap to the vertebrae

388

FAST FACTS

How common: Although everyone experiences loss of bone mass as they age, severe osteoporosis afflicts only 15 percent of men before age 85.

Risk factors: Malnutrition, smoking, heavy drinking, lack of exercise, genetics. Caucasians are more at risk than African Americans.

Age group affected: Increases with age. Most sufferers are elderly, but severe osteoporosis leading to fractures of the spine has been known to occur in men under age 45.

Gender gap: Women are four times more likely to have it than men.

Who to see: Your family doctor, who may refer you to an osteopath or an endocrinologist.

in the spine, causing loss of height, nerve compression or trauma to the sciatic nerve that runs down the spine.

Once you lose bone mass, it can't be replaced. If severe osteoporosis sets in, you are destined to a life of ginger movements and extreme caution.

Easy Strengthening

But why let that happen? For guys there's little reason to develop severe osteoporosis. A well-balanced diet and an active lifestyle will go a long way in preventing bone degeneration. Here's what you can do to prevent the snap.

Be rich in calcium. By far the most common cause of osteoporosis in men is poor diet. Drinking soft drinks and eating potato chips instead of milk and vegetables can help you become fragile before your time.

Milk is the magic elixir for bones since it contains key ingredients they need, particularly calcium, vitamin D and phosphorous, notes Robert P. Heaney, M.D., professor of medicine at Creighton University School of Medicine in Omaha, Nebraska. Don't just put milk in your coffee but drink at least one eight-ounce glass of low-fat milk every day. Cheese and other dairy products should also be part of your regular diet for the same reasons: They are rich in calcium, Dr. Heaney says. Just make sure to eat mainly low-fat varieties.

Keep an eye on food labels because the Food and Drug Administration allows products with high calcium content to say that they may help to reduce the risk of osteoporosis. Calcium is also available in supplements, including some multivitamins; so read those labels to be sure you're getting 1,000 milligrams of calcium a day, the amount recommended by experts.

Also, be aware that salt and protein can cause your body to excrete more calcium than it is absorbing. We're not saying to eliminate the two from your diet, but know that eating an excessive amount of either might affect your bones.

Finally, this cooking tip: When you are making soup stock from bones, pour in a little vinegar. The vinegar helps dissolve the calcium out of the bones and into the broth.

Get plenty of exercise. Exercise is crucial to strong bones, all doctors agree. In fact, studies have shown that weight-bearing exercise actually *increases* bone mass in people who have been sedentary. Weight-bearing exercises include any activity in which you carry your own weight (such as walking, skiing or doing push-ups) or some outside weight (such as when doing yard work or weight lifting). Swimming and bicycling, because your weight is supported, are not weight-bearing exercises.

But the true value of exercise is that it can assure you of remaining active when you get older. "Inactivity is the kiss of death for your skeleton," says Barbara Drinkwater, Ph.D., a research physiologist in the Department of Medicine at Pacific Medical Center in Seattle. As an added bonus, exercise also develops your muscles and improves your coordination.

So take a walk, learn to run, play tennis, climb some rocks, go out and shag some softballs. Anything that gets you moving.

Kick the habits. Okay, you've read this in probably half the chapters in this book. But it needs to be said once again: Don't smoke and cut back on the booze.

It's not yet known why smoking is a factor, but severe osteoporosis is commonly associated with emphysema and chronic bronchitis, both hazards of smoking.

Severe osteoporosis is also an affliction of heavy drinkers, probably because of their poor nutritional habits.

Watch your genes. Yes, severe osteoporosis can be inherited, though the exact genetic causes are still being researched. If your family has a history of osteoporosis, you should be especially careful about following the tips for preventing bone loss.

Watch your head. Dr. Holick has also found an intriguing indicator. He and his colleague, Dr. Clifford Rosen, discovered that men and women who gray prematurely—defined as 50 percent of the hair turning gray by age 40—are as much as four times more at risk of developing severe osteoporosis than men and women who gray at the proper age.

"One of my patients," said Dr. Holick, "a staffer here at the center who began graying in his early twenties, is already suffering the effects of osteoporosis now in his early forties." Dr. Holick says that late graying is not a sign of lower risk, however.

Overweight

Proven Ways to Take Off the Pounds

Generations ago, a corpulent man was an admired man. All that extra ballast attested to his success—proof that he could afford the finer things in life.

Today, admiring glances are more likely to be bestowed upon the fit than the fat. Add to that what we've learned about the health risks of being overweight, and it's not surprising that health clubs are packed with guys trying to whip themselves into shape—or at least get to the point where they can see their belt buckles without a mirror.

There's no escaping the fact that as a man ages, his genes, hormones and slowing metabolism begin ganging up on his gut. "The catch is that while calorie requirements and metabolism are decreasing, most men are eating the same or more and becoming less active," says Robert Kushner, M.D., director of the Nutrition and Weight Control Clinic at the University of Chicago. As a result, we stockpile calories. Which is why in the decade between the ages of 30 and 40 the average man gains about six pounds.

But while a potbelly may become more likely as you age, it's not inevitable. You have the power to get rid of those extra inches—and there's good reason to do it. Lose your potbelly and you'll look better, feel better and have more energy. You'll probably live longer, too.

Fat Facts

The average man walks around with about 30 billion fat cells in his body, and as he gets a little older, they tend to get a little heavier. The National Center for Health Statistics estimates that about one in four American men is obese, defined as being more than 20 percent over their ideal weight.

Carrying around extra pounds does more than keep the large-size clothing industry in business. It also keeps the medics hopping. Compared to their leaner counterparts, obese men have three times the risk of developing high blood pressure, double the risk of high cholesterol and triple the risk of diabetes. They're also more prone to heart disease and cancer. Staying trim can be, quite literally, a lifesaver.

You don't have to lose a lot of weight to reap major benefits, says Judith Stern, R.D., Sc.D., professor of internal medicine at the University of California, Davis. Research shows that overweight guys who drop just 5 to 10 percent of their total weight can cut their risk of heart disease by 20 percent.

This isn't to say that losing weight and keeping it off is easy—*somebody* out there is buying elastic-waist chinos, meal-replacement shakes and *Sweatin' to the Oldies* videos. But weight loss doesn't have to be an impossible undertaking, either. "In most cases all that's needed are fairly small changes in exercise and eating habits," says Susan Kayman, R.D., D.P.H., a dietitian and consultant with the Kaiser-Permanente Medical Group in Oakland, California. "Over time, these can add up to large improvements in how you look and feel."

Fit for Life

In your leaner, meaner days you probably got a lot more exercise than you do now. Even if you weren't a hard-core jock, the combination of gym class, pickup games and the calorie-burning furnace of teenage sexual frustration went a long way toward keeping you thin.

These days, it seems like you spend most of your waking hours behind a desk or sacked out in front of the TV. There just aren't as many opportunities—or as much time—to be active. But even if you're a paper pusher by trade, there are easy ways to get the calories burning.

Get aerobic. Regular aerobic exercise, like biking, running or brisk walking, is probably the most efficient way to burn fat, says Douglas Ballor, Ph.D., assistant professor of physical education at the University of Vermont in Burlington. It doesn't really matter what you do, as long as it gets your heart rate up and keeps it there for at least 20 minutes.

Regular exercise does more than tone the flesh above the belt. Research suggests it can also benefit the equipment down below. In one study 78 healthy but inactive men who began doing aerobic exercise three to five days a week reported having more frequent and better sex. And the more they exercised, the more and better sex they had.

Put on some bulk. Muscle tissue is metabolically far more active than fat. This means that the more muscle you have, the more calories you'll burn, even when you're sleeping. Unfortunately, the average guy loses about six pounds of muscle tissue once he's in his thirties, which seriously cuts into the number of calories burned every day.

To reverse the trend, you should be lifting weights at least three days a week. Whatever routine you choose, be sure not to work the same muscle groups two days in a row—it's important to allow a one-day recovery period between workouts, ex-

FAST FACTS

How common: More than 25 million—or one in four—American men are obese, which experts define as being more than 20 percent over their ideal weight.

Risk factors: Genetics, sedentary lifestyle, overeating, high-fat diet.

Age group affected: Many men begin developing their weight problems in their thirties or forties.

Gender gap: About 25.9 percent of American men are obese, as compared with 22.3 percent of American women.

Who to see: Family doctor.

perts say. That's why some regular gym-going men will typically work their backs and chests on one day, followed by legs and arms the next.

Most important is to find a routine you enjoy and look forward to. Otherwise you won't bother doing it. "The key is to pick something you like, that's enjoyable and that you can do every day," says Dr. Ballor.

Put on your walking shoes. Fitness buffs used to think that if you weren't huffing and puffing at the end of your workout, you weren't burning fat. Not so, says Dr. Ballor. Studies have shown that walking briskly for 20 minutes can confer the same benefits as high-impact aerobic workouts. "Walking is a great exercise," he says. "It's not real stressful for the body and you can do it every day." To burn about 300 extra calories a day, he adds, you need to walk about three miles. You can probably achieve that with a brisk 30-minute walk shortly after dinner each day.

Look for opportunities. You don't need a health club to get your muscles pumping. Instead of circling the parking lot like a vulture looking for prime meat, begin parking farther away and enjoy the walking time. Once you're inside, take the stairs instead of the elevator. Deliver memos by hand instead of e-mail, and don't hesitate to take a walk during your coffee break: It will clear the cobwebs better than caffeine—and you won't be tempted by the doughnuts, either.

Diet No More

If you're like most men, counting calories, on the excitement scale, is somewhere between Christmas shopping and writing your will. But if you're serious about losing weight, you've got to pay at least some attention to what you eat.

This *doesn't* mean dieting, says Morton H. Shaevitz, Ph.D., associate clinical professor of psychiatry at the University of California, San Diego School of Medi-

Healthy Substitutions

It's the old bait and switch. It works for dogs (I'll give you this rawhide bone if you give me back my wing tip), and it can work for you. The next time you find yourself in the kitchen at midnight craving a high-cal, fatty treat, try to salvage your diet by tempting yourself with these leaner alternatives.

- 1 cup roasted peanuts (840 calories, 71 grams of fat)
+ 1 cup raisins (435 calories, 1 gram of fat)

-1 cup premium vanilla ice cream (350 calories, 24 grams of fat)
+1 cup vanilla frozen yogurt (173 calories, 1 gram of fat)

-1 jelly doughnut (289 calories, 16 grams of fat)
+1 bagel with jelly (240 calories, 2 grams of fat)

-1 slice pound cake (220 calories, 10 grams of fat)
+1 slice angel food cake (125 calories, less than 1 gram of fat)

-4 chocolate chip cookies (180 calories, 9 grams of fat)
+4 fig bars (210 calories, 4 grams of fat)

-1 ounce nacho cheese tortilla chips (141 calories, 7 grams of fat)
-1 ounce air-popped popcorn (108 calories, 1 gram of fat)
-10 potato chips (105 calories, 7 grams of fat)
+2 large hard pretzels (125 calories, 1 gram of fat)

-10 peanut M & M's (99 calories, 5 grams of fat)
+10 jelly beans (104 calories, less than 1 gram of fat)

cine, and director of the eating disorders program at Scripps Clinic and Research Foundation in La Jolla, California. "Diets are short-term changes in eating behavior and because they're short-term, all diets fail," says Dr. Shaevitz.

Put another way, going "on" a diet suggests you'll someday go "off"—and probably will end up portlier than you were before.

But there are strategies for losing weight that don't involve dieting—which is why they're much more likely to succeed. Here's what experts recommend.

Trim fat from your diet. It's tough to resist putting extra butter on your roll, or

What's Your Healthy Weight?

If you're old enough to vote and you're still outgrowing your clothes, chances are you're putting on weight. But are those extra pounds actually threatening your health or are they simply a natural consequence of getting older?

To determine your healthy weight, doctors use a scale called the body mass index (BMI). For all but the most-extravagantly muscular it's a good indicator of whether or not you need to lose weight. To calculate your BMI:

1. First, divide your weight (in pounds) by your height (in inches) squared.
2. Multiply the resulting number by 705. You should get a BMI that's somewhere between 19 and 30.

Here's an example. Suppose that Bob is five feet ten inches tall, weighs 180 pounds and is lousy at math. To find his BMI:

1. He gets out his pocket calculator and multiplies 70 × 70 to get his height in inches squared. He then divides the number (4,900) into 180 pounds.
2. He takes his answer, .036, and multiplies that by 705.
3. He comes up with a BMI of 25.

The healthiest BMI for men is between 22 and 24. If your BMI is 28.5 or above, you're overweight. If your BMI has bulged beyond 33, you're seriously overweight.

chewing down that succulent strip of fat that rims a good steak, but the only way to lose weight is to cut back on fat. The reason is simple: One gram of fat has nine calories, while a gram of protein or carbohydrate has only four. So, eating high fat foods will make you fat.

Not surprisingly, while overweight men eat about the same amount as leaner guys, they tend to eat more fatty foods.

Experts agree that no more than 30 percent of your daily calories should come from fat. But don't sweat the math, adds Dr. Shaevitz. Just make it a point to eat less of those foods you already know are high in fat. Cut back on fried foods. Drink low-fat instead of whole milk. Choose lean cuts of meat such as flank steak. Eat more chicken or turkey (without the skin). Eat some meals that are carbohydrate based, like pasta with marinara sauce, rather than steak and potatoes.

Go for the Burn

When you're trying to lose weight, what you put in your mouth is only half the equation. "It's what you expend, not just what you consume, that's really important," says Charles Kuntzleman, Ed.D., adjunct associate professor in the Division of Kinesiology at the University of Michigan in Ann Arbor.

You don't have to be grunting and sweating to burn energy. Everything you do—walking, making love, even sleeping—requires calories. Of course, some activities require more energy than others. If you weigh between 160 and 170 pounds, here's what you'll burn when you're doing the following:

Activity	Calories burned (per min.)
Watching TV	1.33
Engaging in sexual foreplay	1.75
Bartending (on a busy night)	4.08
Mowing the lawn (power mower)	4.41
Mowing the lawn (push mower)	4.75
Having sexual intercourse	5.25
Stream fishing	5.25
Shooting archery	5.50
Bicycling (10 mph)	7.33
Rowing a machine (vigorously)	11.50
Running (7 mph)	12.30
Playing full-court basketball	13.16
Skiing cross-country (9 mph)	17.58
Running (12 mph)	24.40

Don't rush the meal. Men tend to eat as though someone will grab their chow if they don't grab it first. But eating fast can produce more than heartburn. It can also cause your stomach to get full long before the brain knows it, says Dr. Shaevitz. And until the brain shuts off the appetite switch, you're going to keep eating.

To keep your brain and stomach working in tandem, you need to eat more slowly. Dr. Shaevitz recommends setting down your fork or spoon between bites and picking it up only after you swallow. Or when eating Chinese, Thai or Japanese food, use chopsticks, which are guaranteed to slow you down.

Fill up on nutrition. Easy to do: Just add beans, fruits, vegetables and whole grains to your menu. These foods are rich in fiber, low in fat and are chock-full of vitamins, minerals and antioxidants, says Dr. Kayman. In addition to keeping you healthy, fiber is filling, which means you'll be less likely to fill up on fatty foods.

Lay off the add-ons. Bread, pasta, raw vegetables, rice and baked potatoes—all are low in fat and high in complex carbohydrates. But smother them with butter, mayonnaise, sour cream or oily dressing, and you're putting back all the fat calories you've been trying to avoid.

If you're trying to cut back on fatty add-ons but don't want to give them up entirely, check out your supermarket's nonfat offerings. For example, while regular sour cream contains three grams of fat, you can buy a nonfat version instead. Or switch to low-fat condiments, says Dr. Kayman. Instead of putting mayo on your sandwich, for example, use mustard instead. Instead of butter, put salsa on your spud.

Go easy on the alcohol. Some alcoholic beverages have more calories than a rich dessert, says Dr. Shaevitz. Having a mixed drink before dinner and two glasses of wine with dinner can add 500 calories to your meal—about as much as a slice of cherry pie and a bowl of ice cream. What's more, alcohol lowers your blood sugar, which makes you hungrier.

Plan ahead. Keeping low-fat snacks on hand means you'll be less likely to scarf down a candy bar during a weak moment, says Dr. Kayman. "If you know you get hungry midmorning, then bring along fruit, a banana or something that will hold you through to lunch," she suggests.

Penile Trauma

Avoiding the Organ Grinders

It's amazing the trouble a penis can get into. James Sehn, M.D., ought to know. As a general urologist in Manassas, Virginia, "I get to see a little bit of everything," he says. So it didn't shock Dr. Sehn as much as it shocked the rest of the male world when he was called to a local hospital one night to help reattach John Wayne Bobbitt's penis.

In a case that made headlines worldwide, Bobbitt lost his penis to a wife irate from alleged abuse and a sharp kitchen knife. To make a long story short, Dr. Sehn and a plastic surgeon successfully reattached the penis. The Bobbitts became instant, though infamous, celebrities and John and his fully operational organ went on to perform in an X-rated film. Meanwhile, millions of cringing men wondered: Could it happen to me?

Rashes, Ruptures and Rip-Offs

We can't place odds on your movie career, but as far as penile trauma goes, the answer is probably not, says Paul Gleich, M.D., chief of urology at St. Paul-Ramsey Medical Center in St. Paul, Minnesota. "The penis really doesn't get traumatized very often," he says.

In fact, if you're luckless enough to experience that perennial male hazard—a blow to the crotch—the explosive agony you'll feel will most likely come from your testicles, not your penis. The most sensitive penile nerves are at the head of the penis, not the shaft, an area that's rarely hit, says Dr. Gleich. "When there's an impact or injury to the crotch, the penis tends to get moved out of the way—and the testicles get injured instead," he says.

That's pretty cold comfort for most of us. Unlike the arms, legs, fingers, toes or even testicles, we only have one penis; consequently, it's the one appendage we can't bear to think about injuring or even losing. And yet, as long as we have it, there's always the possibility we could bruise it, bend it or break it. And that's no laughing matter. If penile trauma is severe enough, you could be facing impotence, urinary problems or severe blood loss. But knowing what the possible spectrum of damage

FAST FACTS

How common: There are no hard and fast figures on penile trauma, but experts say less than 5 percent of all men are likely to suffer any kind of serious injury to the penis.

Risk factors: Sexual activity always leaves open the possibility of bruises and breaks, particularly when it involves vigorous thrusting or positions where the weight of the partner is bearing down on the penis. Also, men who practice cycling or martial arts are at higher risk of penile trauma than with other sports.

Age group affected: Sexually active men between the ages of 20 and 45 tend to be at the highest risk for penile trauma.

Gender gap: Penile fracture is—no surprise here—strictly a male problem.

Who to see: Urologist.

is—and what can be done about these injuries—might help you deal with it better should the worst arise.

Caught with Your Pants Down?

A common fear—but one of the least common types of trauma among adult men—is that they'll get their penises caught in their zippers. Experts say this happens more with children, but a few hasty adults have been caught on the fly, too. To make sure you're not one of them:

Wear underwear. The easiest way to avoid entrapment is to make sure you have something between you and the zipper, be they briefs or boxers.

Watch the downstroke. Some researchers have found unzipping may be just as hazardous to your health.

Oil up. In some cases liberal application of mineral oil on both zipper and zippee may be enough to unsnag the penis. If this doesn't work, get to a doctor. Unzipping the skin or trying to pry the zipper apart will only make things worse.

Get Bent?

The most frequent type of phallic injury is so gradual you won't even know it—until you begin to notice that your erections are taking a sharp turn.

The problem is called Peyronie's disease, and experts say thousands of men get it every year, even though they aren't sure why. Some doctors think it's a virus that affects the penis; others suspect Peyronie's is a kind of penile arthritis.

Penile Cancer: The Sex Disease You Rarely Hear Of

Penile cancer is not a problem your ever likely to face: It accounts for less than 1 percent of all cancer malignancies in American men. "Even a busy practice might see only one case every two or three years," says Joseph Fowler, M.D., associate professor of dermatology at the University of Louisville School of Medicine/Health Services Center. It's so rare that a number of well-known medical reference texts contain no entries for it whatsoever.

Still, there is reason to be concerned about penile cancer, and it's this: The disease may be caused by a sexually transmitted virus that's also associated with cervical cancer in women. The viral agent in question is human papillomavirus, whose infection rates have been rising sharply. In one study, 33 percent of men who were sexual partners of women with precancerous cell changes in the cervix developed premalignant lesions of the penis.

Penile cancer is easy to see but difficult to distinguish visually from less serious problems. It often takes the form of a red, dime-sized patch similar to what you might see from, for instance, a fungal infection. Sometimes the patch is shiny, other times it's bumpy or crusty. About half the time the lesions itch or hurt. If such problems persist for more than a month, maximum, it's a good idea to see a doctor, who can do a biopsy to determine if the lesions are cancerous or not.

If you have cancer on your penis, you have to get rid of it, period, advises Thomas Stanisic, M.D., a urologist at Affiliated Urology Specialists in Peoria, Illi-

"Peyronie's produces scarring in the erectile chamber—the part that fills with blood to give you an erection—on one or both sides of the penis," explains Dr. Gleich. When you get an erection, the scarred chamber will have a kink in it. "The penis is pushed in the direction of the scarred side and you can get dramatic distortions—almost 90-degree angles in some cases."

If you start to notice a change in the normal curve of your erection, get to a doctor. Treatment can be as simple as vitamin E or anti-inflammatory medication or as complex as surgery on the scar tissue. "But get it looked at as soon as you can," cautions Dr. Sehn. "If you have it for more than a year, it rarely goes away."

Gone Broke?

While an erection might seem like the pinnacle of man's power and potency, it's also a time of vulnerability.

nois. Granted, the picture of someone coming at Mr. Happy with a sharp instrument is, in Dr. Stanisic's words, "The ultimate fear of most men." Still, if you let penile cancer go untreated, the cancer may not be the only thing that has to come off. In cases where lesions penetrate beyond the surface into the structure of the organ, the treatment is sometimes amputation. Fortunately, there are friendlier alternatives for smaller lesions, some of which don't involve cutting of any kind.

The basic tratment is to simply cut away the tumor plus a small amount of tissue around it for good measure, just to make sure no cancer is left behind. Often, this can be done at the same time the biopsy is performed. For men who aren't circumcised, many doctors recommend that the foreskin go as well, to prevent recurrence. Alternative treatments include:

A less invasive operation is daily application of a prescription cream containing the anticancer drug 5-flourouracil (Efudex). One doctor who treated three patients with the drug found it not only got rid of lesions, it kept them from recurring for at least five years. There's been some concern raised about toxicity, but one study found that minimal amounts of the drug enter general circulation when spread on the penis. There is a certain amount of burning and itching, however, says Dr. Fowler. Plus, "You need to watch closely afterward to make sure you killed all the cancer," says Dr. Fowler. "Poor follow-up is dangerous."

"The penis is pretty flexible when it's flaccid, but once it's erect, it's quite brittle," says Dr. Sehn. Too much weight on it, walking into a door, rolling over on it—all are enough to cause penile fracture.

"You'll hear it, too," says Dr. Gleich. "People report hearing a crack. Then their erection goes away pretty quickly." That cracking sound is the lining of the erectile chamber. "When these chambers fill with blood and get hard, they're like an inner tube. And if you put enough strain on them, you'll get a blowout," says Dr. Gleich. By all accounts penile fracture is pretty painful and nasty-looking. "Blood flows under the skin of the penis and it starts to look like an eggplant," says Dr. Gleich. It's not life threatening, but you should get that inner tube patched immediately. Studies show that if you can get the fracture treated within 24 to 48 hours, odds are you'll make a full recovery.

To avoid this break in your routine, be careful moving around dark rooms with an

Priapism: When Big Is Bad

You might think having a permanent erection would put you in the major leagues of lovers. Think again. It just might put you in the hospital. Priapism—a medical condition in which an erection won't go away—is not only painful but potentially dangerous.

"If a man has an erection longer than four hours or so, he should have it examined right away," says Marc S. Cohen, M.D., associate professor of surgery and urology at the University of Florida College of Medicine in Gainesville.

Priapism occurs when blood won't drain from your penis. (It's an inflow of blood that makes it erect.)

Dr. Cohen estimates that most urologists probably see only one or two cases of priapism a year. Yet, despite its relative rareness, many things can cause the painful condition, mostly physical injuries to the penis, scrotum, brain, spinal cord or groin. In these cases—what's generally called high-flow priapism—the physical damage affects your body's ability to regulate the blood flow into and out of your penis.

Other causes of priapism are sickle cell disease, leukemia and reactions to drugs, particularly high blood pressure, psychiatric and illicit drugs such as cocaine. In these cases—called low-flow priapism—it's a deficiency in the blood itself that causes the problem. The low flow allows an erection to occur, but then the blood doesn't drain.

Surprisingly, the most common cause for low-flow priapism is self-injection treatments for impotence, says Durwood E. Neal, Jr., M.D., associate professor of surgery, microbiology and internal medicine at the University of Texas Medical Branch in Galveston.

erection—bumping into a dresser could be enough to fracture your penis. And during intercourse with the partner on top, watch that you don't hit your partner's pubic bone during penetration—most penile fractures are caused by missing the target.

Gone Numb?

An increasingly common form of penile trauma doesn't happen to the penis at all, but to the main blood vessel supplying the penis.

Blunt trauma to the crotch—especially from falling onto the crossbar during bicycling—can damage the artery, cutting off blood flow and causing numbness. Or

In this fairly common treatment, a man is given drugs to inject directly into his penis. The drugs produce a long-lasting erection. The problem is that in 3 to 7 percent of these cases the erections don't go away, resulting in a nighttime visit to the emergency room.

Untreated, priapism can lead to permanent impotence, which is what happens to roughly 50 percent of men who fail to see a doctor fast enough. Even if you're not left impotent, the scar tissue that may develop on the inside of your penis can render you forever less firm and erect.

If you think you have priapism, you have between 12 and 24 hours to act before permanent damage can occur. If you get an erection that won't go away and you have time to spare, try these suggestions. Otherwise, beat feet to the emergency room or call your urologist pronto.

Sit and soak. Sit in a warm bath and try to loosen up. This often relaxes the blood flow in the penis, which will permit your organ to return to normal.

Try to climax. Try to ejaculate, whether through masturbation or with a partner. Since a man often loses his erection after ejaculation, letting nature take its course might ease a sudden case of priapism.

Quaff some cough syrup. Rummage through your medicine cabinet for a cold medicine that contains ephedrine or epinephrine, then follow the directions and take one adult dosage. "That potentially could shrink the blood vessels, which will help cause the erection to go away," Dr. Cohen says. "But the medicine is only a consideration in early cases. In prolonged cases shrinkage of the blood vessels may actually worsen blood stagnation. It's more appropriate to seek professional treatment."

worse, the artery could break. Blood pours into the erection chambers of the penis, creating an uncontrollable erection—a condition known as arterial priapism. According to Irwin Goldstein, M.D., professor of urology at Boston University School of Medicine, roughly 250,000 men are estimated to have impotence as a result of sport-related trauma to the crotch.

"We had a young man once who'd been playing basketball," says Dr. Goldstein. "He went up for a slam dunk, came down, legs spread and landed on somebody's head. Next day, he had an erection that wouldn't go down. We call that slam-dunk priapism."

A Tough Shot

Bitten off by a dog. Stung by a scorpion. Slammed in a car door. Caught in a zipper. Broken during intercourse. Severed by a knife. The perils of penile pitfalls are positively prodigious, purports Irwin Goldstein, M.D., professor of urology at Boston University School of Medicine and a clearinghouse of information on penile trauma. But the worst case he ever saw?

"Gunshot wound," he reports. "The bullet went through one testicle then burrowed its way up the penis and got trapped within the erection chamber." Dr. Goldstein and colleagues operated and eventually got the bullet out. "Six months later he claimed he was potent. That was very impressive," he recalls.

Advice from Dr. Goldstein: "Wear something padded in the crotch area—a jock won't protect the crotch." These measures will only partially protect that artery, so be careful, particularly when cycling. "Buy a bike that doesn't have one of those crossbars," Dr. Goldstein adds, or buy a foam pad for the bar, which you'll find at most bike shops. Make sure you're riding high in the saddle, too.

Did Something Rash?

For no apparent reason a rash or sore might rear its head on the head or shaft of your penis. Many times, these are the sexual equivalent of rug burn—friction from vigorous or poorly lubricated intercourse. But if that rash persists, don't waste any time getting it looked at.

"Penile cancer is always a worry," notes Dr. Sehn. "You always want to be careful about rashes that worsen or if you develop lesions." If the redness lasts longer than a week or you have abrasions that ooze, call your doctor.

Suffered the Unkindest Cut?

Finally, if your penis has been bitten, torn or cut off, you're probably not going to spend any time leafing through this book. But for future reference, should you suddenly be separated from your penis, Dr. Sehn advises a simple, four-step procedure.

1. Put pressure on the wound or tie a tourniquet around the stump.
2. Retrieve the penis if you can (if not, move right on to step 4).
3. Pack the penis in ice.
4. Get to a hospital.

Penis Size

Why You Shouldn't Worry about It

Size doesn't matter. Can you say it?

Okay, here's a tougher question: Do you believe it?

When it comes to penis size, most guys don't, despite the warm, soothing assurances of their partners and the cold, hard facts of science. Fact is, if the Penis Fairy came along and offered us a couple extra inches, we'd be hard pressed to turn him down—no matter what our current measurements were. Because somewhere, in the dim psychological recesses between perception and reality, lurks a vague feeling, an uneasy sense that maybe, just maybe, in our particular case size does matter.

The Long and Short of It

By and large, penis-size problems begin above the neck, not below the waist. Psychologists say we got the itch for more inches as children when we first spied our father's member. Compared to our toddler's tool, Dad was hung like a bear—so we got hung up on size.

"Children don't adjust for scale and make the logical conclusion that Dad's penis is larger because he's an adult," says C. Steven Manley, Ph.D., staff psychologist at The Male Health Center in Dallas. "Some part of that initial perception stays with us." Our shortsightedness can get reinforced in the locker rooms of junior high and high school, says Dr. Manley. "That's where things can become traumatic, because at that age, there's so much competition and intimidation and teasing and locker-room talk," says Dr. Manley. Consequently, he and other psychologists have a full-time job helping men come to terms with their concerns. "It comes down to a self-esteem problem," he says. "And men will often as not hang their esteem on one particular attribute."

If you think you're inadequate, Dr. Manley says knowing the statistics on penis sizes probably won't make you feel any better. But just in case: The average adult penis ranges from four to six inches erect. Length is defined by the distance from the tip all the way to the base of the pubic bone, where the shaft of the penis first

405

Delicate Operations

Members made to measure—that's what a handful of urologists and plastic surgeons are offering men who want nothing short of a bigger, thicker penis.

There are two penile procedures: lengthening and widening. Lengthening involves cutting two ligaments connecting the penis to the pubic bone. The shaft of the penis actually extends far into the body, so cutting the ligaments allows more of the shaft to be exposed. Doctors who have performed the procedure say that the average length gain is about two inches.

In the widening procedure, surgeons remove fat from other parts of the body—usually the pubic area or the stomach—and inject it into the penis. The procedure can double or triple penis girth.

The operations sound too good to be true—and many experts say that they are.

"Penile extensions are really nothing of the kind," says Irwin Goldstein, M.D., professor of urology at Boston University School of Medicine. "It's an illusion—you're exposing more of the shaft you already have." Dr. Goldstein also notes that the snipped ligaments normally help to stabilize erections—without them, things could get wobbly. Moreover, once the ligaments heal, there's a good chance that the shaft will be drawn back into the body—possibly further than when you started. "You could end up with an even shorter penis," Dr. Goldstein warns.

To avoid this, some surgeons are using penile weights after surgery to

emerges from the abdomen—not the pubic hairline as many guys tend to think.

Biologically, the penis only has to be long enough to penetrate and inseminate—just a couple of inches in an erect state would do it. And as far as stimulating your partner goes, the most sensitive parts of the woman's anatomy are in the first third of the vagina.

Granted, there are some cases where a penis can be too short. This is known as microphallus, a type of birth defect that can be effectively treated in infancy. But micro means micro—we're talking less than four inches erect. If you do have this problem, it would be worth your while to see your urologist to determine how to cope with this unusual situation.

maintain the newly obtained length. It's true: Weights specially shaped and designed for penises are worn for several minutes a day, longer as strength builds up over time. While no scientific research has been done on their use, penis weights are being widely tested.

Penile-widening procedures have their complications, too. "It's beginning to be recognized that the fat transfer does not last," says E. Douglas Whitehead, M.D., director of the Association for Male Sexual Dysfunction in New York City. According to Dr. Whitehead, the body reabsorbs most of the transplanted fat. And what isn't absorbed often becomes globular, leaving you with a lumpy penis. Another widening method has emerged that's supposed to avoid this complication. Called the dermal fat graph, it involves placing strips of skin under the skin of the penis. The strips are supposed to be more durable and less likely to lump up, says Dr. Whitehead.

But really, cosmetics are the least of it. In California, one prominent plastic surgeon had to surrender his license after the state medical board received complaints from dozens of the surgeon's hapless patients. They claimed that their penile augmentations left them with pain, scarring and, in some cases, a loss of sensation. The state medical board shut the doctor down as "an immediate danger to public health, safety and welfare."

Finally, the procedures aren't cheap. You can pay anywhere from $4,000 to $6,000 for penile augmentation—and it's not covered by most insurance companies unless there is a health reason to do it, such as trauma or microphallus.

As for the rest of you, here are things you should and shouldn't do to make the most of what you have.

Lose some weight. You may be able to maximize your potential by shedding a few pounds. Many men conceal their true glory under layers of flab, says Irwin Goldstein, M.D., professor of urology at Boston University School of Medicine.

"In particular, there's a fat pad covering the pubic bone at the base of the penis," says Dr. Goldstein. In men with weight problems, that fat pad can cover a good two inches of the penis. "In that case simple weight loss might be all they need," he says.

You can start by limiting fatty foods—particularly red meat and other animal

Member Myths

African-American men are bigger. Caucasian men are smaller. Asians are smallest. The circumference of a man's fist is proportional to his penis width. The size of his shoes has a direct bearing on his penis length.

These and countless other myths have been bandied around locker rooms and barrooms for ages. Irwin Goldstein, M.D., professor of urology at Boston University School of Medicine, has heard them all, but he has never seen any proof. So he set about getting some. At this writing, he's conducting one of the largest scientific surveys of penis size among the races as well as correlations between penile dimensions and the measurements of other body parts. Here are some preliminary results.

Big thumbs, well-hung" remains a myth, as do other old maxims about penis size in relation to other body parts. "For all ages and races, we found no correlation between penis size and arm length, height, weight, finger length or shoe size," says Dr. Goldstein.

African-Americans ARE bigger, at least when flaccid. Dr. Goldstein's research says that, on average, a Black man's flaccid penis is a couple inches longer than a White man's. "There's some truth to the myth," he says.

White men CAN jump in penis size, once they become erect. "We found men whose penises can get as much as four times bigger than when they're flaccid," says Dr. Goldstein. "So we've found that Caucasians are more likely to have small flaccid penises and have significantly larger erections by comparison, whereas African-Americans are pretty sizable to begin with and get just a little bigger when erect."

Asians ARE smaller than the average Caucasian, by as much as an inch, says Dr. Goldstein. But remember, these are flaccid measurements. "Once the blood starts pumping and the penis gets erect, the playing field starts to level out," he says. Indeed, all men are created equal.

products, like eggs and cheese. If you don't exercise regularly, start now. Even mild aerobic exercise—walking or cycling, for example—for 30 minutes three times a week will help. Not only could exercise and smart eating help with penis length, it'll also extend your life.

Can the comparisons. In some ways we haven't progressed beyond our high school years very much. In bathrooms and locker rooms worldwide, guys still make

the male file

Longer is not better.

In fact, a long penis is a downright detriment to the man luckless enough to have one.

"He's more prone to injury, over time he'll have more problems with performance and he may even have problems having children," says Irwin Goldstein, M.D., professor of urology at Boston University School of Medicine.

Why is a matter of simple physics. "Take a branch and a twig. The twig is longer, but the branch is thicker. Which one will break more easily? The twig. That's because longer often means thinner, and the thinner something is, the more easily it snaps when you apply pressure," says Dr. Goldstein.

As with twigs, so with penises. "A long penis is a lot less rigid. It's softer; it's going to have a harder time penetrating a vagina. And the longer it is, the more likely it will buckle or deform over time," says Dr. Goldstein. "No, the best penis is a nice, short, wide one. It'll be much more rigid. It also stretches the vaginal opening more as it enters, which most women report to be quite pleasurable." That's the long and short of it.

surreptitious comparisons between themselves and their fellow men—and come away thinking they don't measure up.

Stop wasting your time, says Dr. Goldstein. "There are certain people who have very long flaccid penises, but they don't change very much during erections," he says. So while other guys might have nine irons in the locker room, if you were to compare yourselves at the peak of engorgement, chances are you'd all be on par. Better yet, you might make theirs look like putters. "The fact is, you don't know. You're comparing yourself to something you'll probably never see—the other guy's erection," says Dr. Goldstein. "So why bother?"

Talk to your doctor. If you don't believe us, ask your doctor. "Most guys are uncomfortable asking, but it's a question I don't mind answering," assures Dr. Goldstein. Doctors see a lot of penises in the line of duty; chances are they can give you a fair estimation of your dimensions. "In most cases the guys who ask are perfectly normal—some are even above average," Dr. Goldstein adds.

Ultimately, the idea is to be satisfied with yourself, not your measurements. If your doctor can't help you feel better about your body, consider talking to a psychologist—someone who can make you feel better about your mind. The more comfortable you are with yourself, the less concern you'll have with your penis size.

Pneumonia

Prompt Care Can Save Your Life

Each breath feels like someone is stabbing you in the chest. When you cough, thick, rust-colored sputum works its way from your lungs to your mouth.

The accompanying symptoms—chills, fever, headache, fatigue—aren't exactly fun either.

Still, the leather-skinned drill instructor within you screams that it's only a cold and you shouldn't let it drag you down.

Be a man. Don't listen to that voice.

You probably have pneumonia, a severe infection of the lungs that strikes about 1.8 million American men annually. It's not a disease to ignore: Pneumonia and influenza, which is often a precursor of pneumonia, kill an estimated 35,000 men each year. Together, this pair is the sixth leading cause of death among American men, according to the American Lung Association.

"Jim Henson, the creator of the Muppets, is a classic example of a guy who delayed getting a diagnosis until it was too late to do anything about his pneumonia," says Ronald Greeno, M.D., co-director of respiratory therapy and pulmonary function at Good Samaritan Hospital in Los Angeles. By the time Henson got to the hospital, he had an overwhelming infection and within a matter of hours he was dead.

"Pneumonia is a killer," Dr. Greeno adds, "but it is very unusual to die of it if you seek medical care in a timely fashion."

The Nitty-Gritty of Pneumonia

Although almost any guy is susceptible to pneumonia, it often preys on men who have weakened immune systems. Smokers, men older than 60 and guys who have health problems such as asthma, diabetes, heart disease, alcoholism, kidney ailments, emphysema and AIDS are particularly at risk, Dr. Greeno says. A recent flu or cold also increases your vulnerability.

When you get pneumonia, phlegm, fluid and other debris clog your airways. This accumulation interferes with the lung's normal ability to remove carbon diox-

FAST FACTS

How common: About 1.8 million American men get pneumonia annually.

Risk factors: Smoking; recent cold or flu; history of disease such as asthma, diabetes, heart disease, alcoholism, kidney ailments, emphysema or AIDS.

Age group affected: Most common among children and men older than age 60.

Gender gap: Men and women are equally susceptible to pneumonia. There are more cases reported for women, however, by a 5-to-4 ratio in a recent year, likely because women consult doctors more.

Who to see: Family doctor or internist.

ide from the body and deliver life-giving oxygen to the blood and tissues, says Julia Schillinger, M.D., a medical epidemiologist at the Centers for Disease Control and Prevention in Atlanta.

In some cases the lining of the lung also becomes inflamed, causing severe pain. This condition, called pleurisy, is a common complication of pneumonia.

"Pleurisy is what causes the pain in pneumonia. The lung itself has no pain receptors," Dr. Greeno says. "I could open your lung and go down into it and you wouldn't feel anything at all. But pleurisy causes a very sharp pain. Unfortunately, you can't immobilize it like a broken ankle because you have to keep breathing." Pleuritic pain is usually relieved with painkillers, like codeine or nonsteroidal anti-inflammatory drugs.

Pneumonia is usually caused by a virus or bacteria, although in rare cases it can be caused by fungi or parasites.

Viral pneumonia is more contagious and usually isn't as severe as the type caused by bacteria. It causes a gradual loss of appetite, slowly rising fever, muscle soreness and a dry, unproductive cough that can develop into a phlegm-producing cough over several days. Antibiotics are ineffective against viral pneumonia, so often the best you can do is make yourself comfortable while waiting out its worst symptoms.

Bacterial pneumonias such as Legionnaire's disease are far more dangerous and usually cause more violent symptoms than viral pneumonia. Men can rapidly develop fevers up to 105°F, shaking chills and mucus-filled coughs.

"Guys sometimes can actually pinpoint their pneumonia to the hour. They actually say, 'Yeah, I first noticed it at 1:30 Friday afternoon when I suddenly developed this sharp chest pain and cough.' Bacterial pneumonia often makes a dramatic presentation like that," Dr. Greeno says.

Unlike viral forms of the disease, bacterial pneumonia is rarely spread by casual contact such as shaking hands. Pneumococcal pneumonia, a common type of bacterial pneumonia, is caused by bacteria that can be found in the nose and throat of healthy people. These bacteria can cause illness if they invade the lungs.

Antibiotics such as penicillin and erythromycin can cure bacterial pneumonias, although some symptoms can persist for weeks.

Caging the Beast

"The truth is most healthy guys who are exposed to pneumonia-causing organisms aren't going to get pneumonia as long as their ability to fight off infections is intact," Dr. Greeno says.

Here are a few ways to ensure that your natural defenses are at their peak.

End the smoke signals. Smoking stuns and eventually kills cilia, the hairlike structures in your airways that help keep your lungs clear of bacteria and other pneumonia-causing organisms, Dr. Greeno says. Smoking also probably disrupts the work of macrophages, immune cells that normally surround and destroy dangerous particles that attack the lungs.

Relieve stress. Stress suppresses your immune system and may make your lungs more vulnerable to pneumonia and other respiratory infections, Dr. Greeno says.

Eat right and exercise. A balanced diet can help keep your immune system on guard. Try to eat at least five servings of fruits and vegetables, six servings of grains, two servings of dairy products and a couple servings of fish, poultry or meat each day.

Regular exercise such as walking 20 minutes a day three times a week also can help keep your lungs healthy, Dr. Greeno says.

Don't infect others. Pneumonia can occasionally be spread by coughs, sneezes and personal contact, like shaking hands, says Dr. Greeno.

And remember—you don't have to have pneumonia to spread the bacteria that causes it. So to minimize your risk of infecting others, cover your nose and mouth when you cough or sneeze and wash your hands with soap and warm water frequently during the day, Dr. Greeno says. Likewise, avoid getting sprayed by other people's coughs and sneezes.

Get a flu shot. Although it doesn't directly cause pneumonia, the flu can alter your immune system so that a pneumonia-causing virus or bacteria can invade your lungs. An annual flu shot can help prevent that, Dr. Greeno says.

Ask about a pneumonia vaccine, too. A one-time pneumococcal vaccine may prevent the most common strain of bacterial pneumonia. It is recommended for healthcare workers who are frequently exposed to pneumonia, men over age 60 or guys who have respiratory diseases such as emphysema or asthma. It generally isn't advised for healthy younger guys since they are less susceptible to pneumonia than older men, Dr. Greeno says. Ask your doctor if the vaccine is appropriate for you.

You Have It, Now What?

See your doctor if you have chest pain, shortness of breath, thick greenish or rust-colored sputum, blue fingers or toes, a temperature higher than 101°F or shaking chills.

If you've been diagnosed with a particularly bad case of pneumonia, you might be hospitalized and given oxygen, painkilling drugs and antibiotics. If you have difficulty clearing phlegm from your lungs, your doctor may perform a nasotracheal suction. During this procedure a flexible tube is inserted into the trachea (windpipe) to help clear the congestion.

But in most cases, you can be treated for pneumonia at home, Dr. Greeno says. Here are a few suggestions that can speed your recovery.

Finish your medications. Men are notorious for not completing their drug treatments, Dr. Greeno says. Yet that is extremely important if you are taking antibiotics for bacterial pneumonia.

That's because during the first few days of antibiotic treatment 90 to 95 percent of the bacteria may be killed and you will begin to feel better. But if you stop taking the drugs, the remaining 5 percent of the bacteria can multiply and you can have a relapse that is more difficult to treat than the original pneumonia since the surviving bacteria are more resistant to antibiotics.

Be an hourglass. Drink an eight-ounce glass of water or juice every waking hour, Dr. Greeno suggests. It will help prevent dehydration and help thin the phlegm so it will be easier to clear out of your lungs and airways.

Don't forget aspirin. Taking two 325 milligram tablets of aspirin or acetaminophen every four hours may reduce your fever and relieve any discomfort, Dr. Greeno says. Nonsteroidal anti-inflammatory medications, like ibuprofen, also work well. Consult with your doctor to see what's best for you.

Warm your chest. To relieve chest pain caused by pneumonia, try using a hot-water bottle or warm heating pad for 20 minute sessions as needed, Dr. Greeno suggests. The heat may relax sore muscles on the chest wall.

Get plenty of rest. Your body needs extra rest in order to recharge the immune system so it can fight off the pneumonia, Dr. Greeno says. He recommends avoiding normal activity until at least 48 hours after the symptoms have disappeared.

But keep moving. Try to sit in a chair while you're awake and get up and walk around for a few minutes every hour, Dr. Greeno says.

It's okay to sleep through the night, but lying in bed all day can interfere with your efforts to cough up mucus and other secretions from your lungs.

Keep coughing. Although it may be painful, coughing helps clear your lungs of phlegm that fuels bacteria growth and reduces the amount of oxygen getting into your blood.

"The cough is a very powerful force," Dr. Greeno says. "It's something that we really can't reproduce mechanically."

If you have difficulty doing it, consider using an over-the-counter expectorant.

Be cautious. While you are sick and in the two to three weeks after you begin to feel better you will be more susceptible to colds, flus and other infections, Dr. Greeno says.

Avoid crowds and people who have known respiratory tract infections, he suggests.

Post-traumatic Stress

Making Peace with Demons

A man watches coverage of the Gulf War on TV and has horrifying nightmares of his own World War II combat experiences in the deserts of North Africa. Another man watches TV coverage of a train crash and is overcome by crying spells and thoughts of suicide, never imagining that this sudden crisis is a delayed reaction to the car accident he was in two years before. A college president is arrested for making obscene phone calls, a seemingly inexplicable aberration until therapy reveals that as a child he was the victim of repeated sexual abuse by his mother.

As disparate as these men's stories may seem, all of them share a common source: post-traumatic stress syndrome. Most of us first became aware of post-traumatic stress after the war in Vietnam, when too many returning veterans seemed incapable of readjusting to society. Since then, researchers have realized that the term applies equally well to survivors of a wide spectrum of human tragedies, from hurricanes and airplane crashes to fires and genocide.

"It started out as a post-Vietnam syndrome and then as a post-rape syndrome," says Chris Dunning, Ph.D., a specialist in post-traumatic stress who teaches at the University of Wisconsin in Milwaukee. "But now we know that any event that produces horror, helplessness or terror can produce the same symptoms."

Shock That Won't Go Away

Anyone can go into shock immediately after being threatened with violent death or witnessing it; shock becomes post-traumatic stress syndrome when the symptoms persist for more than a month. Among the syndrome's most common characteristics is what doctors call hypervigilance, a habit of looking over one's shoulders, constantly on guard against any sudden attacks. Another identifying feature is an exaggerated startle response, meaning someone with post-traumatic stress syndrome is liable to jump at the ring of a telephone as if it were a howitzer that just went off right behind him.

Those with post-traumatic stress syndrome frequently block any memory of the original trauma out of their minds or they distance themselves from it emotion-

415

ally so that they have no feelings connected to the memories. Even then, "trigger" experiences can bring trauma memories flooding back, seemingly from out of nowhere, as if they were being relived. Vietnam veterans have been known to have flashbacks visiting the Adventureland section of Disney World and Florida environs simply because the tropical vegetation there triggered memories of the war.

Not surprisingly, many men with post-traumatic stress try desperately to avoid trigger situations. In doing so, they have a tendency to become socially isolated, which explains why many Vietnam veterans are believed to be living in the woods of Maine and Alaska. The need to avoid horrifying memories can also lead to alcoholism. It has been estimated that between one-third to three-quarters of Vietnam veterans being treated for post-traumatic stress syndrome also have drinking problems.

Resiliency Training

Living in the world today, especially in a big city, you don't have to be a total paranoid to feel sometimes that disaster is lurking around every corner. You may never actually find yourself in a trauma-producing situation, but if you do—or if you already have—there are steps you can take to minimize your chances of developing post-traumatic stress syndrome. The experts call it building up your resiliency to trauma.

Talk it out. Being able to talk openly and frankly about what you've experienced can provide invaluable relief, Dr. Dunning says, often preventing trauma or traumatic stress from progressing into a chronic condition. Don't tolerate those—including yourself—who would diminish the anguish you're going through or tell you to forget about it: Being ignored or feeling blamed in the aftermath of trauma can be devastating. Ask any Vietnam veteran.

Friends and family are the best people to talk with, Dr. Dunning says, but if that isn't possible, find a professional as soon as possible. Groups such as Alcoholics Anonymous and self-help organizations can be of positive value, adds Sylvia Mendel, a senior consultant with the New York City Department of Mental Health, Mental Retardation and Alcoholism Services. She cautions, however, that these groups are only there to help with specific problems related to post-traumatic stress, such as alcoholism and substance abuse, and not the stress disorder itself. No one, she says, should go to a support group expecting anything like professional treatment. "They're therapeutic," she says, "but they're not therapy."

Take control. Perhaps the most frightening aspect of trauma is the complete loss of control over your life. For that reason, taking steps to prepare for a crisis—putting together an earthquake emergency kit, for example, or covering your windows with

FAST FACTS

How common: No hard numbers exist, but some experts estimate that 1 to 2 percent of the U.S. population may have post-traumatic stress syndrome.

Risk factors: Some people develop post-traumatic stress more easily than others, especially those who have been traumatized before. In general, though, if the trauma is bad enough, anyone will develop the disorder.

Age group affected: All age groups can get post-traumatic stress.

Gender gap: Some researchers find men more prone to the syndrome through greater exposure to violence, in war, for example. But they seek treatment less willingly than women, not wanting to show vulnerability.

Who to see: A therapist who is trained to treat trauma and who has experience doing so. Ask your county, city or state mental health clinic for a referral.

plywood when a hurricane approaches—is effective psychologically as well as practically. "Anything people can actually do gives them some sense of control, Dr. Dunning says. "All these things make it less likely that they'll be traumatized."

Give it meaning. Those who recover best from traumatic experiences are often those who somehow manage to find meaning in what happened, Dr. Dunning says. If you can use the tragedy as a spur toward a new commitment, either to a cause or a belief, you're more likely to make your peace with it, she suggests. A classic example of doing just that is offered by John Walsh, who turned his grief over his murdered son, Adam, into a national campaign for child safety.

Getting Treatment

If the aftereffects of a traumatic experience are interfering with your life, you should seek treatment, Dr. Dunning says. You may be reluctant to do so, she adds, because of fear that you will be labeled "crazy". Many trauma victims also suffer from survivor guilt, which causes them to feel even more guilty for needing help. "It's a mental injury that you're not responsible for," she says. "You wouldn't feel guilty about getting treatment for a broken leg. The same goes for trauma."

According to Stuart Kleinman, M.D., president of the New York City chapter of the International Society for Traumatic Stress Studies, increasing evidence suggests that trauma may well be a physical injury that actually alters the wiring of the brain. Although those findings help explain why some symptoms of post-traumatic stress, such as the startle response, are frustratingly resistant to therapy, they do not mean that the syndrome is beyond treatment.

"There are certain symptoms that people with post-traumatic stress will probably have throughout their lives," says Lawrence C. Kolb, M.D., professor emeritus of the Department of Psychiatry at Columbia University in New York City. "But the most serious symptoms decline to the point where they become manageable. I know many people who get along quite well with post-traumatic stress disorder."

Beyond getting treatment, here are some other suggestions for anyone who thinks he may have post-traumatic stress.

Review your routines. You may find some of your old routines comforting because they help restore a sense of order and control. Stick with those. Other routines, however, can provoke flashbacks. Change them. "The most important thing is to avoid the cues that trigger the original trauma," says Dr. Dunning.

Get sober. Alcohol and drugs may provide an illusion of relief, but they only exacerbate the problem by making you less stable than you were to begin with, says Dr. Kolb.

Tell your doctor. If you have post-traumatic stress syndrome and you're planning to have surgery, alert your doctor and your anesthesiologist, Dr. Kolb says. Some anesthetic drugs have been known to provoke traumatic stress flashbacks.

Premature Ejaculation

Taking Your Time on Love's Highway

You're at a stoplight and the kid in the souped-up Chevy next to you is revving his engine and glancing your way.

You try to smile paternally and look away, but then the light turns green. Suddenly you're back in college driving your own speed machine and Pow! You squash the gas pedal like a cockroach, leaving the pimply-faced punk in the dust.

Admit it: Being first is a compulsion for most guys, be it on the road, at the job, in the gym. And what's wrong with that?

Nothing. Except when it comes to sex. Then, always being the first to finish is the last place we want to be. Yet somehow that's where tens of millions of guys are ending up.

"Most men at one time or another ejaculate sooner than they want to. This is an extremely common problem in the men I've seen over the years," confides Marilyn K. Volker, Ed.D., a sexologist in private practice in Coral Gables, Florida.

How Fast Is Too Fast?

Premature ejaculation is mostly a psychological problem, broadly defined as an inability to control the timing of your climax as well as you'd like. Try to get a more accurate medical definition, though, and watch out.

Some experts say it's an ejaculation that arrives less than two minutes after penetration. Others say a premature ejaculation is one that occurs in less than 50 thrusts. Years ago, William Masters, M.D., and Virginia Johnson, of the Masters and Johnson Institute of St. Louis, said a man is a premature ejaculator if he reaches orgasm before his partner more than half the time.

And if this isn't confusing enough, the famous sex researcher Dr. Alfred Kinsey reported years ago that 75 percent of all men ejaculate within two minutes after entering their lover, so by definition 75 percent of us are sexually dysfunctional.

What gives? It boils down to this: Premature is in the eye of the beholder and—in this case—the beholder's partner. What's important is the enjoyment you and your partner get, whether it's measured in hours or nanoseconds.

"Remember, the biological reason we ejaculate is to impregnate females, not for pleasure, so there's no wrong or right," says Marc S. Cohen, M.D., associate professor of surgery and urology at the University of Florida's College of Medicine in Gainesville.

A Premature Primer

Ejaculation occurs in two steps. In step one, you're stimulated to the point where muscle contractions begin mixing ejaculatory fluids with sperm. This concoction, called semen, is then squeezed into a little chamber at the base of your urethra (the tube running through your penis). In step two, rhythmic contractions from muscles near the base of your penis drive the semen up and out of your urethra, usually in several spurts.

This whole ejaculation process occurs because the physical sensations of sex turn on, so to speak, the appropriate switch in the brain. Simply put, the sensations we feel in our penises travel via nerves to our brains, which respond to the appropriate glands with the directive, "Okay, time for action." Voilà, ejaculation.

Although ejaculation seems to be an uncontrollable physical reflex, it's not; there's a mental override. With your mind you can control ejaculation and ejaculation-producing sensations. It's like controlling your breathing while jogging.

You also can control ejaculation physically. With training you can discover your ejaculation triggers—the touches, caresses and kisses that excite you most—and use them to pace your encounter.

Most often, premature ejaculation is the result of bad habits and psychological baggage you've picked up along the way since your sex life began.

"The routine of premature ejaculation may come from a man's first sexual encounters, which probably were something he had to rush through because he was in a situation where he could be caught," says Arlene Goldman, Ph.D., coordinator of the Jefferson Sexual Function Center at Thomas Jefferson University in Philadelphia. "Men without sexual experience may not know what to expect. They may feel anxious about the sensations they will feel, or have performance anxiety."

Nice Guys Finish Last

So now you know there's no real definition of premature. You also know that premature ejaculation isn't a problem unless you or your partner thinks it is. And, you know that if it's deemed a problem, a mental adjustment might be all that's needed to fix it. So where do you start?

With practice, practice, practice.

"Just like you've learned to control your bladder, you can learn to control your ejaculation, and there certainly are many behavioral-conditioning techniques you can use," Dr. Cohen says.

So here are ways to deal with premature ejaculation.

FAST FACTS

How common: More so than most men would care to admit. Some sources estimate 20 to 30 million men suffer from chronic premature ejaculation.

Risk factors: Premature ejaculation generally comes from psychological causes, not physical ones, although some diseases and medications could contribute to the problem. Anxiety can be both a cause and a symptom of the condition.

Age group affected: Affects men of all ages, but often starts in younger men who develop a pattern of premature ejaculation, which builds over time.

Gender gap: Men only.

Who to see: Most likely a sex therapist, since the cause is probably psychological. If you have pain ejaculating or suspect a physical cause or medication-related problem, see a urologist. Some antidepressant medications help men with premature ejaculations. These would often be prescribed by a psychiatrist working in conjunction with a sex therapist or urologist.

Communicate before coitus. Movies, television and advertising tell us we should all be sexual bulls but that's a difficult, if not impossible, image to uphold. And since most of us guys aren't exactly adept at discussing intimate things, like our sexual shortcomings, poor communication with our partners can actually add to our problems. "Good communication is the key to all of this. With good communication a couple can be their own sex therapist," Dr. Goldman says.

Talk with your partner about your sex life. Find out where you're both satisfied and where the trouble spots are. For example, say you've both been bothered by your premature ejaculation. Keeping these feelings inside will only make them worse for both of you, much like keeping anger bottled up makes you feel even angrier. Identifying and discussing your sexual concerns is the first step in curing them.

Try start/stop exercises. In 1955 James Semans, M.D., a urologist at Duke University Medical School, refined a technique for prolonging ejaculation that he learned from a prostitute. Called the start/stop technique, you can do it alone until you are ready to try it with a partner.

Here's how to do it: Wait until you're erect and stimulated almost to the point of ejaculation. Then stop all stimulation and let your urge to ejaculate pass. If you succeeded, wait one to two minutes and then start again with the stimulation, repeating the start/stop process several times to build endurance.

Use the technique to gain awareness of your body and what makes you stimulated. "Try to rate your arousal on a scale of 1 to 10," suggests Dr. Goldman. "Men who ejaculate prematurely often go from 1 to 10 without realizing it." See if you can tell when you have reached 6, she says.

Don't be upset if you fail the first time. Like we said, controlling ejaculation requires practice.

"Just go back and try again later or tomorrow if you fail," Dr. Goldman suggests. "Do this exercise three to four times a week and remember, this technique takes time—usually three to five months—for improvement. It's not something you can do in a week."

Fly solo. Whether alone or with a partner, masturbation can be a great tool when it comes to controlling your climax. "With masturbation a man sees what kinds of touches, strokes and positions maintain his erection," Dr. Volker says.

Use masturbation to identify "hot" touches that turn you on and "cool" touches that aren't as arousing. Then communicate this to your lover. That way, your lover can avoid the hot touches when you're most aroused and pace the encounter by keeping your ejaculation at bay.

Here's another tip: Some men will masturbate an hour or two before having sex because they believe their second erection—and their staying power—is more virile. Though some doctors question whether this is true, a few sex therapists we talked to insist that it has worked for some of their clients.

Do the big squeeze. Developed by Dr. Masters and Johnson, the squeeze technique is similar to the start/stop technique except you or your partner lightly squeezes the tip of the underside of your penis to help hold back the ejaculate. For the best bet, squeeze with your thumb on the top side of your penis and two fingers on the underside.

"What happens is this will push the ejaculate back, delaying ejaculation," Dr. Volker says. "Doing this correctly is not something you get right away, but if both partners learn to do it well, it can actually be a fun part of making love."

Stop being on top. Eschew traditional man-on-top sex positions, because the delicate nerves on the tip of your penis are more fully aroused under these circumstances. Instead, opt for sex while laying on your side, which should help you and your partner last longer. Another good bet for long-distance loving is the woman-on-top position.

Forgo the gizmos. Forget things like delaying creams, which numb the penis as well as the hands or mouth, or so-called aphrodisiacs, like Spanish fly (cantharis), which can be dangerous.

"With these things you rely on something outside of yourself. There are better methods that can enhance learning about yourself and your body. Then you'll feel better about yourself," Dr. Volker says.

Prostate Cancer

Avoiding Trouble below Deck

The prostate is seldom discussed, little heard from. But don't take the walnut-sized gland for granted. When it decides to give trouble, there may be hell to pay.

Of all the parts of a man's body the prostate is the most likely to develop cancer. An estimated 40,400 men die of prostate cancer each year (a figure close to that of breast cancer in women). The death rate is so high partly because the disease is so common: It occurs in 1 in every 128 men between age 40 and 59, with incidence increasing with age. By the time you're in your eighties, your risk of prostate cancer becomes 1 in 8.

It's no wonder that as men have started living longer, prostate cancer rates over the past few decades have gone up. But it's not strictly a disease of old age. "In autopsy studies malignant changes have been found in the prostates of men in their twenties," says Howard I. Scher, M.D., chief of the Genitourinary Oncology Service at Memorial Sloan-Kettering Cancer Center in New York City.

These facts need to be viewed in perspective, however. Most men who have prostate cancer don't die from it; some never even notice it. Two of the hallmark characteristics of prostate cancer are that it develops very slowly and it produces no symptoms until its later stages. What this means is that you could live your entire adult life with prostate cancer and be unaware you have the disease. A full two-thirds of men diagnosed with the disease die of other causes before their cancers ever become life threatening. "The real issue isn't who has it but who is going to be affected by it," says Kenneth Goldberg, M.D., director of the Male Health Center in Dallas and author of *How Men Can Live as Long as Women*.

Risk-Factor Fudging

The prostate is a sex organ, but its duties are strictly back-office: It produces proteins that liquefy semen, then releases the fluid during ejaculation. It isn't yet clear how prostate cancer forms, although your genes appear to play a big role: If a father or brother has it, your risk is double that of the general population. Still, studies linking prostate cancer with a number of behavior-based risk factors suggest there may be ways to stave off the disease or slow its development.

Feed on less fat. Countries with low-fat diets, like Japan, have lower prostate cancer rates than fat-happy Western countries, like the United States. Studies suggest that while fat doesn't cause the disease, it may help trigger its development or speed its growth.

Red meat seems to be a special villain: In one study comparing 120 men who got prostate cancer with 120 who didn't, eating red meat five times a week raised the risk 2½ times compared to eating it less than once a week. One low-fat food worth considering is soy (found in tofu, soy flour and soy milk), which preliminary research suggests may inhibit prostate cancer growth. Other good bets: high-fiber foods, like lentils, tomatoes and peas.

Delight in vitamin D. You get it largely from sunlight or by eating dairy products or fatty fish such as tuna and salmon. Interestingly, populations in latitudes with less ultraviolet rays from the sun get more prostate cancer: the difference between Maine and Florida is nearly 50 percent. The implication is that getting more vitamin D will protect against the disease. This hasn't yet been proven, although a lab test at Stanford University and a human study at Duke University suggest it's true. Bottom line: "There's no sense risking skin cancer from increased sun exposure, but eating a healthy diet will never hurt," says William Catalona, M.D., chief of the Division of Urologic Surgery at Washington University's Barnes Hospital in St. Louis.

Work up a sweat. A Harvard study of 17,719 men found that those who burned 4,000 or more calories a week had a prostate cancer risk that was 47 to 88 percent lower than men who burned less than 1,000 calories a week. It takes a lot of exercise to burn that many calories, at least an hour's worth every day. What explains the effect? It may be that exercisers simply eat better and have less fat.

An Ounce of Detection . . .

While the above measures may help, you can't rely on them to protect you. "There is nothing that has been proven to prevent the disease," Dr. Scher says. If, however, you catch the cancer early, before it spreads outside the prostate gland, there's a good chance you can be completely cured.

The American Cancer Society recommends that all men over age 50 get checked yearly in two ways. First, get a rectal exam, in which a doctor feels the prostate with a gloved finger to detect irregularities. Second, get a blood test that measures prostate specific antigen, a prostate-produced protein whose levels rise when the gland has a problem. High-risk men such as those with a family history of prostate cancer or African Americans should start annual testing at age 40.

FAST FACTS

How common: At least one out of ten men have a lifetime risk of getting it.

Risk factors: Age, family history of the disease, being African American, high-fat diet.

Age group affected: Eighty percent of cases are diagnosed after age 65, though autopsy studies have found that microscopic tumors can start in early adulthood.

Gender gap: Strictly a male problem; women don't have prostates.

Who to see: Urologist. If you're a candidate for treatment, get a second opinion before making any decisions on what's right for you; philosophies on managing the disease can vary considerably from one doctor to the next.

The Treatment Menu

Men diagnosed with prostate cancer have the following options for treatment.

Surgery: If the cancer hasn't spread beyond the prostate, the malignancy often can be cured completely by removing the organ, a procedure called prostatectomy. In a small number of cases the operation leaves patients impotent or incontinent.

Radiation: Ten years after treatment success rates with radiation roughly match those of surgery, although some evidence suggests that after 15 years radiation gains a slight advantage. Best candidates: Older men, who are more likely to experience side effects of an operation.

Hormonal therapy: Reserved for men whose cancer has already spread beyond the prostate, this treatment is administered either with drugs that block male hormones or by removing the testicles, which produce the hormones. It won't cure the disease but may slow it down.

Do nothing: Seriously. The value of treatment depends on your age, overall health and the aggressiveness of the tumor. You may be better off holding tight while closely monitoring your condition. "If you're age 75 and have heart disease and diabetes, the chances of prostate cancer affecting your lifespan are pretty small," says Dr. Goldberg. "On the other hand, if you're 55 and healthy, there's a reasonably good chance it *is* going to affect you."

Prostate Enlargement
How to Stay with the Flow

Every man occasionally has to answer the call of nature in the middle of the night. But it's one of the small indignities of age that this annoyance often becomes . . . well, *more* annoying. Not only do you have to go more often (even during the day), you may feel you're not quite done when you're done. It may be difficult to get things started or to keep them going. And when you have to go, it has to be *right now*.

The problem: Your prostate is growing. Result: This gland, which surrounds the urethra (the tube that urine travels through on its way from the bladder to the penis), is putting the squeeze on your fluid flow. It's a condition known as benign prostatic hyperplasia (BPH).

Why the prostate has a growth spurt during adulthood isn't clear, although it appears to be linked to changes in the amount of testosterone in the blood.

Prostate enlargement eventually occurs in almost all of us, but not every man is affected the same way. For some a hugely enlarged prostate produces no symptoms at all. But in other men even a slight enlargement can cause complete urinary retention, which may lead to kidney problems. "We don't know what makes the difference between those cases," says Robert Cowles, M.D., director of the Atlanta Center for Urology and assistant clinical professor of surgery at Emory University, also in Atlanta. Bottom line: "If you have none of the associated symptoms, you probably don't have a problem," says Dr. Cowles.

Internal Management

There's nothing you can do on your own to keep the prostate from growing. But that doesn't mean you're helpless to control your symptoms. Here are a number of steps you can take to minimize problems.

Nix the nightcap. Avoid not just the hard stuff but *all* fluids before bedtime. "I recommend decreasing fluid intake after 6:00 P.M. and having nothing at all after seven," says Joseph Oesterling, M.D., associate professor and urologist-in-chief at the University of Michigan and director of the Michigan Prostate Center, both in

Ann Arbor. Be particularly wary of alcohol, which relaxes all the body's muscles, including the bladder.

Don't be irritating. At any time of day, avoid drinks that irritate the bladder, making it feel like it's full even when it's not. The primary culprit is caffeine, although some men find acidic drinks, like orange juice, and carbonated beverages, like soda, irritating as well, according to E. David Crawford, M.D., director of the Prostate Center at the University of Colorado Health Sciences Center in Denver.

Put spice on ice. Spicy foods with ingredients like red peppers may also irritate the bladder, and should be avoided.

Shun antihistamines. These drugs simultaneously make the bladder relax and cause the bladder neck that urine flows through to constrict. A fuller bladder with a narrower exit pipe makes urination more difficult.

Give it time. According to Dr. Cowles, about 30 percent of untreated men actually find that their symptoms improve by themselves. The bladder is a muscle, he says, and may strengthen over time to push urine out with greater force.

Engineering Solutions

Still, if symptoms are more severe, or you simply find them overly troublesome, there are a number of options for dealing with the problem.

Clear the pipes. Taking out obstructive prostate tissue surgically is the gold standard of medical treatments, because it's most effective. It results in improved symptoms in 75 to 80 percent of cases. These figures are for a procedure called TURP, or transurethral resection of the prostate. It's a kind of Roto-Rootering of the prostate, and involves no incisions. Instead, a small tube called a rectoscope is slid through the urethra to the prostate, where tissue blockage is electrically cut away, and the passage through the prostate is widened.

It's not a perfect procedure. Complications include impotence (5 to 10 percent of cases) and incontinence (1 percent). TURP takes four to six weeks of recovery.

You won't have trouble finding a capable doctor to do TURP: It's the nation's most common operation after cataract surgery. There are, however, other procedures that are less common but may offer advantages over TURP.

TUIP: That's transurethral incision of the prostate. It's similar to TURP, except that instead of scraping out the prostate, the gland is sliced in one or two locations, making it split open to relieve pressure on the urethra. Its effectiveness is similar to that of TURP, but there are fewer side effects. Drawback: It's not as effective on greatly enlarged prostates. All told, experts, like Drs. Crawford and Oesterling, say it's an underused procedure.

Lasers: Procedures using laser beams to heat away excess prostate tissue can be done on an outpatient basis, with no bleeding, little risk of impotence, incontinence or retrograde ejaculation and only a day for recovery. Short-term results are similar to that of TURP, but because the procedures are still new, they don't have a long track record. "Doctors are still on a learning curve," says Dr. Cowles, who pioneered one form of laser BPH treatment in the United States.

Relieve the pressure. Two drugs are now available to treat prostate enlargement without an operation. Finasteride (Proscar) is touted as the first nonsurgical method for actually shrinking the prostate. It works by blocking an enzyme that converts testosterone into a form that fuels prostate growth. Results are mixed. A study of 895 men conducted at 25 medical centers across the United States found that half the men who take Proscar experience a 50 percent overall reduction in symptoms, which is significant. Still, many men who suffer from prostate enlargement see no effect, says Dr. Cowles.

It's a similar story with the second drug, terazosin (Hytrin), one of a group of drugs known as alpha-blockers. These work by relaxing muscle tissue in the prostate and bladder neck, making urine flow less constricted. In one study Hytrin improved symptoms by 30 percent in 70 percent of men taking it. One advantage Hytrin has over Proscar is that it produces results in a few weeks, while Proscar takes three to six months. But both drugs must be taken for life: Once you stop taking them, prostate symptoms return.

Psoriasis

All about Skin Moisture and Maintenance

Its cause is unknown and its cure is unknown. It's uncomfortable, unpredictable and can be *very* unsightly. Extreme forms of the skin disease psoriasis can even be fatal, as welts can become so extensive that the heart fails in trying to meet their massive demands for blood.

"One encouraging thing that might be said about psoriasis is that it's not contagious," says Eugene M. Farber, M.D., president of the Psoriasis Research Institute at the Stanford University School of Medicine. "It can be a very exasperating disease." Yet in no way should it be thought of as a hopeless one. "We don't have a blanket cure for psoriasis yet, but we do have some ideas of what triggers its flare-ups and how these flare-ups can be controlled," says Dr. Farber. "Everybody can be helped to some degree, the key factor being how much time and effort they're willing to spend in determining what their particular triggers are."

Cells Gone Berserk

Psoriasis is the result of skin cells developing too prolifically for their own good, Dr. Farber explains. Skin cells normally mature and shed in a little less than a month. But with psoriasis this process takes only three to four days, and the cells are poorly formed. The result is a major anatomic traffic jam as skin cells begin to pile up on one another in the form of reddish, scale-covered welts that can itch, sting, bleed and look like living hell.

Nearly any area of the body can fall prey to this cellular mayhem, though the most common sites are the elbows, knees, scalp, fingernails and regions of the genitals and buttocks.

Approximately 2 percent of the population is affected by psoriasis in some form, Dr. Farber says, men and women equally, but Caucasians more so than people of darker complexions, and African Americans least of all. Usually the disease will show itself to some degree by a person's late twenties, though there can be development both earlier and later than that, Dr. Farber says.

There also appears to be a genetic component to this bothersome disease, as approximately 30 percent of the people who are suffering from psoriasis will have a history of the disorder somewhere on their family trees.

As for identifying the disease, the best way is to visit your doctor, who either will be able to make the diagnosis visually or take a small biopsy and have it confirmed in the lab, says David Kalin, M.D., a general practitioner in private practice in Largo, Florida. "Sometimes other conditions such as eczema, contact dermatitis and certain fungal infections can be confused with psoriasis, so it's important to get a professional diagnosis to find out for sure."

Controlling Its Triggers

Once you have been diagnosed, depending on the type and severity of your condition, the rest is pretty much up to you, Dr. Kalin says. There are a number of treatment options, but just as important is identifying and controlling the triggers that cause the disease to act up. Here are the most potent triggers to watch out for.

Emotional stress. It's the catch-22 of psoriasis, says Dr. Farber. "The stress of having the disease can worsen the disease and so can any other sort of emotional turmoil, for that matter." Emotional stress causes nerve fibers within the skin to release a chemical that is a potent psoriasis antagonist, says Dr. Farber. He suggests that people suffering from psoriasis be as calm and objective as possible with that connection in mind.

Physical stress. The rubbing of too-tight pants. A scratch. A bruise. Sunburn. "Anything that traumatizes the skin has potential for initiating a flare-up," says Dr. Kalin. More general affronts to the body such as infections (a strep throat, for example) also can initiate flare-ups. So it's important for people suffering from psoriasis to pay attention to their overall health, Dr. Kalin says.

Medications. Among the drugs that can trigger a flare-up are lithium (frequently prescribed for manic depression), beta-blockers (used to treat high blood pressure), quinidine gluconate (a heart medication), drugs used to treat malaria and ointments containing steroids when used for long periods of time. In some cases even aspirin, acetaminophen or ibuprofen can trigger flare-ups. Check with your doctor if you suspect that some medication could be causing problems for you.

Dryness. During the winter, especially, dry skin can worsen psoriasis, says Bill Fuegy, a registered pharmacist and consultant to the National Psoriasis Foundation. "This can be minimized with proper bathing and moisturizing habits, however," he says. Shower with lukewarm (not hot) water using a mild, deodorant-free soap such as Ivory or Dove. Then pat (don't rub) yourself dry and lightly apply a lanolin- or petroleum-based moisturizer.

It also can help to use an electric rather than blade razor when shaving, Fuegy says, to minimize the risk of cutting or irritating facial skin.

Alcohol. Whether heavy drinking is a cause of psoriasis or simply a symptom of

FAST FACTS

How common: Psoriasis affects approximately 2 percent of the population, but Caucasians more so than Asian Americans, Native Americans and Latinos, and African Americans least of all.

Risk factors: Approximately 30 percent of psoriasis sufferers will have a history of the disease in their families, though the disorder may not appear consecutively in all generations. Severe cradle cap and/or extreme cases of diaper dermatitis during infancy can be harbingers of the disease, and high levels of emotional stress, viral infections, traumas to the skin, alcohol abuse and the use of certain prescription drugs may precipitate the disease.

Age group affected: Signs of psoriasis usually will appear by the late twenties. The disease also can go into periods of extended remission, only to reappear in response to certain environmental triggers mentioned above.

Gender gap: Psoriasis occurs equally among men and women, but men tend to suffer more from lesions in the area of the groin because of the greater friction incurred by their more freely moving sexual parts.

Who to see: Family doctor or dermatologist.

its emotional stress, doctors aren't sure yet. There does seem to be a connection between the two, however, and among men especially. In one study male psoriasis patients who habitually consumed more than 80 grams of alcohol a day (that's roughly five beers or five shots of hard liquor) were found to have significantly worse treatment outcomes than male patients who drank less or not at all.

In another study done in Finland one in three psoriasis patients reported that drinking made their conditions worse while only one in nine patients with other skin disorders (such as dermatitis and acne) reported adverse effects from alcohol.

Some researchers theorize that alcohol may exacerbate psoriasis by aggravating white blood cells. But whatever the mechanism, "Psoriasis sufferers just shouldn't drink—period," states Dr. Farber. "Alcohol is bad for any chronic systemic disorder, but psoriasis especially."

Making the Most of Treatment

Despite the most diligent of preventive measures, psoriasis still can rear its ugly head—and if attacks are severe enough, medical assistance most definitely should be sought. What follows is a list of the therapies that doctors report are meeting with the greatest success. Remember: The one (or combination) that's best for you will have to be decided by your doctor based on your individual situation.

Sunlight. Perhaps the simplest psoriasis remedy is absolutely free, and pretty abundant—regular sunlight. Soaking in the ultraviolet light produced by the sun can lessen psoriasis symptoms. But be sure to regulate the time you spend gathering rays—if you let yourself get a sunburn, you may make the psoriasis worse, and you'll expose yourself to the danger of skin cancer. The best way to give your scales the sun without suffering the consequences is to put sunscreen on all exposed areas *except* the psoriasis spots.

Soaking. To keep your skin comfortable, soak it for about 15 minutes a day with a nice warm bath. To soothe skin even more, add some oil to the water. Adding Epsom salts can help stop itching and remove scales, too. When you get out, pat yourself dry—don't rub.

Moisturizers. While there are plenty of prescription and over-the-counter ointments specially designed to treat psoriasis symptoms, even simple moisturizers can help. Try using lotions or oils with aloe vera or jojoba—these natural ingredients are particularly effective.

Coal tars. Available in both over-the-counter and prescription strengths, coal tar products are good for reducing not just the inflammation of psoriasis but its scaling and itching as well. They're available in ointments, creams, bath oils and even shampoos. Be careful though: They stain fabrics.

Capsaicin. Hot peppers may set your mouth to blistering, but the active ingredient in hot peppers can actually soothe the burning itch of psoriasis. Called capsaicin, this ingredient, when used in cream form, relieved itching—and in some cases even caused clearing of the skin patches—in 66 percent of all cases.

Corticoid creams. Also known as cortisones or corticosteroids, these prescription medications can help reduce the inflammation of acute flare-ups. But if used for too long, they can begin to worsen the symptoms they're designed to relieve.

PUVA. The P stands for psoralen, a light-sensitizing drug taken orally. The UVA stands for ultraviolet light that is administered by special lamps in controlled doses. Therapy generally involves three treatments a week and has proven to be highly effective in approximately 80 percent of cases within about two months.

Anthralin (Anthra-Derm). This prescription cream or ointment comes in preparations for both the body and scalp, but as with coal tars some formulations can stain. It also has the potential for being irritating to normal skin.

Etretinate (Tegison). This prescription drug is a derivative of vitamin A, to be taken orally once a day. It can contribute to bone spurs, dry and fragile skin and high cholesterol, so it's best for extreme cases only and should be used for short periods.

Methotrexate (Mexate). Also a prescription drug to be taken orally, methotrex-

the male file

A man who was undergoing psoriasis treatment at his local hospital stepped outside to have a smoke, lit up—and promptly burst into flames, according to a report in the New England Journal of Medicine.

Luckily, the startled smoker put himself out and suffered no serious injuries. The psoriasis itself didn't cause the patient to spontaneously combust. Rather, doctors discovered that the man had recently had a tar treatment for his skin condition. Because of its high alcohol content, the tar was extremely flammable. The cigarette apparently sparked the flare-up.

ate is like etretinate in that its potential for toxic side effects (to the liver especially) make it appropriate for severe cases and short-term use only.

Vitamin D treatment. Several forms of vitamin D have been proven to scratch the psoriatic itch. In studies conducted by the National Institutes of Health in Bethesda, Maryland, vitamin D in either a capsule or ointment form significantly relieved psoriasis symptoms—more than 90 percent of the time, in some cases.

And now a new form of treatment, vitamin D_3 (Dovonex), seems to be one of the best forms of treatment. Marked improvements have been observed within two to four weeks with topical applications of D_3 ointment made twice daily. The drug has few side effects but must be used continually or symptoms return. Be sure to talk to your doctor about any vitamin D treatment, though—too much of this vitamin can cause serious health complications such as kidney stones.

Antibiotics. Also encouraging has been the success reported by researchers treating psoriasis with antibiotics formulated to eradicate micro-organisms suspected of causing the disease. In one study 50 percent of a group of 126 psoriasis patients experienced complete or near complete remission of their diseases while another 30 percent were improved greatly.

Sexual Addiction

How to Cure the Compulsion

A few years back we watched as Florida's most famous hooker, Kathy Willets of Fort Lauderdale, was tried for prostitution. According to newspaper reports, Willets claimed she had sex with clients as often as eight times a day in her suburban home. But what projected the story to national attention was that her husband, Jeffrey, a sheriff's deputy, arranged it all and watched from a closet.

Willets's arrest and conviction made for the most entertaining newspaper reading this side of the *National Enquirer*. But besides temporarily bumping Elvis and aliens from the tabloid headlines, the story gave sex addiction the limelight.

Three to six percent of Americans are sex addicts, the majority of them men, says Patrick Carnes, Ph.D., clinical director of the Sexual Disorders Unit at Del Amo Hospital in Torrance, California, and author of *Don't Call It Love: Recovery from Sexual Addiction* and *Out of the Shadows*. The condition in men is called satyriasis, coming from the word Satyr, which refers to the Greek deity. (Nymphomania—what Willets claimed but later denied—is sex addiction in women.)

While being addicted to sex may sound stimulating, it's not. "Sex addiction is potato chip sex," says Allen Elkin, Ph.D., clinical psychologist and director at the Stress Management and Counseling Center in New York City. "Like food bingeing, sex addiction can be a dysfunctional, debilitating activity done to relieve anxiety. It should be seen more as a symptom of an underlying problem than anything else."

"Sex addiction is a very real thing," Dr. Carnes adds, "and it can take a large number of forms." You might have a burning need to expose yourself, to use 900 lines for phone sex, to have sex in public places or just to sleep with as many women as you can. "But the reality is, sex addiction essentially is a behavior you don't control," adds Dr. Carnes.

A Profile of the Problem

You probably thought you were a sex addict in your early twenties, when your longing for sex rivaled your appetite for beer. But true sex addiction is like drug addiction, Dr. Carnes says, and they share some key characteristics.

434

The addiction brings pleasure. "Whatever the addiction, it gives pleasure, intensity and reward, which in turn create a dependency," Dr. Carnes explains. "Whether it's cocaine or wearing women's clothing, the result is a rush that addicts relish."

The rush leads to loss of control. "Addicts use their addiction to self-medicate," Dr. Carnes adds. "As well as giving pleasure, the addiction has a calming effect, making them feel better, at least for a period of time. As a consequence the addicts lose control—they engage in the behavior compulsively, that is, having sex when they don't want or intend to."

The addict obsesses over the addiction. "The pleasure and reward sex addicts get from their activities dominate their lives," Dr. Carnes says. "They think about it all the time."

The addiction carries severe consequences. "When the organizing principle of your day is sexual, very little gets done. This may jeopardize many things, including your job," Dr. Carnes says. "Or if your wife learns of your addiction, your marriage could be a throwaway."

As unhappy true examples, Dr. Carnes cites the case of a Florida clergyman who campaigned evangelistically against the evils of pornography but who was arrested for manufacturing pornography; or the case of a successful, wealthy, woman who supplemented her life by working part-time—as a prostitute—and could not stop.

"The whole thing is about power of a sorts—doing the forbidden—and about shame and excitement," Dr. Carnes says. "The addicts may stop whatever it is that turns them on for a time, but eventually they lose control again and binge."

Reasons for the Obsession

Many factors cause sex addiction. Most addicts come from families in which addictions thrive, like alcoholism, compulsive eating, gambling or sex. Most also have a history of sexual or physical abuse—over 80 percent. They also tend to come from families who have negative and rigid attitudes toward sex.

According to Aviel Goodman, M.D., director of the Minnesota Institute of Psychiatry in St. Paul, in a report he wrote for the *Journal of Sex and Marital Therapy*, more than 50 percent of sex addicts have had addiction problems with drugs or alcohol.

Sex addicts frequently suffer anxiety disorders, depression or manic-depression, writes Dr. Goodman.

The need to relieve stress or boost esteem also seems to be a major component, Dr. Elkin adds. "You have to ask what need the addict's behavior is meeting," he says. "He could be using sex to relieve tension or as a quick fix for low self-esteem or the need for love."

Leashing the Longing

Treatment for sex addiction usually occurs after something unfortunate happens.

"Something puts the addict over the line," Dr. Carnes says. "A doctor kills a patient because he's been up all night bingeing on sex, or a businessman loses his marriage when the paper prints a story about his arrest for soliciting a prostitute."

"At some point, addicts realize they're in trouble," Dr. Carnes says. "They have less and less control over the behavior, it's getting more and more risky to satisfy. Like alcoholics, they don't want to face the problem or they pretend it's not a problem until it rears up and kicks them in the face."

So what's the fix? There are two strategies: to prevent further slipups and to prevent relapse. You achieve this through counseling and medication. Here's what to keep in mind when it comes to sex addiction.

Get help with counseling. In many cases there is no home remedy for sex addiction. See a therapist to help determine the right type and length of treatment. If needed, long-term counseling will pinpoint why you're addicted to sex as well as help you deal with it and other addictions.

"Once you know the underlying issue that's driving the behavior, you can generally treat it," Dr. Elkin says. "Counseling helps addicts come to terms with their neurosis or neuroses to develop healthier ways of coping. You try to teach patients to care for themselves or to love themselves so that the behavior is no longer necessary."

"An awful lot of these patients have a history of sexual abuse in childhood," Dr. Carnes adds. "The scar tissue from that is not something you treat with a pill alone. Long-term counseling is an absolute necessity to get these people back on track."

Consider group treatment. One-on-one therapy is one of the preferred treatments, Dr. Carnes says, but support groups are extremely beneficial. Most groups offer therapy based on 12-step programs comparable to those for alcoholics. You also should consider family therapy.

"Therapy that involves the family is especially productive in part because the family is often part of the problem," Dr. Carnes says.

Be prepared: It's not easy. Fighting an addiction is never easy, and with therapy the cure sometimes seems worse than the cause.

"After the grieving period and the shock, addicts generally experience a decline in physical health," Dr. Carnes says. "But the majority of patients get through it, and by the third year have re-established their lives and a relationship with themselves that isn't condemnatory."

FAST FACTS

How common: Sex addiction affects 7 to 14 million Americans, or roughly 3 to 6 percent of the population.

Risk factors: Addictive personality, other addictions such as substance abuse, unresolved emotional problems such as low self-esteem or the scars of sexual abuse.

Age group affected: Starts in the teens; number of cases declines after the age of 40.

Gender gap: Hard to pin down, but more common in men than in women.

Who to see: Sex therapist, addiction therapist or psychiatrist who specializes in sexual disorders.

Try medication. "Anti-obsessional drugs, the antidepressants, like Prozac and Paxil, for example, are very effective—about 80 percent," says Roger Crenshaw, M.D., a sex therapist and psychiatrist in private practice in La Jolla, California.

Antidepressants work by increasing the amount of serotonin circulating in the brain at any given time. Serotonin, a chemical made by the body, slows down the brain's functions and helps you relax.

"The medications help in part because they address the depression of sex addiction since addicts feel so bad about themselves," Dr. Carnes says. "The medications use the body's own chemistry to alter the mood."

"Drugs, like Provera (a female hormone), are also helpful in the same regard," says Dr. Crenshaw. "They take away the drive to engage in the behavior that's at issue."

Another benefit of pharmaceuticals, says Dr. Carnes, is that they might help other mental health problems concurrently. "They're really pretty miraculous at stripping away or significantly relieving the obsession, and since about half of all sex addicts have severe depression, the drugs are very helpful there also," he says.

Sexually Transmitted Diseases

Say No to Unhealthy Erotic Reminders

You wouldn't bungee jump without an elastic cord. You wouldn't skydive without a parachute. So why in blazes would you have sex with a stranger without a condom?

Consider this: Skydiving accounts for about 30 deaths a year. Bungee jumping, less than one. Yet thousands of people are dying each year because of diseases passed on during sex.

There are more than 20 sexually transmitted diseases, or STDs. With the frightening exception of AIDS, which has claimed more than 200,000 lives, few people die from STDs. Even so, they're potentially serious and anything but rare.

Experts estimate that STDs affect roughly 1 out of 20 Americans each year. In one year, adult men contracted 17,977 cases of syphilis, 257,591 cases of gonorrhea and 48,208 cases of chlamydia (statistics for other STDs are not accumulated).

All this despite the fact that STDs nearly always can be avoided.

"STDs are with us and they're not showing any signs of leaving," says Deborah A. Ingram, nursing instructor in the College of Nursing at the University of Florida in Gainesville. "But there definitely are some methods you can use to prevent an STD."

Keeping STDs at Bay

Nature appears to be on the side of males. Although the issue is still largely unresolved, traditional thought has it that a man's body is less likely to be invaded by marauding bacteria than a woman's. That's because a woman's vagina is dark, warm and moist—conditions under which bacteria thrive. Can't say that about a penis. Plus, urination helps flush out whatever gets inside a man's member.

On the flip side, men claim to have far more sexual partners over time than women, putting them at greater risk of exposure. While no one can say definitively whether men get STDs more or less than women, there is absolutely no question that if you have sex, you are susceptible. So here's how to avoid the potential dangers.

Consider abstaining. Life offers few promises, but abstaining from sex pretty much guarantees you won't get an STD. Unless you are in a healthy, monogamous

FAST FACTS

How common: Very. Twelve million people contract a sexually transmitted disease (STD) each year; forty million currently are infected.

Risk factors: Any sexual activity, including oral and digital sex, can put you at risk. Having multiple sex partners, having sex with an infected person and sharing hypodermic needles also increase your chance of contracting an STD.

Age group affected: STDs are most common in younger and middle-age people. Experts estimate that almost half the U.S. population will acquire an STD by age 35. Other statistics show that 86 percent of all STD cases occur between the ages of 15 and 29.

Gender gap: The ratio of male versus female sufferers varies with each disease, and no total statistics exist. A vagina is a better host for germs than a penis, but men have more sexual partners than women. Bottom line: Both get STDs a lot.

Who to see: Family doctor, a physician at a health clinic or a specialist, such as a dermatologist or urologist.

---

relationship, you may want to contemplate sleeping alone until you meet that special someone you think you might have a future with.

Watch the numbers. Obviously, abstention isn't for everyone. A 3,432-person study conducted through the National Opinion Research Center found that more than 50 percent of men claim to have had five or more sex partners after age 18.

Time to face up to facts: The more sexually active you are, the greater your potential risk for contracting an STD. And you don't have to be a Don Juan or have a new partner each week to be at risk, says Robert E. Johnson, M.D., a research scientist with the Centers for Disease Control and Prevention in Atlanta. "For most people it's the fact that they're changing partners once every year or two," Dr. Johnson says.

Count on prescription relief. Since the advent of antibiotics in the 1940s, diseases that had plagued men for centuries suddenly could be cured or controlled. So if you do contract an STD, there's probably no need to take religious vows—just medication.

"Even with most advanced cases of gonorrhea or chlamydia, you can treat them and get good results," Ingram says. "Just don't slip in during the dark of night, get your treatment and disappear," she adds. "You'll need follow-up treatments and blood work" to confirm the treatment has worked.

Condoms 101: Learning about Latex

No glove, no love. Wrap that rascal. If you care, you'll wear.

Sound familiar? You've heard this stuff before, but sorry fella, catchy slogans won't help prevent sexually transmitted diseases (STD). Common sense will.

Wearing a condom is common sense. And while condoms cut your chances of getting an STD better than a Ginsu knife slices through a tin can, they don't guarantee a safe passage to promiscuity.

"We refer to condoms as 'safer sex' because there is no 100 percent guaranteed 'safe' sex," says condom connoisseur Stuart Schlaffman, owner of Condom Kingdom, a condom retail store in Philadelphia.

Nevertheless, there's no excuse not to wear a condom unless you're monogamous with a healthy partner—which means being monogamous for six months and then being retested before "going bare"—or for some perverse reason you have a strong desire to catch a disease.

Men have traditionally complained that condoms reduce sexual sensation, but technology has rendered that excuse obsolete. Today, you can choose among a variety of ultrathins (such as Trojan Very Thin)—condoms so thin you'll hardly know they're there.

"It feels like silky latex. It's not rubbery like a tire, and it also doesn't smell as bad as a normal condom," Schlaffman says.

There's no excuse to be caught without a reserve of rubber, either. Condoms are affordable and easily obtained. At Condom Kingdom, for example, condoms range from $1.50 to $4.25 for a three-pack. You can also get condoms free from most health clinics.

Buy condoms just a short while before you plan to use them, and check the expiration date to be sure you have fresh condoms. Older condoms are more likely to break, and spermicides lose their potency over time. The proper way to store a condom is in a cool, dark place, like a dresser drawer. You're not in high school anymore, so don't pack them in your wallet. The car's glove box is no good either because the temperature extremes inside a car can cause the rubber to break down. Think where you're most likely to use them, and keep them in a place that will be convenient, such as a bedside table or a jacket pocket.

You might be curious about novelty condoms such as flavored or glow-in-the-dark models. But while these can be entertaining, they can't be relied on to protect you from STDs.

Take the test you needn't study for. If you're a mature, responsible, sexually active adult—whether you're 18 or 80—then get tested for STDs. Not only will testing help prevent the potential long-term damage that can be caused by undetected STDs, it will also help ensure you don't inadvertently infect someone else.

"If you've had more than one partner or your partner has had more than one partner, then periodic examinations would be a good idea," Dr. Johnson advises. "It's especially important for men to get tested since men don't always exhibit symptoms."

Private physicians and health clinics routinely test for STDs. Some clinics offer subsidized or free testing for patients unable to shoulder the cost. To detect syphilis or HIV (the virus that causes AIDS), doctors will draw a blood sample. For gonorrhea and chlamydia they'll take a culture from the inside of your penis with a cotton swab. For herpes and genital warts doctors usually give a visual exam, though a culture can be taken from open sores.

"Just remember that tests are not a panacea. The emphasis should be on prevention," Dr. Johnson warns. And remember to ask your partners to get tested, too. It won't do you much good to get a clean bill of health if you're just going to get re-infected again.

Use condom sense. Aside from abstention or healthy monogamy, "a latex condom is the best way to protect yourself," says Katherine A. Forrest, M.D., a medical researcher and marketing consultant in Portola Valley, California.

Latex condoms create a barrier that prevents the passage of microorganisms that cause STDs, Dr. Forrest says. For added protection consider using condoms coated with the spermicide nonoxynol 9 (such as Trojan-Enz), which has been shown to help kill the AIDS virus in laboratory studies.

When choosing a condom, stick with the latex variety, experts say. Skin condoms, which are made from animal intestines, are porous and may not stop STDs from being passed.

Always keep a condom handy, and remember these tips. Put a condom on before any sex act (including oral sex). Roll the condom to the base of your penis. Don't use oil-based lubricants—hand lotions or petroleum jelly, for example—with condoms since they damage the latex. Remove condoms immediately after sex by holding the rim as you withdraw so the condom won't fall off or spill its contents. Use a new condom for each sex act.

Make *her* bag it. These are the 1990s and real men favor equality, so it's not out of the question to discuss with your partner whether she might share the condom-wearing responsibility.

The female condom works like a traditional condom, except in reverse. Rather

Penile Warts: When in Doubt, Check Them Out

Penile warts are the most common sexually transmitted disease, its incidence surpassing even herpes. But while they're a significant threat to women—playing a role in some of the 12,000 cases of cervical cancer each year—they're also harmless and usually painless to us males.

In fact, many guys don't even know they have them because they can often remain too small to be seen without a magnifying glass. Often, they simply disappear without treatment.

But when penile warts grow—raised or flat bumps anywhere along the penis or anal region—it's something few men can ignore. And that's good, because like other warts they're caused by a virus and are highly contagious. While usually transmitted through sex, you can also get them from sharing towels or by picking up the virus on your hands and then touching your penis.

Eradicating penile warts is not a do-it-yourself job (although you can prevent them by wearing a latex condom during intercourse), advises Nicholas G. Popovich, Ph.D., professor of pharmacy practice at Purdue University in West Lafayette, Indiana. Those over-the-counter wart remedies are too powerful for the sensitive skin of your penis. Instead, your doctor will probably prescribe any number of medications or perform cryotherapy, which involves freezing the warts with liquid nitrogen. Another reason to see a professional: What may appear to be a wart may actually be the symptom of a venereal disease or malignant tumor.

than fitting tightly over the penis, it clings to the inner contours of a woman's vagina. The open end provides protection to the outside of the vagina and the base of the penis. A soft, flexible ring at each end of the condom keeps it in place.

"No one is born knowing how to use a condom, so it takes a little practice. They're just about as effective as other barrier devices," says Holly Sherman, spokeswoman for The Female Health Company, which markets the Reality female condom. "As with all condoms, the key is careful and consistent use."

Reality condoms are made of polyurethane, not latex, and appear to be effective in preventing STDs when used properly. Polyurethane is 40 percent stronger than the latex used in male condoms, and does not disintegrate when used with oil-based lubricants.

"The biggest secret is these condoms feel great for men," Sherman adds. "The condom warms up to body temperature, and it's not tight-fitting, so it feels natural. And because an erection is not needed for use, the woman can insert the female condom before lovemaking begins."

The Usual Suspects

In some ways it's easier to guard against an STD than other infectious diseases—at least you know when you're likely to catch it. But you also have to know what you're looking for.

Below are descriptions of some of the more common STDs, like chlamydia and gonorrhea. (AIDS and genital herpes are discussed in their own chapters.)

Chlamydia

Chlamydia is responsible for three to five million new infections a year, making it the most common STD in the United States.

Despite this, "many people don't recognize the name of this STD," says Dr. Johnson. "It's important to get tested for chlamydia since many men won't have any symptoms."

A bacterial infection, chlamydia is spread by sexual contact—it cannot be spread by sharing toilets, kissing, swimming in pools or relaxing in hot tubs. Studies have shown that 25 percent of men with chlamydia have no symptoms at all. If symptoms do show up, it is typically about two weeks after the sexual contact. Symptoms include penile discharge (usually whitish and runny), a burning sensation during urination and, occasionally, swelling of the testicles. Even if you don't show symptoms, the disease spells trouble for men and their partners.

"You can develop epididymitis (an inflammation in the scrotum), which is extremely painful and that can cause scarring, which may leave you sterile," Ingram says.

Treatment for chlamydia consists of oral antibiotics, usually doxycycline (Doryx) or tetracycline (Achromycin V).

Gonorrhea

Commonly known as clap, gonorrhea strikes about 700,000 times a year. The bacteria die easily outside the body, so it's highly unlikely for gonorrhea to be spread by bathtubs, wet towels or by borrowing your best friend's trunks. Occasionally, however, the disease has been spread by objects. Witness the unfortunate sailor who contracted gonorrhea after surreptitiously using his infected shipmate's inflatable plastic doll.

Gonorrhea typically appears within 3 to 5 days, although it may surface in as little as 1 day or in as many as 30. Symptoms in men include penile discharge (usually greenish or yellow) and painful urination. Sometimes the penis head will swell. In as many as 80 percent of women the disease produces no noticeable symptoms.

Gonorrhea can be cured with shots of the antibiotic ceftriaxone (Rocephin) or antibiotic ofloxacin tablets (Floxin).

Syphilis

Syphilis has been around at least since the fifteenth century, so you'd think we'd have learned our lesson by now. Yet in 1990 new cases of syphilis reached their highest point in 40 years.

Caused by bacteria, syphilis could be called the STD of the rich and famous since it's ravaged such notables as Al Capone and the British statesman Lord Randolph Churchill. But you don't have to be famous—or infamous—to catch syphilis. The disease strikes approximately 100,000 Americans each year.

Syphilis is usually transmitted by direct contact with a sore or rash. It's usually passed during sex, but you can also catch it from kissing if there's a sore on the inside of the mouth, or from touching an open sore with your bare hands.

Symptoms progress in three stages. The first stage typically occurs between 10 and 90 days after infection. It's marked by the outbreak of a small, single, painless sore, called a chancre (SHANK-er), that pops up where the bacteria entered your body.

The second stage, which may last several weeks, includes a rash that rarely itches and which generally appears as the chancre fades. The rash often appears on the palms of the hands and soles of the feet, although it can appear elsewhere as well. Other symptoms of stage-two syphilis include fever, swollen lymph glands, sore throat, patchy hair loss and weight loss.

The third stage, which may occur years later, brings the whole, sad act to a close. Symptoms at this stage include paralysis, blindness, heart problems, nerve damage, insanity and even death.

Although syphilis can be treated with penicillin (Pen-Vee K), the antibiotic only kills bacteria—it can't reverse damage already done.

Trichomoniasis

Trichomoniasis (trik-o-mo-NYE-ah-sis) is the Stealth fighter of STDs. Caused by bacteria, it usually goes undetected in men. In fact, some studies suggest that "trich" might be the underlying cause for some chronic cases of male urethritis, an inflammation of the urethra, the tube that expels urine and semen from the body.

So don't feel lucky if your partner recently had trich and you assume you did

the male file

These results show how likely you are to contract a sexually transmitted disease based on your number of sex partners throughout your adult lifetime. The information is based on a national sex survey that examined the sex lives of 3,159 people, 45 percent of whom were men.

Bacterial Diseases (gonorrhea, chlamydia, syphilis, etc.)

Partners	Percent ever infected
1	about 1
2-4	about 3
5-10	about 11
11-20	about 21
21 or more	about 28

Viral Diseases (genital warts, genital herpes, hepatitis B, HIV/AIDS)

Partners	Percent ever infected
1	about 1
2-4	about 2
5-10	about 3
11-20	about 11
21 or more	about 13

not. In a study of 447 men at the University of Washington School of Medicine in Seattle, researchers found that 22 percent of men whose female partners were infected had the disease themselves.

Symptoms of trich that *may* appear include irritation on the inside or outside of the penis, as well as a slight discharge and burning sensation when urinating. Treatment usually consists of one oral dose of metronidazole (Flagyl).

Crabs

Crabs are pubic lice—small, flat-bodied bloodsuckers that you can see with a magnifying glass. (They look like tiny scabs to the naked eye.) About one million people get crabs each year, mostly from skin-to-skin contact with someone who has them. You can catch crabs during sex. You can also get them from towels or other personal belongings, or even by sitting on an infested toilet seat.

Symptoms—itching in the pubic or groin areas, accompanied by the appearance of small, blue bite marks—often appear about five days after exposure. You can treat crabs with over-the-counter medications or shampoos (such as A-200) that you apply directly to your pubic area. "Treat it the way the package says, then make sure you dry clean or wash all your linens and underwear in a hot washer and hot dryer," says Dr. Forrest. "Make sure everyone you live with does the same." Items that can't be washed can be put in a sealed plastic bag for two weeks. This starves the lice. Big items, like couches, can be cleaned with bug sprays containing disinfectants.

Chancroid

Chancroid is a bacterial disease that causes genital ulcers. Although painful, it is quite rare, with about 4,000 new cases occurring in this country each year.

You can get chancroid by touching an open sore. Unfortunately, avoiding the sores can be tricky since they may be hidden out of sight inside the rectum or vagina. The symptoms, however, which typically appear in four to ten days, can be hard to miss. First, there's a tender bump at the spot where the bacteria entered the body. After a couple of days the bump becomes a soft, tender, ragged sore that is often filled with pus. Chancroid is easily treated with pills of the antibiotic erythromycin (E-mycin) or with a shot of the antibiotic ceftriaxone.

Shaving Problems

Scraping Away Irritation

Shaving off those first few chin hairs is a male rite of passage almost up there with losing your virginity. And, truth be told, the first shave in some ways is more satisfying.

Yet at least half of us learn quickly that physical pain accompanies any psychological pleasure of standing bare chested before a steamy mirror with a shaving-cream beard and sharp steel in hand. Skin can be an enemy, waging a dermatological battle each time we take up the razor.

For the sensitive—or the hasty—each scrape of the blade can raise welts and bumps. Nicks get flagged by bloody scraps of toilet paper. Rashes pop up, as mysterious as they are painful. Scars from shaving miscues make women ponder your chin wound rather than your eyes.

These are all obstacles that can be cut down to size. You have dozens of options—certainly more than your ancestors did, who used stones, seashells and bronze knives each morning. In the past century and a half we've gotten the safety razor, disposable blades, exotic electronic shavers and musk-scented shaving cream. The perfect, hassle-free shave may be as close as your medicine cabinet.

Hair-Raising Problems

All too often it's not shaving itself but how you shave that causes problems. If you have tender skin, why insist on shaving as close as possible? Unless you treat your facial hair with the proper respect, it's going to object strenuously to any attempt to cut it off. Here are a few problems you face that go beyond the nick or scratch.

Ingrown hairs. These are most common among African Americans, but anyone who has curly hair is at risk, says Jerald L. Sklar, M.D., a dermatologist in private practice in Dallas. If you have ingrown hairs, some of your facial hairs twist down when they grow. When you shave, you sharpen the tip of the hairs, making it easier for them to pierce the skin and re-enter it on the way down. Your body, not recognizing the hairs after they have pierced the skin, fights the invaders off, leading to infected bumps.

Barber's itch. This is a bacterial infection in the beard area, says Paul Lazar,

M.D., professor of clinical dermatology at Northwestern University Medical School in Chicago. It was named after the barbers who passed the bacteria around by using contaminated equipment. It occurs when a skin injury—such as a cut or nick—allows bacteria to hone in.

Warts or acne. These make it almost impossible to reach shaving nirvana. Shaving not only irritates these protrusions, but it can lead to infections, says Dr. Sklar.

Skin discoloration. This can occur if you are shaving too closely. That irritates the skin and produces excess skin pigmentation, says Dr. Sklar.

Hair Today, Gone Tomorrow

The key to the perfect shave is preparation. That means putting your beard, razor and environment in perfect order, says Dr. Sklar. That's something your grandfather's barber understood whenever he swathed grandpa's face in steamy, hot towels a couple of minutes before he started scraping.

You can treat your beard with the same loving care, and you don't need a barber's chair and a razor strop to do it. Here are the steps to follow to make your shave as pleasurable as you always wanted it to be.

Choose the right razor. Electric shavers and blade razors were built to do different things, so they give different kinds of shaves, says Dr. Lazar.

If you want a close shave, choose a blade razor. If you want a meticulously close shave, choose a twin blade over a single blade. Replace the blades regularly—how often depends on how thick your beard is, how often you shave and how well you prepare your beard—usually once every five to seven shaves. Dull blades, after all, are more likely to nick your face.

If you need a shave that's not as close—and you might if you have sensitive skin, suffer from ingrown hairs or have acne or warts—choose an electric shaver. The latter doesn't remove any skin, reducing irritation and thus aggravation. Another point of personal preference: choosing between a rotary electric, where there are two or three cutters behind a spring-mounted guard, or a foil-head, which features a thin, flexible screen over the cutting head. Studies show the two types cut about the same;

the male file

Your chin and upper lip have about 385 whiskers per square inch, and they grow at a rate of about an inch every eight weeks. At that rate, each square inch of chin will generate more than two miles of stubble over 50 years.

FAST FACTS

How common: Virtually everyone who has ever toted a razor has learned—the hard way—that skin can get surly first thing in the morning.

Risk factors: African-American and other men with very curly hair are more susceptible to ingrown hairs. Men with sensitive skin also get irritated more easily. Nearly one out of five men younger than 35 say shaving irritates their skin.

Age group affected: As soon as you start to shave, you're eligible.

Gender gap: Women have their own set of shaving problems (and they don't even include borrowing their significant others' razors). If you think it's difficult to shave under your chin, try shaving under your armpit.

Who to see: Most men can solve their shaving problems themselves or by talking to their barbers. More serious problems, like ingrown hairs or infections that require antibiotics, require a dermatologist.

---

the rotary is more traditional, while the foil-head is the newer arrival.

Remember, there is no right or wrong choice; there is only what makes you comfortable. Experiment, and base your decision on things like whether you need the convenience of an electric, whether your skin is too delicate for blades, even whether your motor skills are operational first thing in the morning.

Then there's the cost question. An electric shaver can run upwards of $100, but might last for years; a pack of disposable blade razors is a couple of bucks, but you'll be buying them continuously.

After you've made your decision, give it a couple of days to see how it feels. Don't cut and run just because the first shave with your new blade turns your face red or because your new electric shaver leaves too much stubble.

Get wet with a blade. Blade beards love water—the more, the better, says Dr. Sklar. Soak your face with warm water for at least five minutes, wrapping your face in a warm washcloth. Or drench it during the morning shower. The hairs will swell and stand up, and they'll be ripe for the cutting.

Get dry with a shaver. Shavers need a dry, stiff face to work on, something that will stand up to the machine's cutting edges, Dr. Sklar says. If your face is wet and sweaty, you not only won't get a good shave but you'll irritate your skin.

Prepare the surface. Blade men can choose between soaps, gels or creams; razor aficionados have fewer choices. Dr. Lazar says this is truly a personal preference— use what feels best. Keep in mind that gels reduce friction more but cost a little more, while soap costs the least. Electric shaver preparations—like Lectric Shave—are usually necessary only when you can't get your skin dry enough naturally.

Take your time. Haste makes waste, and when you're talking about shaving, what you waste is skin and blood. Don't rush with either a blade or electric razor, says Fred Wexler, the director of research for the Warner-Lambert Shaving Products Group, makers of Schick and Wilkinson blades and razors. If you're done shaving while there's still steam on the mirror, you probably haven't taken long enough.

Shave with the grain. This can be difficult, especially in hard-to-reach and hard-to-see places. But shaving with the grain reduces skin irritation, swelling, redness and pain. For a really close, smooth shave, repeat the routine a second time. This removes the small rubble that you might have missed on the first go-round.

Skip the alcohol. Aftershaves are not a medical necessity, but there's something about a good, stiff slap of a skin bracer that seems to make the perfect shave that much more refreshing. Don't use things with alcohol or witch hazel—unless you want to run around the bathroom shrieking in agony. Check the aftershave ingredients; many popular preparations contain alcohol but sensitive skin alcohol-free formulations are also available.

the male file

Barber Denny Rowe works fast. In 1988 he shaved 1,994 men in 60 minutes with a safety razor in Herne Bay, England, taking an average of 1.8 seconds per volunteer and only drawing blood four times. Fellow barber and Brit Tom Rodden of Chatham shaved 262 men in 1993 with a straight-edge razor, averaging 13.8 seconds per man. He drew blood only once.

Shingles

How to Prevent an Unhappy Return

To everything there is a season, as it says in the Good Book, and diseases are no exception to the rule. Childhood is the time to itch with the chicken pox virus, and later in life to suffer the slings and arrows of shingles.

Actually, chicken pox and shingles are caused by the same bug—varicella-zoster, a type of herpes virus. Long after the chicken pox rash has faded into itchy memory, the virus remains, snuggled in among nerve cells.

The immune system keeps it in check for years, usually several decades. But then, for some unknown reason, the virus rides again out to the surface of the skin, where it causes a beltlike rash (the name shingles comes from the Latin cingulum, which means girdle or belt), often accompanied by blisters, itching and pain, sometimes severe.

Who's Susceptible

"There's no way to predict who will get shingles, and there's no way to prevent it," says Marilyn Kassirer, M.D., director of the Pain Management Team at the Veteran's Administration outpatient clinic in Boston. The risk is particularly high, however, for anyone whose immune system has been weakened by AIDS, certain cancers and other diseases.

Although the varicella-zoster virus can stage its comeback at virtually any time, the risk grows progressively steeper with age, quite possibly because the immune system loses some of its punch with passing years.

Of the 200,000 to 300,000 cases each year, senior citizens get a lot more than their share. According to the *New England Journal of Medicine*, after age 50, 5 in 1,000 will get shingles; by the time you reach your eighties, the rate has doubled. The disease hits men and women at about the same rate and with the same symptoms. Live long enough, in other words, and the odds rise that the virus you met in childhood will come back to haunt you. It's been estimated that 40 percent of men who have had chicken pox will eventually get shingles.

451

Pain That Persists

Shingles is no picnic. It typically begins with pain and itching and is often accompanied by fever and fatigue. Then red blisters appear, usually on one side of the chest or waist. The blisters crust over in ten days to two weeks and the attack is over. Most people never get another.

For 10 percent of sufferers, however, their episodes aren't so easy to forget. In those cases shingles is like a horror story with a very long sequel—a painful condition called postherpetic neuralgia, or PHN, that can last months or even years.

The cause of PHN is unknown, but the pain—sharply stabbing, deeply aching, generally nasty and often relentless—is legendary. Often, it takes the form of lasting hypersensitivity in the area where the blisters were—a light touch, even a breeze, can trigger it. The red rash and persistent pain have earned shingles the nickname "a belt of roses from Hell."

Like shingles, PHN discriminates against the elderly. If you get shingles in your thirties or forties, your chance of PHN is negligible. But if your over-60 father gets it, it's even money. There's only one surefire way to avoid shingles: Don't get chicken pox. Too late? Probably. An estimated 95 percent of Americans have been infected by the time they reach adulthood.

You can't catch shingles from someone with an active case. But if you or your children never had chicken pox, then stay away from the shingles sufferer. The varicella-zoster virus is contagious, and shingles blisters are full of them. Direct exposure can easily bring on chicken pox. And remember—chicken pox is far more serious in adults than in children.

Preventing—or Limiting—an Outbreak

For the most part over-the-counter anti-inflammatories, like aspirin or ibuprofen, are enough to control the pain of a shingles outbreak. But there is little medicine available to attack the disease directly.

The antiviral prescription drug acyclovir may reduce the risk of PHN. The emphasis is on "may." According to Neal Penneys, M.D., professor of medicine at St. Louis University Health Sciences Center, clinical trials haven't proven it, but anecdotal evidence suggests that the drug can tip the odds. And given the stakes, even a possible advantage is worth the effort.

It has been well-established, moreover, that oral acyclovir can shorten the course of the shingles episode itself, cutting days off the time from blisters to crusting. But it must be started right away. "Get to the doctor quickly, within 24 hours after the lesions appear," Dr. Kassirer urges. "After that, it's unlikely to do much."

Prompt action is absolutely vital, she adds, when the shingles rash appears on

FAST FACTS

How common: From 200,000 to 300,000 new cases are reported each year in America. An estimated 40 percent of people who have had chicken pox will get shingles during their lifetime.

Risk factors: To get shingles, you first had to have chicken pox. After that, age is the key factor. Diseases that strike the immune system (AIDS, lymphoma) also raise the risk.

Age group affected: The vast majority of people who get shingles are over age 50.

Gender gap: None. Men and women get shingles at the same rates.

Who to see: An internist or family doctor can treat uncomplicated shingles. Dermatologists have more expertise in the area. The pain of postherpetic neuralgia may require referral to a neurologist or pain management specialist.

the face. If the virus travels along certain cranial nerves, loss of vision is a real threat. In this situation, the doctor will probably prescribe high, intravenous doses of acyclovir.

Beyond acyclovir nothing is likely to have much effect on the length and severity of a shingles outbreak.

Treating shingles with steroid drugs, like prednisolone, is controversial because they suppress immune activity and may worsen the infection. Dr. Penneys prescribes it—very carefully—in combination with acyclovir, when pain is unusually severe.

Other Hands-On Help

Some other things to be done when shingles emerge include:

Be old-fashioned. Lotions, solutions and similar measures—what Dr. Penneys calls old-time dermatology—can also ease some of the discomfort. An over-the-counter astringent solution, like Domeboro, can help dry out oozing lesions; cool compresses, cornstarch and baking soda also give relief.

Use common sense. Don't scratch the itch, of course. That delays the healing and spreads the virus. Get some rest so your body can fight the virus. And as mentioned, take a painkiller, like aspirin, acetaminophen or ibuprofen if the pain is getting to you. Plus, keep a positive attitude as best as you can. Sooner or later the pain will be gone.

Get prescribed. For PHN sufferers there are a battery of drugs—tranquilizers, anti-inflammatories, anti-convulsants, antidepressants (particularly amitriptyline), even the ulcer drug cimetidine—that can help relieve the agony in some cases, Dr. Kassirer says.

Get spicy. Two unlikely additions to the arsenal for PHN are capsaicin, an extract of red pepper, and good old-fashioned aspirin, applied topically.

Capsaicin is available in an over-the-counter cream (Zostrix) and a stronger prescription formulation. It works on the nerve endings, depleting them of substance P, a chemical that carries pain impulses. Zostrix should only be used after the lesions are gone, however.

A paste of aspirin, applied to the painful area, also appears to work directly on the nerve endings. Pain relief lasting two to four hours in people with either shingles itself or PHN was reported by Robert B. King, M.D., professor of neurosurgery at State University of New York, Syracuse College of Medicine. He used aspirin dissolved in chloroform, which probably isn't available at your local drugstore. For an effective homemade treatment try crushing two aspirins in a few tablespoons of Vaseline Intensive Care Lotion, Dr. Kassirer suggests.

Deaden the nerves. When these methods fail to quell the pain, there's heavy-duty anesthesia such as injections to deaden the nerves for a time. "In medicine the basic premise is, the more options there are, the less likely anything is wonderful," says Dr. Penneys. "I use everything."

Let time heal all your wounds. If nothing else works, there's time. In most cases, says Dr. Penneys, the pain of PHN gradually gets better on its own.

Sick Building Syndrome

Finding an Indoor Pollution Solution

If your office building had an ignition system, it could probably be launched into orbit and serve nicely as a space station. That's because skyrocketing energy costs have caused engineers to seal off the buildings they design as tightly as possible from the outside environment.

The idea—to conserve heat in the winter and air-conditioning in the summer—is a good one, but there's a catch. The air in your office might have pollutants in it that you'd rather be flushed out the window, pollutants that are believed to cause the array of illnesses and allergies that have come to be called sick building syndrome.

The specific causes of sick building syndrome have proven hard enough to pin down that some researchers still believe it's more of a psychological than physical malady. But Bill C. Wolverton, Ph.D., an environmental research scientist and consultant and president of Wolverton Environmental Services in Picayune, Mississippi, isn't one of them. Literally hundreds of chemical by-products of various types have been found in office environments, he says. They range from copy machine chemicals to gases given off by the glues and fibers in carpeting. From formaldehyde emitted by particleboard shelves to cleaning solvents and air fresheners. From insecticides and paint fumes to insulation dust. From molds and mildew to cigarette smoke, not to mention the carbon dioxide exhaled by you and your fellow workers.

Any one of those elements alone may not be present in levels high enough to cause problems, Dr. Wolverton and others believe, but if you mix them all together and combine them with lousy ventilation, you have all the ingredients for a potentially dangerous toxic stew. "There's no mystery to me why sick building syndrome is happening," Dr. Wolverton says. "When you have an environment like that, how could it possibly be healthy?"

An Irritating Workplace

One of the problems in diagnosing a sick building is that many of the symptoms it causes are common enough to be mistaken for other problems including colds, allergies and the flu. Signs to watch for include irritated eyes, stuffy nose, sore throat, headache, drowsiness and fatigue. What distinguishes sick building syndrome from those sorts of illnesses is that it lasts. "Don't assume if you're sneezing or coughing or having chest congestion for a couple of weeks that it's okay," says Thomas Godar, M.D., chief of pulmonary disease at St. Francis Hospital in Hartford, Connecticut.

You may have to play detective to determine whether you have an indoor pollution problem where you work. Here are some important clues to watch for.

Keep a log. If you're having symptoms you suspect may result from sick building syndrome, the first thing to do is to track them, says Dr. Godar. Do your symptoms fade at the end of the day or over the weekend or while you're on vacation? Are the symptoms more pronounced when you work in a particular section of your building? Keeping a record in writing may help if and when the time comes to take your complaints to a supervisor.

Take a poll. The second step in your detective work is to find out if the people you work with are experiencing symptoms, too. "You can begin to get a kind of baseline sense of where the problem occurs," says David Mudarri, Ph.D., who works with the indoor air quality division of the Environmental Protection Agency in Washington, D.C. "Find out if it's localized to you and your area or if it extends to other floors."

Look for trouble. Although many of the problems that can cause sick building syndrome may be hidden behind walls or inside heating ducts, many other causes are fairly obvious if you look for them. "Sometimes a very simple probing can pay off in a big way," says Alexander Chester, M.D., a sinusitis expert who is in private practice in Washington, D.C.

Start with the ventilation system—investigations by the National Institute for Occupational Safety and Health have found inadequacies in ventilation in more than 50 percent of all sick building cases. Try holding a ribbon up to the air ducts in your office to see if a healthy stream of air is coming out. Be sure as well that your

the male file

In the average 100-person office, here are the most frequent excuses for taking sick days and the average number of days these reasons eat up a year: flu (76 days); muscle sprains (30 days); fractures (23 days); colds (21 days). According to one survey by the National Center for Health Statistics, the average man takes 4.3 sick days, the average woman 5.5 (excluding time off to give birth).

FAST FACTS

How common: No one is sure exactly how many "sick" buildings there are, but the National Institute for Occupational Safety and Health has investigated more than 1,500 cases in the United States over the past 20 years or so, and that's a fraction of the number of complaints it's received.

Risk factors: New or remodeled buildings that are poorly ventilated and overcrowded. Overcrowded buildings with moisture and growth of fungi or bacteria in indoor surfaces or in the ventilation systems.

Age group affected: Anyone working in a sick building can develop sick building syndrome.

Gender gap: A majority of those complaining of sick building syndrome are women. Researchers believe that's because women tend to report illnesses more quickly, but it may also reflect the fact that women still hold more clerical jobs than men—and that workers with clerical jobs usually don't have private offices.

Who to see: A family doctor or an otolaryngologist can help with specific symptoms. For information on how to address a sick building problem, call the Indoor Air Quality Information Clearinghouse hotline at 1-800-438-4318.

ducts aren't blocked by file cabinets, room dividers or other obstructions. Exhaust ventilation is especially important in rooms that house copy machines; smoking areas should have their own exhaust ducts.

Follow your nose. Bad smells can provide vital clues to the sources of indoor air pollution. Is the air stale? Overcrowding a workplace can result in an overload of carbon dioxide, Dr. Wolverton says, and stingy building managers have been known to cut the amount of fresh air circulating in a building to unsafe levels. Are there chemical fumes drifting past your desk from the janitor's supply closet across the hall? You may want to ask that a better storage area be found. If your office is filled with the smell of car exhaust or chow mein, try to track down where your building's ventilation system is drawing in outside air. Next to a loading dock or the local Chinese take-out joint is not an ideal location.

Be especially suspicious of moldy smells. According to Mark Mendell, Ph.D., an epidemiologist with the National Institute for Occupational Safety and Health in Cincinnati, researchers looking for the most likely causes of sick building syndrome increasingly are focusing their efforts on fungi and bacteria coming from moist surfaces somewhere in the building.

Humidify at work. The air in tightly sealed office buildings is usually dry—so dry that it can easily irritate your eyes, nose and throat. That irritation makes you more susceptible to the further irritations of pollutants in the air. A humidifier can help, Dr. Chester says.

But humidifiers need to be cared for if they are not to become a problem themselves. Clean it daily, replace the water regularly, turn it off at night and only use distilled water, Dr. Chester suggests. Otherwise, the humidifier will turn into a source of mildew and indoor pollution, too.

Humidify at home. To help soothe irritated nasal passages, Dr. Chester suggests inhaling some steam, either by holding a hot cup of water under your nose or standing in the bathroom with the hot water on in the shower.

Go back to basics. Two of the lowest-tech methods for combating indoor air pollution are also among the most effective. The easiest is to open your windows if they'll open.

Another is to add a little greenery to your office. "I would get as many houseplants as you can grow and put them around your personal breathing zone," Dr. Wolverton says. "The more the better." Two to four plants per 100 square feet are recommended.

Again, some caveats: Overwatering can cause spilling and thus mold. One solution is to put a saucer under the plant to catch excess water and then discarding the overflow. Also consider topping the soil with a half-inch of aquarium gravel to prevent mold from growing on wet, air-exposed soil.

Practice diplomacy. If you decide to take your concerns about indoor pollution to your boss, your cause will be better served if you can avoid a confrontation. According to Dr. Mendell, many studies have found that sick building syndrome is exacerbated by work stresses. Those studies are borne out by the personal experience of many experts in the field, including Dr. Godar, who have seen cases of sick building syndrome unnecessarily prolonged because of skepticism and mistrust between managers and workers.

Sinusitis

Opening the Taps

At first you were just a little stuffy, but each passing day has brought new misery: a pounding headache, a copious flow of mucus and enough pressure between your eyes that you briefly wonder if your head might explode.

Just a cold? Probably not. Any cold that lasts longer than a week and is accompanied by symptoms like headache or discolored mucus has probably set the stage for a separate infection of your sinuses. Doctors call this sinusitis, and it affects about 14 million men every year (that's nearly one in every six). In fact, it's the number one health complaint in the United States, says Edmund Pribitkin, M.D., an otolaryngologist at Thomas Jefferson University Hospital in Philadelphia.

A Headful of Trouble

The sinuses consist of eight hollow cavities inside the skull. No one's sure what they do, but researchers speculate they may play a role in lightening the skull, adding resonance to the voice, fighting off infection and warming and moistening incoming air before it hits the lungs.

The sinuses normally secrete up to a quart of mucus a day, which passes through the nose and traps dust particles, bacteria and other irritants. Then it flows down the back of the throat and into the stomach, where acids destroy any dangerous invaders.

When the nasal passages get irritated, however—this can be caused by allergies, smoke, air pollution or an infection caused by colds or flu—the sinuses increase mucus production. At the same time, swelling in the nose makes it difficult for mucus to drain. The result is that excess mucus backs up and becomes a prime breeding ground for bacteria, which in turn may cause sinusitis, says Gailen D. Marshall, M.D., Ph.D., director of the Division of Allergy and Clinical Immunology at the University of Texas Medical School in Houston.

"Any time your nasal passages are clogged long enough, you will get a sinus infection," says Dr. Marshall. "The question isn't whether you'll get it, but when."

As tender tissues inside the sinuses become inflamed, they can press on nerves leading to other parts of the face, causing throbbing headaches, painful pressure behind the eyes, cheek pain and even toothaches. There may be a prolific flow of yellowish, foul-tasting mucus.

In most cases sinusitis isn't serious and may go away on its own after about three weeks. But there have been cases where it persisted for months or even years. In severe bouts the infection can spread to nearby parts of the head, including the eyes and brain. And very rarely, sinusitis can lead to permanent damage or life-threatening ailments such as meningitis.

Breathing Easy

Once you have sinusitis, your doctor will probably give you antibiotics to clear up the infection, says Dr. Marshall. A better bet is to prevent it from occurring in the first place. This means trying to keep the sinuses open and draining at the first sign of trouble. Here's what experts recommend.

Take evasive action. Obviously you can't dodge every virus and allergy-causing particle out there, but by stopping congestion before it occurs, you can vastly reduce your risk for sinusitis, says Dr. Pribitkin.

Getting a flu shot in the autumn is perhaps the best and easiest thing you can do to prevent seasonal infections, he says. It's also important to wash your hands frequently during the day because many viruses are transmitted by hand-to-mouth or hand-to-nose contact.

Men with hay fever are particularly prone to sinusitis. If you're one of them, staying indoors in the early morning and afternoon, which is when most airborne pollens take wing, will help keep your sinuses clear. In addition, using an air conditioner will help filter out allergy-causing particles before they reach your lungs.

Head to the drugstore. Once congestion strikes, your priority should be to keep the mucus flowing. "The first line of therapy is to take a decongestant coupled with a pain reliever," advises Dr. Pribitkin. Over-the-counter medications such as pseudoephedrine (Sudafed) and oxymetazoline (Afrin Nasal Spray) are very effective at clearing away congestion.

When using sprays, however, it's important to use them for no more than five days. If you use them longer, rebound congestion—in which you'll develop more stuffiness than you had before—may occur. Men who have heart problems, high blood pressure or insomnia should check with their doctors before using any decongestant, Dr. Pribitkin adds.

Make your own spray. Rather than using a powerful decongestant, you can make your own nasal spray by mixing one-quarter teaspoon each of salt and baking soda in eight ounces of warm water, and then sniffing a handful every hour or so,

FAST FACTS

How common: About 14 million men get sinusitis annually.

Risk factors: Nasal congestion, usually caused by allergies, colds and flu, or physical obstructions such as polyps in the nose or sinuses.

Age group affected: Sinusitis can occur at any age, although it seems to be most common in men under age 35. It may be that younger men are more susceptible to colds and allergies than older guys.

Gender gap: Men and women are equally prone to sinusitis.

Who to see: Start with your family doctor. You might get referred to an otolaryngologist or allergist.

suggests Dr. Marshall. This will help reduce congestion by clearing mucus and soothing inflamed membranes. "It approaches your normal pH and won't scald the nose the way some medications do," he says.

Get steamed. Perhaps the quickest way to break up congestion without taking drugs is to breathe a snootful of steam, says Dr. Marshall. Taking a long, hot shower is one way to do this. Another is to drape a towel over your head, lean over a pot filled with hot water and inhale away. Your nose, incidentally, shouldn't be anywhere close to the surface of the water. "Some people literally boil their noses—it's incredible the burns I've seen," Dr. Marshall says.

Give up the smokes. Smoking dries the delicate membranes in the nose and throat, which makes them more susceptible to marauding viruses and subsequent irritation, says Dr. Pribitkin. This is why smokers usually get more colds—and sinus problems—than nonsmokers.

Eat spicy. Studies have shown that eating hot peppers or other spicy foods—many of which contain a fiery chemical known as capsaicin—will really turn on the nasal taps and get the mucus flowing.

Drink plenty of water. Experts say you should drink at least eight eight-ounce glasses of water each day. Drinking lots of water will help to dilute mucus in your nose and sinuses and keep it flowing freely, says Dr. Marshall.

Keep your feet on the ground. If you have a severe case of sinusitis, it probably isn't a good idea to fly. Pressure changes during the flight can cause tremendous pain and damage your sinuses, says Eric G. Anderson, M.D., a family physician in La Jolla, California.

Check your progress. If you suspect your sinuses aren't getting better despite two or three days of home care, try this: Go into a darkened bathroom, stick a penlight in your mouth, close your lips around the penlight and look in the mirror, Dr. Anderson suggests. The reddish glow from the penlight should penetrate equally into your cheekbones. If one side of your face appears less red than the other, then your sinuses are probably still clogged and you should see a doctor.

You also should consult a physician if you have a fever of 101°F or higher, increased facial swelling, severe headaches that aren't relieved by aspirin or acetaminophen, increased yellow or green nasal discharge, nosebleeds, vision changes or feel a pain between the ridge of your nose and a lower eyelid.

Restore the Flow

In most cases sinusitis is readily cured with oral antibiotics such as amoxicillin. Once you begin taking these drugs you'll probably start feeling better within a day or two. But don't do the typical male thing and stop taking your medication the minute you're feeling better, Dr. Pribitkin warns. It's critical to finish the entire prescription—usually about two weeks' worth—to prevent any hardy bacterial survivors in there from making you sick all over again.

If your sinuses are in a perpetual stage of uproar—a condition doctors refer to as chronic sinusitis—you may need surgery to clear away scar tissue or correct structural defects such as a deviated septum that interfere with mucus drainage, says Dr. Marshall. In the past these procedures often required extensive surgery and lengthy hospital stays. But with a modern technique called endoscopic sinus surgery—in which tiny surgical instruments are inserted through a narrow tube inside a nostril—many nasal surgeries can be completed in less than an hour.

"It can be done as an outpatient procedure and the discomfort is usually minimal," says Dr. Pribitkin. "A lot of people are able to have the surgery and go back to work within a few days."

Skin Cancer

Shining Light on the Superficial Tumor

Skin cancer is a rare beast. Not in the sense that few people get it; in fact, it's the most common of all cancers, with about one million new cases every year. Rather, skin cancer is rare in that it's so plain to see. Tumors and—this is important—the growths and lesions that *lead* to tumors make themselves obvious on the outside of the body.

It's one reason why skin cancer is so infrequently deadly: It tends to be caught early and treated. In fact, the most lethal form of skin cancer, melanoma, doesn't even make the American Cancer Society's top ten list of annual cancer killers.

Another reason skin cancer causes relatively few deaths is that the vast majority (some 97 percent) of cases aren't melanoma at all but are the much less-threatening kinds known as basal cell carcinoma and squamous cell carcinoma.

So, should you be concerned about skin cancer? You bet.

"The most important reason to prevent and treat it is that if you don't, it will just continue to grow larger, and if it's on the head—where a lot of skin cancers are—in a worse case scenario, it could spread into the brain or cause paralysis of the face," says Martin Weinstock, M.D., Ph.D., associate professor of dermatology at Brown University School of Medicine and director of the Moles and Melanoma Unit at Roger Williams Medical Center, both in Providence, Rhode Island. And you can't ignore the fact that people *do* die from skin cancer: 7,000 a year from melanoma and 1,000 from nonmelanoma. Significantly, *twice* as many men get skin cancer as women.

Get Off the Sol Train

Virtually all skin cancers are caused by one thing: exposure to the sun, whose ultraviolet rays damage the skin. Eliminate sun exposure and skin cancer usually isn't a problem. Of course, fully following that rule would mean living like a cloistered monk—and even monks get outside now and then. The real trick is to minimize exposure when you are in the sun.

For a full range of protection options, you need remember nothing more than Slip, Slop, Slap—the name of a national program in Australia, where skin cancer rates have skyrocketed in recent years. What to do.

Slip on a shirt. When possible, wear clothes made from tight weaves, which block more of the sun's rays.

Slop on some sunscreen. For best protection, use creams with a sun protection factor of 15 or more. Reapply at least every two hours, even if you're not swimming: Sunscreens come off with sweat.

Slap on a hat. Preferably a hat with a three- to four-inch brim, which will shade particularly vulnerable areas like the tops of the ears, the back of the neck and the top of the forehead.

Beyond these basics, however, there are a number of other steps you can take to reduce your exposure.

Look for the short shadow. Ultraviolet radiation is most intense at midday, when fewer rays get absorbed by the atmosphere before hitting your body. The standard recommendation is to avoid sun exposure between 10:00 A.M. and 3:00 P.M., although dermatologists note that even in the late afternoon—between 3 and 4—ultraviolet doses are still substantial, especially in summertime.

Don't be dim. Stay protected on less-than-bright days: The sun is just as damaging to skin when it's clouded by overcast skies as on sunny days. What's more, shade doesn't offer complete protection if reflective surfaces such as sand, snow, concrete, glass or water are bouncing rays onto your skin.

Check your prescription. A number of drugs increase the skin's sensitivity to ultraviolet radiation. Be especially protective of skin if you're taking antibiotics such as tetracyclines (Monodox) and sulfonamides (Azulfidine), diabetes medications such as sulfonylureas (Glipizide) or psoriasis treatments, like psoralens (Oxsoralen).

Back off on fat. In a study of 76 people with nonmelanoma skin cancer, those who cut back the fat content of their diets to 20 percent of calories had more than three times fewer new precancerous growths than people who ate a typical high-fat diet.

Spot Checking

Since spotting skin cancer is so important to treating it, it's vital to recognize problems when you see them. Any kind of new growth or change in the skin should be considered suspect, but what you're looking for differs depending on the type of cancer involved. For nonmelanoma be on the watch for:

- Small, smooth, shiny or waxy lumps, which may sometimes bleed or turn crusty.
- Flat, red spots that can be scaly, crusty or smooth.
- Firm, red lumps.
- Rough, scaly, red or brown patches on sun-exposed skin.

FAST FACTS

How common: It's the most common form of cancer (though far from the most deadly), with roughly 500,000 new cases every year among American men.

Risk factors: Sun exposure, light-colored skin or hair or a tendency to burn easily.

Age group affected: Skin cancer is brought on by long-term exposure, so it often doesn't show up until after age 60. But plenty of people still get it in their thirties and in the 25 to 29 age group. Sun exposure during one's youth has a significant bearing on rates of cancer later.

Gender gap: Rates in men are almost twice that of women, for a number of reasons: Men are out in the sun more, expose more of their bodies outdoors and have shorter hair.

Who to see: Dermatologist.

Look especially on the head and neck. That's where 80 percent of basal cell carcinomas are found, and it's also where tumors that spread tend to pop up most often in men.

As a rule, you can wait about a month before seeing a doctor about a suspicious-looking area. "The issue is that it's something that doesn't heal," says Dr. Weinstock. "Give it a little time."

For the more dangerous melanomas, the thing to watch is moles. To identify problems, look for the ABCD symptoms.

Asymmetry: One side of the mole looks different from the other.

Border irregularity: The edges of the mole are ragged, blurred or uneven.

Color: The shade varies from one part of the mole to another.

Diameter: The mole is bigger than a pencil eraser.

Don't wait if you find these patterns. When melanoma is caught early, it's 90 to 99 percent curable.

Skin Erasers

If you do have melanoma, the solution is simpler than the diagnosis. "Melanoma is always excised, no matter where it is," says Warwick Morison, M.D., associate professor of dermatology at Johns Hopkins University School of Medicine/Francis Scott Key Medical Center in Baltimore. That means it's cut out, usually with some space around the edges to spare. No other treatment is considered as simple, effective or protective against recurrence.

For nonmelanoma, however, there are a number of options that are especially attractive for areas that are either difficult to reach or would be noticeably scarred with conventional surgery, or which are particularly responsive to alternative methods. The choices:

Electrosurgery. Usually used on basal cell carcinomas, the cancer is scooped out with a special instrument called a curette, then the area is zapped with an electrical device to kill remaining cancer cells. Advantage: for fair-skinned people, less scarring than with conventional surgery.

Freezing. Liquid nitrogen is sprayed on the growth, killing the cancer, which then flakes off, leaving a white scar.

Mohs' technique. The tumor is shaved away in thin slices, which are examined under a microscope for evidence of cancer. Benefit: No more tissue than necessary is removed.

Photodynamic therapy. In this experimental approach, tumors that absorb an injected drug are killed when a special wavelength of laser light activates the drug.

Radiation. Skin is showered with x-rays, which kill cancerous cells at the surface while leaving healthy cells deeper down relatively unscathed.

Topical drugs. The anticancer prescription drug 5-fluorouracil (Efudex) can clear up abnormal precancerous growths, usually producing inflammation during treatment, but leaving no scars.

"The reasons for using one method over another vary from case to case," says Dr. Weinstock.

Smoking

Quitting Is Just a Puff Away

You've heard it all before. Smoking has been linked to lung cancer. Throat cancer. Heart disease. Wrinkles. Ulcers. High blood pressure. Hernias. Emphysema.

In fact, the tobacco industry may be the only group left that still maintains that smoking won't kill you. That should tell you something.

And yet, as of the last detailed accounting, 28 percent of men in the United States still smoked. The average number of cigarettes a day: 21.6, or more than a pack.

But there's good news. More than half of U.S. males who had ever smoked categorized themselves as former smokers, meaning tens of millions have already peeled the tobacco monkey off their backs.

Quitting smoking is not only possible but the side effects are positively glorious. Your lungs clear up. Your food tastes better. Your breath won't scare away dogs and small children.

Above all, you'll live longer, says Alfred Munzer, M.D., past president of the American Lung Association and co-director of pulmonary medicine at Washington Adventist Hospital in Takoma Park, Maryland.

So what's the catch?

It's that smoking is addictive, both physiologically and psychologically, says K. Michael Cummings, Ph.D., director of the Smoking Cessation Clinic at the Roswell Park Cancer Institute in Buffalo. That means quitting is harder than just flushing your butts down the toilet and getting on with your life.

Says Dr. Cummings: "You have to be persistent, and you have to realize there is going to be backsliding, but that the backsliding won't stop you from quitting."

No Butts about It

Smoking's physical addiction is the fault of nicotine, as addictive a drug as anyone ever ingested. The nicotine hooks you just as surely as its more disreputable cousins—heroin and cocaine, says Jack Henningfield, Ph.D., chief of clinical pharmacology research at the Addiction Research Center at the National Institute of

Drug Abuse in Baltimore. "Your brain gets hungry for it," says Dr. Henningfield.

Nicotine gives smokers a high, a quick jolt that surges through the bloodstream in a matter of seconds. Smokers can develop a tolerance for nicotine, which means they have to smoke more to get the same high. That's how you go from puffing behind the garage as a kid to a two-pack-a-day adult.

Then there's the psychological addiction. For many smokers, taking a drag has become second nature, just like breathing or blinking. One pack of cigarettes can turn into 150 to 200 puffs a day, seven days a week, 52 weeks a year, says Dr. Cummings.

You have a cigarette when you get up in the morning. You have a cigarette after dinner. You have a cigarette while you're waiting in line at the drive-in window at the bank. You have a cigarette in your hands and you're not quite sure how it got there—it's just there.

Getting Your Kicks

Kicking the habit requires a double-edged attack. Just when you think you have the physiological addiction under control, the psychological addiction can undermine all your hard work, says Robert Robinson, D.P.H., associate director for program development at the Office on Smoking and Health at the Centers for Disease Control and Prevention in Atlanta. You also must decide you want to quit. "There are a whole range of reasons you can choose from to quit smoking. Select the ones that will motivate you," says Dr. Robinson. If you don't want to quit for yourself, Dr. Robinson encourages smokers to quit for the ones they love. Find the reason that makes the most sense to you, and make the decision.

Once you've made the firm decision, there are dozens of methods, from nicotine patches to self-help books to friends who can provide you with the social support you need, to kick the habit for good. Here are some guidelines to keep in mind.

Take each day one day at a time. If this process works for alcoholics, it will work for you, says Dr. Cummings. Worry about not smoking for that one day, and not for the rest of your life. The latter is an intimidating and self-defeating process—sort of like dropping out of school forever if you don't do well during milk-and-cookie time in kindergarten.

Besides, it gets easier the longer you stay away from the butts, says Dr. Cummings. It takes three to five days to purge the nicotine from your system and about a month for the worst of the withdrawal symptoms to go away (even if you're such a heavy smoker that you find yourself lighting up while you brush your teeth in the morning). That means that for just three weeks—from the time the nicotine leaves until the time withdrawal ends—you may feel cravings, anxiety, nausea, cramps, depression or dizziness.

Change your environment. Every smoker does thousands of things that enable

FAST FACTS

How common: Approximately 46 million adult Americans smoke, and 1 million quit every year. The number of smokers has declined by 1.1 percent a year since 1985; in fact, there are equally as many people who have quit smoking—46 million—as there are people who smoke.

Risk factors: If you don't start smoking as a teenager, you probably won't ever start. The Surgeon General's 1994 report on smoking and health says advertising appears to increase the odds teenagers will start since it makes smoking seem cool.

Age group affected: If you're a man between the ages of 25 and 44, you're more likely to smoke than anyone else.

Gender gap: In 1983, 35.1 percent of all American men and 29.5 percent of all women smoked. A decade later only 28 percent of men smoked, and the women's figure declined to 23 percent. In fact, more than half of all men who have ever smoked have quit, 51.9 percent by the last count.

Who to see: You can quit on your own, and millions have been successful. But your chances of success increase if you see a physician or a therapist. There are no guarantees, but if you're motivated enough to see someone, chances are you're motivated enough to quit for good, says Robert Robinson, D.P.H., associate director for program development at the Office on Smoking and Health at the Centers for Disease Control and Prevention in Atlanta.

him to smoke, whether it's picking up matches at a restaurant or arranging his schedule at work to sneak in 15 minutes to go outside for a nicotine fix. That's part of the psychological addiction.

The way to beat it is to think about the things you do that lead up to lighting up, and then don't do them. Don't keep any ashtrays in the house. Have that afterwork brew some place other than your local bar, where smoking is part of the atmosphere. If you always have a cigarette with your coffee after dinner, give up the coffee and try going for a walk instead. If you always have a cigarette after sex, try making love in the shower. Says Cummings: "Change your routine and alter your habits, and you're not as likely to light up."

Taper off. Of course it's hard to quit cold turkey. If it was easy, you wouldn't be reading this. That's why you might want to try stepping down gradually instead of going mano a mano with your habit, says Dr. Robinson. First, if you're smoking two packs a day and the thought of giving it all up at once is out of the question, work your way down to ground zero gradually. Instead of 40 cigarettes a day, try 20, then

Secondhand Smoke

Secondhand smoke isn't as deadly as smoking itself, but it's deadly enough.

"Secondhand smoke is, in fact, dangerous, and those who don't think so are fooling themselves," says Alfred Munzer, M.D., past president of the American Lung Association and co-director of pulmonary medicine at Washington Adventist Hospital in Takoma Park, Maryland. "If you're not concerned enough about your own health to quit smoking, then you should quit because of what you're doing to the health of the people around you."

The scientific evidence is mounting to support this once-controversial issue. Studies show that men who don't smoke face an increased risk of heart disease and cancer from passive smoking. Several doctors examining mortality data found that nonsmoking men who marry a smoker have a significantly higher risk of nasal cancer, for example. And at least one researcher estimates that passive smoking increases the U.S. coronary death rate among people who have never smoked by up to 70 percent.

Your smoking also endangers the people around you. Women who have never smoked face a 30 percent higher risk of lung cancer if they marry a smoker, according to one study. But your partner isn't the only person your smoking affects. After examining the scientific evidence over the last decade, at least one researcher concluded that paternal smoking contributes to increased respiratory diseases, inflammation of the middle ear and other health problems during fetal growth, infancy and childhood.

10. Second, try switching to a lower-nicotine cigarette. Both methods wean your body off the nicotine gradually, reducing the shock to your system.

That's the philosophy behind nicotine patches and nicotine gum. The patch (one brand is Nicoderm, available by prescription) attaches to your body, usually on the arm, and releases regular amounts of nicotine into your system. The gum (such as Nicorette, also available by prescription) is less controlled. You can increase the flow of nicotine by chewing harder. How successful are they? Studies show a wide variance—from almost no difference in one trial to a five-times better chance in another, according to a report from the University of Wisconsin Medical School in Madison. But overall, doctors estimate that, for the typical guy, gums or patches double the success rate. The success of the patches and gums also varies depending

the male file

Why stop smoking?

Within 20 minutes:

—Blood pressure, pulse rate and the body temperature of hands and feet return to normal.

Within 8 hours:

—Carbon monoxide level in blood drops to normal.

—Oxygen level in blood increases to normal.

Within 24 hours:

—Chance of heart attack decreases.

Within 48 hours:

—Senses of taste and smell start to return to normal and are noticeably enhanced.

Within two weeks to three months:

—Circulation improves.

—Lung function increases up to 30 percent.

Within one to nine months:

—Coughing, sinus congestion, fatigue and shortness of breath decrease.

—Overall energy level increases.

Within 1 year:

—Risk of coronary heart disease drops to half that of a smoker.

Within 5 years:

—The lung cancer death rate for an average former smoker (at one pack per day) decreases by almost half.

—Risk of stroke is reduced to that of a nonsmoker within 5 to 15 years.

Within 10 years:

—Chance of lung cancer death is similar to that of a nonsmoker.

—Precancerous cells are replaced.

—Risk of cancer of the mouth, throat, bladder, kidney and pancreas decreases.

Within 15 years:

—Risk of coronary heart disease is that of a nonsmoker.

on what else you're doing to quit. The University of Wisconsin study discovered that patches by themselves are a lot less effective than patches used in conjunction with other forms of therapy.

Practice the four Ds. Dr. Cummings recommends this to all of his patients.

When you feel like a smoke, *delay*. Think of something else, like why you decided to quit. Breathe *deeply*, counting to ten slowly while you do it. This helps reduce stress, and stress helps to bring on the craving like washing your car brings on a downpour. *Drink* water, at least six to eight eight-ounce glasses a day. This helps flush the nicotine out of your system. *Do* something else. When you feel like a drag, you can chew gum, tap a pencil or crack your knuckles. Almost anything will help you pass the time until the craving passes.

Keep a smoking diary. Okay, it's not a guy thing. But a diary can help you become more aware of your smoking patterns—the times you smoke only because it's a habit and the times you smoke because you genuinely feel a craving, says Dr. Henningfield. Each time during the day that you feel like taking a puff (and before you do), write down the time, what you're doing and how badly you want a drag (on a scale of 1 to 3, with 1 for the worst craving and 3 for the mildest). Once you figure out which cigarettes are smoked because you always smoke at that time—those that get a 3 on the craving scale—you can cut them out of your day.

Snoring

Stopping the Nocturnal Noise

The next time you're rudely awakened in the middle of the night with a sharp elbow to the ribs followed by a head-splitting harangue about your snoring, calmly tell your bedmate to count her blessings. After all, you're no Melvyn Switzer. Then again, there can be only one true champ.

When it comes to the dubious distinction of world-class snoring, Switzer, of Dibden, Great Britain, is the mouth that roared. One night in 1992 he was recorded snoring at 92 decibels—a level about midway between heavy traffic and a rock concert—to claim the mark that still stands in the Guinness Book of World Records. How a man could create such a cacophony without knowing it is one of life's great mysteries. As Mark Twain pointed out: "There ain't no way to find out why a snorer can't hear himself snore."

Snoring through the Ages

If you've ever shared a room with a few buddies, you know that snoring isn't exactly rare. And the problem only gets worse the older you get. Between the ages of 30 and 35 about 20 percent of men snore compared to 5 percent of women. By the time we hit 60, about 60 percent of men are sawing logs. Just in case you're smugly thinking that at least *you* won't have to put up with the noise, think again. By the time they reach their sixties, 40 percent of women also are snoring. Now there's something to look forward to.

Snoring occurs when tissues in the upper airway that are taut during the day relax during sleep. As air passes through the narrowed channel, it causes the tissues to vibrate like the reed in a bass saxophone. What you lack in pleasing pitch, you probably make up in volume.

Snoring usually gets worse as a man ages because the muscles and other tissues in the throat, like those elsewhere in the body, become less firm, says James D. Frost, M.D., a sleep specialist and professor of neurology at Baylor College of Medicine in Houston. Being overweight can also pump up the volume as the neck and throat accumulate more noise-producing tissue.

In some cases snoring is a symptom of more serious medical problems such as

473

nasal polyps or sleep apnea, in which a man stops breathing during sleep. More often, snoring isn't a problem at all—at least not for the one snoring. "I saw one man whose wife had moved out of the bedroom 15 or 20 years before he came to see me," says Dr. Frost. "The reason he finally came in was the neighbors complained—and that was with the windows closed."

Turning Down the Volume

If your nocturnal noisemaking has landed you in the domestic doghouse—or worse, on the couch—it's time to change your tune. Here are some steps you can take to revive that golden oldie "In the Still of the Night."

Roll over. When you sleep on your back, the tongue falls backward into the throat, partially blocking airflow and causing snoring, says Edmund Pribitkin, M.D., an otolaryngologist at Thomas Jefferson University Hospital in Philadelphia. "That's why your wife is always knocking you in the side to get you to roll over," he says. Sleeping on your side or stomach will usually reduce, if not eliminate, the racket.

Play bed tennis. You don't need the racket, just the ball. When it's sewn into a pocket stitched to the back of a T-shirt or pajama top, it makes it almost impossible to roll over on your back while you sleep, says Dr. Pribitkin. "It usually doesn't eliminate the snoring, but it can make it softer."

Keep the pounds down. Although thin men also snore, the problem is more common and usually more severe in those who are overweight. After all, the weight you gain doesn't accumulate only on the hips, but on the neck and inside the throat as well. "They're usually out of shape so the muscles in the back of the throat are weak and more likely to collapse," Dr. Pribitkin explains.

Keep regular hours. Being tired is a common cause of noisy snoring, says Dr. Frost. In part, this is because the more tired you are, the more the muscles in the throat are going to relax during sleep. In addition, going to bed exhausted means you'll spend more time in deep sleep, which is when loud snoring usually occurs. Keeping a regular schedule can at least help keep the volume down, he says.

Cut down on drinking. Consuming alcohol at bedtime reduces the normal muscle tone inside the throat, which makes airway collapse that much more likely, says Dr. Frost. "A lot of guys go off on hunting trips and the alcohol flows freely," he says. "They come to see me after their buddies tell them that they can't come hunting anymore because of the snoring."

Nix the sleeping pills. Like alcohol, taking sedatives relaxes muscles in the upper airway. If you must take them, ask your doctor which types are least likely to jump-start the snoring.

FAST FACTS

How common: About half of all adults snore occasionally. In one study 19 percent of people of all ages said they snored nearly every night.

Risk factors: Sleep apnea, fatigue, sleeping on the back, using alcohol or sleeping pills.

Age group affected: Snoring occurs at all ages, but is most common after age 60.

Gender gap: Snoring is more common (and usually more severe) in men. Doctors believe this is because men, who are larger than women, have more tissue in the neck and throat. They're also heavier, which means there is more downward pressure on the airways. As a result, it's harder for the airways to stay open during sleep.

Who to see: For extreme cases, you might be referred to an otolaryngologist, neurologist or a sleep/pulmonary expert.

Don't dry out. Moist air reduces snoring. "Dry air exacerbates it, so using a humidifier is helpful," says James Perl, Ph.D., a psychologist in private practice in Boulder, Colorado, and author of *Sleep Right in Five Nights.*

Butt out. Smoking cigarettes irritates membranes in the nose and throat, causing mucus to be secreted. At the same time, it causes tissues inside the nose to swell, which also turns up the snoring volume. So if you haven't already quit, here's yet another reason to kick the habit.

Keep your head up. Most men can make themselves snore less by sleeping in a more upright position, experts say. Some men resort to sleeping in an easy chair. An easier way is to prop up the head of the bed about six inches by putting books or bricks under the legs, says Dr. Pribitkin.

Stop Snores at the Source

If, despite your best efforts, snoring continues to disturb the domestic peace, your doctor may recommend more aggressive treatments.

There are a number of medications—including antidepressants and mild stimulants such as caffeine—that are occasionally used to help reduce both the frequency and volume of snoring, says Dr. Pribitkin. They do this either by increasing muscle tone in the upper airway or by decreasing the amount of time a man spends in deep sleep, which is when the loudest snoring typically occurs. While the drugs are usually somewhat helpful, they won't eliminate the problem, says Dr. Pribitkin.

Sleep Apnea: Finding Rest for the Weary

The word "apnea" means "without breath," and that's exactly what happens when you have sleep apnea. Men with this condition may stop breathing dozens or even hundreds of times a night. Each time, they partially awaken as the body desperately struggles for air. "Fatigue, depression, irritability and moodiness are very common in these men," says Karl Doghramji, M.D., associate professor of psychiatry and director of the Sleep Disorders Center at Thomas Jefferson University Hospital in Philadelphia.

Research suggests the problem may be far more common than was previously thought. A study involving 602 middle-age men and women found that 4 percent of men and 2 percent of women suffered from severe sleep apnea resulting in excessive sleepiness during the day, says Dr. Young, who led the study. In addition, 24 percent of men and 9 percent of women suffered from a milder form of disrupted nighttime breathing, the health impact of which is unclear.

The surest sign that you may be suffering from sleep apnea is "an uncontrollable sleepiness during the daytime," Dr. Young says. Men with this condition "cannot fight off the need to fall asleep during the day. Against their will, they need to take a nap."

It's normal for muscles in the back of the throat to relax and partially collapse when you sleep, says Edmund Pribitkin, M.D., an otolaryngologist at Thomas Jefferson University Hospital. For most guys, this causes nothing worse than a little snoring. In men with sleep apnea, however, the airways may close so much that air can't get through. The resulting apnea, or lack of air flow, can last from about ten seconds to more than a minute.

In addition, they often cause side effects, including a dry mouth and disturbed sleep. As a result, they're rarely used for long, he says.

A newer, more effective technique is called continuous positive airway pressure, or CPAP, in which a jet of air blows into a face mask during sleep. The increased pressure inside the mask forces the upper airway to remain open, which reduces or even eliminates the snoring, says Dr. Frost. Not everyone is enthusiastic about wearing a mask, of course, so this technique isn't for everyone.

"The sleeping brain has a choice to make here: Does it want to go on sleeping and not breathe, or wake up and breathe?" says Dr. Young. "And the organism chooses to breathe over sleep."

In most cases the awakenings are so brief that the man doesn't remember them the next morning. "Believe it or not, people can have literally hundreds of apneic events a night," says Dr. Pribitkin. Sleep studies have shown that some men spend more of their nights not breathing than breathing.

Just because you snore doesn't mean you have sleep apnea. But if you're always feeling run down or your snores are setting off seismic alerts, then you should probably get a checkup. Without treatment sleep apnea can be extremely dangerous, says Dr. Doghramji. "The decreases in oxygen are linked directly to heart rhythm disturbances," he says. "In addition, apnea patients have a higher risk of hypertension, not only during the apnea but during the day as well."

If you share your bed with someone, your partner may be able to help you figure out if you have sleep apnea. If your snoring is interrupted by periods of silence followed by gasps and snorting, you're definitely a candidate.

If you sleep alone, set a voice-activated tape recorder by your bed and let it run all night, Dr. Young suggests. In the morning listen for the pattern of snoring followed by silence followed by gasps for breath. If you hear it, see your doctor.

If the problem is severe, you may need surgery, medications or other treatments in order to correct it. But if your case is not severe, applying the tips for snoring will also help control sleep apnea.

Another option is to have surgery to remove some of the tissue that's causing all the noise in the first place. With lasers, surgeons are able to zap away tissue a little bit at a time. The results are impressive, with about 85 percent of men being cured of snoring and an additional 13 percent showing some improvement, says Dr. Pribitkin. "A person can have the surgery done in the office and go back to work the next day," he says. "It's very effective."

Sore Throat

An Easy Act to Swallow

Finding out what's causing your sore throat is like pointing a finger at the reason behind the national debt: There's no single culprit to blame—and not much chance of escaping it either.

"Sore throats are part of being human. If you're breathing, you're going to get one occasionally," says Eric G. Anderson, M.D., a family physician in La Jolla, California.

That's not particularly comforting when it's *your* throat that feels like it's on the business end of a lit match. But considering what your throat goes through, it's almost surprising that we don't get sore throats more often.

An Easy Target

Overuse—whether from yakking with friends at Friday night poker or belting out Italian arias in the shower—will often leave your throat red and raw. Sore throats can also be caused by allergies, air pollution or breathing in cigarette smoke. Even heartburn—caused by an upwelling of stomach acid into the esophagus—can light your throat on fire.

Perhaps the most common cause of sore throat pain is infection. Unlike other parts of the body, the throat is directly exposed to airborne viruses and bacteria, says Greg Grillone, M.D., an otolaryngologist and director of the Voice Center at Boston University Medical Center.

"One of the primary ways that viruses and bacteria get into our bodies is through the nose and mouth, and both of those openings lead into the throat," Dr. Grillone explains.

Although the throat is normally well-protected against microbial onslaughts, sometimes your resistance is low—because of fatigue, for example, or poor nutrition. The resulting infection can be a tough act to swallow.

You should always see a doctor if your sore throat is accompanied by a rash, earache, discolored mucus, high temperature (over 100°F), chest pain or shortness of breath. In most cases, however, sore throats can be eased—or prevented—with simple home treatments. Here's what doctors recommend.

FAST FACTS

How common: Virtually every man will get a sore throat at some time in his life.

Risk factors: Sore throats frequently accompany upper respiratory infections like a cold or flu. Smoking, allergies, air pollution or excessive yelling or talking can also make your throat sore.

Age group affected: Sore throats can occur at all ages. If you're over age 40 and have a sore throat for more than a week, you should see a doctor to make sure it's not something more serious.

Gender gap: Because more men than women smoke cigarettes, they also get more sore throats.

Who to see: Family doctor or otolaryngologist.

Crank up the humidity. Air conditioners and home heating systems dry the air, which can make your throat feel scratchy and irritated, says Bradley M. Block, M.D., a family physician in private practice in Winter Park, Florida. Occasionally opening a window about an inch when using your air conditioner will help boost humidity to comfortable levels, he says. Or plug in a humidifier to replenish soothing, moisture-laden air to your throat's tender tissues.

Grab the aspirin. "If a guy who is otherwise feeling fine has what seems to be a minor sore throat, then taking two aspirin or acetaminophen tablets up to four times a day may relieve the discomfort," Dr. Anderson says. An alternative to swallowing the tablets is to crush and then mix them in six ounces of water, gargle with the mixture and then swallow the gargle.

Reach for the lozenges. When sore throats strike, over-the-counter lozenges containing a mild anesthetic such as benzocaine may help you cope until the pain and swelling subside, Dr. Anderson says.

Lozenges made from slippery elm, available in health food stores and some drugstores, will also help soothe irritated tissues.

Taste sweet relief. Putting a dab of honey on the back of your tongue will cause the thick, soothing liquid to glide across your irritated throat like a slow-moving waterfall, Dr. Anderson says.

Log some pillow time. The energy it takes to fight a sore throat has been likened to taking a 40-mile hike with a 40-pound backpack. To help your body fight off the infection, you have to rest, says Hinda Greene, D.O., an internal medicine and emergency medicine physician at Cleveland Clinic Hospital in Fort Lauderdale, Florida.

Getting even one extra hour of sleep a night may be all you need, she adds.

Let the liquids flow. Drinking at least one eight-ounce glass of water every hour will help relieve swelling and keep the raspy areas lubricated, Dr. Greene says.

Take some tea. Gargling with tea—brewed at double strength and allowed to cool to lukewarm temperature—once every 15 minutes will provide fast relief. "Tea contains tannic acid, which helps soothe the throat," says Dr. Greene. "It won't kill any germs, but it can help your throat feel better."

Snort some salt. Plunging your nose into a saltwater solution and sniffing the fluid so it drips down the back of your throat may provide fast relief, says Dr. Anderson. Gargling can also help, although sniffing may be better because it allows the fluid to penetrate farther into the throat, he says.

To make the solution, mix one level teaspoon of salt in a six-ounce glass of warm water. Bend over a sink, pour some of the water into your cupped hand and sniff up a small amount. Dr. Anderson recommends sniffing salt water three times a day for three days. Then taper off to once or twice a day until your throat starts feeling better.

Let others do the cheering. Yelling is hard work, and your throat deserves some R and R. So while you're recovering from a sore throat, give your voice a break. Cut back on talking, singing, cheering, even whispering, Dr. Grillone says.

Go easy on the hooch. If you're recovering from a sore throat, it's advisable to lay off of alcoholic beverages completely. It can exacerbate the soreness and the inflammation of the throat.

Pack it in. Smoke—whether it's from your own cigarette or secondhand from someone else's—will quickly irritate and inflame the throat's lining. Smokers are far more likely than nonsmokers to have chronic throat irritation, says Bruce Campbell, M.D., an otolaryngologist at the Medical College of Wisconsin in Milwaukee.

Think zinc. One study found that zinc gluconate tablets can help relieve sore throat and other cold symptoms. To be effective, however, they have to dissolve slowly in your mouth; chomping and swallowing won't help. "The trick is to let the dissolved zinc bathe your throat for a while," says Donald Davis, Ph.D., a researcher at the Clayton Foundation Biochemical Institute at the University of Texas at Austin.

Keep up your strength. Good nutrition helps fuel your immune system when you need it most, says Dr. Greene. She recommends eating at least five servings a day of fruits and vegetables, six servings of whole grains, two servings of dairy products and two servings of fish or poultry.

If your throat is so sore that you can't bear to swallow food, try drinking four to five cans of liquid nutritional supplements such as Meritene or Gainer's Fuel 1000 or instant breakfast drinks such as Carnation Instant Breakfast. In addition, increase your intake of clear liquids, like tea, apple juice or water.

Elevate your bed. If you typically wake up with a sore throat—and it's not sore at other times of the day—you may be suffering from acid reflux, an upsurge of throat-searing stomach acid that occurs during sleep. Adjusting your bed frame so the head is elevated four to six inches higher than the foot will put gravity on your side and help keep the acid down, Dr. Campbell says.

Look for yeast. Some guys will occasionally get a sore throat after engaging in oral sex. If this happens to you, you may have a yeast infection, says Dr. Anderson.

He recommends using a shaving mirror to examine the inside of your mouth and throat. If you see what appear to be small white patches of wet tissue paper stuck in your cheeks, mouth or throat, you could have an infection and should see a doctor. Fortunately, yeast infections like this are rare and typically occur in men who already have weakened immune systems.

Sperm Problems

Breeding Healthy Habits

You'd think that evolution would have favored a method of human conception that was easy, efficient and fail-safe, but it ain't necessarily so. Consider these numbers.

From puberty until old age a man's testicles produce about 50,000 sperm each minute. An average ejaculation contains 200 million of the little tadpoles. That should be more than enough to take care of business, yet once deposited in the female's vagina, only 400 sperm ever reach the vicinity of an egg. And of those, only one has even a 15 percent chance in any given month of actually hitting the target.

With those odds, it's a miracle anyone gets pregnant. Make the odds even tougher by throwing a glitch of some kind into the works and you have one of the more wrenching dilemmas a couple can face: infertility.

If you and your mate have been having unprotected sex for more than six months and still haven't conceived, you have what the doctors define as a fertility problem. There are three main areas of concern if the problem's yours, or partly yours: the number of sperm you're ejaculating (your sperm count), the shape of your sperm (their morphology) and the ability of your sperm to swim in a prompt and orderly fashion toward their goal (their motility). Every man's sperm count varies from month to month, and every man is going to have plenty of sperm that are deformed or that don't move properly. In fact, if 60 percent of your sperm are normal on all scores, you're doing fine.

Born to Breed

Much of what determines your breeding power is out of your control, fixed by genetics, but there are steps you can take to enhance the health of your sperm.

Look for trouble. You may be able to tell if you have the leading cause of male infertility—a varicocele—with a quick self-examination, according to Eugene Stulberger, M.D., a specialist in male infertility at St. Barnabas Medical Center in Livingston, New Jersey. A varicocele is an enlarged blood vessel in the scrotum. It impedes the flow of blood there, causing the temperature of the testicles to rise enough to damage sperm.

FAST FACTS

How common: Between two million and three million men in the United States are thought to have some sort of sperm problem.

Risk factors: Injuries to the testicles, poor health habits, genetics.

Age group affected: Although men can father children well into old age, fertility gradually declines beginning at about age 40.

Gender gap: Approximately 15 percent of all couples have fertility problems. About 50 percent of the time, the man is partially or fully responsible.

Who to see: Urologist who specializes in male fertility problems.

To locate a varicocele, stand up, preferably after a shower, when your testicles are warm and thus hanging loose from your body. Because of the structure of the veins in the testicles, varicoceles are far more likely to occur on the left side than the right, says Marc Goldstein, M.D., professor of urology and director of the Center for Male Reproductive Medicine and Microsurgery at the New York Hospital–Cornell Medical Center in New York City. Feel in the scrotum above the testicle and look for a soft, mushy "bag of worms." Straining downward as though trying to have a bowel movement may cause a varicocele to bulge out, making it easier to detect.

If you do detect one, don't worry. It's easily corrected with a short operation performed in the hospital or in an outpatient clinic, according to Dr. Stulberger.

Hang loose, stay cool. The testicles hang free from the body of the human male for a reason: If they're going to produce sperm, they need to remain about four degrees cooler than body temperature. Heat-avoiding techniques listed by Dr. Goldstein include staying away from long, hot baths and hot tubs, wearing loose-fitting underwear and pants and, if you're very overweight, losing weight so that your testicles aren't surrounded by fat.

Watch your diet. Although research hasn't confirmed it definitively, many doctors feel men may enhance the health of their sperm by consuming certain vitamins. Larry L. Lipshultz, M.D., professor of urology at the Baylor College of Medicine in Houston, stresses the importance of adequate vitamins C and E and beta-carotene, because they're "scavengers" of oxidants, which are naturally produced toxic elements that can damage sperm. Dr. Goldstein also recommends the mineral zinc, which is beneficial for the prostate, where the seminal fluid is produced.

The best way to get these sperm-protecting nutrients into your system is by eating at least two fruits and three vegetables a day. Dr. Goldstein also recommends a multivitamin/mineral supplement containing at least 20 milligrams of zinc.

Take it easy. Another commonsense suggestion many doctors offer their patients is to deal effectively with stress, which would include exercising moderately. "Stress affects the whole body," says Dr. Goldstein, "so it would surprise me if it did not have an impact on fertility."

Quit smoking, period. Nicotine lowers your sperm count and damages sperm's morphology and motility, according to Machelle Seibel, M.D., medical director of the Faulkner Centre for Reproductive Medicine in Boston. Studies have also shown that male smokers' sperm are less able to penetrate eggs than nonsmokers' sperm; that pregnancies conceived by men who smoke are more likely to miscarry than pregnancies conceived by nonsmokers; and that smoking causes chromosome damage in sperm that could potentially be passed on to children in the form of birth defects or cancer.

Stock up on C. If you're still battling to quit smoking but haven't yet taken your final drag, you might want to consider vitamin C supplements. One study at the University of Texas Medical Branch at Galveston compared the ejaculate of heavy smokers who took vitamin C supplements to that of puffers who didn't. The men taking the supplements not only had 34 percent more sperm, but the little rogues were noticeably healthier and more mobile. The supplements that were taken dished up 1,000 milligrams of vitamin C a day—that's equivalent to 13 white or 11 pink grapefruit, more than most of us are likely to get in our diets.

Ban the booze. Alcohol not only decreases sperm production, according to Dr. Goldstein, it can also worsen the effects of a varicocele. He advises cutting back to two drinks a week.

Watch your exposure. Lead and radiation have been shown to have at least temporary effects on male fertility, according to Dr. Lipshultz. Check your drinking water to be sure it's lead-free, although significant exposure through drinking water alone is unlikely. Also, when you're having x-rays, make sure the protective apron covers your testicles.

Peruse your prescriptions. Some medications for high blood pressure, inflammatory bowel disease, ulcers and gout have been linked to male infertility. So have some antibiotics. Safe alternative drugs are usually available. Ask your doctor.

Sports Injuries

Teaching Your Body Teamwork

On the sporting fields of youth, we all learned the value of teamwork. Coaches drilled into us the importance of every player's role, regardless of size or position. And we knew if any player didn't do his part—or tried to do too much—it could cause a setback for the entire team, maybe even cost us the game.

Well, consider your body as a sports team: A collection of professional nerves, ligaments, muscles, vessels, bones and a brain working together for a common goal, be it the next touchdown or the next set of reps on the circuit trainer. Each of those body parts plays an important role in reaching that goal. When one part doesn't play that role—or tries to do too much—you could end up injured. And if you don't train properly, your team could lose some serious yardage in the big game of health and fitness.

Making a Joint Effort

Most men think of sports injuries as something you get from full-contact rugby, but you can easily suffer one during a leisurely nine holes of golf or a moderate workout at the gym, too.

"The fact is, most sports injuries are noncontact injuries," says Fred Allman, M.D., director of the Atlanta Sports Medicine Clinic. "They mostly come from overuse of a specific part of your body, improper technique or undertraining." More often than not, these injuries occur around the body's numerous vulnerable areas, like the joints—ankles, knees, hips, shoulders and elbows especially. There, the cartilage, ligaments, tendons and muscles all are making sure this bone is connected to that bone. It's a complex junction that can be thrown out of whack without much provocation.

"Take the knee, for example," says Dr. Allman. "With the quadriceps and the hamstrings there, you have muscles that protect the knee joint, that absorb force. But if the muscles are weak, the force is absorbed by the underlying tissue, then by the bone itself." In other words, everything is connected. Once one part goes, the rest can go down like bowling pins—and take you along with them.

485

The Muscles: Stay Warm and Loose

With a little teamwork and a good game strategy you can condition your body's systems against injury. The first place you should focus on is the muscular system and underlying connective tissues—the ligaments and tendons that anchor the muscles to each other and your skeleton. These players are the cornerstone of your team; they do most of the work and take nearly all of the punishment during physical activity. Here are some methods for training your body to go the distance, along with some simple remedies in case you have to drop out of the game. For more details see "Muscle Aches and Pains" on page 362.

Warm up before a workout. Regardless of your chosen sport or form of exercise, take at least five minutes beforehand to warm up.

"Your muscles are cold when you start to exercise," points out Gary Gordon, D.P.M., director of the running and walking program at the University of Pennsylvania Sports Medicine Clinic in Philadelphia. If you start playing or exercising too vigorously, those cold muscles and tendons could snap like brittle sticks of gum. "Do some light exercise for five minutes first—something like biking or walking or jogging," suggests Dr. Gordon. This gets blood flowing through the tissues more, literally warming them up and making them more flexible.

Stretch out. Once you've warmed up, you'll be supple enough for a little stretching. "Otherwise, you'll have tight muscles. They'll have to work harder—and they'll end up fatiguing faster," says Dr. Allman. These stretches can be as simple as touching your toes or reaching for the ceiling. For more elaborate stretching exercises check your local gym or sports facility, which usually posts such information. And when you're finished with whatever activity you're pursuing, don't forget to do a little homestretch before you hit the showers.

"It's almost more important to do your stretching after your workout," says Dr. Gordon. "It not only keeps your muscles supple, but also prevents soreness the next day." When you do stretch, take your time. Short or jerky stretching motions will do ligaments and tendons more harm than good, so stretch slowly and fully, giving the muscles and underlying tissues plenty of time to extend.

Get in training. Regardless of what sport you play, don't rely on it as your sole form of exercise. For at least 20 to 30 minutes two to three times per week, get off the field and into the gym. "The best way you can protect yourself from most sports injuries is through strength training and exercise programs," says Mike Nishihara, director of athletic development for the National Institute for Fitness and Sports in Indianapolis, and a strength and conditioning specialist.

"With strength training we're talking about a relatively modest number of repetitions of fairly significant weight, be it machine or free weights," says Bob Cantu,

FAST FACTS

How common: Virtually every man who exercises will suffer some type of sports injury.

Risk factors: Guys who suddenly get on an exercise kick—after being a couch potato for months—are most likely to try to do too much too soon. In general, any man who doesn't train or exercise properly for his particular activity will tend to get injured.

Age group affected: Active men between the ages of 20 and 40 suffer sport-related injuries the most.

Gender gap: Because of an overly aggressive attitude toward sports and exercise—and the sheer number of male-dominated sports—men suffer sports injuries at least twice as much as women.

Who to see: Family doctor, sports physician, exercise therapist.

M.D., past president of the American College of Sports Medicine and a sports physician in Concord, Massachusetts. Dr. Cantu suggests working on the 7-11 principle: Start at a weight that you can lift at least 7 repetitions. "When you get to 11 reps, increase the weight by about five pounds and lift that for as many reps as you can. If you can't do more than seven, then go back and increase the weight by only two or three pounds," says Dr. Cantu.

The point is to strengthen connections in your body. That way, ligaments and tendons will be less likely to tear during high-speed twists and turns. Plus, you want to condition all the muscle systems in your body equally, not bulk up. "In fact, that would hurt you in sports where you need fine motor control, like baseball or the racquet sports," warns Dr. Cantu.

Accentuate the abs. And when you do work out, be sure to pay special attention to your abdominal muscles.

"Most guys don't work these out enough," says Nishihara. "But you use your abdominals in almost every activity there is." Try to work a few extra crunches or situps into every workout. "Stronger abdominals will not only help your performance, they'll also help prevent lower back injuries, too," Nishihara adds.

Go through the motions. Be fluid in your exercising or sporting techniques. Avoid short or jerky motions. Since these create shock waves that your body has to absorb, you're causing unnecessary wear and tear—particularly to joints and connective tissues. Before you begin your activity, ask an expert—be it the head trainer

(continued on page 490)

Casualty Chart

From the ground up, here's a rundown of the most common sports injuries, plus some quick tips for avoiding the agony of defeat—or just plain agony.

Injury	How You Get It	How You Avoid It
Foot swelling	Running, walking	Wear shoes with good arch support or orthotic inserts
Ankle sprain	Basketball, running, racquet sports	Keep ankle strong and flexible; Run on even surfaces
Achilles tendinitis	Running, walking	Wear shoes with proper heel support; Stretch regularly
Shin splints	Running, walking	Strengthen lower leg muscles with heel and toe raises; Run on soft surfaces
Knee strain	Running, cycling, swimming	Strengthen knee and thigh muscles with stretching and weight training; Wear cushioned shoes
Pulled hamstring	Basketball, racquet sports, running, cycling	Warm up hamstring muscles with leg curls
Groin pull	Basketball, running, skating	Side and hip stretches; Avoid sudden lateral moves where practical
Back strain	Basketball, racquet sports, cycling, golf and situps	Stretching; Stomach crunches to strengthen abdominal muscles
Shoulder pull	Baseball, racquet sports, golf, swimming	Stretching; Strengthen shoulders with rowing exercise
Elbow tendinitis	Baseball, racquet sports, golf, swimming	Use proper technique and equipment; Wrist curls to strengthen elbow muscles; Brace or splint to support previous injuries

How to Treat It

Rest, ice, anti-inflammatory painkillers; Do toe exercises such as scrunching a towel with your toes

Wear a brace or high-top sneakers for support of previous injuries; Rest, ice, compression, elevation

Rest, ice, over-the-counter painkillers

Rest, ice, over-the-counter painkillers

Rest, ice, compression, elevation

Rest, ice, heat

Rest, ice, heat

Rest, ice, heat; See a doctor if there is any numbness or tingling

Rest, ice, over-the-counter painkillers

Rest, ice, over-the-counter painkillers

at the gym or your club's golf pro—to watch your biomechanics, or the fluidity of your form. A sports doctor will also be able to give you a physical that will include a full biomechanical evaluation.

Got pain? Abstain. If you feel any pain during an exercise, be it a sharp tingling or a constant throbbing, stop what you're doing.

"The concept of 'no pain, no gain' is all wrong," says Dr. Cantu. "Soreness after an exercise is one thing. But if you're feeling pain during an exercise, then it's absolutely essential to stop and figure out what's wrong before you make the injury worse," he says.

Get wild about R.I.C.E. If you do pull, strain or sprain something, you'll know it pretty quickly. Symptoms like throbbing, swelling and tenderness are all classic signs of a sports injury.

Ironically, swelling is actually your body's idea of helping the injury. "Once there's an injury, the body sends in blood and fluids to begin repairs," says Dr. Allman. But swelling often is an overreaction that makes you feel anything but swell. Unless it's kept to a minimum, inflammation reduces your mobility and can keep you sidelined even after the pain of the injury goes away. But you can alleviate swelling by making it harder for the body to send in the fluids.

"The classic remedy is R.I.C.E.—rest, ice, compression and elevation," says Stephen Nicholas, M.D., associate team physician for the New York Jets professional football team and associate director of the Nicholas Institute of Sports Medicine and Athletic Trauma. Besides the obvious need for rest, ice shrinks swelling; compression—in the form of an elastic bandage, for instance—keeps blood and fluids from rushing into the injured area, preventing even more swelling. Finally, elevating the injured area above your heart stops swelling even more. "Do this for a couple of days," says Dr. Nicholas. And don't try to exercise the injured area. "You'll just make it worse, and turn a two- or three-day recovery time into two or three weeks."

Ask for anti-inflammatories. In addition to the R.I.C.E. method you can dull some of the pain with anti-inflammatories, like aspirin or ibuprofen. "Two tablets a couple times a day should help with the pain, as well as reduce swelling at the site of the injury," says Dr. Nicholas.

Turn up the heat. For muscle spasms—a common result of overworking the muscle—apply a little heat. "Moist heat is best," says Dr. Nicholas. "Wrap a warm, wet towel or a heating pad around the area." Keep it there for ten minutes and repeat as needed. Caution: Do not use heat if you have a significant amount of acute swelling. "That will just make the inflammation worse," says Dr. Nicholas.

The Skeleton: Bones Need Exercise, Too

No amount of stretching and toning will do you much good if your muscles and connective tissues don't have a solid foundation. That's where the skeletal sys-

Shoeing Injury Away

Clothes may make the man, but shoes make or break the athlete.

That's a fact often lost amid commercials that emphasize name brands, professional athletes and whether or not the shoes pump up or light up. In this world of $100 footwear sooner or later we have to wonder whether our flashy sneaks will really improve our performance any more than the old canvas high-tops we wore as kids.

Actually, they will—assuming you buy them for the right reasons. "Some of the features of these shoes are gimmicks, it's true. But good shoes are vital to avoiding injury and maintaining a peak level of performance," says Gary Gordon, D.P.M., director of the running and walking program at the University of Pennsylvania Sports Medicine Clinic in Philadelphia.

The key features to bear in mind, Dr. Gordon says, are not the pump-action of the shoe, nor its space-age design. Rather, there are two, and only two, crucial issues: support and shock absorption. Without these your body will bear more stress during exercise, something to avoid in any activity.

If your activity involves a lot of running and walking, Dr. Gordon suggests looking for a runner's shoe with loads of shock absorption in the tread. If there's lots of stopping and starting, as in basketball or volleyball, it's especially important to have both support and shock absorption. Dr. Gordon suggests a high-top shoe to support your ankles, but be sure it absorbs shock well, too.

Finally, you should change your shoes every four months—sooner if you work out every day. "You won't see it, but the shock-absorbing material in the shoe will break down by then," says Dr. Gordon. "When your shoe doesn't absorb impact anymore, that force will start taking a toll on your body."

tem comes in. Like any good foundation, the bones in your skeleton should be plenty strong and solid. But even the best-laid foundation can sometimes crack under too much pressure. Where your bones are concerned, sports injuries break down into two categories: the contact fracture and the stress fracture.

"Most fractures have obvious signs," says David Janda, M.D., director of the Institute for Preventative Sports Medicine in Ann Arbor, Michigan. "Of course, there will be pain and limited mobility, and chances are you'll notice something is obviously crooked." In that case, try not to move the suspected fracture too much and get to a hospital.

Stress fractures are trickier to spot. As the term suggests, stress fractures are brought about by repeated stress and force being applied to the bone. "Ultimately, the force overpowers the bone, and it will crack," says Dr. Janda. "But it may not be readily apparent." So here are some tips for dealing with potential fractures—and strengthening your foundation overall.

Call for calcium. To begin with, make sure you're getting plenty of calcium, an important mineral for strengthening bones—most guys need about one gram per day. You can find calcium in virtually any dairy product. One cup of nonfat yogurt, for example, will give you almost half your daily calcium requirement.

Exercise your bones. Weight-bearing exercise—for the legs, that means any exercise in which you are on your feet—helps strengthen bones by building up bone mass. So if all of your exercise is done on a weight bench, your leg bones might not be as built up as they should be to absorb tackles in a football game.

Wear a helmet. Skull fractures are about the most dangerous of breaks—and thanks to an increasing interest in high-velocity sports, like cycling and skating, they're unfortunately becoming more common. In bicycling alone, experts reckon you're four to seven times more likely to suffer a serious head injury if you're not wearing a helmet. So wear one.

Spot stress indicators. Stress fractures cause more pain than swelling, says Dr. Janda. "If you feel a constant, steady pain—not soreness—about an hour after an activity, get it looked at," he says. Common areas for stress fractures include the feet and legs, since bones there absorb a force equivalent to three times your body weight every time you run.

Bone up on rest. The good news about a stress fracture is that you probably won't need a huge, cumbersome cast. The bad news is you will need to rest that bone. Experts say you should avoid any exercise with it for a couple of months. After that, your doctor can give you a support brace or bandage to help the injured bone while you resume your favorite sport.

Circulation: Having a Good Heart

Most men don't think of their hearts and blood vessels as potential candidates for a sports injury, but they can be. If it's not in shape, your cardiovascular system can make you weak and expose you to sports injuries elsewhere in the body.

"If your system isn't trained to deal with the metabolic demand of exercise, you're looking at a host of problems, from high blood pressure to a heart attack," says Dr. Nicholas. Of course, anyone with existing heart and circulatory problems shouldn't be doing any exercise without his doctor's supervision. Otherwise, here are some tips for toning your ticker.

Adopt aerobics. Probably the best thing you can do for your heart is an aerobic workout for a minimum of 20 minutes three times a week. "The ideal aerobic exercises for your cardiovascular system are those that are rhythmic and nonstop," says Dr. Cantu. "Swimming, cycling, jogging—even brisk walking—are good examples."

Forgo fat. If you want to be a lean, mean, fightin' machine, focus on the "lean" part. Eat fatty foods sparingly. Otherwise, large amounts of fat and cholesterol can build up in your arteries, restricting blood flow and creating coronary disease—the biggest killer of men around.

Quit smoking. If you smoke, stop it. In addition to causing cancer, smoking decreases oxygen flow to the body, will drastically cut into your athletic performance and puts an enormous strain on your heart.

Breathing: Lungs That Last

Your lungs are just as important as your heart—without oxygen we can't live, let alone exercise. As with other parts of your body, you can train your lungs to do a better job and help you stay in the game longer without getting winded.

Take a deep breath. Aerobic exercise is as good for the lungs as it is for the heart, says Dr. Cantu. "Any exercise that causes you to breathe deeply—but not so deeply that you can't still carry on a conversation—is good."

Don't swallow—inhale. When you're doing that deep breathing, make sure you're inhaling the air. If you're gulping it like a fish, then you're swallowing air, which does nothing to train your lungs. Plus, you'll probably develop a sidestitch— that white-hot pain you sometimes feel in your sides from working out too hard. That won't help your game average either.

Go for a dip. In addition to your usual workout, throw in a half-hour of swimming now and again. You get plenty of aerobic benefits, plus, working out in the water will help you increase your lung capacity even more.

Be alert to asthma and allergies. Many men can develop exercise-induced asthma, a devilish respiratory problem that leaves you gasping for breath any time you start a vigorous activity. Other signs of asthma include dizziness, shallow breathing and a dry, hacking cough when you exercise.

"This kind of sports-induced ailment is not something to deal with on your own—you really need to see a pulmonologist or an allergist," says Dr. Janda. Most bouts of exercise-induced asthma can be controlled through prescription medications that open asthmatic airways. Since allergies often can trigger asthma attacks, an allergist also can help you determine what you're allergic to, so you can avoid exposure before or during a workout.

Digestion: Food Makes the Athlete

Regrettably, unless your name is Popeye, there are no miracle foods for building up muscles or instantly giving tendons the tensile strength of bridge cables. Nevertheless, your diet is an important part of avoiding sports injuries.

"If you don't have a healthy diet, it's going to affect every part of your body," says Becky Zimmerman, R.D., staff dietitian at The National Institute for Fitness and Sport in Indianapolis. "Your muscles won't have enough fuel, your cardiovascular system won't work as well, your body won't be as strong and you'll be more susceptible to injury."

That diet should include plenty of grains, fruits and vegetables, with only a modicum of meats and dairy products. And athletes may benefit from particular emphasis on these forms of fuel.

Count on carbos. Complex carbohydrates are the preferred gas to put in your tank on a daily basis. "We need the calories from complex carbohydrates to fuel the muscles as well as make repairs," says Zimmerman. Cereals, rice and pasta are terrific examples of carbohydrate sources.

Ask for antioxidants. Many fruits and vegetables contain antioxidants, vitamins and minerals that help neutralize cancer-causing particles as well as improve circulation. "Antioxidants may even reduce recovery time from injuries," says Zimmerman. You'll find antioxidants in most plant foods including a variety of fruits, vegetables and whole grains. Good choices include dark green and orange vegetables and fruits, like squash, peppers, carrots, citrus fruits, peaches and—Popeye had the right idea—spinach.

Drink heavily. Drink fluids often and early; before, during and after exercise. "A lot of people don't drink enough fluids when they work out," warns Dr. Gordon. Because you're sweating out so much fluid during exercise, that puts you in danger of dehydration, which will lead to fatigue, cramps, dizziness and potential injury. Experts recommend drinking 8 to 12 eight-ounce cups of fluid a day. "The bulk of that should be water," says Zimmerman. During exercise drink a half-cup for every 10 to 15 minutes of activity.

And during your activity, avoid any beverages that contain caffeine or alcohol. "These are natural diuretics—they'll cause you to lose even more fluid," says Dr. Gordon. Plus, alcohol's judgment-impairing effects make it that much easier for you to fall prey to a sports injury that will put you off the team—and maybe even bench you for good.

Stress

What to Do When It's Hammer Time

As an angry young man in 1964, John Lennon complained, "It's been a hard day's night, and I've been working like a dog." Every stressed-out guy knows the feeling. But as a middle-age husband and father 16 years later the former Beatle was singing a different tune. In "Beautiful Boy," one of the last songs he recorded before he was cut down by an assassin's bullet, Lennon sang, "Life is what happens to you while you're busy making other plans."

"It's a wonderful line," says Stephan Rechtschaffen, M.D., president of the Omega Institute in Rhinebeck, New York, which teaches healthy relaxation techniques. What Lennon came to realize is the central point espoused by physicians and psychologists who work with patients whose lives have blurred into a hard day's night of unrelenting stress: You have to live in the present. With all due apologies to President Bill Clinton, Fleetwood Mac was wrong. You *should* stop thinking about tomorrow. Because that's what causes 99 percent of today's stress, says Dr. Rechtschaffen.

"In the present moment there is no stress," he says. It's only when we start worrying about what else we have to do and what others will think about what we're doing that we feel stressed out.

Defining the Terms

"One definition is that stress is simply energy, but it's more energy than you can use now," says Neil Fiore, Ph.D., a psychologist in Berkeley, California, and author of *The Now Habit: A Strategic Program for Overcoming Procrastination and Enjoying Guilt-Free Play*. "Technically, then, when you have the appropriate level of energy in the present, there is no stress."

Most men suffering from stress are either overly anxious about the future or shackled by past failures and disappointments. To keep their bodies' natural stress-response systems from overheating, they must free their minds from the guilt and regret of the past or potential dangers in the future, and focus on what they can do now, Dr. Fiore says.

Everyone has stressors—things that make them uptight—in their daily lives. A

Burnout: How to Keep the Flames Alive

It's hard to even remember now, but years ago, you took the job because you wanted to make a difference. You may be a lawyer or a police officer; a doctor or a nurse; a teacher or a journalist; a minister or a social worker.

Now, that youthful idealism has been replaced by stinging sarcasm and constant complaining. You're often late for work, and when you do show up, you spend much of your time daydreaming. Feelings of hopelessness and help-lessness overwhelm you. Day after day, you go through the motions in what you now see as a meaningless job.

You're burned out. And it probably happened so gradually, you don't even realize it. "It's a slow bleed," says Ronald Nathan, Ph.D., professor of family practice at Albany Medical College in New York and author of *Coping with the Stressed-Out People in Your Life*. "Sometimes, people who are burning out think, 'If I just work harder and do a little more.' It's sort of like, 'Walk on the water one more time.' And that can be very self-defeating."

Stephan Rechtschaffen, M.D., president of the Omega Institute in Rhinebeck, New York, which teaches healthy relaxation techniques, says idealis-tic people are especially prone to burnout because they are inherently unhappy with the way things are in the present. "They start with a strong belief that they can change the future. And that's a very positive, wonderful human trait. But it's not very accepting of the way things are right now," he says.

Because the present moment never measures up to their idealized version of the future, they grow tired and disillusioned. "You're going to burn out," Dr. Rechtschaffen says. "You have to burn out."

The difference between being stressed out and burned out is when hope and energy disappear, Dr. Nathan says.

"The shift occurs when there's no longer that excitement and hope that you're going to overcome it," he says. "It's really giving up on the show. It's the shift where you're not fighting anymore. You have nothing left to give and you're exhausted."

Dr. Nathan says nurturing the self with the stress management techniques outlined in this chapter can help bring someone back from burnout. The key, Dr. Rechtschaffen says, is for a burnout victim to make peace with the present. "People have to be able to accept the fact that the present moment is the way the present moment is," he says.

FAST FACTS

How common: Up to 90 percent of office visits to primary-care physicians stem from stress-related complaints, some experts believe. Surveys have found that nine out of ten American adults experience "high levels of stress" at least once or twice a week, with more than a quarter complaining of stress on a daily basis.

Risk factors: One in four of us are "genetically predisposed" to abnormally high stress responses. Perceived pressures from society, parents, children, mates, employers all can generate stress.

Age group affected: All age groups are affected. Studies have shown middle-aged men are particularly prone to hypertension and sudden death from heart attack as a result of stress.

Gender gap: Stress afflicts everyone, but experts say men tend to have fewer coping skills to deal with it.

Who to see: If stress is interfering with your home or professional life, see your family physician, psychiatrist, or a psychologist.

demanding job or obnoxious boss. Tight deadlines. Tighter finances. Family obligations and problems. Car troubles. Junk mail. Telephones, fax machines and beepers. But stress isn't an outside force that invades your life. "Stress comes from within," says Richard E. Collins, M.D., director of the Heart Institute in Omaha, Nebraska.

"Some people can have a lot of stressors, but not really experience stress because of how they perceive those stressors and how they respond to them, adds Jennifer Abel, Ph.D., a psychologist with Psychiatric Consultants in St. Louis.

Not everyone reacts—either physically or mentally—to stressful situations in the same way. From a psychological viewpoint, Dr. Collins says it is helpful to think of stress as a hammer. "Some people are made out of glass, and when it strikes, they're permanently destroyed. Some people are a piece of wood. When the hammer strikes, they're dented, it leaves a mark, but it's survivable. The third type of person is basically a pillow. (The hammer) strikes, but the pillow fluffs up and is ready to take the next strike."

The good news, Dr. Collins and other experts say, is that how people manage the psychological impact of stress is primarily a learned response. "It can be unlearned," he says.

Shocking the Monkey

What most of us experience as stress is perfectly natural. The human body, when it perceives a threat, reacts by releasing stress hormones—particularly adrenaline—into the system. The body goes on red alert for danger, and it makes no difference whether that danger is an oncoming train or a fast-approaching deadline. "It's not as though we're facing immediate physical harm, yet our bodies keep responding as though we are," says Ronald Nathan, Ph.D., professor of family practice at Albany Medical College in New York and co-author of *Coping with the Stressed-Out People in Your Life.* "That's why we get stress-related disorders."

Stress exacts a terrible toll on the human body. It has been linked to virtually every modern malady, from acne to the common cold, from temporomandibular disorder to sperm problems, from high blood pressure to sudden death from heart attack. Some people have a "genetic predisposition" to overreact when confronted with stressful situations, says Dr. Collins. Their bodies send out abnormally high levels of stress hormones and their coronary arteries constrict, cutting down the flow of blood to their hearts. Their pulse rates increase and their blood pressure rises.

"One in four of us really overreacts and sends out a four-alarm fire signal when there's really just smoldering embers," Dr. Collins says. "They're walking around with an adrenaline high and they never come down off of it. It's kind of like those studies in the 1950s, where we shocked the bottom of a monkey's cage and then stopped doing it. The monkey goes in the back of the cage, scanning the environment, waiting for the next shock that never happens. But he eventually withers up and dies of coronary heart disease because he's constantly under the threat of stress."

You don't have to let stress make a monkey out of you. Here are some ideas to help you become de-stressed, instead of increasingly distressed.

Focus on the big picture. You're on your deathbed. As you look back on your life, what are your final thoughts? "I wish I had made more money, and I wish I had worked harder." Or, "I wish I had spent more time with my family and more time fishing." Dr. Abel asks some of her stressed-out patients to ponder the deathbed scenario to help them figure out what really matters in their lives. "Just about everybody will say, 'Gee, I think that on my deathbed I would be thinking, I wish I spent more time fishing and spent more time with my family.' That sometimes will help people do more of those things, and that will reduce their stress."

There's no point waiting until your life is almost over to figure out how you want to live it. Make that your top priority, says Dr. Rechtschaffen. "If you have absolute clarity about who you are, what you want and what you need to do to get there, then you have a clear perspective about what's important in your life," Dr. Rechtschaffen says. Take time to write down your priorities and what you like to do.

the male file

Caffeine in large doses can be lethal. Having ten grams—about 100 cups of coffee—in four hours can kill the average person.

Know the time. If you feel like there aren't enough hours in the day, it's time to look at what you're doing with them. Write out a schedule for a full week, covering all 24 hours each day. Mark out the hours for sleep, commuting, work and necessary chores, such as shopping and doing laundry. What's left is *your* time. The question is how you're using it. Be honest. How much television do you watch? Get a realistic picture of how you spend each day, and then pull out your list of priorities and things you like to do. Compare the two lists and see if the way you're using your time reflects your priorities.

"I talk about the importance of fighting for time to be with your kids for half an hour, time for yourself to exercise for an hour, time for yourself to read for half an hour, time for yourself to have a decent, civilized meal without interruption for at least half an hour, three times a day," advises Dr. Fiore.

The schedule is only meant to be a snapshot that shows what you're doing with your time. Don't fall into the trap of trying to devise the perfect schedule, with every minute of every day accounted for. Life doesn't work that way. Setting an inflexible schedule will only lead to more stress when unforeseen events occur.

Don't play G.I. Joe. The U.S. Army, in its highly successful advertising campaign, exhorts us to "Be all that you can be." Hogwash, says Dr. Fiore. "You cannot be all that you can be at every given moment," he says. "And that actually becomes counterproductive. My message to some of my stressed-out clients is you don't have to be all that you can be. You don't have to have everything that you want. You don't have to have fun. You don't need to be optimizing every moment of your time."

Don't bite off more than you can chew. It may be a cliché, but it's true. "If you have a list of things you have to do this week, don't try to get them all done the first day," says Dr. Abel. "I think that's what people try to do. They think about everything they have to do in the whole week on the first day of the week. Break it down into reasonable steps of one day at a time."

Exercise. Walk. Jog. Play tennis. The important thing is to do something to flush those stress hormones out of your system. Exercise burns off the adrenaline released into your system and releases endorphins, natural chemicals that relieve pain and produce a feeling of well-being. Studies have shown exercise to be one of the most reliable stressbusters.

Don't be a stress magnet. In a sense, stress is contagious. If you're living or working with a stressed-out person, Dr. Nathan warns, "their stress can become your stress." And the way men respond to stressed-out people often serves to escalate the problem. If someone yells at you, you yell back. Next time try to be a calming influence. If your boss is agitated and screaming at you, Dr. Nathan says, try asking softly, "Can you run that by me again more slowly?" That demonstrates that you recognize the importance of what the boss is saying, while helping defuse a potentially volatile situation.

And the next time someone comes to you with a problem, don't act like Mr. Know-It-All and tell them what they should do. Dr. Nathan advocates a different approach: Listening without giving advice. "Avoid trying to fix things for everyone else," he counsels. You may think you're doing your boss or friend a favor by telling them what to do, but in reality, you're undermining their sense of competence. "Being a sounding board is much more effective than giving them the solution," Dr. Nathan says. "It has to be their solution or else they won't do it."

Use your imagination. You're trying to concentrate on the job in front of you, but all of the other tasks piling up in your in-basket keep taunting you. Try this technique, courtesy of Dr. Abel: If you use a computer, close your eyes and imagine that the list of things you have to do is on the screen. Then, visualize them fading out, one by one, except for the top one, which is highlighted. That is the only job that stays on the screen. Focus on it.

Or, if the computer image doesn't work for you, visualize everything you have to do written on balloons you hold in your hand. Then, slowly let go of each balloon until you only have one left—the one thing you want to do at that time.

Take a six-second tranquilizer. When the telephone rings, most of us dive for it. Instead, use the ringing as a cue to relax, Dr. Nathan says. Wait six seconds, or about two rings, before picking up the phone. During those precious moments take a deep, relaxing breath and think of a word such as "calm" or "relax." Then, imagine yourself as a rag doll, completely relaxed and limp in your chair. Now you're ready to answer the phone. Using this "six-second tranquilizer" offers you a break from stress every time the phone rings. But it doesn't have to be cued to Alexander Graham Bell's invention. You can obtain instant stress relief while waiting in line for a cashier or while stopped at a red light or stop sign.

Forget the power lunch. Use mealtimes as a break from the daily grind. Before eating take a moment to say a prayer or just sit quietly so you shift out of your work mode and actually take the time to enjoy your food.

Limit your worrying. You may not be able to completely eliminate worry, but you certainly can limit the amount of time you spend doing it. "For people who have a lot of realistic stress and who need to really spend some time thinking about these things, what I will do is help them to postpone worry," says Dr. Abel. At the end of the day set aside a half-hour to think about all of the things that are causing you stress. During that time, Dr. Abel says, "Jot down a bunch of solutions, no matter how far-out they are." Then, choose one or more of the solutions to take action on. If you find there is nothing you can do about a problem, that raises a perfectly logical question: Why worry about it?

Drive slower. Dr. Rechtschaffen confesses he would "fax myself between the house and work" if he could. Fortunately, he can't—and neither can you. So don't view your morning commute as wasted time. Slow down and think of it as your time, Dr. Rechtschaffen says, a chance to be with yourself and enjoy the company.

Be a homeboy. When you get home from work, shower or change clothes to signal a clean break from the office, Dr. Rechtschaffen recommends. It's kind of the same idea as having a highball—only healthier.

Lay off the booze and junk food. After a long day at work many of us flop down in an easy chair, crack open a cold beer and start munching chips. That's a big mistake. "We're drugging ourselves," Dr. Fiore warns. "We're drugging ourselves with junk food, with TV, with alcohol. And it becomes a vicious cycle."

Tune out. If you're wondering where the time goes, it may be getting zapped by cathode rays. "If you look at 35 hours a week of TV, you realize you're watching somebody else be creative, rather than creating something for yourself," says Dr. Fiore. "If you're able to keep your TV viewing under 5 hours a week, you have a lot of extra time. You can find 15 or 20 hours to learn to play the piano or the guitar, or to learn Italian or to do a number of things that can be enhancing and enriching."

Make eating a happy time. Add a joke du jour to the dinner menu. Don't allow your evening repast to become a nightly gripe session about what went wrong that day. "This day and age, the table at dinner becomes a stress pot," Dr. Collins says. "Everyone comes to the table bringing their stresses of the day. Pretty soon your digestive tract is grinding away and no one's happy. We try to, at our table, have everyone bring a joke or have some humor. It's a very important way of uncoupling stress."

Let leisure suit you. Don't fill every waking moment with something you must do. As Dr. Collins puts it, "Leisure time has become stressful in our lives." Do something relaxing and noncompetitive, whether it's reading, meditating or taking a walk. "You need leisure time in order to be productive," says Dr. Fiore. "I love the paradox in that statement."

Meditate. The best way to shut down an overactive stress-response system is to meditate, says Dr. Collins. "Yoga, tai chi, all of those things that are related to self-understanding, I think, are essential."

Check out certified yoga schools in your area, recommends Dr. Collins. Or look for stress management courses offered at hospitals.

Retreat. Go on a weekend retreat in the country. Leave your watch at home. Slow down and take time to explore your emotions and feelings for a change. You'll come back rested and renewed.

Take a vacation. If you thought *National Lampoon's Vacation* was a documentary film, you may need to change your approach to your own summer getaways. The point of a vacation is to relax and get away from the pressures of the office and daily life. Too many men trade their hectic, stressful jobs for hectic, stressful vacations, says Alvin Baraff, Ph.D., a clinical psychologist and the founder of MenCenter, a counseling practice in Washington, D.C. The typical take-no-prisoners executive gets up at dawn to see every sunrise, visits every museum and historical site in the guidebook and takes more pictures than a photographer for *National Geographic*. "He comes back from vacations more tired than when he left," says Dr. Baraff.

This time, try slowing down. Sleep late. Read a good novel. And don't try to see everything. "Whatever you wind up seeing," says Dr. Baraff, "will be more than what you've seen."

Stroke

Avoiding a Brain Breakdown

Actor Raul Julia will always be remembered as the vigorous, sensuous Gomez Addams from the *Addams Family* movies. He danced with reckless abandon and brandished his fencing rapier with lightning speed. Yet, at only 54 years of age, Raul Julia died from the complications of a stroke.

Julia's death was a shock. But that he died of a stroke is not. Stroke is the third leading cause of death in the United States, preceded only by heart disease and cancer.

Think of stroke as a heart attack of the brain—a "brain attack," as the experts say. Like a heart attack, a stroke is quick, unexpected and often deadly. As a man, your chance of getting a stroke is 30 percent greater than that of a woman. Only 40 percent of men who suffer a stroke die, however, compared to 60 percent of women.

How Strokes Happen

As with heart attacks, most strokes are not illnesses. Rather, they're the body's response to something else, often the narrowing of arteries from a buildup of cholesterol.

There are two kinds of strokes. The first, called an ischemic stroke, occurs when a blood clot interrupts blood flow in the brain, or when blood flow to the brain is dramatically reduced because of the narrowing of an artery that feeds the brain. Ischemic strokes account for roughly 70 to 80 percent of all strokes.

The other type of stroke, a hemorrhagic stroke, occurs when a blood vessel in the brain ruptures. Hemorrhagic strokes are the more lethal of the two.

Symptoms for each are about the same: weakness; numbness in the face, hands, arms or legs; slurring of speech or inability to understand what people are saying to you; blindness in one eye; and dizziness.

Doctors say that when someone is diagnosed with a stroke, "time is brain." This means that the faster the blood flow is restored or the hemorrhage stopped, the more brain function will survive. The more you know about stroke, the sooner you'll seek help if you or someone else is having one.

"There's a lot of optimism about strokes. You can identify the risk factors to see if you're at risk for stroke," says Patricia Grady, Ph.D., deputy director for the National Institute of Neurological Disorders and Stroke in Bethesda, Maryland.

Moreover, many risk factors are in your control. "The brightest scientists in this country agree that up to 80 percent of all strokes can be prevented. We know what's causing them and we know how to prevent many of them," says Marjorie G. Anderson, Director of Communications for the National Stroke Association in Englewood, Colorado. "When it comes to strokes, the onus is on the individual. Knowing the risk factors and warning signs isn't enough. You need to call 911 if you experience them, because it's a medical emergency."

What You Need to Know

Here are some of the most common risk factors for strokes.

Factors you can't control.

• Age. As a rough estimate, risk for stroke doubles every decade after 55.

• Diabetes. Diabetes can weaken blood vessels, boosting your chance of stroke by 40 percent.

• Gender. Men are 30 percent more likely to have strokes than women. (But remember we're less likely to die.)

• Heart attack. If you have atrial fibrillation, a condition in which the heart beats irregularly, your risk of stroke is four to six times higher. Atrial fibrillation occurs frequently in men who've had a heart attack.

• Heredity. "If you have a history of heart disease in the family, that's a clue that you should be closely followed by a physician," Dr. Grady says.

• Race. African Americans are 60 percent more vulnerable to fatal and disabling strokes than Whites.

• Stroke two. If you've had a stroke before, your chances of having another are increased by ten times.

Factors you can control.

• Cholesterol. Having a high cholesterol count may increase your chance of having a stroke. Total cholesterol ratings over 200 are considered a risk, but your doctor can tell you more.

• Diet. Diets high in fat help clog your arteries, particularly the life-giving vessels that feed blood to your brain.

• Sedentary lifestyle. If you never get your blood moving with exercise, fat particles conglomerate like the spices in an unshaken bottle of Italian salad

FAST FACTS

How common: Stroke is the third leading cause of death for people in the United States. About 550,000 people suffer a stroke each year, most of them men. About 150,000 of those people die each year, roughly 60,000 of whom are men.

Risk factors: Involuntary: age, gender, race (Blacks are more at risk), diabetes, previous stroke, heredity, previous heart attack. Voluntary: high cholesterol, high blood pressure, diet, being overweight, smoking, heavy drinking, lack of exercise.

Age group affected: Men over age 55 are at an increased risk, and their chance for stroke doubles every decade thereafter.

Gender gap: Men are 30 percent more likely to have a stroke than women, but less likely to die.

Who to see: Emergency room physician ASAP, then a neurologist.

dressing. When this happens the fat builds up in your arteries, reducing blood flow and increasing your chance of stroke.

• Smoking. It increases your chance of getting a stroke by 70 percent. "The number of cigarettes you smoke is directly related to the narrowing of your blood vessels," Dr. Grady says. "If you stop smoking, you can't reverse damage already done, but you can prevent more damage from occurring."

• Blood pressure and weight. Having high blood pressure, more than about 140 over 90, increases your chance of stroke. Ditto for being overweight. Both can be modified through diet and exercise.

Striking Out Strokes

It's pretty clear that to diminish the risk of a stroke you should address the six factors above that are within your power. Here are more specific tips.

Watch your red. A high red blood cell count means a greater blood clotting factor, and a blood clot in the wrong place causes an ischemic stroke. Knowing where your cells stand is a good defense.

"After, say, age 50 and beyond, it is a good idea to have yearly physicals, which will usually include some blood work to measure your blood cell count," Dr. Grady says.

Improve your diet. Eating too much fat and not enough fiber can lead to heart disease and the breakdown of arteries, veins and blood vessels. So avoid fatty snacks, like candy bars. Instead of eating fatty or greasy foods, emphasize grains, vegetables and fruits. Cut your meat eating back to three times a week. Fish oils are good for you, so include some mackerel, haddock and cod in your diet.

"Remember that a cholesterol glob doesn't know the difference between a heart attack and a stroke. If your lifestyle is causing problems for your heart, it's probably causing problems for your brain, too," Anderson says.

Exercise more. Walk when you can. Jog. Bicycle. Have fun. Moderate exercise for about 30 minutes at least three times a week makes for a healthier heart and better circulation. It also helps reduce your chance of stroke by lowering blood pressure and cholesterol.

No ifs, ands or butts. "Quitting smoking can result in a dramatic decrease in risk," Dr. Grady says. Research shows that quitting for five years brings your risk of having a stroke down close to the same level as someone who's never smoked.

Drink only in moderation. Alcohol in moderation might be good for you. One or two drinks a day actually can decrease your chance of heart disease and stroke. But overdoing it is asking for trouble.

"Some experts are finding strokes are more likely associated with binge drinking and drinking excessive amounts of alcohol, so keep it to no more than two drinks a day," Anderson says.

Take an aspirin a day. Studies have shown that one aspirin taken daily can help reduce clotting, which could reduce your chance of stroke. But don't think aspirin is a panacea.

"There's a lot of controversy about this, but many physicians will agree that taking one aspirin a day or every other day doesn't do any harm for most people," Dr. Grady says. "If you're going to do this, it's better to talk to your doctor first."

Consider Mac the Knife. Let's say years of fast food, beer binges and shunning exercise have clogged your arteries worse than five o'clock traffic clogs a city highway. There's still hope. Consider an operation called a carotid endarterectomy, which clears the arteries in your neck, thus preventing decreased blood flow and stroke. Doctors check if your carotids are clogged by listening to the blood flow in your neck. They also can perform a sonogram for a more accurate reading.

The carotid endarterectomy's role in prevention seems extremely promising, based in part on two studies her institute has supported, says Dr. Grady. In the latest study, conducted between 1987 and 1993, researchers followed 1,662 people from 39 Canadian and American medical centers. Every person had carotid arteries that had been reduced by more than 60 percent in diameter. Overwhelmingly, the patients who received the procedure had a reduced rate of stroke. The results were so encouraging that doctors participating in the survey were asked to re-evaluate the patients who did not receive the treatment.

A Precursor to the Crash

A stroke hits suddenly and without warning—usually. But in one in ten stroke cases a transient ischemic attack (also called a TIA or ministroke) will precede a major stroke by about a week. The symptoms are the same: weakness, dizziness, numbness, slurred speech or the inability to understand what people are saying. The symptoms of a TIA almost always clear up after several hours.

"A TIA is an important warning signal. A wake-up call. A signal that you have a problem and need to see your doctor," Dr. Grady says. "Even if you have a TIA, you might be able to prevent a stroke from following."

If you have a TIA, go to a hospital immediately. While 10 percent of strokes are preceded by a TIA, about 40 percent of TIAs are followed by a stroke.

What to Expect

When a patient with symptoms of a stroke arrives at the hospital, a doctor immediately assesses the vital signs (heart rate, blood pressure, respiration rate) and examines for evidence of brain injury.

The doctor will also seek fast answers to several key questions.
• When did the event begin?
• Could this be something other than stroke, like a seizure?
• If it is a stroke, is it secondary to something else life threatening, like a heart attack?
• Is it a hemorrhagic or an ischemic stroke?
• What area of the brain and which vascular regions (for example, carotid arteries) are affected?

"These questions are important to help determine immediate treatment options," says Gregory Albers, M.D., director of the Stanford Stroke Center and associate professor of neurology and neurological sciences at Stanford University Medical Center. "For instance, if the stroke is ischemic, it may be appropriate to administer an anticoagulant, or blood-thinning, drug. But if it's a hemorrhagic stroke, blood-thinning medications could be dangerous."

To help answer these questions, doctors typically order up a picture of the brain (CAT scan or magnetic resonance imaging), imagery tests of blood vessels and a routine blood test.

If the stroke is because of a hemorrhage, blood pressure will be carefully controlled and in some circumstances, surgery may be recommended. If it's ischemic, tests will be done to look for the cause of the blocked vessel.

Stroke patients typically have a hospital stay of about one week. Survival rates are 70 percent or better, depending on the type of stroke and how much damage was done. Permanent damage can range from none to marked disability.

During your hospital stay doctors are going to watch for poststroke complications such as fluid on the brain (edema), spasms in the blood vessels (vasospasm), fever and signs of further stroke. They'll also watch for what paralysis remains after your treatment has taken hold.

Coping with the Crash

Two out of three people who have a stroke need some sort of rehabilitation after they're released from the hospital. Problems may range from difficulty in speaking to severe paralysis, so you'll probably be sent to a rehab center.

The key to poststroke rehab is getting the brain to recircuit its wiring so that other brain cells take over from the damaged ones in telling your muscles what to do. Some cells are dead but others are just injured and within months they're starting to function again. Rehab is for retraining your brain on how to move your body.

Doctors and therapists know that at first you're going to get exhausted even thinking about therapy. But the sooner you get into rehab, the better your chances are of regaining what you've lost. The more you work at it, the more you'll regain.

Rehab even helps with paralysis, perhaps the most debilitating effect of stroke. "Even when regaining the use of a paralyzed limb is not possible," Anderson says, "rehab could teach the survivor ways to adapt to their disability."

Remember that nobody knows what you can do after a stroke. A doctor may have said you'll never use your arm again or that you'll need a wheelchair; a year later you could be throwing baseballs or jogging.

"The brain has a much greater capacity for recovering and assuming new functions than was previously thought," Dr. Grady says. "You see some patients recover and you think, 'How can they do that?' But they do. It's very encouraging."

Sunburn

Why You Need Shelter

You wake to a brilliant sunny Saturday and eagerly consider the possibilities: the beach, bike riding, volleyball, a picnic.

As soon as you step outside, you'll be hit by ultraviolet radiation from the sun that within minutes could start wreaking havoc inside your skin. Cells break, blood vessels leak, tissues swell and possibly, deep down, a cancer begins.

Alarmist rhetoric from pale and pimply doctors? Sorry. No matter how much you want to believe otherwise, all research shows that tanned skin is damaged skin, and sunburned skin is even worse for you.

"It is possible for one very bad sunburn to initiate changes in skin that result in skin cancer," says Rodney Basler, M.D., a dermatologist and assistant professor of internal medicine at the University of Nebraska Medical Center in Omaha. "The norm, though, is a lifetime of unprotected sun exposure for developing skin cancer."

Getting the Burn

Virtually all light-skinned people experience sunburn at some time in their lives from direct exposure to the sun or from its light reflected off water, snow or sand. For some the injury of sunburn will be a mildly painful reddening of the skin—a first-degree burn—that fades in a few days. For others it will be a fiery, excruciating, blistering, skin-peeling ordeal that lasts weeks. For a rare few, severe sunburn can require hospitalization.

Even when the pain of sunburn has faded, however, its cancer potential lingers. Sunburn appears to suppress the immune system and could increase susceptibility to disease. Repeated burns cause degenerative changes that speed up aging and produce wrinkled, leathery skin.

More importantly, chronic exposure to the sun causes damage to skin-cell DNA and can produce cancerous and precancerous skin lesions. And, a history of frequent sunburn increases the risk of melanoma, the most dangerous of these cancerous skin lesions.

Melanoma is the "most rapidly increasing malignancy of all malignancies," says Vincent DeLeo, M.D., associate professor of dermatology at Columbia University's

509

St. Luke's–Roosevelt Medical Center in New York City. "The ozone's not doing it. It's people's search for the golden tan that's causing it."

Your body tries to protect itself against further sun exposure by tanning, or producing a pigment called melanin, which absorbs ultraviolet (UV) light. Generally, the more an area has been tanned, the more intensely it will tan after each new exposure. But tanned skin is not healthy skin; it's already been damaged. Further tanning produces further damage. "There's no free lunch and no safe tan," says Dr. DeLeo.

People with darker skin color have more built-in protection against the sun because they have more efficient melanin-producing cells. But they can still suffer sunburn from prolonged exposure.

Sunburn and its symptoms can also be made worse by the interaction of UV light and certain kinds of prescription and over-the-counter drugs. These include many antibiotics, various anti-cancer compounds, diuretics, acne medications, heart medications and high blood pressure drugs. You should consult with a physician about possible interactions between the sun and medications you're taking.

Avoiding Red

The first step is the hardest: becoming convinced that a tan is not good for you and that burns are serious business. That's not easy: Society considers a golden tan a symbol of health and vitality. But all those doctors aren't making up the scare talk. Excessive sun on skin means trouble, and you should avoid it.

We know you're not always willing to stay out of the sun. After a long winter indoors, sun on the skin can be a blessed thing. So here are some steps you can take to minimize sunburn problems.

Fry in the off-peak hours. The best way to prevent sunburn is to know when the sun's rays will be the most intense. Sunburning rays are strongest when the sun is overhead. If you are going to be in the sun, try to do so before 10:00 A.M. or after 3:00 P.M. when the sun's light has to travel through more atmosphere to reach you and UV light is decreased.

Also, many local newspapers and TV shows carry the National Weather Service and the U.S. Environmental Protection Agency's experimental UV index as part of their weather reports. Look at the index to find out how long you may safely stay outside based on the weather, location, season and your ability to tan.

Cover up. If you're going to sun yourself, at a minimum, wear a hat to protect your tender scalp. A brimmed hat is even better since it will protect your eyes, too. In addition, invest in a pair of UV-resistant sunglasses. Yes, they might cost more, but they're far cheaper than cataract surgery, which you run the risk of facing someday without them.

FAST FACTS

How common: Anyone who bares skin to the sun is vulnerable, and most everyone gets burned at some point in their lifetime.

Risk factors: Prolonged exposure of skin to direct or reflected sunlight, roughly between the hours of 10 A.M. and 3 P.M. Fair-skinned people are at greatest risk.

Age group affected: Men of all ages get burned. More serious skin problems linked to sunburn are cumulative, meaning the more you get burned, the more susceptible you are to other skin diseases.

Gender gap: None.

Who to see: Family doctor if sunburn is severe and symptoms include blistering, weakness, confusion or convulsions. Also if you are taking medications that might increase sensitivity to sunlight.

When you do want to cover your body more fully, be aware that not all fabrics are equal in their abilities to filter out UV light. Some thin or loose-weave fabrics can let enough sun through to leave a mosaic burn on your skin. And many fabrics when damp provide little or no protection. Try shopping at outdoor-clothing suppliers for cool, loose-fitting garments made of fabric especially designed for sun protection.

Use sunscreen. Before gardening, bike riding or starting any kind of prolonged outdoor activity, get in the habit of putting on sunscreen, especially during peak sunburn hours. Sunscreens contain chemicals that absorb UV light before it can damage skin. The products are rated on the sun protection factor (SPF) scale. Dermatologists consider an SPF 15 to be the minimum acceptable protection. This will allow the average man to stay in the sun 15 times longer than normal without burning.

Coat exposed areas liberally and thoroughly; avoid those telltale and painful red splotches on missed spots. Be aware that sweating, wiping off with a towel or prolonged immersion in water can erode your protection. Reapply the sunscreen at regular intervals. And be sure to slap some on your kisser—men are a lot more susceptible to lip cancer than their lipstick-wearing female counterparts.

Also, buy a sunscreen that filters out two types of ultraviolet light, UVA and UVB. UVB is the main culprit in sunburn, but UVA, which penetrates more deeply into the skin, is thought to be involved in other kinds of skin damage. Ironically, doctors say, exposure to UVA is on the rise. The reason? People stay in the sun longer with sunscreens that block only UVB or contain less UVA block. And, they say, the use of UVA tanning machines is increasing.

Feeling the Burn

If you're turning red, get out of the sun immediately. "The skin never forgets," says Thomas A. Gossel, Ph.D., a registered pharmacist and dean of the College of Pharmacy at Ohio Northern University in Ada. "Any amount of exposure to the sun is potentially damaging."

If within a few hours you see severe reddening or blistering or you experience weakness or convulsions, get medical help right away. But if your sunburn appears to be more moderate, there are some things you can do to help you through it.

Cool off. The tried-and-true remedies are still among the best for dealing with the immediate heat and pain of mild to moderate sunburn. A cool compress or bath—the water should be body temperature—provides temporary relief. Never use ice water or place ice directly on your burned skin. Over-the-counter hydrocortisone creams or anesthetics containing lidocaine or benzocaine also help.

Moisturize. Cooling and soaking sunburned skin can give temporary relief, but they can also make the skin turn dry in the long run. So after you cool it down, smooth on some bath oil and then lock it in a minute later with skin lotion or moisturizer.

Dose up. Aspirin–two to three tablets every six hours for up to two days–may block the inflammation involved in sunburn. Ibuprofen is also recommended. Follow the dosage instructions on the bottle.

Toss a salad. Some sunburn victims swear by home remedies that include slices of raw potato or cucumber applied to the burn area, gauze soaked in cool milk or cool extract of boiled lettuce, a tepid bath that's had a cupful of white vinegar added to it or a bag of frozen peas wrapped in a towel and strapped to the hot spot. If it works for you, then consider it good medicine.

Teeth Grinding

Give Your Jaw a Rest

In movies, in sports, in the barroom, it is the stereotypical action of the hard, angry man. In real life it is either a foolish habit of nervous men or an innocent nocturnal problem. Either way, it's no good for you.

We're talking about clenching the jaw and grinding the teeth—dentists call it bruxism. Most bruxing takes place when we're fast asleep. For that reason many teeth grinders aren't even aware they have the habit unless their mate or their dentist tells them about it.

Researchers believe that bruxism is an inherited behavior—if your mom or dad is a bruxer, chances are you will be, too. Stress, however, is the trigger that sets the habit in motion. "Often these people are working two or three jobs and faced with significant life challenges," says John D. Rugh, Ph.D., professor of orthodontics at the University of Texas Health Science Center in San Antonio. "They're really pushing hard."

Serious teeth grinders can damage fillings or grind right through a tooth's outer coating of enamel. That exposes the softer inner part of the tooth, causing the nerve to die. Clenchers are more apt to strain their jaw muscles, causing facial pain, headaches or, some dentists believe, dislocation of the jaw joint.

Grinding to a Halt

Given that teeth grinders are genetically predisposed to brux, is there anything they can do to eliminate the habit? Not much, according to Dr. Rugh. "It's like an ulcer," he says. "It's something you have to learn to manage the rest of your life."

The most common treatment dentists prescribe is a night guard, a molded, protective plastic shield that fits over the top or bottom teeth. Some dentists may feel it necessary to grind or cap the teeth to modify a bruxer's bite, although in most cases it's rarely needed, says Andrew S. Kaplan, D.D.S., director of the TMJ/Orofacial Pain Clinic at Mount Sinai School of Medicine of the City University of New York in New York City.

If bruxing is causing severe damage, muscle relaxants or even antidepressants may be prescribed to temporarily reduce the tension that's causing the problem in the first place. But that's the extreme case. There's plenty you can do to manage your bruxism before it ever goes that far.

Play it cool. Since stress exacerbates bruxism, do what you can to reduce your stress. "Take a stress reduction class," suggests Richard Price, D.M.D., a clinical professor of dentistry at Boston University's School of Dentistry and an adviser to the American Dental Association. Dr. Kaplan has found that biofeedback treatments can help teach patients to identify situations that provoke stress and to relax when they arise.

Stretch it out. Like any group of muscles, jaw muscles can be loosened up with exercise. John Dodes, D.D.S., lecturer in the Department of Dental Medicine at the State University of New York School of Dental Medicine in New York City, recommends simple stretching exercises such as opening your mouth moderately wide in sets of ten with your fist under your jaw for pressure.

Scratch the stimulants. A simple way to reduce the tension in your body is to cut stimulants such as coffee or tea out of your diet, Dr. Rugh says.

Sleep around. You can sometimes reduce your nighttime bruxing simply by sleeping in a different position. John C. Brown, D.D.S., past president of the Academy of General Dentistry, suggests asking your mate to monitor what position you're sleeping in when you're grinding. Try shifting to a different position—onto the other side or onto your stomach if you grind while sleeping on your back—and see if the bruxing subsides. Use pillows to keep propped in the most desirable position.

Soothe the pain. For temporary relief of sore jaw muscles, take ibuprofen or aspirin, Dr. Kaplan says. You can also apply moist heat to the jaw, he adds, either with a wet washcloth or a hot pack, or simply let the shower run on your face for a few minutes. Don't let the water get so hot that it burns your face, though.

FAST FACTS

How common: Studies show that 80 percent of men periodically clench or grind their teeth. Only about 5 percent, however, brux enough to hurt themselves.

Risk factors: Heredity, stress, fillings that are rough or protruding, poorly fitted dental work.

Age group affected: People of all ages grind and clench, although it usually isn't until they reach their twenties or later that the effects start causing problems.

Gender gap: Men and women grind their teeth about equally, although some dentists believe men are more likely to put up with any pain bruxism causes without seeking treatment.

Who to see: Dentist.

Testicular Cancer

Beating the Young Man's Disease

When John Kruk returned to his former baseball team, the Philadelphia Phillies, after completing treatment for testicular cancer, which included removal of one gonad, he had a T-shirt made that read, "If you don't let me play, I'm taking my ball and going home."

It's not every cancer you can make light of without being depressingly macabre, but upbeat outcomes are typical of testicular cancer for the simple reason that of all malignancies, male or female, it's one of the easiest to cure. Still, that didn't help another young professional athlete, Brian Piccolo, a running back for the Chicago Bears in the late 1960s. He died of the disease in 1970 at age 26, inspiring the book and movie *Brian's Song*.

The difference between the two cases is telling. First of all, since Piccolo's time enormous progress has been made in treating testicular cancer. "When I was a medical resident 20 years ago, the cure rate was 20 to 30 percent, and we thought we were doing pretty well," says Michael Warren, M.D., chief of the Division of Urology at the University of Texas Medical Branch in Galveston. "Now it's 85 to 90 percent."

Second, as Kruk's T-shirt attests, people aren't as squeamish about publicly discussing explicitly male problems as they were back when Piccolo died. This openness is perhaps the most crucial development because testicular cancer is virtually symptomless. That puts the burden on men—especially young men, who are most at risk—to be educated about it and actively seek to find it.

Search and Destroy

There is no better way to keep testicular cancer at bay than to examine yourself for signs of its presence at least once a month, and ideally once a week. "You can't emphasize the testicular self-exam enough," says Dr. Warren. "It clearly makes a difference and it's very easy to do."

The exam is best done when the testicles are relaxed and loose, which is why most doctors recommend performing it just after taking a warm shower or bath. Taking one testicle at a time, gently roll it between your thumb and first three fin-

515

gers until you've felt the entire surface. A healthy testicle will be about the consistency of a hard-boiled egg: smooth and firm, but not hard. If you feel lumps or areas of hardness, find one testicle to be larger than the other or experience any pain, you may have trouble. (Tumors can be felt when they get to be about the size of a pea—a small growth.) The exam takes about 30 seconds.

A number of problems can feel like testicular cancer but aren't; if you find something, don't get overly alarmed at first. "Twenty to 30 percent of the men I examine turn out to have an abnormality but not a significant problem," says Richard D. Williams, M.D., professor and chairman of the Department of Urology at the University of Iowa College of Medicine in Iowa City. The main point is to see a doctor immediately: Even if the problem is benign (fluid buildup in the testicle, for example), you'll want to relieve your anxiety and if necessary, fix the problem.

Your doctor may do a number of mild tests to determine whether or not you have cancer. He'll hold a light to the testicle (the light will pass through mere fluid but not through a tumor). He may do an ultrasound to get a better picture of what's there. He may also order a blood test, looking for various proteins whose levels rise in response to a tumor.

Killing the Cancer

If it's cancer, you have to get rid of it. "Surgery is what all patients start with," says Dr. Williams. The surgery in question is called orchiectomy—removal of the testicle. It's not an appealing option, but it's highly effective, isn't complicated and has few side effects other than discomfort (one of the more common is numbness on one side of the scrotum, which generally clears within six months.) If a tumor is caught in its earliest stages, surgery alone may be all that's required.

If, however, the malignancy has spread to lymph nodes in the abdomen or, worse, to the lungs, follow-up treatment may be needed. What that treatment is depends on the nature of the tumor and how far it has spread. One class of tumor, seminoma, for example, is highly responsive to radiation (whose side effects include nausea and lack of appetite). Another class of tumor, nonseminoma, is less responsive to radiation and is also more aggressive, so doctors may instead prescribe a regimen of chemotherapy (side effects include loss of hair, nausea and possible sterility). In some cases, the favored option is a second surgery, this time to remove small tumors from the lymph nodes. The silver lining in all of these dark-sounding options, however, is that the disease is highly responsive to the weapons used against it. There is no point at which a physician would write you off as completely incurable, notes Dr. Warren.

FAST FACTS

How common: Not very, overall. Only about 6,600 new cases (about 1 percent of all male cancers) are diagnosed each year in the United States.

Risk factors: Most concern childhood testicle problems, particularly an undescended testicle, which raises risk 2½ to 40 times that of the general population. Also: White men are more at risk than Blacks.

Age group affected: While uncommon among men in general, testicular cancer is the *most* common malignancy diagnosed in men between ages 20 and 35. Tumors are rare after age 40.

Gender gap: Strictly male.

Who to see: Urologist.

A Word about Prevention

There appears to be little you can do to prevent testicular cancer. Diet, for example, which mediates the occurrence of many other types of cancer, hasn't been shown to come into play here. The primary risk factor isn't a behavioral matter at all: Men whose testicles never fully descended from the body into the scrotum during fetal development are at higher risk. (If the problem is fixed in early childhood, as is often the case, risk may be significantly reduced.) There are, however, a few things that doctors tenuously say may help. These are:

Exercise more. In a study conducted in England, men who exercised 15 hours a week or more had a substantially reduced risk of testicular cancer compared with men who didn't exercise at all. And men who were seated ten or more hours a day had a 71 percent greater risk than men who were seated less than three hours a day.

Still, these are extreme comparisons, only a few studies have established this link and many doctors on the front lines are unconvinced it's important.

Avoid estrogen exposure. Researchers have suggested that increased exposure of pregnant women to various types of the female hormone estrogen may be the cause for a wide range of male reproductive problems developed in the womb. From that hypothesis it may make sense to avoid estrogen, says Marc Goldstein, M.D., professor of urology and director of the Center for Male Reproductive Medicine and Microsurgery at the New York Hospital-Cornell Medical Center in New York City. You might, for example, cut back on beef and milk or eat a high-fiber diet, which helps the body quickly excrete contaminants. But this is speculation. Says Dr. Goldstein. "As far as special measures go, self-examination is far more important."

Testicular Problems

Preventing Agony below the Belt

If there's one thing that would make Rambo, G.I. Joe and Hulk Hogan cry like babies, it'd be testicular pain.

Who among us doesn't cringe at the thought of the family jewels in danger? It hurts just thinking about crotch-catching a line drive or getting in the way of an unfriendly knee.

Testicular problems aren't just generated by errant blows, however. A long list of conditions from infections to broken internal plumbing can generate pain in the testicles or scrotal area.

Despite the natural tendency to curl up in a fetal position and pray testicular pain passes, doing so isn't a good idea, because some conditions, like torsion, require immediate attention.

"Most men are real funny when it comes to these things. They won't even tell the nurse what's wrong—they just want to talk to me," says Durwood E. Neal, Jr., M.D., associate professor of surgery, microbiology and internal medicine at the University of Texas Medical Branch in Galveston. "But it's important to swallow your pride and see the doctor, especially since so many of these things are fixable."

A Kick in the Pants

When it comes to testicular trauma, they don't call it trauma for nothing. Any guy who's been kicked, pricked, whopped or bopped below the belt knows it's traumatic. But what happens, and why does it hurt so much?

Truth is, the damage from a blow usually isn't as bad as it feels. Because the testicles move about inside the scrotum, they usually bounce back, so to speak, without ever sustaining serious injury. When their mobility doesn't protect them and serious injury does occur, the usual result is a rupture or *hematocele*.

As for why testicle blows hurt so much, that's a different story. According to Dr. Neal, these blows are so painful because the testicles are connected to nerves in a different way from, say, your hands.

When nerves around muscles get tweaked, the pain is very specific to the location—a necessary function for dealing with the external world, explains Dr. Neal.

518

FAST FACTS

How common: Depending on the cause, testicular problems can range from the common to the rare. Infections, for example, are fairly common causes of testicular pain, while torsion is somewhat of a rarity.

Risk factors: The causes of several testicular problems remain unknown. But if infection is the problem, it's likely you got the bacteria from sex. Not using a condom and having sex with multiple partners or with someone whose sexual history you're unsure of puts you at risk.

Age group affected: Men of all ages.

Gender gap: Men only.

Who to see: If pain from a blow doesn't end within an hour or if you are hit with sudden sharp pain that doesn't go away, get to your family doctor fast. For more complicated problems, see a urologist.

But when internal organs get hit, the pain tends to be deeper and more widespread. In the testicle's case a blow causes pain throughout the abdomen that can be accompanied by sweating, nausea and dizziness.

"If I reached into you and pinched your bladder or your intestine, you would not perceive it as a pinch, you'd perceive it as visceral discomfort," Dr. Neal adds. "Remember that the testicles are visceral organs that have migrated outside the body. Pain for them is different."

Use Dr. Neal's "hour rule" if you receive an agonizing shot below the belt: If the pain hasn't subsided in an hour or so, see a doctor fast. You might have a rupture or torsion, which means you could be in danger of losing a testicle.

Meet the *Cele* Family

We'll call these testicular problems celes because their names end with that suffix. The word *cele* refers to a noncancerous tumor, a swelling or some type of problem with a body cavity, and when it comes to ticking off your testicles, all these definitions can apply.

Except for hematoceles, which occur mostly from physical injuries, many of these conditions develop for no apparent reason. They're just part of the problems that come with a man's plumbing.

Here are the common celes to watch out for.

• A *varicocele* is a varicose vein in your scromatacord, a collection of nerves, arteries, veins and lymphatic channels that run to and from the testicle.

"It may or may not be something you notice, though sometimes it feels like a dull pain or a dragging sensation, or even like a bag of worms inside the scrotum," says Marc S. Cohen, M.D., associate professor of surgery and urology at the University of Florida College of Medicine in Gainesville. The feeling often subsides after lying down.

• A *hydrocele* is a collection of fluid, usually in the membrane lining the inside of your scrotum. A hydrocele may go unnoticed, but it may feel like a dull ache or a sensation of heaviness in the scrotum. "Because a hydrocele surrounds the testicle, it may mask an underlying condition," says Dr. Cohen.

• A *hematocele* is a hydrocele, except that the pooled fluid is blood. It's often painful because it's usually caused by physical damage, like a blow to the testicles. You can use a flashlight in a dark room to help spot a hematocele in your scrotum. "Unlike other hydroceles, light won't pass through a hematocele," explains Dr. Cohen.

• A *spermatocele* is a sperm-filled cyst growing on or near your testicular tubes. Most times you won't even know it exists unless you feel it during a testicular self-exam. "Though it's usually not painful, a spermatocele is what causes guys to joke about having a third testicle," Dr. Cohen says. "It feels like a round ball above your testicle. A spermatocele lights up under a flashlight in a darkened room."

A Painful Twist of Fate

Torsion is probably the most painful of testicular problems. It occurs when one of your two spermatic cords twists in on itself, cutting off the blood supply. These cords normally hold your testicles like a piñata in your scrotum. Unless untwisted, the testicle will die a slow and painful death, swelling to the size of a grapefruit before shrinking to the size of a pea.

"Your testicle is like any other body part that needs blood. When the blood is choked off, the testicle will swell, inflame, then atrophy," says Dr. Neal.

Torsion mostly occurs in teens and children, but it can occur in adults. It sometimes happens when your testicles are jostling around during athletics, when you're wearing tight-fitting underwear or even when you're sleeping.

But regardless of how torsion begins, it must end with a trip to the doctor. If you think you have torsion, don't delay—you have only four to eight hours before facing permanent damage.

Infectious Fiends

Infections are a common cause of testicular pain in adult men. Lots of things can cause infections, with the biggest culprit being bacteria acquired through a sexually transmitted disease. Here are the common infections that can make your testicles testy.

• *Epididymitis* is inflammation of the epididymis—spaghetti-like tubes inside the scrotum that are coiled up behind each testicle and store and carry sperm. The infection is usually characterized by swelling of the epididymis and feelings of pain—sometimes severe pain.

Several things can irritate your epididymis. In younger and sexually active men the cause frequently is a sexually transmitted disease. In older men and men who aren't sexually active, a urinary or prostate infection is usually at fault. And in physically active men, particularly weight lifters, epididymitis can occur when pressure on the back causes fluid from the prostate and epididymis to back up when you strain.

• Bacterial infections of the urinary tract, kidney or prostate can cause pain in your testicles and even the whole groin area. Often treated with antibiotics, these infections are sometimes accompanied by painful urination, lower back pain or fever.

• *Orchitis* is inflammation of the testicles themselves. It's usually caused by bacteria and is marked by swelling, heaviness and pain of the testicles.

• Sexually transmitted diseases are common causes for testicular pain. The worst offenders are gonorrhea and chlamydia, which can cause orchitis as well as penile discharge and painful urination.

Easing the Pain of Your Privates

You can't do much when it comes to treating testicular pain yourself, so leave treatment to the experts. Nevertheless, here are some tips on preventing and alleviating the agony.

Give it a lift. Elevate a swollen scrotum by lying down with a pillow under your butt. If you have an infection, like epididymitis, this will ease the pain. Also try wearing a jockstrap or briefs-style underwear for added support—it gives the same effect. Be warned that if torsion is marauding your manhood, the pain will probably worsen when you give yourself a lift.

Ice is nice. Try an ice compress on swollen testicles to alleviate pain and reduce swelling. But be warned that ice also might increase the pain of torsion.

"If you put an ice compress on your testicles and suddenly the pain gets worse, it's a pretty gross indicator that you have torsion," Dr. Neal says. "Of course, you don't want to rule out torsion if the pain doesn't worsen with ice."

Try sticking ice cubes in a plastic bag and wrapping the bag in a hand towel, since applying ice directly to delicate scrotal skin can be damaging.

Try the hot stuff. If ice isn't doing the trick, then try heat to ease the pain and swelling. Place a heating pad wrapped in a towel or a warm compress on your painful privates.

"Heat sometimes helps, like ice, but remember neither is going to cure the problem. You might feel a little better, but you still need help," Dr. Cohen warns.

Fight the inflammation. Stop swelling and pain by taking an adult dosage of any over-the-counter anti-inflammatory, like aspirin or ibuprofen.

Bag it. Since sexually transmitted diseases are common causes of testicular pain, use common sense and wear a condom during sex, especially if you're having sex with multiple partners or are unsure of your partner's sexual history. Putting your manhood under wraps might be the easiest thing you can do to prevent testicular pain—and an unwanted sexual souvenir.

Testosterone Problems

Is It a Man's World?

In one of the most unforgettable and disturbing scenes from director Stanley Kubrick's classic movie *A Clockwork Orange*, Malcolm McDowell chases a woman through her home brandishing a ridiculously large, sculpted phallus—and then bludgeons her to death with it.

In the eyes of testosterone's detractors the history of the world can be viewed in a *Clockwork Orange* hue. These experts believe that "testosterone poisoning," as it has been called, can help give a lad, in the words of the movie, a taste for the old ultraviolence.

"That's ridiculous," replies Adrian Dobs, M.D., associate professor of medicine and director of the Endocrinology and Metabolism Clinical Studies Unit at Johns Hopkins University in Baltimore. "There's no data that criminals have higher testosterone levels."

Such a debate rages over many of the medical issues surrounding testosterone. From how the male hormone affects a man's actions to how much is too little or too much, there is not a whole lot of consensus. One thing is pretty clear though, and it's probably what matters to you most: There are few medical problems directly related to testosterone levels in men.

The Hormone Debate

One of those who has investigated the possible link between testosterone and violence is James M. Dabbs, Jr., Ph.D., professor of social psychology at Georgia State University in Atlanta. After studying levels in men guilty of violent crimes, he concluded that, on average, higher testosterone was associated with more violent crimes. He also says that there is a connection between the male hormone and what he terms "unruly behavior."

"Testosterone is certainly a risk factor for bad things," says Dr. Dabbs. "It may sometimes lead to good things, too, but it certainly is a risk factor for misbehavior."

The notion that testosterone is somehow inherently evil and responsible for the world's woes, not to mention world wars, completely baffles Dr. Dobs and other medical researchers.

Indeed, testosterone puts the man in mankind. Without it, there would be no male of the species. The sex hormone starts pumping midway through fetal growth, guiding the development of a penis and testicles. At puberty a flood of testosterone is released, turning boys into men. The hormone spurs the growth of sex organs, hair and sexual function.

To those who believe there is too much testosterone in the world and that we might be better off stemming the flow, Dr. Dobs offers this wry observation: "It certainly wouldn't do much for the population. If you take away men's libido and ability to get an erection, we're really in bad shape."

Ebb Tide for Testosterone

The real problem, according to Dr. Dobs and other experts, is not too much testosterone, but too little. As you age, usually between your fifties and seventies, your testosterone level may drop dramatically. The natural process has given rise to the concept of "male menopause"—one Dr. Dobs and other experts dispute. "There's no such thing as a real male menopause," Dr. Dobs says. "Menopause, by definition, is this rapid drop in sex steroids that occurs in women. If men have anything like that, it's a very gradual decline. I think the term is really misused a lot."

Most men won't notice any appreciable change in their sexual appetite or general health as they age from year to year. "There's a broad threshold of what is considered normal," says Laurence A. Levine, M.D., director of the Male Sexual Health Program at Rush-Presbyterian-St. Luke's Medical Center in Chicago. "Over time, many men's testosterone levels decline by as much as half or more without having an effect."

Throughout your life testosterone ebbs and flows. In general, you wake up in the morning with the hormones raging and then they fall off during the day. Your testosterone level can decline by half or more over the course of a day and still be perfectly normal, says Anthony E. Karpas, M.D., director of the Institute for Endocrinology and Reproductive Medicine in Atlanta.

How much is enough? That's hard to say. The mean level is about 500 nanograms of testosterone per deciliter of blood, Dr. Dobs says. But men can check in anywhere from 300 to 1,100 nanograms and still be considered normal, says Dr. Karpas. When your testosterone level goes below 300 nanograms, you may need to give it a boost, experts say.

"We don't measure testosterone enough on men," says Dr. Dobs, who is conducting several studies into the hormone's potential health benefits. "I think the condition is underdiagnosed." Studies have indicated, Dr. Karpas says, that as many as 20 percent of men over age 50 may be hypogonadal, meaning they have

FAST FACTS

How common: The testosterone levels of most men decline as they age. It's estimated that about 20 percent will drop to abnormally low levels.

Risk factors: Aging, infections, injuries to the testicles, pituitary gland problems, testicular tumor, amputation of both testicles.

Age group affected: Most experts believe testosterone levels begin to decline after age 50, with the drop becoming steeper after age 60.

Gender gap: Women, whose sex drive is also fueled by testosterone, have about one-twelfth to one-tenth as much of it in their blood as men do. One to 3 percent of women have androgen disorders, which include high amounts of testosterone or other androgens that cause excessive hair growth. Testosterone plays a key role in women's sex drive as well as men's, and some studies support the claim that decreased androgens can reduce sexual desire among women.

Who to see: Since a flagging libido can result from any number of ailments, it's a good idea to start with a family doctor, who can look at the big picture. The next stop would be a urologist or endocrinologist.

abnormally low testosterone levels. "It's a lot more common than people think," says Dr. Karpas.

There is nothing you can do naturally to boost your testosterone level. Moderate exercise may help, but that idea still falls in the chicken-and-egg category. "Do men with high testosterone levels tend to exercise more or do men who exercise more have higher testosterone levels?" Dr. Karpas says. It is believed that stress, fatigue, lack of sleep and alcohol can lower levels.

Serious testosterone deficiencies do occur in men in their forties and younger, but it's rare, says Richard Spark, M.D., assistant clinical professor of medicine at the Harvard Medical School and author of *Male Sexual Health*. It's also probably an indication of a medical problem that needs attention. The most likely causes, he says, are damage to the testicles, such as an injury or testicular tumor; a viral infection, such as the mumps; or some problem in the pituitary, the gland that sends hormonal signals to the testicles to produce testosterone.

When To Test

There are some signs that may indicate a need for you to get your testosterone level tested. They are:

Loss of libido. The question isn't whether you can get up for sex. It's whether you even *want* to. "Sex drive seems to be more important than sex function," Dr. Karpas says. He recalled asking one patient who had come in for possible testosterone replacement if there was anything wrong with his sex life. The man replied, "No." So Dr. Karpas asked him when the last time was that he had sex. "Two years ago, but it doesn't bother me," the man told him. "Obviously, that's a lack of sex drive," Dr. Karpas says. "If somebody truly has a lack of sex drive, not having sex really doesn't worry them that much."

Going soft, part I. If you do get the urge, but can't achieve or maintain an erection, your testosterone tank may be running low.

Feeling run-down. Men with abnormally low testosterone levels often complain of feeling weak, tired or fatigued. There's a major drop in their energy levels and abilities to function throughout the day, Dr. Dobs says. This can be accompanied by a decline in mental sharpness as well, says Dr. Karpas.

Going soft, part II. Low testosterone levels are being studied because of a suspected link with increased belly fat and decreased bone and muscle mass. Other telltale signs are thinning of pubic, underarm or facial hair and a loss of weight, says Rahmawati Sih, M.D., a geriatrics fellow at the St. Louis University Medical School.

Filling Your Tank

Men diagnosed with hypogonadism are candidates for testosterone replacement. At present, hormone levels can be boosted through a patch attached to the scrotum or injections. Experimental forms include tablets, pellets inserted under the skin or patches attached to nonscrotal skin. Considerable research is being conducted to determine whether hormone replacement therapy for men offers wide-ranging health benefits. Studies have indicated that testosterone may help build muscles, strengthen bones, guard against heart attacks, slim potbellies and whet sexual appetites.

But there is no indication that boosting testosterone in men who already have normal levels will do any good. Just the opposite. It may create dangerous side effects, chief among them is stimulating the growth of pre-existing prostate tumors. "Testosterone therapy is only warranted when there's a bona fide testosterone deficiency," says Dr. Spark. "In the absence of a deficiency it will do men harm."

The reason: If your testosterone level is in the normal range, taking extra doses of the hormone will temporarily reduce your own natural production. "It's not going to bring up the level," explains Dr. Dobs. "You're just going to have the same level. But you're going to be dependent on this medication to get it, as opposed to your own body making it."

Among men with low testosterone there is no indication that boosting levels will bring out the beast in them. Even researchers who have linked high-testosterone levels to unpleasant behavior say that social factors play a significant role in how men act. "If you go to a group of Quakers or Amish people, I suspect they have just as many high-testosterone members as anybody else does," says Dr. Dabbs. "But they don't behave that way."

Dr. Karpas says he has seen nothing but positive results from testosterone enhancement. "If anything, they seem to feel better and become more motivated," Dr. Karpas says. "I see a lot of their wives as well, and I have yet to have a report that they didn't like the way it made their husbands behave. In fact, most of the wives are extremely happy."

Thyroid Disease

Unsticking the Throttle

Imagine hurtling down the highway, watching the miles whiz by, your vehicle perfectly balanced on the edge of the speed limit. Suddenly, a short in the system damages the cruise control and you start picking up speed. The engine is racing, the chassis is shaking and you're careening out of control.

On the other hand, maybe the cruise control just shuts down. Your speed drops and eventually you shudder to a stop in the middle of the road.

In a car you could prevent either situation with a quick kick of the pedal, putting you back in command. Unfortunately, when the vehicle in question is your body, that cruise control—better known as the thyroid gland—governs a lot more than speed.

"Virtually all the processes in the body are affected one way or another by the thyroid," says David Cooper, M.D., director of endocrinology at Sinai Hospital in Baltimore and co-author of *Your Thyroid*. And Dr. Cooper means everything, from how fast we think to how often our bowels move. Essentially every cell in our bodies is tuned to respond to thyroid hormones secreted by that gland in our throats. When the thyroid malfunctions, the effects are bodywide.

Time was, thyroid problems were common, in large part because of a lack of iodine in our daily diets. Iodized salt changed that. Today most thyroid diseases do not have a known cause, although many are the result of hereditary conditions or, more rarely, direct exposure to radiation. On balance, men don't have to worry about thyroid disease nearly as much as women, who are about ten times more likely to develop thyroid problems. But that still leaves more than a half-million men who suffer from thyroid diseases—and many of them may not even know it.

"If you have a thyroid problem, there's really nothing you can do on your own to prevent it from occurring," admits Brian Tulloch, M.D., clinical associate professor of endocrinology and metabolic diseases at the University of Texas Medical School at Houston. Nothing except learn more about catching problems in their early stages. Then your doctor can guide you toward any one of the highly successful therapies being used to treat temperamental thyroids.

FAST FACTS

How common: Thyroid problems affect less than 1 percent of American adult men.

Risk factors: Most thyroid problems can develop for seemingly no reason—most are because of hereditary problems. In some instances exposure to direct radiation can cause thyroid ailments.

Age group affected: Thyroid problems can occur at any age but are most common in men over age 65.

Gender gap: Women are ten times more likely to develop thyroid problems than men.

Who to see: Family doctor, endocrinologist.

Spotting a Grave Problem

At first glance most men probably wouldn't mind having an overactive or *hyper* thyroid. "People with hyperthyroidism have lots of energy," says Peter Sigmann, M.D., associate professor of medicine at the Medical College of Wisconsin in Milwaukee. "A lot of them think it's great—at first."

An overactive thyroid gland puts you on the fast track to burnout. "You won't be able to sleep. Your bones and muscles will eventually weaken. You're also more likely to have a heart attack," says Dr. Sigmann. Besides an energy surge or insomnia, watch out for heart palpitations, intolerance to heat, general muscle weakness or shortness of breath—all are classic signs of an overactive thyroid and should be treated by a doctor immediately.

Hyperthyroidism is most commonly caused by Graves' disease, when your body suddenly decides the thyroid is a foreign invader and dispatches antibodies to attack it. Instead, the antibodies only overstimulate the thyroid and, consequently, you. When this happens, the best way to shut it down is by taking radioactive iodine.

Now radioactive *anything* may sound pretty dangerous. But experts agree the procedure is safer than the other alternatives. Drugs, for example, can slow down the thyroid, but they don't cure the problem and they have various side effects. And part of the thyroid can be surgically removed, but that is expensive and risky. That leaves the option of radioactive iodine. "Because the thyroid absorbs the iodine, the radiation concentrates only on the thyroid—it won't harm any other part of the body," says Dr. Sigmann. But the radiation will keep the thyroid from acting up again.

From Surge to Slump

Meanwhile, for some men, the thyroid isn't acting up but is slowing down. *Hy-po*thyroidism, or an underactive thyroid, is one of the easiest thyroid problems to treat, but it's also one of the hardest to spot.

"A lot of times, hypothyroid problems are mistaken as general signs of aging," says Dr. Cooper. "People just think they're slowing down, but they don't have to be."

So pay attention to extreme mental and physical fatigue for no apparent reason, intolerance to cold, muscle cramps, dry or brittle hair and dry skin. These are common signs of hypothyroidism, and a simple blood test can prove it.

"After that, the treatment is very simple," says Dr. Cooper. "You just take a thyroid hormone replacement tablet every day. It's one of the most commonly prescribed medications in the world." And the quickest way to get back up to speed again.

Lumps and Bumps

We all know what it feels like to get a lump in our throat, but if you can actually see that lump, chances are it's a thyroid problem worth getting looked at.

Probably the hardest lump to miss is a goiter. Your thyroid gets so large it can cause a sizable bulge in your throat. Goiters can be the result of an over- or underactive thyroid, or even a tumor. Either way, rather than walking around like a bullfrog, you're better off getting to a doctor to find out exactly what's causing the goiter.

Other lumps and bumps are trickier to spot, considering where the thyroid is located.

"If you feel your throat, you'll know there are a lot of bumps and rough spots already there," says Dr. Sigmann. No one wants to embarrass himself in front of his doctor by mistaking the Adam's apple for a thyroid tumor, so Dr. Sigmann says to look before you leap. "While you're shaving, just look in the mirror, under your chin," he says. Look for any unusual swelling. Swallow a couple of times. "If a lump moves in the lower part of your neck when you swallow, then it's likely related to the thyroid," says Dr. Sigmann.

And if you have reason to suspect the worst, remember that most thyroid tumors are benign. "You should still get it looked at," advises Dr. Tulloch. "Thyroid cancer is relatively rare compared to other diseases, but there's always that chance."

Finally, as you get older, the odds of developing thyroid problems will increase. That's why the thyroid specialists recommend that men over the age of 50 be screened annually for thyroid function. Otherwise, you'll run a greater risk of burning out before your time—and most men would find that hard to swallow.

TMD

No More Jaw Pain

It's the start of another daily grind. You wake up tense, your mind already focusing on the business of the day. At work you call a few clients, the phone jammed between your head and shoulder while you type on the computer. Later, nervously chewing on your pen, you go over the notes for the big meeting. Outside the conference room door you straighten your shoulders, grit your teeth and saunter in. On the way home your head is pounding, as usual, but it wasn't such a bad day. In fact, everything is clicking right along. Including your jaw.

Many of your daily habits at work and at home can lead to temporomandibular disorder, or TMD, a mouthful of a name that describes a head full of pain and discomfort. You get TMD when your jaw joint becomes damaged through injury or overuse. The more you work the joints, the more the bones grind against each other, causing pain and damage.

If you have frequent headaches, muscle aches in the head and neck and a telltale clicking sound every time you open your mouth, chances are you're the one out of every ten American men who has TMD. But that doesn't mean you can't get rid of it.

Why Good Joints Go Bad

TMD usually starts with an injury—even a minor one—to the jaw or head. "With men, that most often means trauma as a result of a sports injury or auto accident," says Brendan Stack, Sr., D.D.S., director of the National Capitol Center for Craniofacial Pain in Vienna, Virginia. The joints controlling the jaw get damaged, and Dr. Stack says men add insult to the injury by, well, just being men.

"The men who get this problem are your basic Type A personalities: intense guys who have a lot of stress," says Dr. Stack. In fact, they have so much stress that nine out of ten TMD sufferers will make their problems worse by grinding their teeth in their sleep, a condition known as nocturnal bruxism. "They'll wake up sore and tense because they've been working their jaw all night," says Dr. Stack.

You can alleviate that problem by getting a mouthguard designed by your dentist. It might feel weird the first few nights you wear it to bed, but Dr. Stack says it's one of the most important things you can do to keep the jaw joint from eroding.

531

Taking TMD in Stride

That John Wayne saunter you've adopted may help you make an impression when you walk into a room, but it's not helping your jaw any.

Foot specialists are finding that the way we walk can actually cause muscle and joint pain elsewhere in our bodies—and directly affect problems like temporomandibular disorder (TMD), says Howard Dananberg, D.P.M., a podiatrist in private practice in Bedford, New Hampshire. The key is something called referred pain—when pain starts in one part of the body but is felt elsewhere, say, in your jaw.

"If your limbs aren't correctly in position when you walk, muscles in the rest of your body—your trunk and head—are going to compensate for that," says Dr. Dananberg. That overcompensation could eventually translate into muscle strain, pain and TMD. People who sway from side to side or saunter when they walk are prime targets for this kind of referred pain. If you think you suffer from this foot-and-mouth connection, Dr. Dananberg recommends seeing a podiatrist who specializes in gait analysis—he'll be able to tell if your walking style is potentially harmful. Usually, the problem can be treated with an orthotic—a specially designed insole to help swing your gait back to normal.

"The clicking is the first sign of erosion," he warns. "After that the jaw will lock every once in a while—eventually it could lock up completely and you won't be able to open your mouth very much." Granted, it takes a while to reach this stage—sometimes one or two months, sometimes as much as 20 years. But if it happens, you may be facing surgery to realign the jaw.

Avoiding the nightly grind is only half the battle. "Your average go-getter does all kinds of things to make the TMD worse," says Dr. Stack. So here are some daytime tips to make sure the only thing that clicks in your head is the lightswitch for your next bright idea.

Quit the bad habits. Any overuse of the joint possibly will make the TMD worse, says Harold T. Perry, D.D.S., Ph.D., professor emeritus of orthodontics at Northwestern University Dental School in Chicago and editor emeritus of a dental medical journal that focuses on TMD problems. And the quickest way to overuse the jaw is by excessive chewing. "Nonfunctional oral habits—chewing pens, clenching pipes or cigars between your teeth, and lip and cheek biting may perpetuate or accentuate your TMD symptoms," says Dr. Perry.

Don't get chewed out. It's also a good idea to avoid chewy foods, says Dr. Stack. "Bagels, taffy or thick cuts of tough meat are particularly bad," he says, and should be avoided until you get your joint in order.

Hang up the phone. At work most men like to do two things at once, such as making a phone call while jotting notes or working on the computer. With our hands full most of us tend to pinch the phone between our head and shoulder. "Holding the phone that way is just plain bad," says Dr. Stack. Not only are you pushing your jaw to one side, you're also talking and straining your neck and shoulder muscles—a TMD triple whammy. Dr. Stack's advice: "Get a head set." Your office should be able to order one for you, or you can buy one for less than $100 at most office-supply stores.

Make a palm tree. While it's true that overworking your jaw can make TMD worse, certain jaw exercises can make it better—or even eliminate the clicking. Try these two to three times a day.

• Rest your elbow on a table and place your palm under your chin. Apply slight resistance to your palm, then open your mouth about ¼ to ½ inch and close slowly. Don't open so wide that your jaw clicks or hurts. Start with five and work up to ten repetitions.

• Put your right palm under your chin, fingers covering your right cheek. Move your lower jawbone slightly to the left and back to the center for ten repetitions. Repeat with your left hand and move your jaw to the right.

Give yourself a warm, wet one on the cheek. For a temporary soother, warm, moist heat in the form of a towel or heating pad can help you unclench those jaw muscles. Apply the heat for about 15 to 20 minutes twice a day—usually first thing in the morning and right after work, when you're likely to have jaw problems the most.

Escape the clenches. It's completely natural for most men to grit their teeth or set their jaws when they concentrate on a specific task. But Dr. Perry says this can be as bad as clenching your teeth all night. So train yourself out of the habit.

"If you have a wristwatch alarm, set your watch every hour—or every 15 minutes," says Dr. Perry. "When it goes off, don't stop what you're doing, but let that beep serve as a reminder. Let your shoulders, neck and jaw relax. Pretty soon, you'll get into the habit." Just remember—it's okay to be slack-jawed at work.

Type A Personality
Take Yourself off the A-List

Nice guys finish last. Idle hands are the Devil's workshop. If you want something done—and done right—you have to do it yourself. And it had to be done yesterday.

If these hackneyed phrases are part of your life's creed, you probably need to cut yourself some slack. "Nope, can't do that," you protest. "I'm just not the type."

Oh, yes you are.

Type A personality is a clinical, psychological term, but it gets used pretty freely these days as a synonym for being intense and high-strung. Some men even consider it a compliment, a description that speaks well of their motivation, ambition and willingness to take on difficult tasks.

But the Type A man has a darker side, too. Nice guys may finish last, but Type A guys never seem to finish at all—they're in a constant race, driven by boundless impatience, frustration and more than a little anger, speeding towards a checkered flag they can never hope to reach. If your life is one big game of Beat the Clock— and you have a nagging sense that you're losing—chances are you're on the Type A team, too.

You're not alone. A full 75 percent of all American men have Type A characteristics, and it's slowly but surely hurting them.

"Type A personality is a sickness. A Type A man really has only one approach to everything, and that's full-speed ahead. This approach has serious health consequences. A person who fits the pattern ought to seek help," says Meyer Friedman, M.D., director of the Meyer Friedman Institute in San Francisco and co-originator of the concept of Type A, which he also refers to as hurry sickness.

The Type A personality was identified by Dr. Friedman after studying the effects that mental stress had on the human heart. In his research men who were always impatient, extremely aggressive, competitive and quick-tempered were three times as likely as their mellower counterparts to develop heart disease. Type A personalities also suffer more than their share of migraine headaches, high blood pressure, ulcers, irritable bowel syndrome—even certain types of cancer were more prevalent in Type A people.

Getting from Point A to Point B

Type A's share certain specific characteristics that aren't good for them: They are very self-critical, set extremely high goals and tend to blame themselves for failures. But experts don't think men are born with these traits—they learn them.

"Type A's often suffer from a real sense of inadequate unconditional parental love," says Dr. Friedman. That kind of environment is prime breeding ground for feelings of hostility and worthlessness. "Type A's never—and I mean never—feel they're giving enough or working enough or doing enough; they always feel inadequate," Dr. Friedman adds. And so men compensate in later life, looking for challenging situations that offer struggle and a chance for high achievement, which makes them feel better about themselves. Or so they think.

"The problem is, Type A men blame themselves for everything that goes wrong when they don't reach those high goals," says David Jenkins, Ph.D., professor of preventive medicine and community health at the University of Texas Medical School at Galveston. "This mind-set can lead to careless and even self-destructive behavior. For example, Type A personalities are about 3½ times more likely to have an accident of some sort, are more likely to break a bone or get a divorce, than Bs," he says.

That's right, there's a Type B personality—characterized by solid feelings of self-worth and an easygoing attitude toward life. Type B men are usually better adjusted, even-tempered and still successful in their personal and professional lives. If you're Type A, it's enough to make you want to throttle them. But you don't need to. Because even if you've been programmed from birth to be an A, you can still be a B.

"It's a matter of what we call behavior modification, where you slowly learn to alter your way of thinking," says Harrison Madden, Ph.D., chairman of the Department of Psychology at California State University, Fresno. "The idea is not to develop a completely different personality, but just to modify your behavior enough to minimize the harmful effects of a Type A personality."

Becoming a New Man

Sometimes modifying your personality requires the help of a qualified behavioral psychologist. But by and large, learning new ways to react to day-to-day chal-

the male file

Laughter has been shown to reduce stress and induce relaxation, but adults laugh only an average of 15 times a day—children laugh an average of 400 times a day.

FAST FACTS

How common: About 70 to 75 percent of all men have some Type A personality traits.

Risk factors: Men who didn't receive unconditional love when they were growing up tend to develop hard-driving, competitive, hostile personality traits.

Age group affected: Although the Type A traits develop in childhood, the results become more pronounced when men hit their professional years.

Gender gap: Almost twice as many men fit the Type A profile as women.

Who to see: Psychologist specializing in Type A behavior modification.

lenges and annoyances is up to you. It sounds impossible, but then, if you have Type A tendencies, you should have no problem volunteering for an impossible task. As it happens, there are plenty of exercises and drills experts recommend to help Type A men change their behaviors. Here are a few to get you started.

Work up a sweat. Since there's a mind-body connection at work here, pay some attention to that body and exercise it. One study at the University of Manitoba in Winnipeg suggests an association between Type A men's ability to reduce the harmful effects of their behavior and their participation in moderate exercise on a treadmill. Type A stress causes us to produce all sorts of hormones that our bodies need in crisis situations. But when we react as though we're in a constant crisis—a hallmark of type A's—the stress hormones can build up to toxic levels, leading to health problems, like heart disease and cancer. In the study, exercise helped burn off those stress hormones. And exercise also improves the fitness of your heart and lungs, making you better able to deal with the daily annoyances and stressors.

Just don't go overboard. Dr. Jenkins points out that it would be just like a Type A guy to turn a morning jog into an Ironman run.

Wait a minute. Severe, foot-stomping, teeth-gnashing, horn-blowing impatience over the slightest delay is one of the chief characteristics of Type A personality. And it's a killer—you become a pressure cooker, and the self-generated stress pushes your blood pressure up and deteriorates your health bit by bit.

Dr. Friedman says you should learn to cope with everyday delays, so start by putting yourself in a deliberate holding pattern now and again. For example, one drill he recommends is looking for the longest line at the grocery store, making a point of standing in it and then—the tough part—making a point of relaxing by finding distractions or daydreaming instead of being irritated or impatient.

"Turn it to your advantage," he says. "Think of it as an opportunity to collect yourself. You could even consider it an opportunity to meet new people." Try this about every other trip to the store to get your behavioral shift in gear.

Take the long way home. If there's a scenic route to and from work, take it at least once a week. If you use public transportation, give yourself a few minutes to do a little walking or window-shopping before you head for the bus stop or subway. Not only will the change of scene calm you down, you'll probably avoid the traffic snarls or crowded public conveyances that usually raise your ire.

Sit still. Plunk a chair in front of a window or on the porch and sit in it. Don't bring work with you; don't write letters; don't reach for the phone; don't have the TV on in the background. Dr. Friedman says Type A's try to do too many things at once. So do one thing for a change: Sit and look out at the world; resist the urge to be a participant in it. For the next few minutes you're just a spectator.

Get time on your side. For Type A's, time is the enemy, but Dr. Friedman says you can make it your ally. "Type A's tend to look at things minute by minute, which can be very stressful. Type B's, on the other hand, succeed by focusing on long-term goals," he says. "We say it's a matter of setting your goals by a calendar, not by a stopwatch."

Start by modifying your schedule. For example, if you're always rushing out the door in the morning, set your alarm to go off 15 minutes earlier. "You'll have more time to dawdle and it could have an impact on the rest of your day," Dr. Friedman says.

Making changes to your daily schedule might seem insignificant at first, but if you keep it up, you might even be able to avoid being typecast for the rest of your life.

Ulcers

Stopping Acid Attacks

You know a couple of guys who have ulcers. Your brother, the surgeon. Your buddy over at the stock brokerage. The guy down the hall in marketing.

It doesn't surprise you, really. They're all workaholic, work-till-you-drop maniacs who are now paying the price with those gnawing, burning holes in their insides. You figure you're in the clear since ulcers aren't likely to bother mellow fellows like yourself. Right?

A few years ago, the medical establishment probably would have agreed. But recent research shows that the ulcer equation is more complex than was previously thought. While having a Type A personality may play some role, the cause of ulcers is more likely to be something quite different: bacteria. Plus, other factors such as alcohol and certain medicines can also be involved.

Still, there's a lot you can do to reduce your chances of getting an ulcer. What's more, there are new treatments that will not only help ease the pain but in many cases cure the condition as well.

Equal Opportunity Pain

An ulcer is simply a sore that forms when powerful stomach acids begin burning through the lining of the digestive organs. The majority of ulcers occur in the duodenum, the portion of small intestine that's nearest to the stomach. The remainder, called gastric ulcers, form in the lining of the stomach itself.

Most ulcers aren't life-threatening, but they can be incredibly painful, causing gnawing, burning pain in the gut. In more severe cases, they can also cause internal bleeding, which typically turns the stool nearly black.

Every year about a half-million people will develop an ulcer. In addition, about four million ulcers will reappear in people who have previously been diagnosed. It used to be that more men than women had ulcers, but the gap seems to have closed. In fact, in adults under 45, slightly more women than men report having ulcers.

What's Eating You?

For a long time researchers proclaimed stress to be the prime ulcer-inducer. Smoking, heredity and even type O blood were thought to be other causes.

But new findings suggest that while stress and these other inducers may make existing ulcers worse, they probably play little or no role in causing them, says David Alpers, M.D., professor of medicine and chief of the Division of Gastroenterolgy at the Washington University School of Medicine in St. Louis.

Rather, a bacterium called *Helicobacter pylori*, which resides between the lining of the digestive tract (the epithelium) and its overlying mucous layer, is probably a key factor in causing ulcers to form. Studies have shown that 75 to 80 percent of people with gastric ulcers and 90 to 100 percent of people with duodenal ulcers are infected with *H. pylori*.

The bacterium is difficult to avoid. In Western countries studies have suggested that between 40 and 60 percent of adults at age 60 are infected with *H. pylori*. In the United States, Hispanics and African Americans have a higher rate of infection than Whites. Yet for reasons that aren't clear, only about 10 percent of those with the bacteria in their systems actually develop ulcers, says Dr. Alpers.

Presumably, *H. pylori* sets the stage for ulcers, while other factors—like stress and the others mentioned above—may cause them to eventually appear.

Apart from bacterial infection, the other leading cause of ulcers is the regular use of anti-inflammatory medications. Over-the-counter drugs like aspirin and ibuprofen or prescription drugs like indomethacin (Indocin) reduce the body's production of prostaglandins, chemicals that are needed to help protect the stomach and intestine from injury, says Dr. Alpers. The regular use of these medications may increase the risk of developing an ulcer tenfold.

Playing Your Cards Right

While ulcers can be readily controlled with medications (which we'll discuss in a bit), a better bet is to prevent them from occurring in the first place. Here's how.

Quit smoking. Studies have shown that smoking decreases the production and release of the chemicals that protect the lining of the stomach and intestine. Smokers get more ulcers, take longer to heal and suffer more recurrences than nonsmokers.

Don't overdo the libations. While heavy drinking has been linked with an increased risk of ulcers, a moderate amount of alcohol isn't likely to cause problems, says John Kurata, Ph.D., associate adjunct professor at the University of California, Los Angeles, and director of research and health policy at San Bernardino County Medical Center. He adds, however, that some experts feel that drinking at the same time you're taking aspirin may cause problems, so be careful not to mix the two.

FAST FACTS

How common: An estimated one in ten men will develop an ulcer during his lifetime.

Risk factors: Infection with *Helicobacter pylori*, use of anti-inflammatory medications.

Age group affected: Most common in adults over age 60.

Gender gap: Under age 45, women have ulcers at a slightly greater rate than men. Between the ages of 45 and 64, men have the edge.

Who to see: Internist, gastroenterologist.

Pick your pills carefully. Since aspirin, ibuprofen and similar painkillers, known collectively as nonsteroidal anti-inflammatory drugs (NSAIDs), are hard on the gut, you're better off taking acetaminophen, which is less likely to cause problems, experts say.

Keep the dose low. If you do need aspirin or a similar drug to control pain, at least start with the lowest possible dose that will provide relief, says Mark Feldman, M.D., vice-chairman of the Department of Internal Medicine at the University of Texas Southwestern Medical Center in Dallas. If you're taking one or more of these medications regularly for a chronic condition like arthritis, it's best to do so under a doctor's supervision, says Dr. Feldman. In some cases the doctor may recommend a prescription substitute that will be easier on your insides.

When Pain Strikes

Although ulcers often can be prevented, experts estimate that about one in ten men will develop an ulcer at some time in his life. So if the pain's already begun, here's what doctors recommend.

Start with an antacid. These over-the-counter medications provide a quick, inexpensive way to control an ulcer's symptoms, says Dr. Alpers. There are dozens of antacids to choose from, but most contain aluminum, calcium, magnesium, sodium, magaldrate or a combination of these ingredients. All are effective but may cause mild side effects. You may have to try several kinds before finding the one that's best for you.

Turn off the acid tap. When antacids don't help, your doctor may recommend that you take prescription medications to reduce the amount of acid in the stomach. Most common are the H_2-receptor antagonists—H_2-blockers, for short. Drugs such as ranitidine (Zantac) or cimetidine (Tagamet), taken one to four times a day, can reduce stomach acid secretions by up to 80 percent, healing most duodenal ulcers within four to eight weeks.

Other drugs that can help reduce acid include famotidine (Pepcid), nizatidine (Axid) and omeprazole (Prilosec). Sucralfate (Carafate) improves the body's natural defenses against acid by forming a protective coating over the ulcer. But while all of these drugs can help ulcers heal, they don't really attack the underlying cause. As a result, says Dr. Alpers, the ulcers often come back.

Go after the source. Once you begin having pain, your doctor may want to run tests to see if you're infected with *H. pylori*. If you are, the next step may be to take antibiotics. Studies have shown that the bacteria can be eradicated in 90 percent of those who undergo "triple therapy"—treatment with two antibiotics plus a drug called bismuth subsalicylate (found in Pepto-Bismol), says Dr. Kurata.

In one study, less than 5 percent of those given the triple therapy saw their ulcers return. By contrast, more than half of those treated with H_2-blockers alone had relapses within 12 weeks. Top experts now agree that when a man has an ulcer and is also infected with *H. pylori*, treatment with antibiotics may be his best bet.

Not all men need to undergo the therapy, adds Dr. Alpers. Even if tests show you're infected with the bacteria, you may not need treatment at all if you don't have an ulcer or have no symptoms, or if the symptoms have another explanation, he says.

Try to reduce stress. While stress may not cause ulcers, it can exacerbate one you already have, says Dr. Kurata. Reducing your stress levels—with exercise, yoga, meditation, biofeedback or just reducing your workload—can help keep the problem in check, he says.

Add some comfort. If you're taking medications that are causing stomach upset, like aspirin or ibuprofen, your doctor may advise combining them with another drug, misoprostol (Cytotec), that can help protect cells in the intestinal tract.

In a study of 420 patients with osteoarthritis, more than 12 percent of those taking NSAIDs developed ulcers. In those taking the anti-inflammatory drugs plus misoprostol, the ulcer rate dropped to less than 5 percent.

Get follow-up advice. Once you've been diagnosed with an ulcer, it's important to get regular checkups to make sure it's healing properly—or hasn't gotten worse, says Dr. Kurata. In addition, research into the best ulcer medications is ongoing, so you'll have to stay current with state-of-the-art developments.

Urinary Problems

How to Go with the Flow

You probably haven't thought about urinary problems since kindergarten, when the top issue was making it through naptime without soaking the floor.

But urinary control problems aren't just for kids. Millions of men have them. And we're not talking about the long line to the bathroom at the ballpark.

If you don't know much about the demons that can plague your privates, you're not alone. Some urinary problems are relatively rare and little talked about. But don't think ignorance is bliss. Problems of the urinary system can lead to dangerous complications if untreated, and some apparently minor pains can be symptoms of more serious problems.

A Primer on the Plumbing

Here's what you need to know: The urinary system removes excess fluid and liquid waste from your body. It consists of the kidneys, bladder, ureters (tubes from the kidneys that bring urine to the bladder) and urethra (the tube that carries urine out of the body.)

In the kidneys, tiny filters called nephrons remove waste from the blood. They then move the waste through the ureters to the bladder. When enough accumulates, it sends a signal for you to expel the fluid through the urethra. On average, you excrete 1½ quarts of urine a day. Healthy urine is clear to pale yellow and consists mostly of water and urea. Other components include sodium chloride (salt), phosphoric acid and sulfuric acid.

Here's what can go wrong and what you can do about it.

Incontinence: When You Lose Control

Incontinence is the lack of bladder control. Approximately six million men in the United States are incontinent.

Incontinence is not a disease. It's a symptom of some underlying condition. It ranges in severity from feelings of urgency to leakage to complete loss of control. Causes include a bladder muscle that doesn't work properly, an enlarged prostate,

Dribbling off the Court

It's okay to dribble on the basketball court, but it's not okay to dribble on your pants, especially if we're talking about urine.

Yet some guys have this problem when they urinate. They think they've finished urinating, but a little bit of urine trickles out onto their trousers or underwear when they're tucking themselves away. This dribbling is not incontinence (lack of bladder control) and it's not penile discharge, per se. But it is annoying—and it is easily corrected.

For the most part urine dribbling is a result of poor urination habits, weak muscles or both. Here are some tips on stopping the trickle.

Give it room. Pull your pants far away from your penis, and don't try to urinate by pulling your penis over the top of your underwear. Use your fly, that's what it's there for. By not giving your penis enough room to urinate, you slow the flow of urine through your urethra, the small tube that expels urine. As a result, urine that isn't expelled dribbles out when you tuck yourself away.

Milk your urethra. After you finish urinating, apply some gentle pressure behind your scrotum with one hand and coax out any remaining urine. This is where the widest part of your urethra is, the part where urine tends to pool in men. Gentle pressure might be all you need to get rid of those last few drops.

Control with Kegels. Kegel exercises can help you strengthen the muscles in your pelvis, which will give you better urinary control. To do these exercises, slowly and tightly squeeze the muscles you normally use to stop the flow of urine. Then release. Do three sets of five daily for a week. Then gradually add 5 repetitions to each set, working up to 30 repetitions, three times a day.

nerve injuries, surgery and certain diseases, like multiple sclerosis or diabetes.

Incontinence "is absolutely devastating to men," says Katherine F. Jeter, Ed.D., executive director of Help for Incontinent People, a nonprofit consumer organization in Union, South Carolina. "Incontinence for men is terribly emasculating. Men don't just want the problem under control, they want it cured."

Incontinence could be your body's way of saying there's trouble elsewhere, so consult your doctor if you experience a problem. Meanwhile, here are some tips to keep in mind.

Check what's in your medicine cabinet. If you're suddenly dogged by incontinence, check your medications. Some medicines, including cold medications, antidepressants and muscle relaxants, can affect urinary control.

Plan the pit stops. You may be able to gain more urinary control if you map out a pit-stop plan. Urinate according to a regular schedule each day—every hour, for example—and gradually build up time so that you are able to postpone the need to go for two to three hours at a time. Dr. Jeter says this technique works by building bladder endurance, much like gradually increasing your running distances helps you train for a marathon.

Start a urine log. Record urination information on paper, including the day and time of every pit stop, how much you expelled, how much liquid you drank over the course of the day and whether your leakage was small, medium or large.

"I need to know this to know what's going on," explains Jacques G. Susset, M.D., clinical professor of urology at Brown University School of Medicine in Providence, Rhode Island. Dr. Susset suggests keeping the log for three periods of 24 hours.

To measure the flow, pee into an empty milk carton. Along the carton's outside edge—before it's full—mark off one-ounce increments, like a measuring cup, so you'll know at a glance how much you've expelled.

Give 'em a squeeze. Kegels are exercises that strengthen the pelvic floor muscles, including the muscles that control urine flow. Squeeze for a few seconds the muscles you use to stop the flow of urine, then let them relax. Do three sets of five daily for a week. Then gradually add 5 repetitions to each set, working up to 30 repetitions, three times a day. This should help in strengthening the pelvic floor muscles and may help control your bladder, Dr. Jeter says.

Bladder Problems: Rare but Pesky

As medical conditions go, bladder problems are relatively rare. Yet some of the more pesky—and dangerous—bladder problems hit men more than women. Below are three bladder problems you should know about and tips on what to do for them.

Bladder cancer: Although uncommon, bladder cancer isn't dead, and as a man you're three times more likely to get it than a woman. The average age of diagnosis is 65, but an unhealthy lifestyle today could increase your chances later on. Smoking accounts for 50 percent of bladder cancer cases in men.

"Cigarette smoking is insidious. You may not get problems until 30 or 40 years later," says Perry W. Nadig, M.D., clinical professor of urologic surgery at the University of Texas Health Science Center in San Antonio.

Symptoms include frequent and/or urgent urination and, in advanced stages, bone pain. The hallmark symptom is blood in the urine. It's present in 85 to 90 percent of the cases.

"My main advice is anyone who passes blood in their urine without any other symptoms should immediately seek a doctor to rule out malignancy," says Emil A. Tanagho, M.D., chairman of the urology department at the University of California School of Medicine in San Francisco and co-author of the medical text *Smith's General Urology*.

Doctors treat bladder cancer with surgery, chemotherapy, radiotherapy and other measures. Although you can't do much yourself once cancer is detected, you can take precautions to decrease your risk of contracting it. Here's how.

Quit smoking. "The toxic products of smoking are excreted through the urine, and these chemicals bathe the bladder for years," Dr. Nadig says.

Know the risks. Exposure to chemicals causes 15 to 35 percent of all bladder cancer cases in men. The culprits include benzidine, beta-naphthylamine and 4-aminobiphenyl. They're found in the chemical dye, rubber, petroleum, leather and printing industries. If you're unsure whether or not you're exposed to these chemicals, find out before your bladder tells you the hard way.

Bladder stones: Experts estimate that 95 percent of all bladder stones occur in men. Symptoms include blood in the urine, frequent urination, pain, chronic urinary tract infections and dribbling.

Bladder stones are not too common nowadays—not as common as, say, kidney stones. But they may indicate an underlying medical condition.

Here's how to keep one from developing.

Water it down. Drinking lots of water helps retard the growth of urinary stones, be they in the bladder or kidneys. Dr. Nadig says men who have a history of stones should drink at least eight eight-ounce glasses a day.

Watch ol' yellow. The color of your urine varies with whatever you've consumed. But if you're not getting enough water, then you'll see bright yellow urine, a sign that it's too concentrated. "This especially is important in the summer or when you're working outdoors because of dehydration," Dr. Nadig says. "If you've had stones, keep your urine from getting yellow."

Empty the tank. Fully empty your bladder when you urinate, and if you drink frequently, make sure to urinate frequently, too. This prevents the chemical compounds in urine from binding. By drinking lots of fluid and passing all your urine, "you'll be washing out the stone crystals rather than giving them a chance to form together," adds Dr. Tanagho.

Bashful bladder: A bashful bladder is when you're unable to pee in public. It's a psychological problem rather than a physical one, yet bashful bladders can traumatize guys who like concerts, football games or other events where urinating in close quarters is common. Although bothersome, bashful bladders aren't usually dangerous. Here's how to fix the problem.

FAST FACTS

How common: More than six million men have incontinence problems. Major medical problems are far rarer.

Risk factors: Smoking and working with certain industrial chemicals put you at risk for bladder cancer. Prostate enlargement and similar problems put you at risk for incontinence and other disorders. Promiscuity can put you at risk for a urinary tract infection caused by a sexually transmitted disease. Psychological causes can prompt bashful bladder syndrome.

Age group affected: Urinary conditions can affect men of all ages. Men over age 50 and men with prostate problems suffer more from incontinence and other urination disorders. Younger men have more infections because of sexually transmitted diseases.

Gender gap: Men and women both can have urinary problems, but some conditions, like bladder cancer and bladder stones, almost exclusively affect men.

Who to see: Urologist.

See the pros. First see a urologist to make sure there's no physical cause for your bladder's shyness.

Stall for time. Yup, this is an obvious one. Instead of vainly trying to use a urinal, wait for a stall. For busy rest rooms, strategically plan your pit stops to avoid rush hours, like the intermission between a play or halftime at a football game.

Consider drugs. One drug that's been used for patients with bashful bladders is urecholine (Benthanechol), which stimulates bladder emptying. Since it's not always effective, talk to your doctor about this and other options.

See also Kidney Stones, Sexually Transmitted Diseases

Varicose Veins

The Benefits of Good Legs

On the scale of men's medical worries, varicose veins rank pretty near the bottom. We tend to think of "road map legs" as a women's thing, and one that won't surface till late in life.

While it's true that varicose veins are more than twice as common in women, the problem is so widespread—an estimated 30 to 60 percent of American adults have it—that it still affects quite a few guys.

And although varicose veins grow progressively worse with age, they often start early. "I see it in men in their twenties, thirties and forties," says Conrad Goulet, M.D., director of the Guylaine-Lanctot Clinique in Palm Beach Gardens, Florida.

Where do they come from? The veins in the lower body are lined with valves that help blood return to the heart against the pull of gravity. "When the wall of the vein becomes slack, the vessel dilates and the valves don't close entirely," says Dr. Goulet. "Blood flows backward and pools in the veins." The same process in smaller vessels creates little webs of "spider veins."

An American Thing

While a lot of men are willing to ignore varicose veins even when they're unsightly, a lot of others can't. In fact, up to half of the people who seek medical care report occasionally being bothered by distressing symptoms, like aching, swelling and night cramps, which are just as likely to afflict men as women.

What's more, varicose veins needn't be big, blue and bulging to cause distress. Small veins early in the course of the condition can cause considerable pain, too. Even spider veins generate painful symptoms 50 percent of the time, Dr. Goulet says.

If your legs ache, blame your parents. Between 80 and 90 percent of people with varicose and spider veins report that it runs in their families, says Dr. Goulet. Or blame your job: Occupations that require long periods of standing or sitting carry an increased risk.

As common as varicose veins are hereabouts, the majority of people across the globe—in developing countries, in particular—rarely get varicose veins. And this is

548

FAST FACTS

How common: An estimated one- to two-thirds of American adults have varicose veins. According to a U.S. Health Survey, it's the seventh most common chronic disease. All counts are rough, however, since men often don't see a doctor when a minor case breaks out.

Risk factors: Advancing age, prolonged standing at work, family history.

Age group affected: Varicose veins are progressive. They're seen in 20-year-olds (and even children), but grow more common with age.

Gender gap: The incidence of varicose veins is roughly five times as great in women than in men.

Who to see: Dermatologists, vascular surgeons and phlebologists (vein specialists) treat varicose veins. It may be best to get more than one opinion.

hard to pin on genes. While Africans are rarely afflicted, African Americans get them as often as white Americans, suggesting lifestyle plays a role.

By the time you see varicose veins, the process has been underway for some time, says Brian McDonagh, M.D., founder of Vein Clinics of America in Schaumburg, Illinois. "It's a condition that's out of sight for most of the time it's developing. What you see is the tip of the iceberg."

For Virtuous Veins

The same measures can make varicose veins less likely to appear at all or slow them down and relieve discomfort once they've started to develop.

Exercise. "Walking, biking . . . anything that promotes good circulation in the legs will prevent the formation of varicose veins and relieve symptoms," says Dr. Goulet. Leg muscle contractions help return blood to the heart against the pull of gravity. Not only does exercise give veins an active assist while you're doing it, tighter muscle tone adds continual support.

Fiber up. "You don't want to be constipated," says Dr. Goulet. "When you strain on the toilet, pressure in the abdomen gets transmitted to the veins of the legs." It has been suggested that diet is the critical factor that makes varicose veins a rarity in much of the world. Make sure you eat enough fiber and drink enough water to keep bowel movements soft.

Slim down. If you're overweight, your legs—and their veins—must bear the burden, Dr. Goulet points out.

Work out smart. Avoid heavy weight lifting, which also heightens pressure from the abdomen downward. If you do abdominal exercises, like sit-ups, keep your legs elevated at a 30-degree angle, Dr. Goulet advises.

Be supportive. Medical support stockings, which are most snug at the ankle and progressively looser higher up on the leg, aid vein circulation more effectively than the department store variety, Dr. McDonagh says. For these, you need a prescription.

But Dr. Goulet believes that store-bought, nonprescription support hose are usually adequate if your varicose veins are fairly small. It's best to go with professional caliber, however, if your work demands a lot of standing or sitting.

Cool it. Heat causes veins to open up, bringing more blood to the legs and keeping it there. "Avoid very hot baths and showers," says Dr. Goulet. "A Jacuzzi is okay once in a while, but not on a regular basis."

Shun the sun. Sunburn on your legs breaks down the supporting fiber of the veins and makes them less elastic. Just sunbathing, for that matter, dilates veins and promotes blood pooling.

Put your legs up. Particularly if they ache at the end of the day after you've been on your feet, sitting or lying with your legs higher than your buttocks should reduce swelling and ease pain quickly, Dr. Goulet says.

Sleep on a slant. Elevating your legs while you sleep is especially helpful if varicose veins are advanced, but may promote comfort at any stage, Dr. Goulet says. There are drawbacks: If you're prone to heartburn, this position will make it worse.

Strip and scar. When the discomfort is more than you're willing to put up with, or your veins have deteriorated to the point where poor circulation causes ankle ulcers or other circulatory complications, more active measures may be called for. Taking action relatively early in the game may, for that matter, prevent more veins from going bad. There are two procedures to eliminate severely affected varicose veins: "stripping" surgery and sclerotherapy.

Both take the affected vein out of action—stripping by surgically tying it off and physically removing it, and sclerotherapy by injecting a chemical that scars the vein and makes it shrivel and die.

This step is less dire than it may sound, since the veins have become thoroughly useless by this time anyway, Dr. McDonagh points out. "There's no blood passing through them anymore . . . they're like sausages filled with blood." Deeper veins have already taken over their duties, so removing them is "like weeding a garden."

No treatment, however expertly it's done, is entirely painless, and because varicose veins are chronic and progressive, the very same symptoms may reappear when other veins become involved, according to Dr. Goulet. Be wary of exaggerated claims about "permanent" and "breakthrough" techniques, the Federal Trade Commission warns.

Vasectomy Problems

They're Rare and Usually Avoidable

Matthew, a book editor in Pennsylvania, was 30 years old when he decided to have a vasectomy. He was about to move in with his girlfriend, and she had an 11-year-old boy and an 8-year-old girl. The idea of not having to worry about birth control was appealing, and Matthew felt he had all the fatherhood responsibilities and joys he needed with the instant family he was about to inherit.

"Kids, whether they're from your genes or somebody else's genes, are just kids," he says. "I felt no driving need to pass on my genetic legacy to the world."

Matthew is the first to admit he didn't research his vasectomy as carefully as he should have. He picked a urologist's name out of the telephone book. The guy turned out to be a bit of a jerk; he disapproved of Matthew's decision and tried to talk him out of it. When Matthew insisted, the doctor agreed to do the procedure, but to this day Matthew wishes he had done his homework better (as you'll soon find out).

Fortunately, Matthew's experience is rare. Most men who have vasectomies walk away as very satisfied customers. But there are some things you should know if you are considering the procedure for yourself.

Fast and Final

Vasectomy is one of the most common surgeries in the world, and one of the most effective: It successfully prevents pregnancies more than 99 percent of the time. It's also quick. The surgery takes about 20 minutes.

For something so fast, the effects of a vasectomy are long-lasting, whether you want them to be or not. "You should consider it permanent contraception. Vasectomy reversal is highly successful in getting the sperm back into the ejaculate, but the chance of having a pregnancy as the result is about 60 percent," says Marc Goldstein, M.D., professor of urology and director of the Center for Male Reproductive Medicine and Microsurgery at the New York Hospital-Cornell Medical Center in New York City. "The sperm may not function normally because of tissue damage from the vasectomy."

More worrisome to many men these days, especially those who have already had their vasectomies, may be the reports that a link had been found between vasectomies and prostate cancer. Two studies from the Harvard Medical School claimed to have found evidence of such a link, causing a major stir in medical circles. Other studies before and since have found no association, and the World Health Organization, National Cancer Institute and the National Institutes of Health in Bethesda, Maryland, have concluded, judging from the evidence gathered so far, that the cancer connection is unlikely.

Research continues, but most doctors feel the prostate cancer scare—like an earlier scare that vasectomies might contribute to coronary artery disease—ultimately will prove to have been unfounded.

Cut and Run

So, you've decided to sever your sperm connection. What should you expect on the big day?

To start with, your doctor may give you a painkiller so that you're floating by the time you lie down on his table. Once you're prone, your scrotum will be shaved, if the doctor hasn't asked that you take care of that before you arrive. Next comes a shot of local anesthetic administered in the scrotum, which may sting for a few seconds. That's the last pain you should feel for the remainder of the procedure.

The goal of a vasectomy is to sever two spaghetti-like tubes, called the vas deferens, that lie close beneath the surface of the scrotum. They carry sperm from the testicles to the seminal vesicle, a small holding tank just behind the bladder, where it mixes with the semen that's ejaculated during orgasm. That's why after the vasectomy you'll still ejaculate semen, but it won't have any sperm in it.

To get to the vas, the doctor makes an incision in the scrotum (some doctors make two incisions, one on each side), ranging from about a quarter-inch to a half-inch long. He fishes each vas out of the scrotum with a pair of tongs and snips them in two. The ends are either tied off or cauterized with a battery-operated tool that resembles a soldering iron. For Matthew, that was the strangest moment of the surgery. "There's nothing that quite compares," he says, "to the sound of sparks and the smell of burning flesh coming from between your legs."

The incision is closed with a dissolvable stitch and you're done. You may be asked to spend a little time resting before you leave, and it's a good idea to have someone drive you home. Most men will feel little discomfort when the anesthetic wears off, although the groin area will be sore to the touch, according to Randy Pritchett, M.D., a urologist at the Virginia Mason Medical Center in Seattle. He suggests you stay off your feet the rest of the day and take it easy for a day or two after

FAST FACTS

How common: Between 400,000 and 550,000 American men a year have vasectomies. Of these, fewer than 2 in 100 will experience any kind of complications.

Risk factors: None.

Age group affected: The typical vasectomy candidate is in his mid- to late thirties, but any man past puberty is eligible.

Gender gap: For every five men who opt for surgical contraception, there are eight women who do, too. Since the female's works are harder to get to than the male's, her surgery (a procedure called tubal ligation in which the fallopian tubes are tied) is riskier and more expensive. And in contrast to a vasectomy, the only way to find out that the operation was not successful is that the woman becomes pregnant.

Who to see: Urologist, family doctor or general surgeon.

that, which is why Friday tends to be the great American vasectomy day.

By Monday you should be ready to return to work, Dr. Pritchett says, although he doesn't recommend you do any heavy lifting for a week. That's about how long it should take for the tenderness to fade completely.

Doing It Right

The chances that you'll develop complications such as infection, internal bleeding or serious bruising are slim, less than 2 percent, according to Joel S. Feigin, M.D., associate professor of family medicine at the Robert Wood Johnson Medical School in New Brunswick, New Jersey, and clinical director of The National No-Scalpel Vasectomy Center in Phillipsburg, New Jersey.

Matthew, unfortunately, was in that minority. "My legs turned black and blue for three inches on either side of my genitals, including my penis," he says. "I was in a lot of pain for at least a week." That, Matthew concedes, was probably the price he paid for picking a doctor out of the phone book.

Here are some tips for avoiding his fate.

Ask your wife. To find a doctor experienced in doing vasectomies, Dr. Pritchett suggests asking your wife or female friends to poll their obstetricians or gynecologists. And don't forget to ask your prospective doctor how many vasectomies he performs. "If the answer is less than a dozen a year," Dr. Pritchett says, "I'd stay away from him."

Finding a doctor experienced in doing vasectomies can help you avoid an un-

wanted pregnancy as well as physical discomfort. The tiny percentage of vasectomies that fail usually do so because the snipped ends of the vas deferens haven't
been adequately sealed. Dr. Pritchett says the failure rate can vary from 1 in 1,000
procedures to 1 in 100, depending on the method of blocking the tubes.

Take time to flush. Although it's perfectly safe to resume your sex life a week or so
after your vasectomy, don't assume you'll be shooting blanks. "It takes most men
about two months to flush their old sperm out of the system," Dr. Pritchett says. Use
another form of contraception until two semen analyses have shown the coast is clear.

Cool it. When you get home from the doctor's office, it's a good idea to keep
your scrotum chilled with some ice for a few hours to minimize swelling. An ice
pack or some cubes in a plastic bag work fine, Dr. Pritchett says, although he recommends applying the ice over your pants instead of directly on the genitals. "I don't
want them to freeze," he says. "One patient fell asleep and woke up with frostbite,
and that's worse than the surgery."

A Kinder Cut?

The cutting edge in the vasectomy biz is the no-scalpel technique. Developed in
China in the mid-1970s, no-scalpel vasectomies were introduced here in 1986.
They've been gradually catching on ever since, and AVSC International (79 Madison Avenue, New York, NY 10016) has a list of about 500 American physicians
trained to perform them.

The difference between a no-scalpel vasectomy and the regular kind is that the
doctor gets to the vas deferens by using a specialized instrument to make a tiny
opening in the scrotum instead of making an incision. Because it's a less-invasive
procedure than the traditional vasectomy, the risk of complications with the no-
scalpel technique is significantly smaller, says Dr. Feigin. Since there's no need for a
stitch, the wound heals more quickly, without a scar. There's also less bleeding, less
postoperative pain and a quicker recovery.

If all this is true, how come everybody isn't laying down the scalpel in favor of
the newer technique? Advocates like Dr. Feigin say the old-fashioned way is so simple that a lot of doctors feel they needn't bother learning an alternative. From the
patient's standpoint, though, Dr. Feigin feels there's a distinct psychological as well
as physical advantage. Anything that keeps a knife away from a man's testicles, he
says, can be considered a plus.

Vision Problems

Getting the World in Focus

You work in front of a computer. Play under the glare of tennis court spotlights. Travel your world gazing through a dirty windshield and try to learn about it squinting at too-small type in the newspaper.

No wonder your eyes say "nay," with their itching and aching, burning and blurring. But don't blame vision problems solely on your active lifestyle—there's also life itself: Being exposed to smog, smoke, sunlight and even the "wrong" kind of light-bulbs can poop out your peepers faster than a biker's bachelor party.

The Test of Time

Father Time also gives your baby browns the blues. "Changes in your eyes and your vision are a normal part of the aging process," says Hunter Stokes, M.D., vice chairman of the ophthalmology department at the University of South Carolina Medical Center in Columbia. "As you get older, your eyes just don't work as well as they did when you were younger."

The clearest evidence of this is presbyopia, or aging eyes. It happens to most guys around age 40, when the eye lens starts to get less flexible. The result: Close-up vision starts to get fuzzy and out of focus, and you notice that your arms are too short to read a newspaper. If you've never worn glasses, it's usually a time to start. If you have been wearing glasses, it usually means bifocals.

Aside from presbyopia, most long-term vision problems are usually inherited, but age has made them worse. If you need corrective lenses for nearsightedness, far-sightedness and astigmatism, the smart money is betting that you're following a family tradition. But as you get older, you may need a stronger prescription—once again, because the lens loses some of its flexibility.

High-Tech Hassles

But you can't blame the headaches, focusing problems and double or blurry vision just on the family tree.

"The typical work environment can certainly cause a lot of eye stress—and video display terminals are one of the leading causes," says Jay Cohen, O.D., associ-

Fine-Tuning Your Workstation

Since high-tech computers can cause vision problems, here are some tips on reducing glare at your workstation.

Darken your environment. To compensate for the brightness of your computer screen, the American Optometric Association (AOA) recommends you dim surrounding lights to about half the level of normal office lighting. It's also wise to attach or install an antiglare device or filter that carries the AOA Seal of Acceptance if your video display terminal does not already have one, advises Alan Reichow, O.D., associate professor of optometry at Pacific University in Forest Grove, Oregon. He also recommends wearing darker clothing, which doesn't cause annoying reflections off the computer screen.

Choose the right screen. If you're in the market, choose one with amber or green letters—the easiest on your eyes. Screen size isn't important, but letter size is: Capital letters should be at least one-eighth-inch high.

Adjust accordingly. According to AOA guidelines, your screen should be 20 to 26 inches from your eyes, with the top of the screen slightly below eye level and tilted away from you between 10 and 20 degrees. You should sit, with feet flat on the floor and elbows bent between 90 and 100 degrees.

ate professor of optometry at the State University of New York College of Optometry in New York City. "That's because when you look at a sheet of printed paper, there's an immediate change from the white of the paper to the black of the letters—the borders are very well-defined, which is easy on your eyes. But with a computer screen, you're looking at letters that have a bright center and get dimmer at the edges. The eyes have a great deal of trouble focusing when you don't have an exact edge, which causes eyestrain."

Of course, there are other environmental factors—both indoors and out. Humidity, pollution, smoke, even your diet all play a role in the short-term eye fatigue that can lead to long-term hassles. Here's how to minimize those woes.

Lighten up. A 60-year-old may need six times as much light as he did at age 20 to perform the same task. But it's not just a question of how much you need. "The *kind* of light also plays a role," says Dr. Cohen. "Fluorescent lighting (the most popular kind in offices) produces a lot of glare, which causes a lot of eyestrain."

Another problem: Even though fluorescent lights appear to be "on" all the time, they actually flicker about 60 times a second. Although unnoticeable, this fatigues the brain, causing headaches, according to research by Robert A. Baron, Ph.D., an

FAST FACTS

How common: More than half of us wear glasses or contact lenses, and almost everyone who has ever worked with a computer screen has felt eye fatigue and irritation.

Risk factors: Heredity, the type of work you do and environmental factors. Using computers, exposure to smoke, pollution and sunlight also play a role, as does indoor lighting and lack of humidity.

Age group affected: Nearsightedness, farsightedness and astigmatism almost always develop in children, while presbyopia becomes more common the closer you get to age 40.

Gender gap: Nearsightedness is less prevalent in men than in women. But beyond that, there is little difference in eye problems between men and women. Men have a higher rate of trauma from accidents and injuries.

Who to see: There are three types of eye specialists: An ophthalmologist is a doctor who treats eye diseases; an optometrist is a doctor who examines the eyes for health and visual ability; an optician is a technician who fills prescriptions for glasses and other corrective eyewear.

industrial psychologist and professor at Rensselaer Polytechnic Institute in Troy, New York. Better: If you can, use table lamps or other incandescent lighting.

"No matter what type of lighting you have, sometimes just changing the color of the bulb can reduce eye stress and make people more comfortable," adds Dr. Cohen. "Most bulbs are either 'cool white' or 'warm light.' You're better off with warm bulbs, which have shades of reds and yellows as opposed to the blues of cool whites, because they better duplicate natural sunlight."

Take a break and focus. Whether you're working in front of a computer, reading or performing other intense "near" tasks, any kind of long-term intense gazing can cause visual fatigue resulting in vision problems. Many experts recommend that you stop what you're doing every 15 minutes or so and refocus on something far away for a few seconds, says Alan Reichow, O.D., immediate past chairman of the American Optometric Association's sports vision section and associate professor of optometry at Pacific University in Forest Grove, Oregon. This way, you'll relieve or avoid spasms in the eye muscles responsible for close-up focusing.

Get your vitamins. Studies show that certain vitamins and nutrients can help minimize the damaging effects of eye overuse and environmental factors that can cause vision problems. Foods rich in vitamin C and beta-carotene, such as carrots, squash, melons and other yellow-orange fruits and vegetables, lead the list, accord-

Machismo Means Injury

While most eye problems are equally divided between the sexes, men suffer eye trauma far more than women.

"It's because men are more macho, and as a result, they're not as careful as women in taking the proper safety precautions," says Jay Cohen, O.D., associate professor of optometry at the State University of New York College of Optometry in New York City.

Guys being guys, here's what you need to know.

• To remove a foreign body, such as a particle of wood, metal or stone, listen to Mom: Don't rub it! Instead, blink several times—often that's enough to dislodge it. If blinking doesn't work, lift the upper lid over the lower lid and try blinking again. This allows eyelashes of the lower lid to brush the inside of the upper lid, discharging the speck. If this still doesn't help, keep your eye closed and see a professional.

• For scratches and burns, see your eye doctor. While ultraviolet burns and scratches rarely lead to permanent blindness, recovery will be quicker (a few days) with the aid of doctor-prescribed drops. Chemical burns, meanwhile, should be treated as an emergency.

• Black eyes and other "pops" should be treated with an ice pack. Leave it on for 15 minutes, off for 15 minutes and continue this routine for about an hour. The coldness constricts blood vessels in the eyelids and reduces swelling.

ing to a study of 5,000 people at the University of Wisconsin-Madison.

"And there's some exciting research with vitamin B_{12}," adds Dr. Cohen. "A Japanese study found that there was a major improvement in eyestrain and other problems in computer workers who got vitamin B_{12} injections compared to those who did the same work without the B_{12}." His advice: Eat plenty of lean meat and fish, which are good sources of this nutrient.

Follow the bouncing thumb. An optometrist can work with you to develop a specific regimen of eye exercises, says Mark Greenberg, O.D., chairman of the sports vision section of the American Optometric Association. While these exercises may not correct all hereditary eye woes, they might help ease some vision problems caused by environment or lifestyle factors.

the male file

The muscles that operate the lens of your eye move an average of 100,000 times a day to focus, making them the hardest working muscles in the body. To give your legs an equivalent workout, you'd have to walk 50 miles a day. The average rate of blinking is once every five seconds—or 6.25 million times a year.

One exercise often prescribed to offset aging eyes is to hold out your thumb at arm's length. Move your arm in circles and figure eights, fully extended at first and then closer in. This helps keep your eye muscles fully flexed.

Only about 15 percent of practicing optometrists are qualified in vision therapy—the name for these exercises, says Dr. Cohen. To find one in your area, contact the College of Optometrists in Vision Development, P.O. Box 285, Chula Vista, CA 91912, or the Optometric Extension Program Foundation, 2912 S. Daimler St., Santa Ana, CA 92705.

Humidify your surroundings. A heated room has only about 15 percent relative humidity—as dry as Death Valley. That can cause eyes to become red and irritated, which can affect vision (if only temporarily). "If your eyes are red and irritated, you need to make a conscious effort to blink several times a minute," says Dr. Cohen. "But it's also a good idea to increase the humidity of your environment. Get a humidifier or add more plants to your home or office to increase humidity." Another good way to boost humidity is to place shallow pans of water near radiators or other heating sources.

Have a good cry. Besides blinking, another way to keep eyes well-lubricated is to have a good cry. But if you're not in touch with that warm and sensitive side, keep a bottle of preservative-free artificial tears handy and follow the package directions—especially if you do a lot of computer work, says Dwight Cavanagh, M.D., vice-chairman of the Department of Ophthalmology at the University of Texas-Southwestern Medical Center in Dallas. That's because staring at a screen all day or doing other eye-intensive work can dry out eyes, and the tears help replace the moisture that you lose—without the "rebound" effect of some commercial eye drops. But stick with only those products labeled preservative-free or nonpreserved because preservatives can damage your eyes.

Warts

Be a Prince, Not a Toad

Over the ages toads have figured prominently in discussions about warts. "I've had guys swear that after they've handled frogs, they've gotten warts," says W. Steven Pray, R.Ph., Ph.D., professor of pharmaceutics at Southwestern Oklahoma State University School of Pharmacy in Weatherford.

Since males are associated with toads from childhood—toads and snails and puppy dog tails, as the saying goes—it's probably best to dispel the myth once and for all. Warts come solely from strains of the human papillomavirus (HPV), not toads.

"Almost everybody seems to have had warts at one time or another," says Dr. Pray. Doctors have no idea why, in some cases, the same wart can last forever. A survey by the American Podiatric Medical Association shows men and women get warts in equal numbers; some people suffer with hundreds that never seem to go away and others get one or two in a lifetime.

"It probably has something to do with whether or not you have a strong immunity," says Alvin Zelickson, M.D., clinical professor of dermatology at the University of Minnesota Medical School. "That's why you see warts more often in young kids than adults. Adults have built up a better resistance."

Understanding Warts

Warts are benign skin tumors that grow when your body's natural defenses refuse to do battle with the virus that causes them. "For some reason your body doesn't fight back," says Dr. Pray.

About the only way to prevent warts is to avoid contact with someone who has them. But even then, prevention is tricky. Books, clothing or wooden objects can shelter the invisible virus.

Because of its long incubation period, it's quite possible to contract the virus in May and not see the wart until November. Different strains of the HPV cause different types of warts that can appear just about anywhere you have skin. The most prevalent, according to Dr. Pray, are common warts, flat warts and plantar warts. Though these warts share some characteristics—most have tiny black dots where the blood vessels have coagulated—they usually look quite different.

Most noticeable are common warts, raised flesh-colored bumps that are found on the hands or other areas of the body. Much less remarkable are flat warts, slightly raised gray or yellowish brown bumps found on the face, neck or legs. Even easier to miss are plantar warts, found on the bottom of the feet, since they're often mistaken for calluses until they become painful.

Warts are usually harmless nuisances that you can treat on your own, but they occasionally become painful, and it is not always safe to assume you can correctly diagnose and treat them. "There are so many other things that it could be," says Dr. Zelickson. Other possibilities include precancerous or cancerous lesions.

Grinding the Bump

One more reason to consider seeing a doctor if you have warts in sensitive or prominent places: The most common over-the-counter treatment for warts, salicylic acid, can eat into healthy tissue if misapplied. Use it on your face and it might cause permanent scarring or damage your eyes. Better to have a professional deal with it. That said, if the wart is on a less sensitive, easily accessible part of the body, you can safely and effectively treat yourself with salicylic acid gels or liquids, as long as you follow the directions on the label.

Though your immune system may be strong enough to defeat the wart virus on its own, allowing the lesion to disappear without treatment usually takes months. Leaving a wart untreated means running the risk of spreading it to other parts of your body, to your loved ones or strangers. Scratching, biting, poking or playing with the wart is enough to cause it to ooze. If the fluid then comes in contact with any mild cut—either on your body or someone else's—the virus can be transferred.

"I've seen people with warts on their tongues and lips because they've bitten at warts," says Dr. Pray. "As long as you have even one, it has the potential to spread. So get rid of it."

Ideally, you want a treatment that eliminates the wart quickly and painlessly, leaves the skin flawless and prevents recurrence. Of course, that treatment doesn't exist. "This is a very successful virus," says Dr. Pray. "It can stick around for 40 years." He agrees with many dermatologists that the simplest, least traumatic treatment should be tried before more painful approaches—freezing with liquid nitrogen or applying electrical current to them—are used.

How to Handle Warts

Here's some help in dealing with common and plantar warts.

Check your feet. Most people rarely look at the bottoms of their feet. "Early recognition is very helpful in treating warts," says Glenn Gastwirth, D.P.M., deputy executive director of the American Podiatric Medical Association.

Plantar warts usually start as painless dark spots. If they appear on a part of your foot that doesn't bear weight—the arch, for example—they tend to grow outward and look fleshy. If, though, they appear on the weight-bearing part of the foot, the growth tends to get implanted, becomes hard and resembles a small, imbedded kernel. Walking causes the wart to dig itself in deeper and deeper.

Destroy it. "You're not going to cure a wart," says Dr. Gastwirth. "All treatments depend on various types of destruction." Any over-the-counter preparation with salicylic acid (Compound W, DuoFilm, Occlusial HP, Transversal) can be effective, but they require some diligence. And if you have an infection, poor circulation or diabetes, don't use salicylic acid at all.

How to apply? First, soak the wart in warm water. Then, using a pumice stone or emery board, sand the surface until the dead skin is gone. Then apply just enough salicylic acid to cover the lesion. Repeat the process twice daily until the wart is gone, which could take as long as 12 weeks.

Patch it up. Some over-the-counter preparations come in patch form. Trim the patch to the size of the wart, wear it while sleeping and remove it during the day until the wart is gone. If the treatment becomes painful, if the wart seems unyielding or if you suspect you have another sort of growth, see a physician or podiatrist.

Try some natural alternatives. A long list of alternative cures have proven successful for some people. They include breaking open a capsule of vitamin A and squeezing the liquid directly onto the warts once a day; applying a paste made from crushed vitamin C tablets and water; wrapping the wart snugly with medical or first-aid tape and leaving it there around the clock for at least three weeks, with changes only for cleanliness; even using hypnosis or imagination to will the wart away. Ask your doctor for his recommendation.

Don't spread it around. Since most warts don't hurt, "people figure they'll leave it alone or pick at it," says Dr. Gastwirth. If you scratch it, the virus can get under your nail and out pops another wart. Then you may have to undergo the difficult and painful process of removing part of the nail to get rid of the growth.

Warts around fingernails and knuckles often prove to be most painful since they tend to break open easily. Remember, an open wart is likely to be infectious, so treat it as you would any other contagious disease. Wash your hands every time you touch it. Don't allow anyone else to use your towels.

See a doctor. If over-the-counter methods fail, you need something more powerful. Only a doctor can remove the more stubborn growths, and even then, the process can require multiple office visits. "A wart is like an iceberg," says Dr. Zelick-

FAST FACTS

How common: Afflicts nearly everyone at some time in their lives.

Risk factors: Coming in contact with one of the strains of human papillomavirus that triggers the growth of warts.

Age group affected: Warts are most prevalent among teenagers and tend to diminish with age.

Gender gap: Men and women suffer equally.

Who to see: Consult your family doctor for diagnosis of genital or painful warts if over-the-counter remedies have failed or if you have any doubt about the growth's cause. See a podiatrist for warts on the feet.

son. "What you see is just the top." In other words, Dr. Zelickson explains, some doctors don't get it all on the first go-round.

Cautery is the most common office treatment. The doctor applies a local anesthetic to the growth and then kills the wart with what looks like a wood-burning gun. The treatment can be painful and leaves an open sore that must heal. One study showed that 86 percent of the warts treated with controlled, localized heat therapy disappeared over the course of one to four applications. Of those, none regrew during a 15-week follow-up period.

Cryosurgery, also performed by a physician, destroys the growth with cold instead of heat. Though it leaves no open wound, the procedure may result in blisters if the doctor freezes too much of the surrounding tissue.

Protecting the Feet

Finally, here are a few extra tips for keeping your feet clear of plantar warts.

Shower with your shoes on. Because plantar warts always attack your feet, shoes are your best defense, especially if you're in an unfamiliar bathroom. Since you don't know what the guy before you at the Marriott had, it makes good sense to spend a couple bucks on a pair of thongs and never let your feet touch the ground. Same holds true for any time spent at water theme parks.

Keep your feet dry. Moisture helps keep the virus alive, says Dr. Zelickson. If you wear sneakers, wing tips, loafers—any shoes that don't allow your sweaty feet to breathe—make sure you keep your feet powdered and your socks clean.

Wrinkles

Why Smooth Is Better

Consider the finely creased faces of Clint Eastwood, Sean Connery, Kris Kristofferson. If these well-weathered Romeos can follow their facial furrows straight to the hearts of women half their age, why should the rest of us worry about a few wrinkles here and there?

Two reasons, actually. Unless your face is as finely crafted as theirs, the only effect your "character lines" will have on young women is to get you called sir sooner than you'd like. More importantly, there can be health problems associated with those seemingly innocuous smile lines, especially if you find them developing before their time.

"The two greatest causes of facial wrinkles in men also are two of the greatest risk factors for developing skin cancer—being fair skinned and spending a lot of time in the sun," says Gerald Imber, M.D., a Manhattan plastic surgeon and assistant professor of plastic surgery at the New York Hospital-Cornell Medical Center in New York City. "What this means is that any man who finds himself developing a lot of wrinkles, and especially if it's at an early age, definitely needs to question whether he might be doing so for reasons that also could be increasing his risks of this potentially serious disease."

Avoiding the Creasing

This isn't to say that all causes of wrinkles invite skin cancer. But the message is clear: A smooth face has a better chance of being a healthy face, and probably even a more attractive face. So why not do what you can to wear one? Here's how.

Shun the sun. A tan might look healthy, but it's anything but. "Tanned skin is damaged skin, and this holds true whether a tan is gotten at the beach, on a ski slope or in a tanning booth," says New York City dermatologist and dermatologic surgeon Karen Burke, M.D., Ph.D.

The tanning rays of the sun break down collagen—the protein responsible for giving skin its wrinkle-resistant elasticity. In addition, the sun can damage the genetic makeup of skin cells, substantially increasing their chances of becoming precancerous or cancerous, Dr. Burke says.

Worse yet, as the skin attempts to protect itself from damage, it thickens and becomes leathery. "There's no question that the sun is the number one cause of wrinkles *and* skin cancer that men face today," says Dr. Burke.

So cover up. Wear a sunblock with an SPF (sun protection factor) of at least 15 (and preferably 25) year-round, Dr. Burke says. Wear sunglasses to prevent squinting—the major cause of "crow's feet" in men who spend a lot of time outdoors. To be doubly safe, you might also consider wearing a wide-brimmed hat when outside, Dr. Burke says, especially if your mane has been on the wane. Not that wrinkles should be of major concern on a balding head, she says, but skin cancer can be. Put some of that sunscreen on the backs of your hands while you're at it, she says.

Don't be a boozer or butthead. A fondness for alcohol can pickle your skin, and so can smoking, says Dr. Imber. Heavy drinking can damage the liver in ways that can impair the body's ability to maintain healthy skin. It can also cause facial swelling the morning after, which can make skin more wrinkle prone. "Skin is much like rubber in that the more times you stretch or bend it, the less elastic and, hence, more prone to wrinkling it becomes," Dr. Imber says.

This is why smoking also is such a "kisser-krinkler," explains Dr. Burke. In addition to damaging skin from the inside by causing blood vessels to constrict (thus starving skin of oxygen and other vital nutrients), smoking causes wrinkles from the outside thanks to all the facial contortions it requires to inhale.

"Just watch the face of a smoker sometime and you'll see," Dr. Burke says. "The lips pucker, the eyes squint, the brow furrows. Over time these contortions are the very stuff of which wrinkles are made. Smoking abuses facial skin externally and internally alike."

Wash, don't lay waste. Abusive, too, believe it or not, can be some of the heavy-handedness we guys tend to employ when scrubbing ourselves, says Jerome Z. Litt, M.D., assistant clinical professor of dermatology at Case Western Reserve University School of Medicine in Cleveland. You don't want to be washing your face like you would your car tires, he says. Go lightly, using cool or lukewarm water and a soap that's mild, such as Cetaphil, Neutrogena or Dove. "The problem with scouring your face is that you risk removing essential oils that work as natural moisturizers," he explains. "Your goal should be to remove surface dirt, not skin itself."

This isn't to say that a good scrubbing once a week or so can't do some good. "It can help to keep the skin smoother and younger looking by helping to remove dead skin cells, almost as a kind of mild chemical peel," says Richard Glogau, M.D., clinical professor of dermatology at the University of California, San Francisco. Use a sponge or washcloth that has some abrasiveness to it, or try one of those cleansing creams that contains a fine grit that you may have noticed being used by the significant other in your life. Apply a moisturizer afterward to reduce irritation and bingo, your own "facial."

Keep moist. No, moisturizers can't help cure wrinkles, or even do much to prevent them, but they can help mask them, says Stephen Brill Kurtin, M.D., assistant professor of dermatology at Mount Sinai School of Medicine of the City University of New York. "Moisturizers help keep the skin plumped up with water, which can give an appearance of greater smoothness," he says. "This is why moisturizers are best applied after you've washed or showered. The moisturizer acts as a sealant to keep in the water that has in fact come from the bathing."

Change your weight slowly. Excess body fat can keep facial wrinkles "inflated," says Dr. Burke. This isn't to suggest you should strive to keep whatever extra padding may be upholstering you, but rather that you should approach weight loss gradually so that your skin can have the time it needs to "downsize" along with the rest of you, she says.

Eat for healthy skin. What you put in your face can be as important as what you put on it, says Dr. Burke. "More and more we're finding that certain nutrients known as antioxidants may be of value in preserving healthy skin because of their ability to reduce damage to collagen and other cellular membranes caused by free radicals," she says.

Free radicals are molecular misfits within cells (caused by sun exposure as well as the aging process itself) that increase the risks of wrinkles and skin cancer. "Studies show that diets rich in antioxidant nutrients appear capable of preventing much of this oxidative damage within skin cells," Dr. Burke says.

Vitamins C and E, beta-carotene and the trace mineral selenium appear to be the most potent antioxidants to date, Dr. Burke says, so try to get them in your diet. Fresh fruits and vegetables are your best sources of vitamins A and C. Dr. Burke also recommends taking 400 international units of vitamin E and 100 micrograms of selenium daily (available in health food stores either as L-selenomethione or brewer's yeast). Decent food sources of selenium are whole-grain cereals and breads, saltwater fish and poultry, while vitamin E can be gotten in small amounts in wheat germ, whole-grain products, vegetable oils and green leafy vegetables.

Ironing Out the Wrinkles

Can existing furrows be erased? That depends on how "deep" they are and how badly you want to do the erasing, says Melvin Elson, M.D., medical director of the Dermatology Center in Nashville. For very fine wrinkles such as those around the eyes, good results are being achieved with Retin-A cream, a prescription medication that needs to be applied daily, Dr. Elson says. Retin-A does have some side effects, however, so talk to your doctor before using.

FAST FACTS

How common: Most men will begin to show at least some signs of facial wrinkling by their midthirties. One's propensity can vary, however, depending on risk factors and genetics.

Risk factors: Being fair skinned, a history of sun exposure, smoking, excessive alcohol consumption, frequent squinting. Fair-skinned men of Celtic heritage tend to wrinkle most readily, African Americans the least. "The darker your complexion, the more wrinkle resistant you will tend to be," says Gerald Imber, M.D., a Manhattan plastic surgeon and assistant professor of plastic surgery at the New York Hospital-Cornell Medical Center in New York City.

Age group affected: Men in their midthirties and above.

Gender gap: Men are less prone to wrinkling than women because of several factors. They have skin that is 10 to 15 percent thicker; because of this extra thickness, their skin contains more collagen, which gives skin its elasticity. Men also benefit from shaving, which helps keep the skin (of the cheeks at least) smooth by scraping off skin cells that have died. Men also enjoy a slight buttressing effect from their whisker hairs that helps keep skin around the cheeks from sagging as early as a woman's.

Who to see: Cosmetic dermatologist for wrinkling; plastic surgeon for sagging skin (such as jowls or chin).

Fine wrinkles also can be treated with chemical peels performed by a dermatologist, he says. More than 14,000 of these procedures are done annually on men, according to the most recent statistics compiled by the American Academy of Cosmetic Surgery (AACS).

For more serious facial gullies such as smile lines, furrows on the forehead and ripples on the neck, more involved surgical procedures usually are required, Dr. Elson says. One option is the proverbial face-lift where small sections of skin are removed so that remaining skin can be pulled tighter. Nearly 7,000 of these operations are performed each year on men, according to the AACS.

If that seems like too much of a stretch, however, deep wrinkles also can be "inflated" with injections of collagen or, sometimes, fat removed from other areas of your own body. Neither technique is cheap, however, and results can vary. All things considered, you're best off doing what you can to avoid the Spencer Tracy look in the first place, Dr. Elson says.

Index

Note: <u>Underscored</u> page references indicate boxed text and tables.